Internal Fixation of the Spine

Wei Lei • Yabo Yan
Editors

Internal Fixation of the Spine

Principles and Practice

Springer

Editors
Wei Lei
Department of Orthopedics
Xijing Hospital
Air Force Medical University
Xi'an, Shaanxi
China

Yabo Yan
Department of Orthopedics
Xijing Hospital
Air Force Medical University
Xi'an, Shaanxi
China

ISBN 978-981-16-1561-0 ISBN 978-981-16-1562-7 (eBook)
https://doi.org/10.1007/978-981-16-1562-7

This Springer imprint is published by the registered company Springer Nature Singapore Pte Ltd.
The registered company address is: 152 Beach Road, #21-01/04 Gateway East, Singapore 189721, Singapore

Foreword by Gending Dang

Principles and Practice of Spinal Internal Fixation Systems is a monograph focusing exclusively on spinal internal fixation techniques. Though the content of the book is concise and focused, its approach is systemic and comprehensive. The book is laudable in its making full use of pictorial content and illustrative cases, making the reading and learning process intuitive and visually appealing. The authors have spared no efforts and are innovative in bringing to fruition a professional reference book that meets the needs of current clinical practice and has great reference and practical value.

The value of any new technology lies in its applicability. The more widely and universally applied a technology, the more it can play its role in promoting transformation and progress of the real world. In this sense, the development, application, and widespread dissemination of new technologies are equally important. At present, in the application of spinal internal fixation systems, orthopedic surgeons face the problem of how to optimize and rationally apply an internal fixation system. Meanwhile, they also tackle the issue of how to fully understand, master, and apply these new technologies so that these technologies are practiced in wider areas in order to enhance the treatment of patients. Therefore, the publication of this book is of practical significance.

A good book is like a handy tool dedicated to readers. I fully believe that readers will benefit from reading *Principles and Practice of Spinal Internal Fixation Systems* and thereby improve their skills in the use of spinal fixation systems.

Beijing, China

Gending Dang

Foreword by Yan Wang

I am greatly honored to have the opportunity to write the Foreword for *Principles and Practice of Spinal Internal Fixation Systems*!

This monograph is a witness to as well as a natural outcome of the remarkable development in spinal internal fixation techniques over the past two decades in China. It contains more than seven hundred pages of useful and practical contents, over 1500 images, more than 30 illustrative cases, and numerous caveats. The monograph is the culmination of the teamwork led by Professor Wei Lei, which fully reflects the contemporary understanding and treatment concept of spinal internal fixation techniques by spine surgeons. The authors not only unreservedly detail the operative techniques of spinal internal fixation but also highlight potential pitfalls during the operation. The book is full of illustrations, and intraoperative and radiological images, and, especially through these exquisite images, the authors simplify our understanding of complicated operative procedures by visualizing abstract concepts and by presenting both two-dimensional and three-dimensional images to the readers. This is a landmark monograph in the application of spinal internal fixation techniques.

The successful writing of this book is the result of Professor Wei Lei and his team's long-term commitment to the study on the diagnosis and treatment of spinal diseases as well as their research and development of new spinal internal fixation devices. For many years, they have led clinical developments by clinically oriented innovations. They have focused on identifying, analyzing, and solving problems in their clinical work and have been awarded numerous national and international PCT invention patents. They have successfully applied expansive pedicle screws and bone cement augmented pedicle screws in spinal internal fixation.

I am very pleased to see that the many years of clinical experience of Professor Wei Lei and his clinical team are presented in the form of a book. This is a classic and practical textbook. It is a must-have companion for the new generation of spine surgeons to improve their operative techniques.

Beijing, China — Yan Wang

Acknowledgments

It has been my long-cherished wish to write a truly practical and somewhat artistic reference book on the applications of spinal internal fixation systems. Today, with the launch of *Principles and Practice of Spinal Internal Fixation Systems*, I am filled with joy and thankfulness, as the book marks the culmination of my twenty years of clinical services as an orthopedic surgeon. I am greatly indebted to several of my great teachers who have provided guidance and teaching at critical junctures of my life and setting me on the right path.

I would like to express my thanks to my middle school teacher Mrs. Jingfeng LIN whose patience, care, and emphasis on the importance of knowledge in career life have ever since motivated me to lead a purpose-driven life. She has instilled in me the values of ideal, life goal, endeavors, self-respect, kindness, and generosity. She has led me to the shiny path of pursuing my ideals in life.

I am also forever indebted to my university instructor, Mr. Ruyi TANG, who taught me to always think from a different perspective and think dialectically. He has shaped my rigorous and open mindset. I fought under him during the border war and the war experience as an army surgeon, which has taught me to be thankful for and respect life, has become part of my cherished memory. Until this very day, he is still my mentor in the philosophy of life.

I am also grateful to my medical professor, Dr. Yupu LU, who personally went to see the chancellor of the medical university to allow me to shadow him as an orthopedic surgeon. His professionalism and truth-seeking attitude have deeply influenced me. His kind and straightforward personality has deeply attracted me. His strict requirements and meticulous care have laid a solid foundation for me to develop good work and living habits and strive to be a good doctor. He is the initiator of my medical career.

I would also like to express my thanks to my graduate tutor, Professor Yaotian HUANG, who recommended me for directly doing doctoral studies. His scientific attitude of being honest and seeking truth from facts has guided me to pursue scientific research and motivated me to continue to develop and dare to transcend. He made me determined to become a research-oriented and innovative surgeon. He is the leader of my exploration of medical mysteries.

Finally, this book is dedicated to my teachers and friends who have encouraged and took pride in each progress and achievement of mine. I will carry forward the excellent qualities and profound knowledge of my teachers and pass them on to the students so that our common cause keeps ever improving and moving forward!

Introduction

The aims of this book are to familiarize young spine surgeons with the surgical anatomy of the spine, train their three-dimensional thinking, and help them gain mastery of operative techniques of the spine. Meanwhile, we aim at sharing our practical clinical experiences with the readers and introduce the use of clinically effective spinal internal fixation devices.

The book consists of seventeen chapters, in the order of the cervical vertebrae, thoracic vertebrae, and lumbar vertebrae. The book describes in detail the application of 16 major spinal internal fixation systems in the treatment of spinal degeneration, trauma, and malformation. The book covers the clinical indications and contraindications of internal fixation systems, surgical steps of each operative procedure, clinical vignettes, intraoperative considerations and clinical pearls, and postoperative management.

The main features of this book are: (1) it is rich in information and contains both textual and pictorial contents with a total of 1500 high-resolution images; (2) the book clearly delineates the relationship between the implant and its surrounding important anatomical structures by using a large number of high-quality sectional images of vertebral specimens along with three-dimensional images; 3) the book graphically describes commonly used spinal internal fixation techniques; and 4) for each internal fixation system, clinical vignettes and intraoperative pitfalls and clinical pearls are provided. All anatomical images and radiological images in the book were completed by the authors, and all cases in the book were provided by the authors.

The authors would like to thank Jing CONG, Xin ZHANG, Rui HU, Jianxiong ZHU, Ruohui ZHAO, Ran SHENG, Xiaoliang HU, Mei GUO, Wei LU, Ye LU, and Shining LI for their assistance and support in the writing of this book. We are particularly grateful to radiodiagnostic experts Professors Jing REN and Yi YI, especially Professor YI. Most of the three-dimensional reconstructed CT images in the book have been the hard and gifted work of Professor YI, which contribute enormously to the appeal of this book.

Contents

Technique and Application of Atlas Internal Fixation

1

Yi Cui and Wei Lei

Abstract

The developmental history of the internal fixation screw and the different methods of atlantoaxial fixation were briefly introduced in this chapter. Furthermore, the anatomy of the atlas and the corresponding measurement parameters were introduced. The different screw entry points and surgical techniques of C1 lateral mass screws were introduced in detail, and the VERTEX internal fixations were introduced in two cases. Finally, the precautions in the process of C1 lateral mass screw placement are summarized.

Keywords

Atlas · Atlas internal fixation · C1 lateral mass screw · Screw entry points · Atlantoaxial fusion

1.1 Atlas Internal Fixation: A Historical Perspective

Atlas fixation technique was developed to meet the needs of reconstruction of atlantoaxial stability. It has undergone the development of the wire technique, the laminoplasty technique, and the lateral mass technique. Milestones in the development of atlas fixation techniques include Gallie technique [1] (Fig. 1.1); Brooks-Jenkins technique [2] (Fig. 1.2); Dickman method [3], also called Sonntag technique (Fig. 1.3); Halifax technique [4] (Fig. 1.4); Jeanneret and Magerl technique [5] (Fig. 1.5); Goel technique by Goel and Laher [6] (Fig. 1.6); Harms and Melcher technique [7] (Fig. 1.7); and Tan's technique [8] (Fig. 1.8).

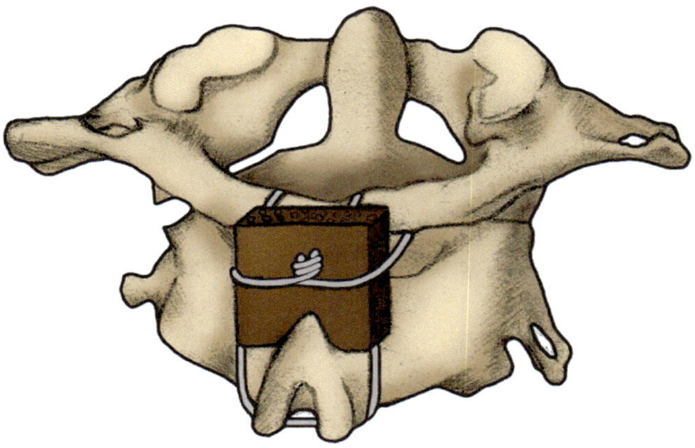

Fig. 1.1 Gallie technique for atlantoaxial fusion

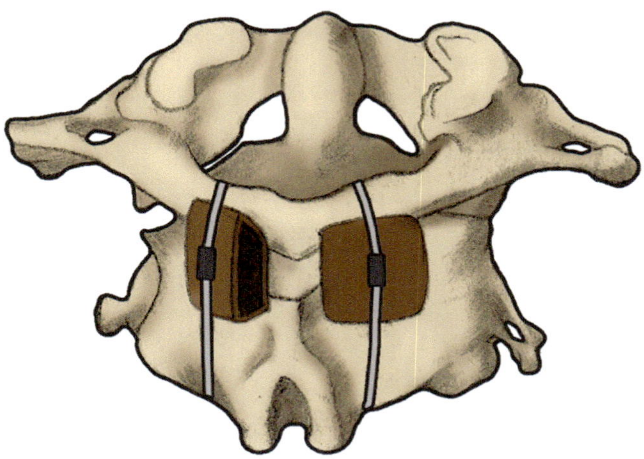

Fig. 1.2 Brooks-Jenkins technique for atlantoaxial fusion

Y. Cui
920th Hospital of Joint Logistics Support Force of PLA, Kunming, China

W. Lei (✉)
Department of Orthopedics, Xijing Hospital, Air Force Medical University, Xi'an, Shaanxi, China
e-mail: leiwei@fmmu.edu.cn

W. Lei, Y. Yan (eds.), *Internal Fixation of the Spine*, https://doi.org/10.1007/978-981-16-1562-7_1

Fig. 1.3 Sonntag technique for atlantoaxial fusion

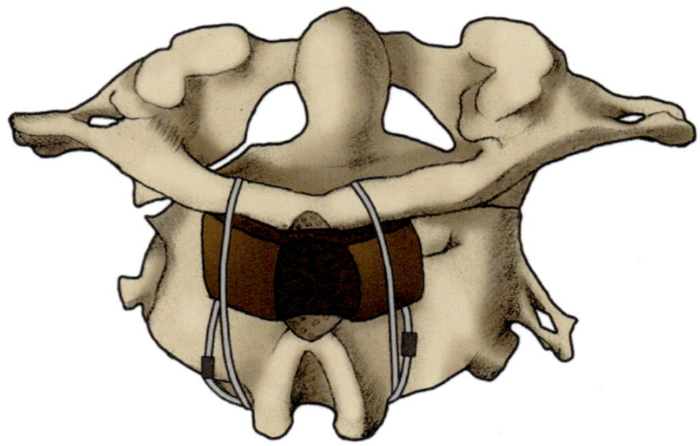

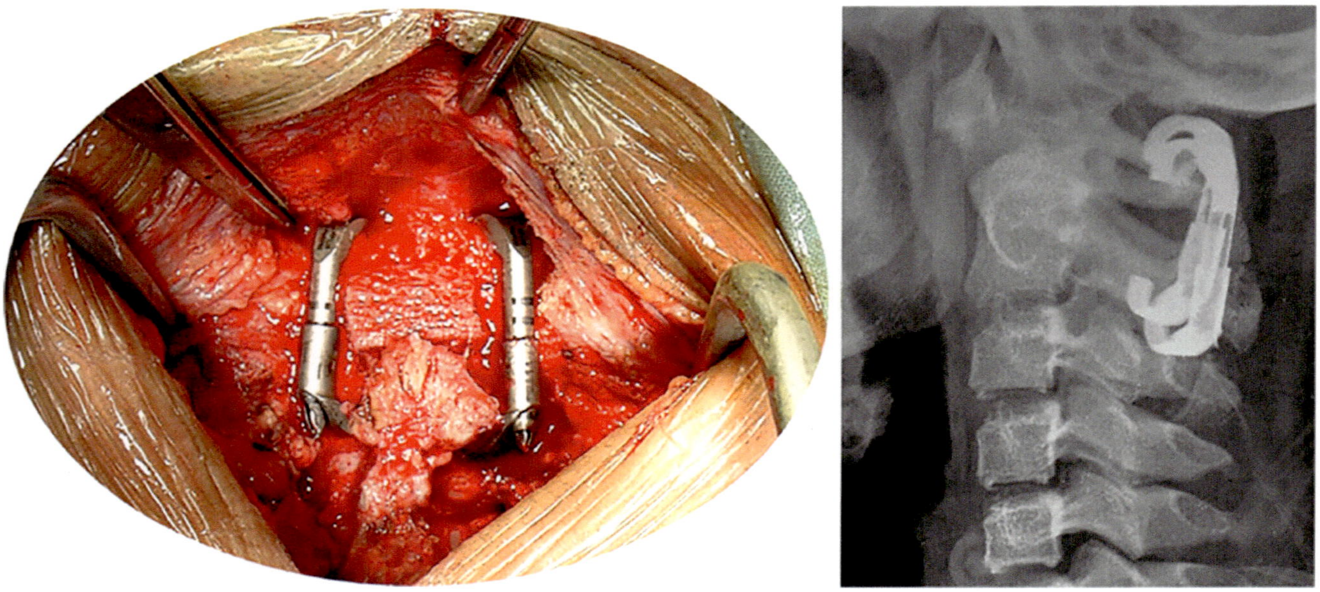

Fig. 1.4 Halifax technique for atlantoaxial fusion

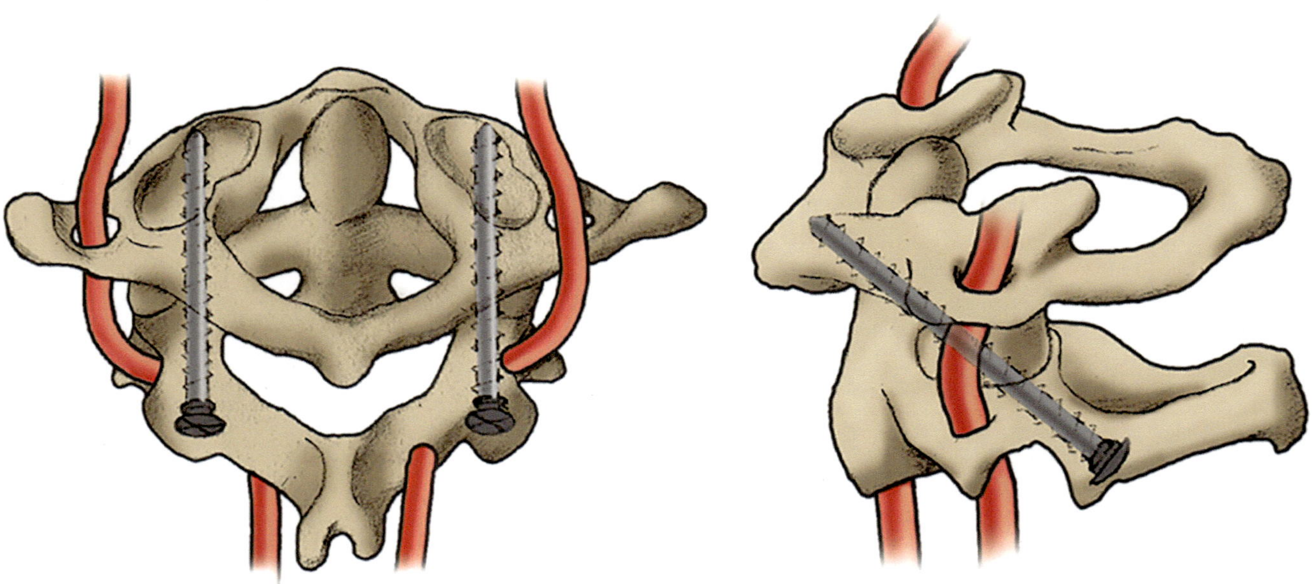

Fig. 1.5 Magerl's transarticular screw technique for atlantoaxial fusion. (*Left*) Posterior view. (*Right*) Lateral view

1.2 Atlas Anatomy

The atlas consists of an anterior and posterior arch connected by two lateral articular masses, forming a ring that pivots about the odontoid process. It lacks a vertebral body.

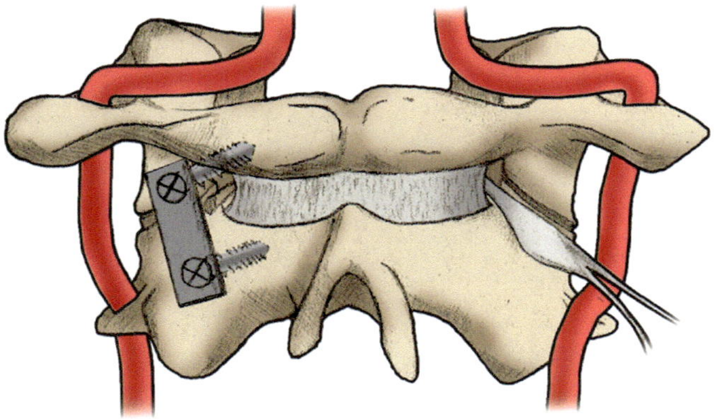

Fig. 1.6 Goel technique for atlantoaxial fusion

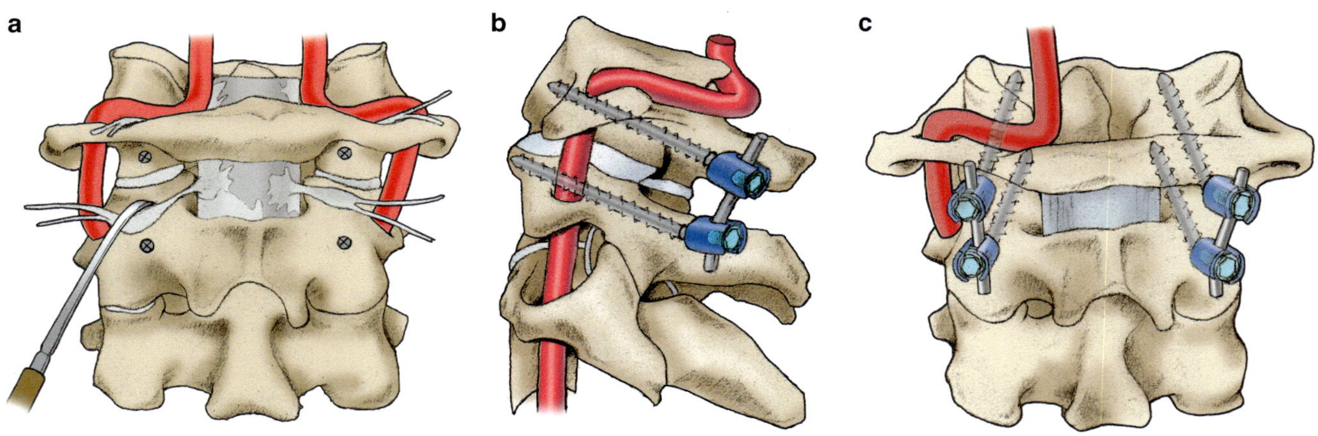

Fig. 1.7 Harms and Melcher technique for atlantoaxial fusion. (**a**) Posterior view of the upper cervical spine showing the location of the entry points in C1 and C2. (**b**) Lateral view. (**c**) Posterior view

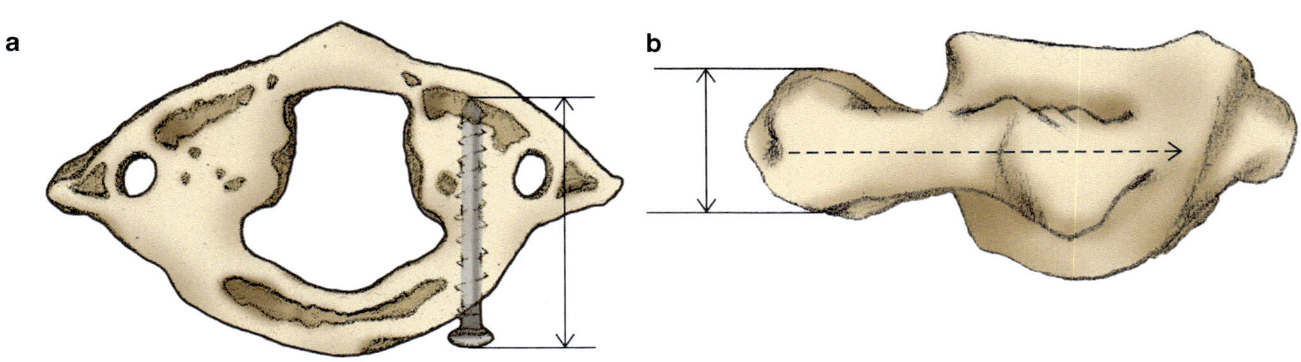

Fig. 1.8 Tan's technique for atlantoaxial fusion. (**a**) Axial view; (**b**) Lateral view

1. Measurement of the transverse section (Fig. 1.9)
2. The anterior view of C1 (Fig. 1.10)
3. The posterior view of C1 (Fig.1.11)
4. The lateral view of C1 (Fig. 1.12)
5. The sectional view of screw entry site in the lateral mass

Screw entry site via the posterior arch lateral mass (Figs. 1.13, 1.14, and 1.15):

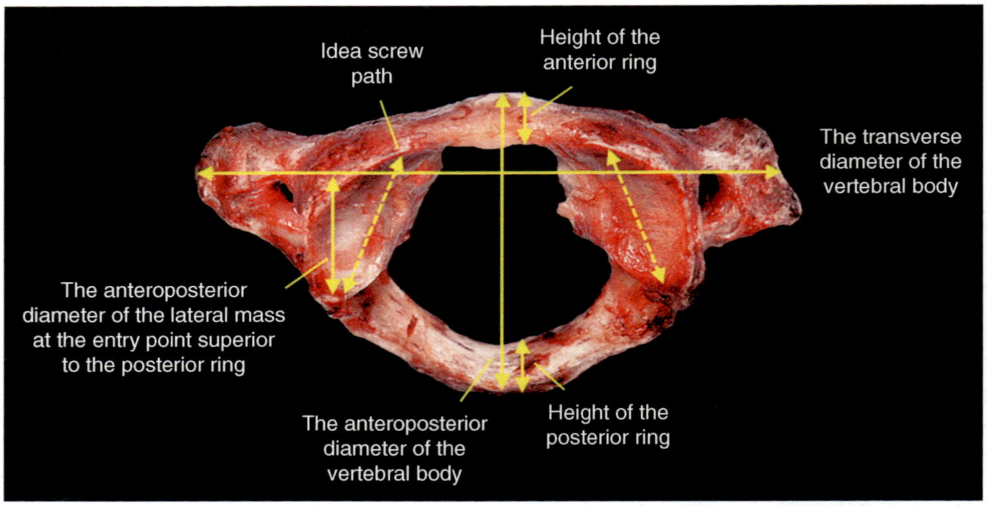

Fig. 1.9 The superior view of the atlas. The axial image shows the screw entry site on the lateral mass and direction of screw entry (forming a 5°–10°angle with the sagittal plane)

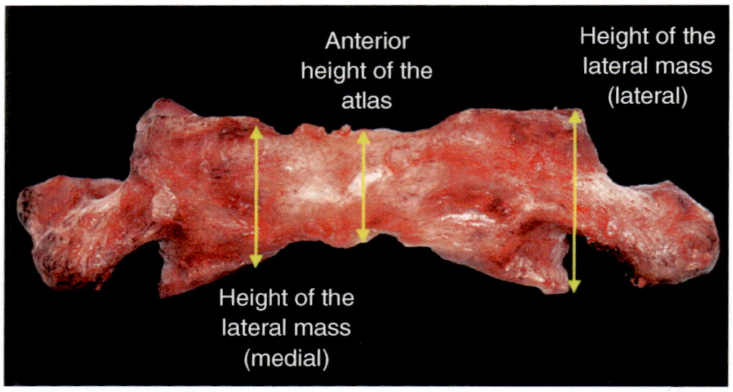

Fig. 1.10 The anterior view of the atlas. The height of the lateral mass in the medial border is 8.81 ± 1.46 mm; the height of the lateral mass in the lateral border is 18.01 ± 2.33 mm [9]

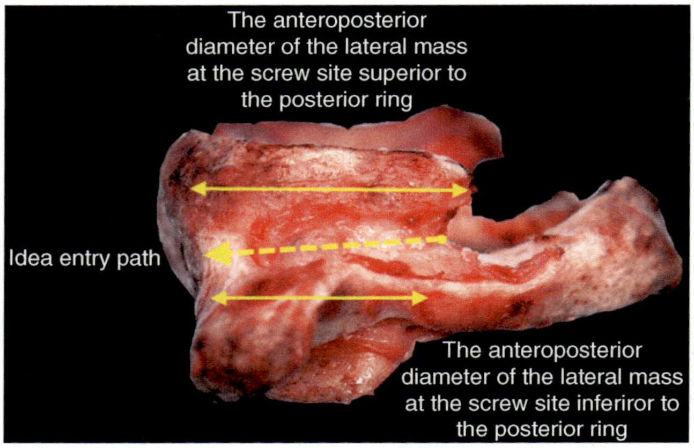

Fig. 1.12 The lateral view of the atlas. The ideal entry path can be seen in the lateral view (at a caudocephalad angle of 10–15°). Note that the entry site is located at the junction of the posterior ring and the lateral mass

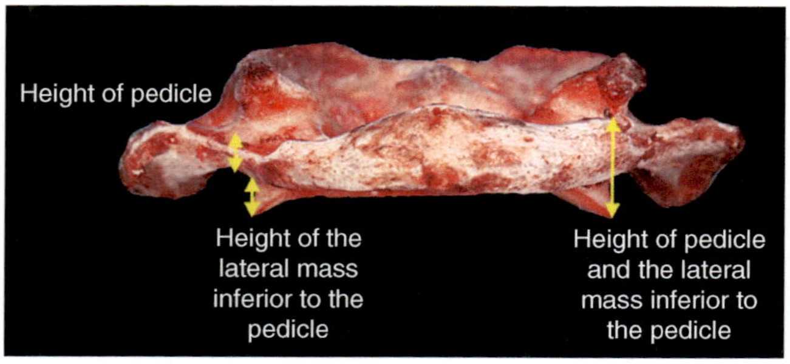

Fig. 1.11 The posterior view of the atlas. The vertebral artery courses through the groove and overlaps with the posterior arch of the atlas in the posterior view. The pedicle height is 4.80 ± 0.93 mm; the pedicle width is 9.82 ± 1.48 mm [9]

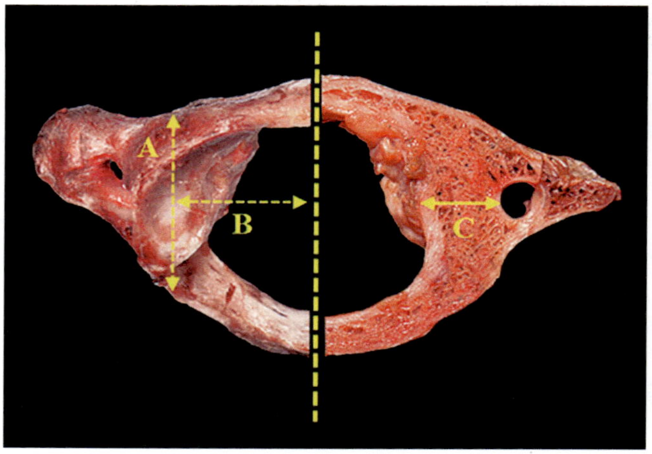

Fig. 1.13 Dimensions of the lateral mass of the atlas. (*a*) The distance between the entry site and the anterior edge of the lateral mass is 28.01 ± 1.35 mm in the right and 27.98 ± 1.24 in the left; (*b*) The distance between the entry site and the middle line is 13.82 ± 1.05 mm in the right and 13.81 ± 1.06 mm in the left; (*c*) The width of the lateral mass is 8.27 ± 1.63 mm in the right and 8.24 ± 1.62 mm in the left

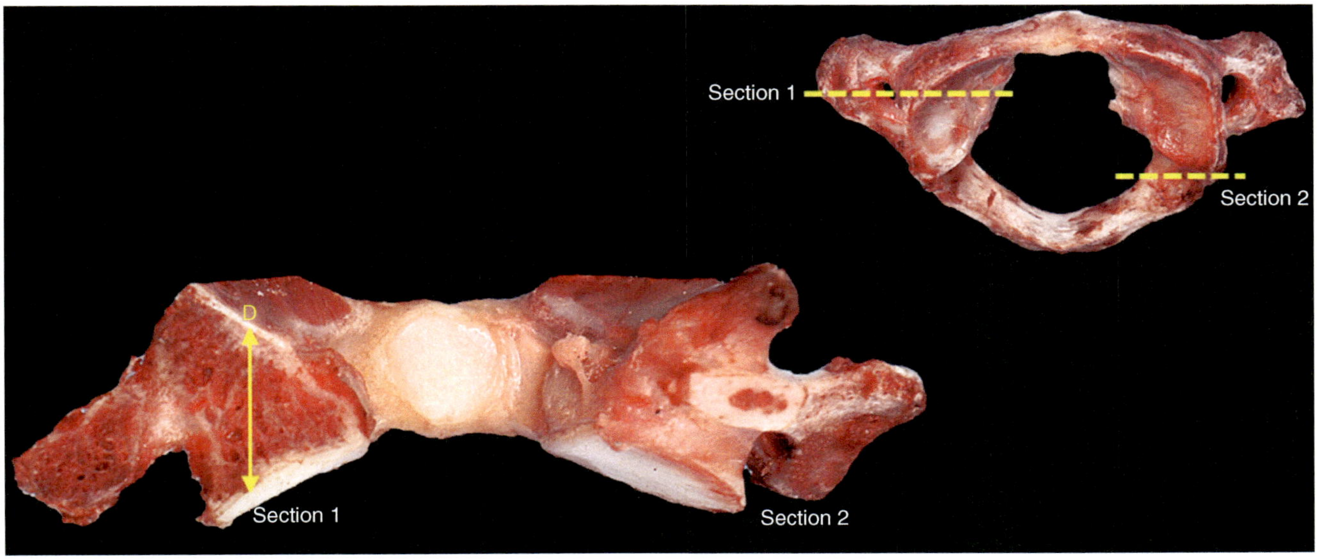

Fig. 1.14 Dimensions of the lateral mass of the atlas. (*d*) The height of the lateral mass is 10.24 ± 0.80 mm in the right and 10.22 ± 0.80 mm in the left

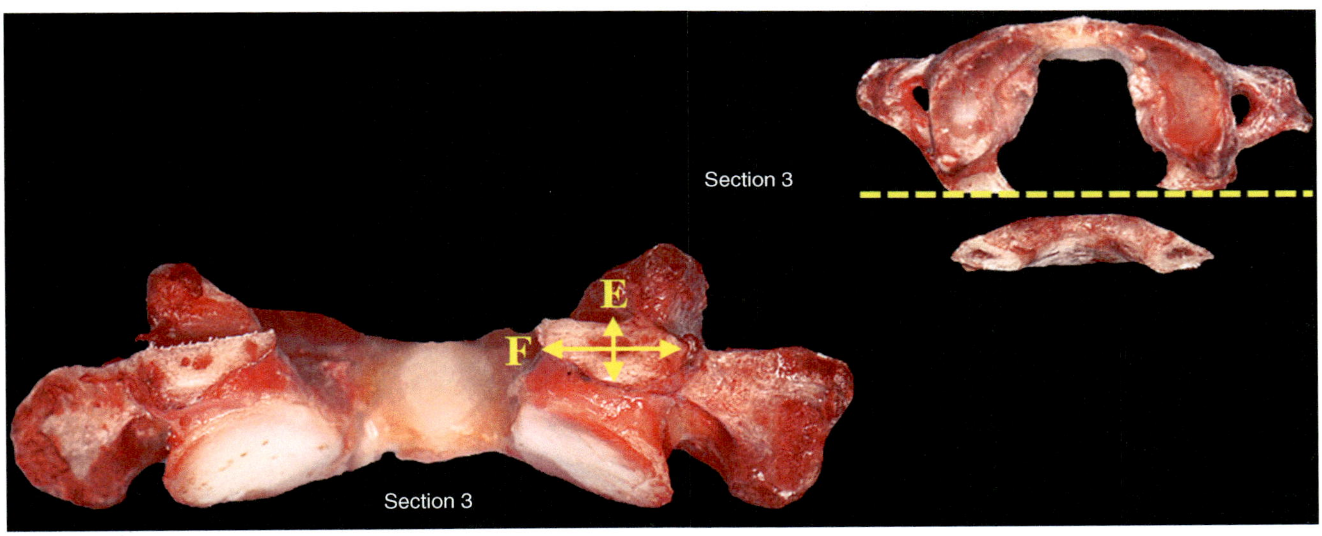

Fig. 1.15 Dimensions of the pedicle of the atlas. (*e*) The pedicle height is 4.62 ± 1.06 mm in the right and 4.56 ± 1.12 mm in the left; (*f*) The pedicle width is 9.63 ± 1.51 mm in the right and 9.69 ± 1.36 mm in the left

1.3 Key Points of Atlas Lateral Mass Screw Technique

1.3.1 Determining Screw Entry Points in the Lateral Mass of the Atlas

Anatomically, the atlas is peculiar as it has neither a vertebral body nor a vertebral lamina. Therefore, the vertebral pedicle does not exist anatomically.

There are two entry methods (methods A and B) for screw placement in the atlas (Figs. 1.16, 1.17, and 1.18).

Method A is a clinically commonly used fixation technique for screw entry into C1 lateral mass via the posterior arch and the isthmus.

In **method B**, the screw is directly inserted along the longitudinal axis of the lateral mass of the atlas at the transition zone between the inferior border of the posterior arch and the posterior border of the lateral mass of the atlas. Because the

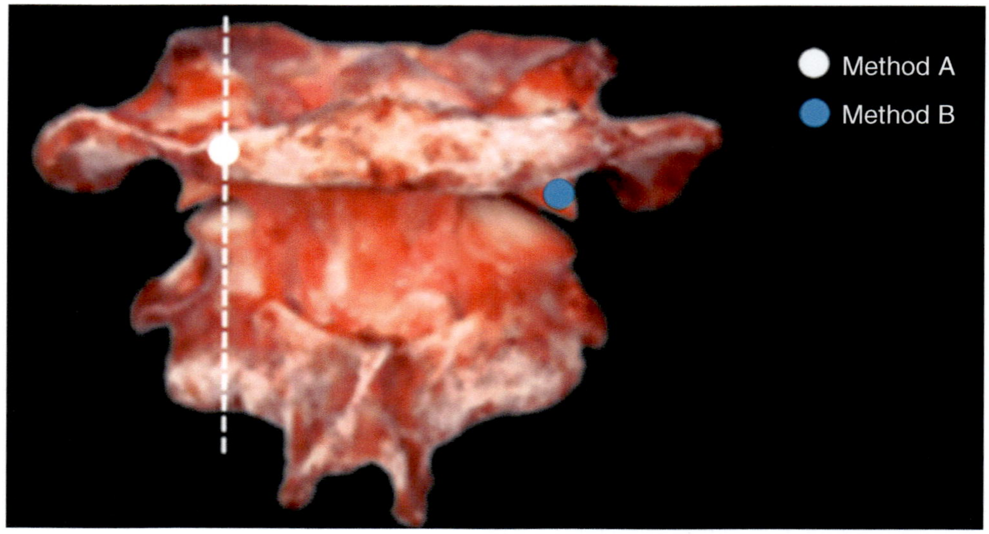

Fig. 1.16 Two methods of screw entry

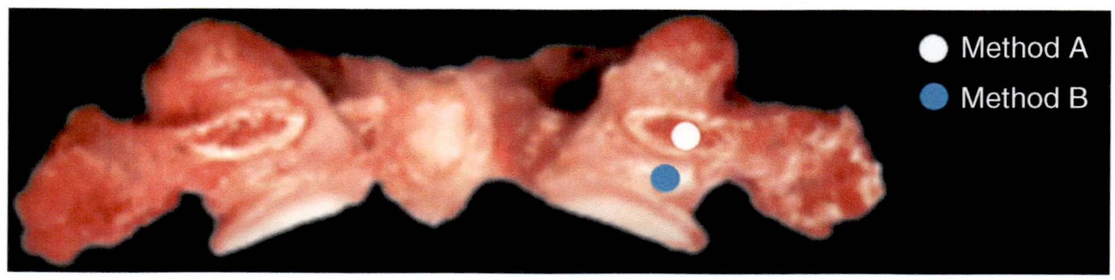

Fig. 1.17 Comparison of two screw entry sites

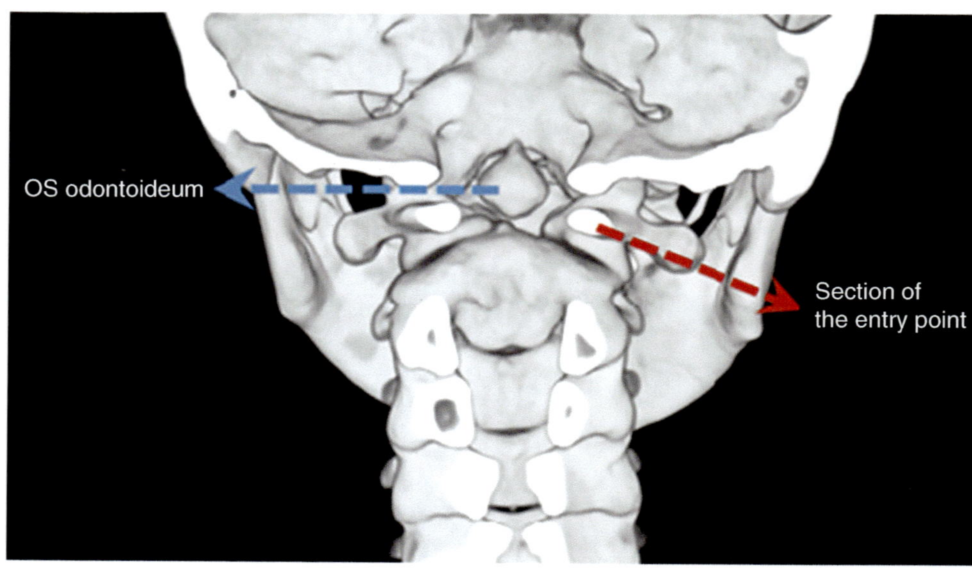

Fig. 1.18 An illustrative case with free dens showing the pedicle section

vertebral vein and C2 nerve roots run across the entry path, nerves and blood vessels may be inadvertently injured intraoperatively, leading to profuse bleeding; however, hemostasis is difficult to achieve (Table 1.1).

1.3.2 Entry Angle for a C1 Lateral Mass Screw

6. Method A: The entry angle for a lateral mass screw via the posterior arch of the atlas (Fig. 1.19)

Table 1.1 Comparison of methods A and B

	A	B
Via the posterior arch of the atlas	Yes	No
Exposure of the atlantoaxial venous plexus	No	Yes
Volume of blood loss	Smaller	Larger
Possibility of vertebral artery injury	Higher	Lower
Screw length	Longer	Shorter
Level of difficulty	Greater difficulty in preparation of screw entry path	Greater difficulty in exposure of screw entry points

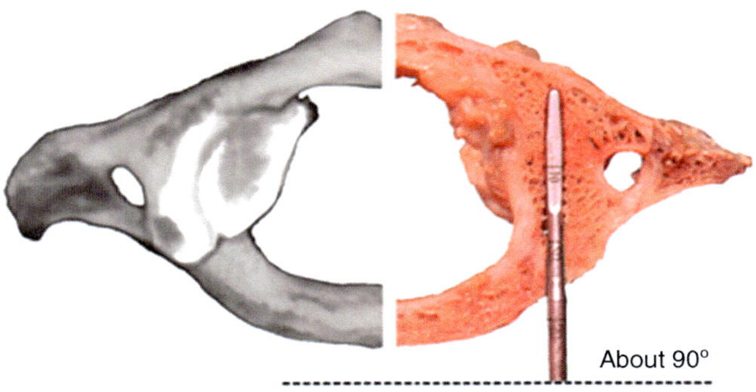

Fig. 1.19 Screw entry angle

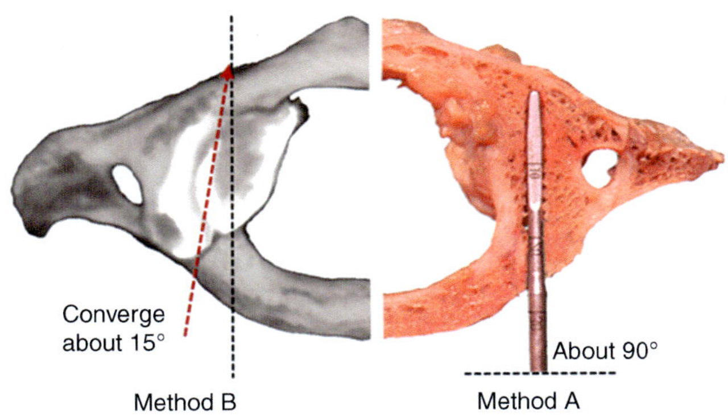

Fig. 1.20 Screw entry angle

7. Method B: The entry angle for a screw with direct entry into the lateral mass (Fig. 1.20)

The screw is situated in the lateral mass of the atlas, at a distance of 3–4 mm from the superior facet of C1 with a medial inclination of 15°.

1.3.3 Depth of C1 Lateral Mass Screws

1. The screw is inserted for an approximate depth of 25 mm into the lateral mass of the atlas.
2. Diameter of C1 lateral mass screws: The diameter of the most commonly used lateral mass screws is 3.5 mm.
3. The length of screw inside the bone in method A is longer than that of method B.

1.4 Surgical Steps (Method A)

1. A mill is used to disrupt the cortical bone at the screw entry point (Fig.1.21).
2. A screw hole is drilled using a drill bit (Fig. 1.22).
3. Drill depth is increased using a 3.5-mm drill bit with drill guide (Fig. 1.23).

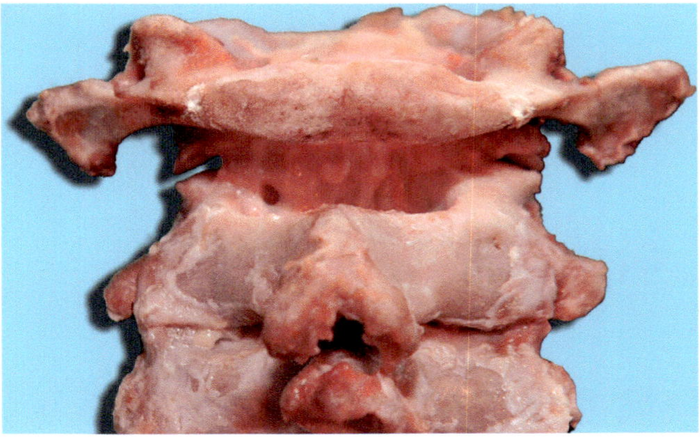

Fig. 1.21 A mill is used to disrupt the cortical bone

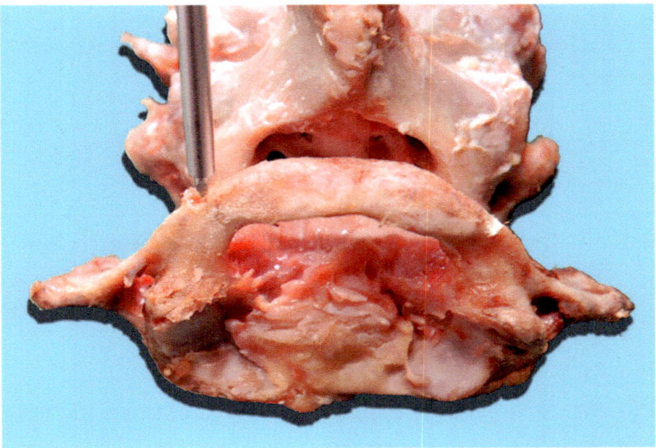

Fig. 1.22 A screw hole is drilled using a drill bit

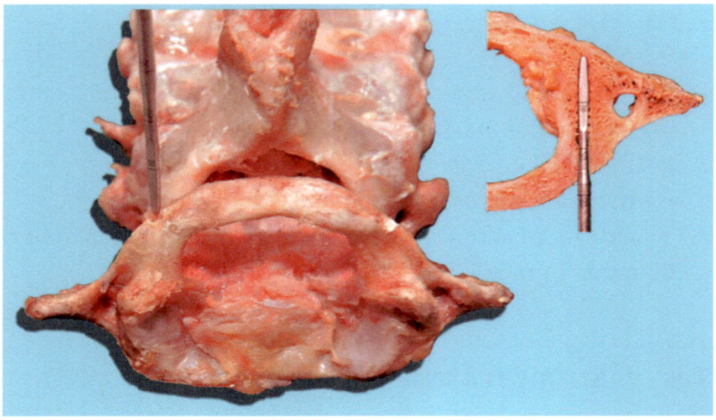

Fig. 1.23 Increasing the drill depth

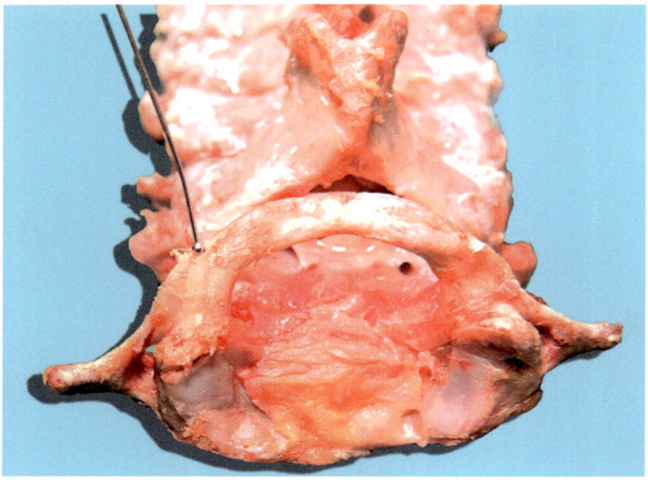

Fig. 1.24 Probing the screw path

4. The screw path is then probed (Fig. 1.24).
5. The screw path is tapped (Fig. 1.25).
6. The screw is implanted (Figs. 1.26 and 1.27).
7. Section at the screw path of a C1 lateral mass screw (Figs. 1.28, 1.29, and 1.30).

Posterior arch of the atlas/section of screw entry site

1.5 Imaging Features of Standard Pedicle Screws of the Atlas (Figs. 1.31, 1.32, 1.33, 1.34, and 1.35)

Case 1

Patient: A 54-year old female complained of traumatic neck pain with limited mobility for 25 days.

Diagnosis: C2 odontoid fracture (Fig. 1.36).

Surgery: VERTEX internal fixation with bone graft and fusion (Figs. 1.37 and 1.38).

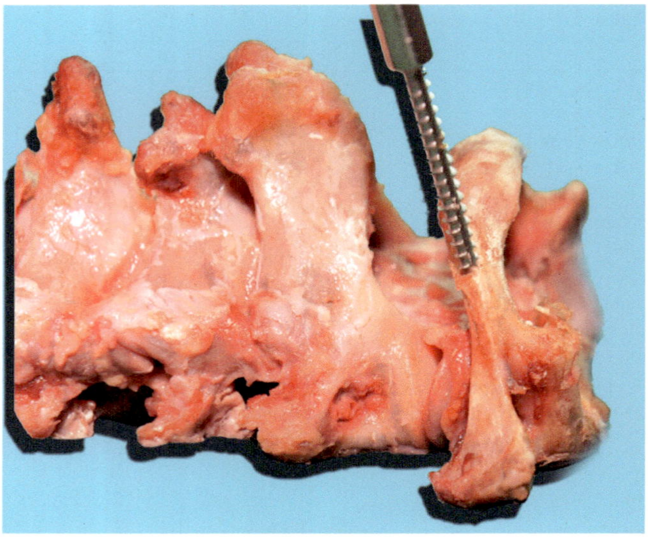

Fig. 1.25 Tapping the screw path

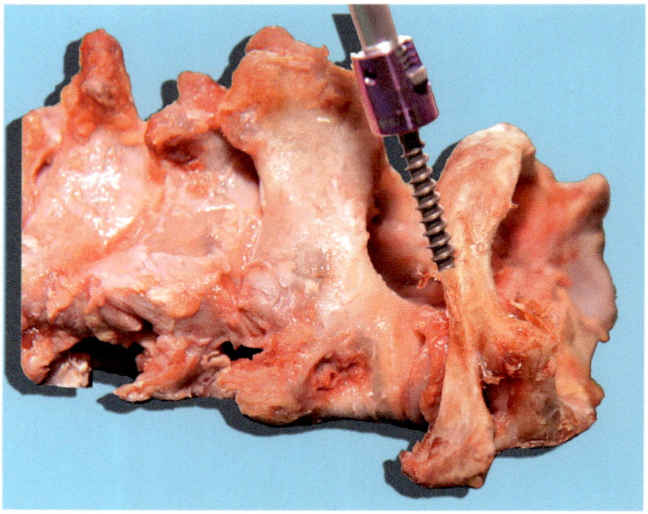

Fig. 1.26 The screw is implanted

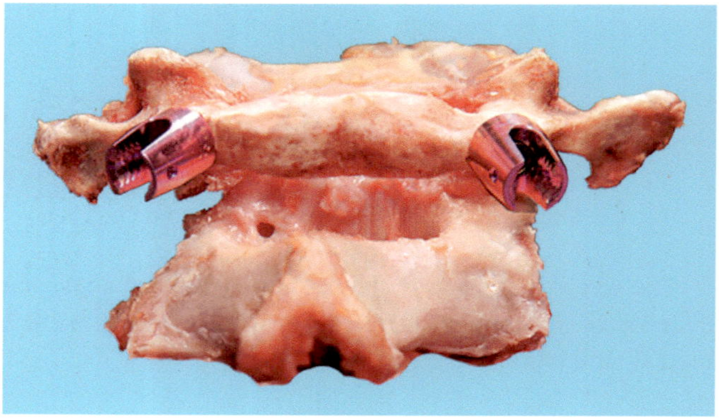

Fig. 1.27 The contralateral screw is implanted

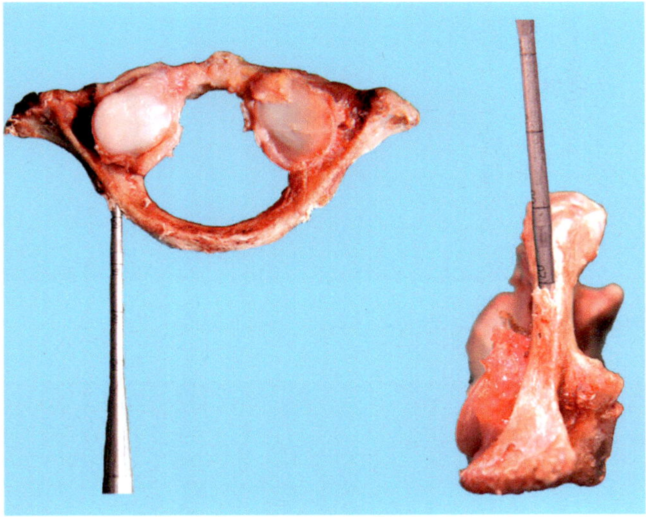

Fig. 1.28 Lateral view of the screw path

Case 2

Patient: A 40-year-old female complained of cervico-occipital pain for 5 years

Diagnosis: Congenital odontoid malformation and C1–C2 dislocation (Fig. 1.39).

Surgery: C1–C3 open reduction via the posterior, VERTEX internal fixation, iliac crest bone graft and fusion (Figs. 1.40 and 1.41).

Caution: Simple instability of C1–C2 only requires stabilization by reduction. When atlantoaxial or foramen magnum decompression is not required, C1 and C2 segments should be chosen for stabilization. In this patient, C3 was stabilized (Fig. 1.41), which is beyond the aforementioned segments to be stabilized. In addition, stabilization should not be extended to the occipital bone.

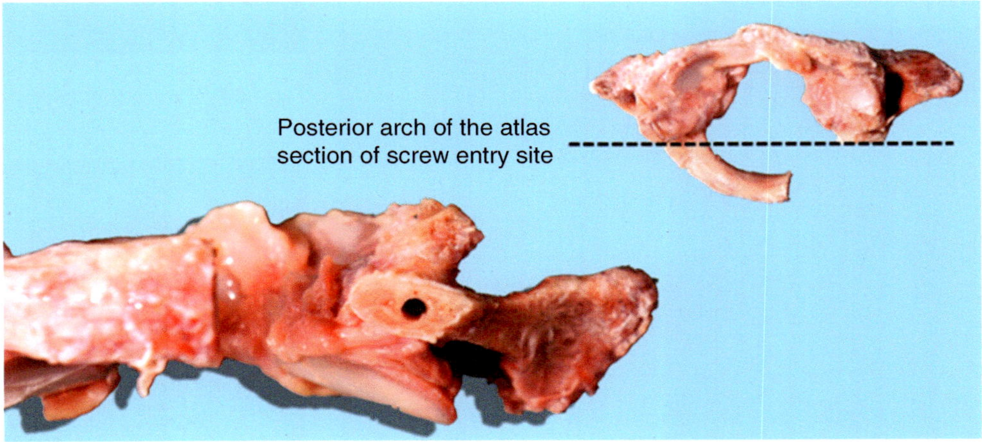

Fig. 1.29 Sectional view of the screw path

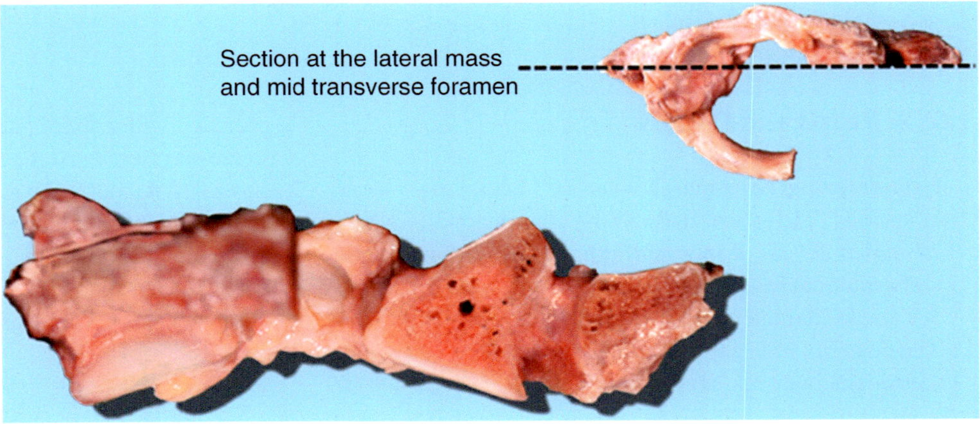

Fig. 1.30 Sectional view of the screw path in the lateral mass

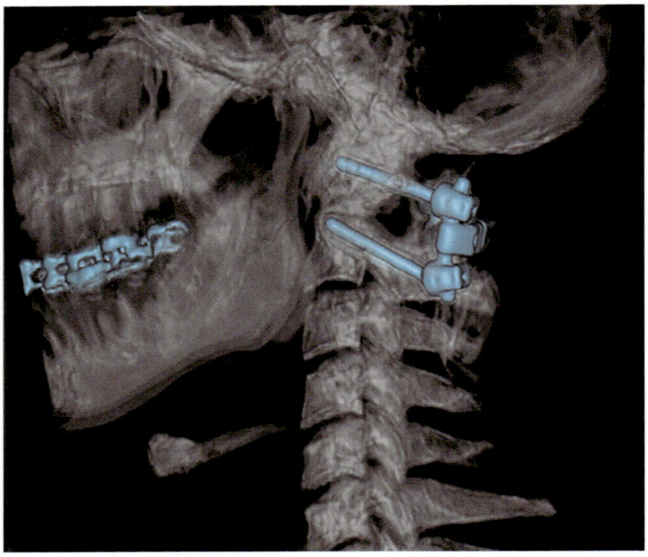

Fig. 1.31 Lateral view of atlantoaxial fixation

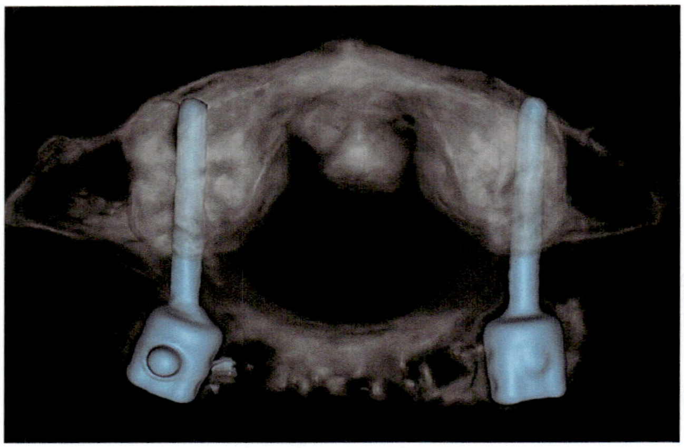

Fig. 1.32 The superior view of C1 lateral mass screw

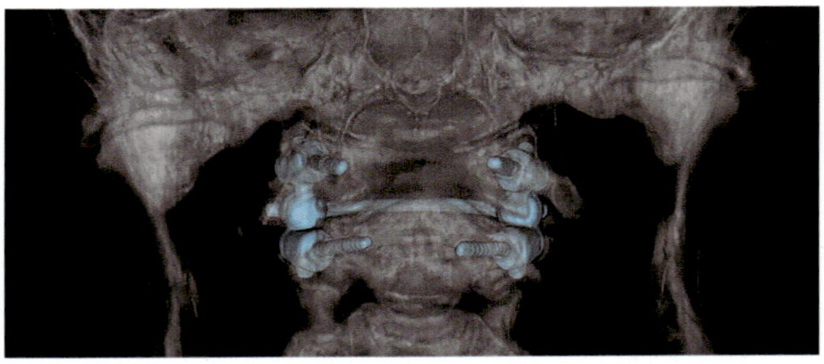

Fig. 1.33 The anterior view of atlantoaxial fixation

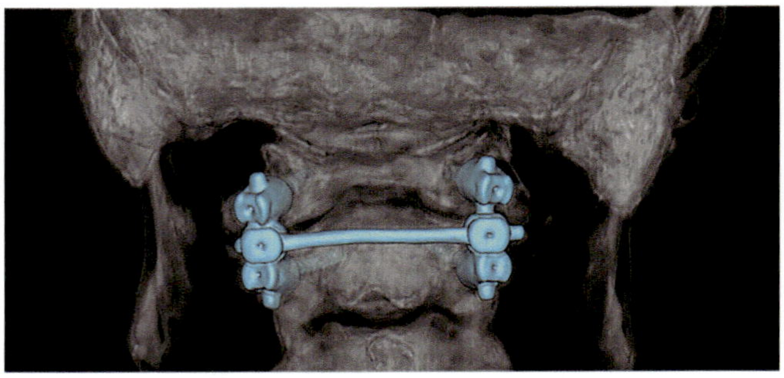

Fig. 1.34 The posterior view of atlantoaxial fixation

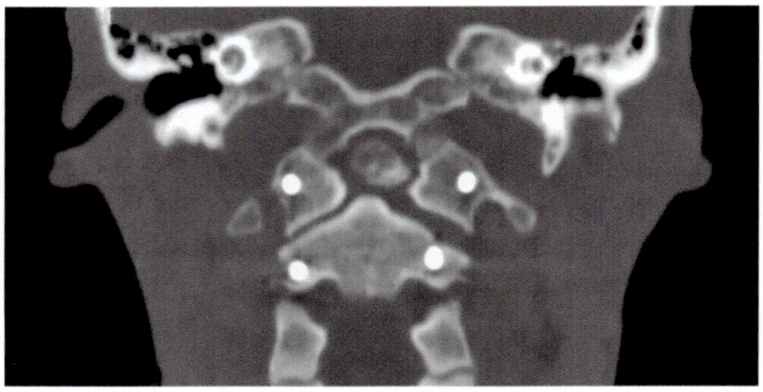

Fig. 1.35 The coronal section view of Atlantoaxial fixation

1.6 Pearls and Pitfalls

1. Caution should be exercised when a C1 lateral mass screw is inserted. The lateral mass of the atlas is approximately 27 mm in length, 8 mm in width, and 10 mm in height, and anatomical studies have demonstrated that a screw of 3.5 mm in diameter is safe.
2. The posterior arch and lateral mass of the atlas have scant cancellous bone and are solid. The screw path should be prepared with caution, and use of a tap is recommended to prevent rupture of the screw path.
3. Lateral to the posterior arch of the atlas runs the vertebral artery, and inferior to the posterior arch travels the venous plexus and inside is the cervical spinal cord. A surgeon should be familiar with regional anatomy and avoid injury to the nerve roots and vessels during operation.

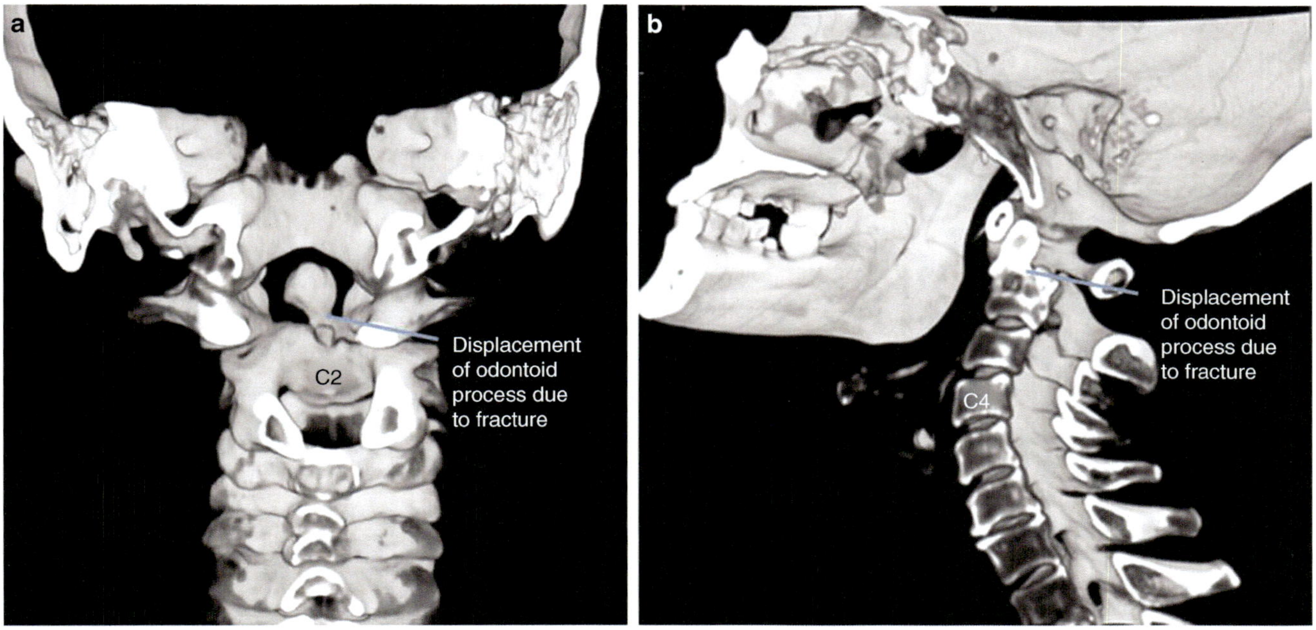

Fig. 1.36 Three-dimensional (3D) CT reconstruction. Split coronal (**a**, *posterior view*) and longitudinal (**b**, *lateral view*) 3D CT reconstruction images of the spinal canal

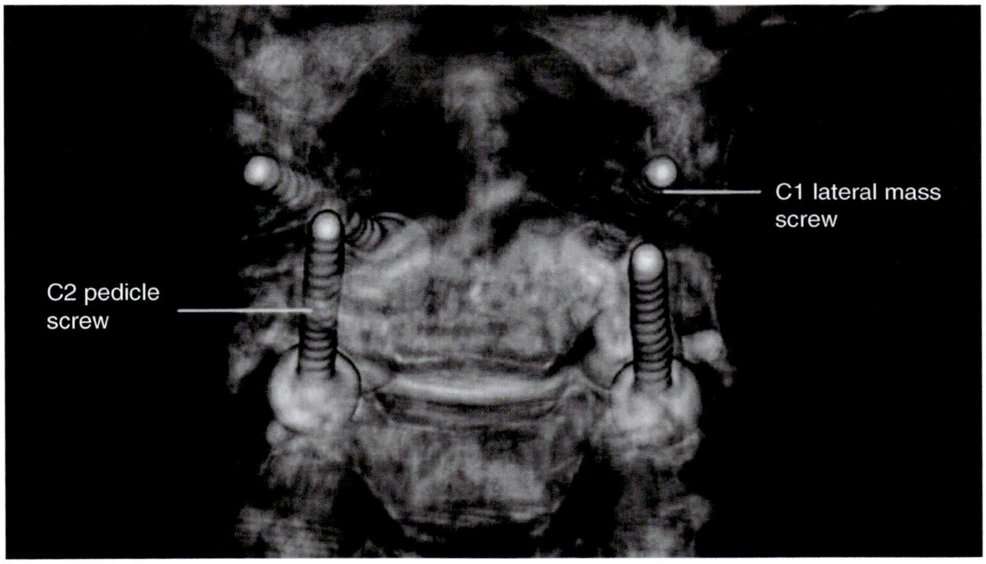

Fig. 1.37 Location of internal fixation (*anterior view*)

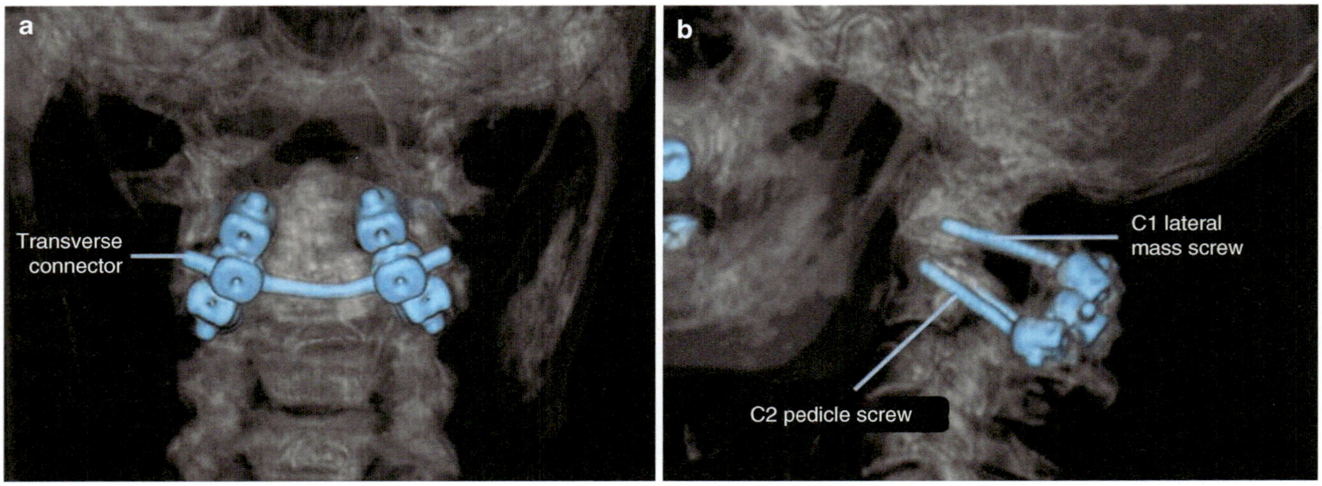

Fig. 1.38 Location of internal fixation. (**a**) Posterior view; (**b**) Lateral view

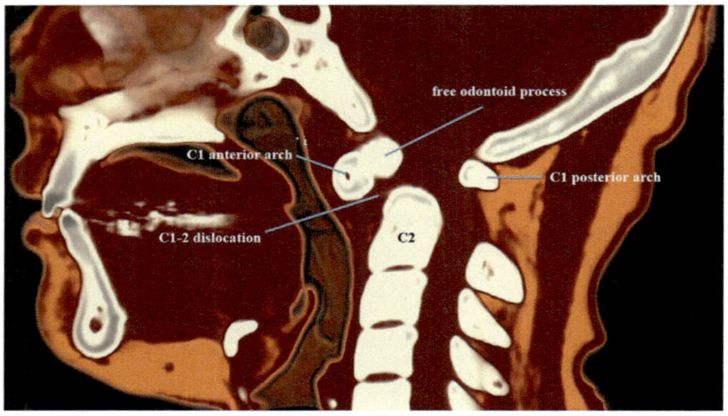

Fig. 1.39 Image of the spinal canal (*sagittal view*). C1 anterior arch; free odontoid process; C1–C2 dislocation; C1 posterior arch

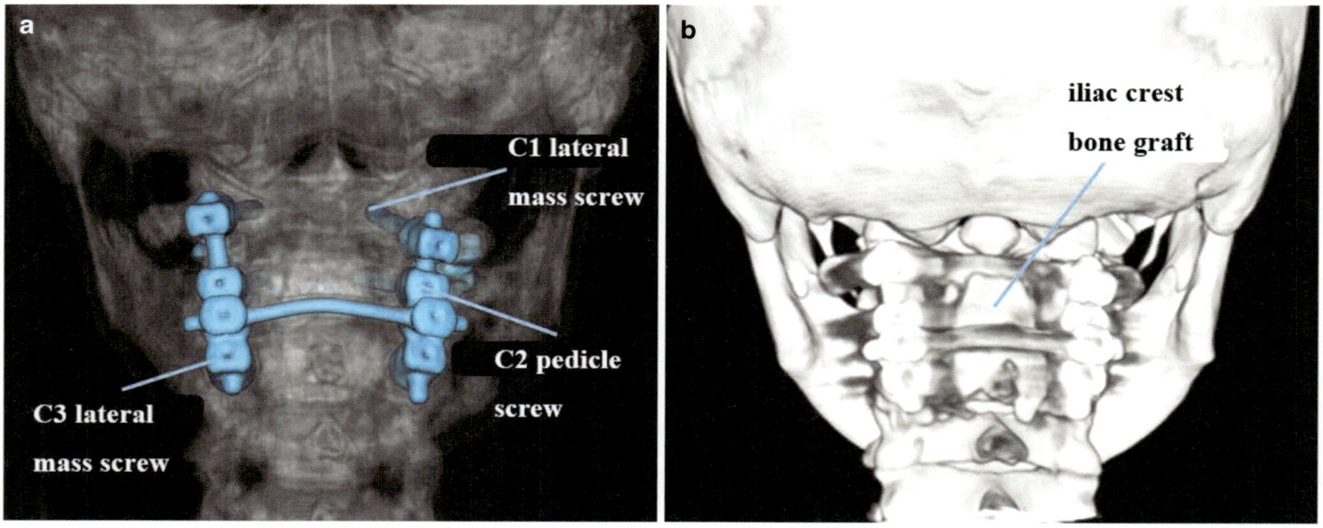

Fig. 1.40 Postoperative 3D reconstruction. (**a**) Location of internal fixation (*posterior view*); (**b**) Location of internal fixation (*posterior view*); (**c**) Position of C1 lateral mass screw (*horizontal view*); (**d**) Location C2 pedicle screw (*horizontal view*)

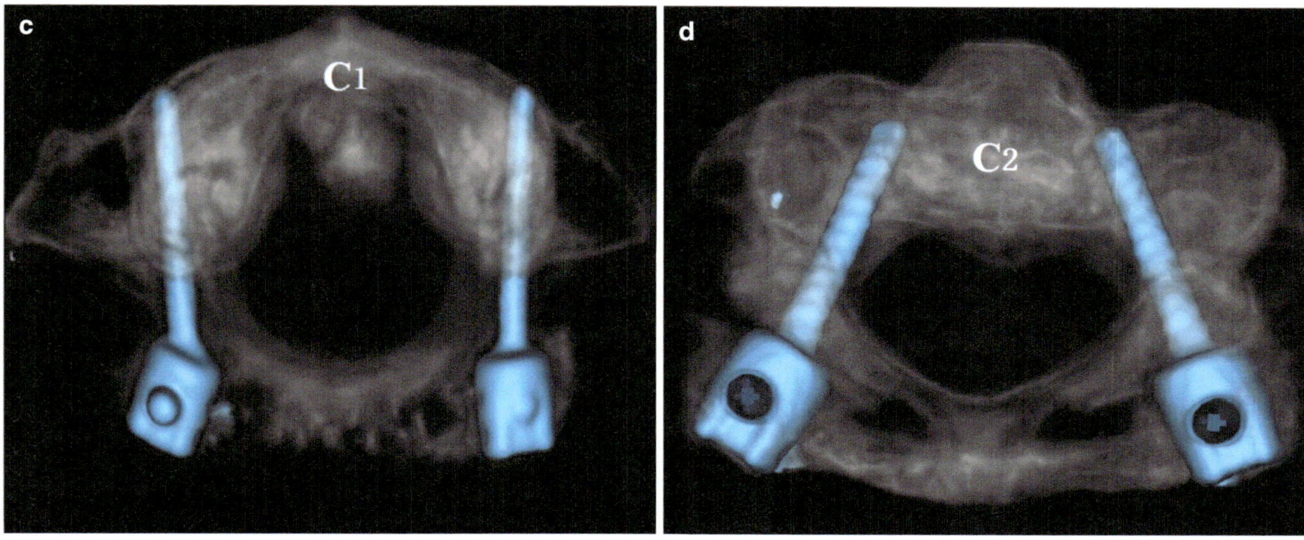

Fig. 1.40 (continued)

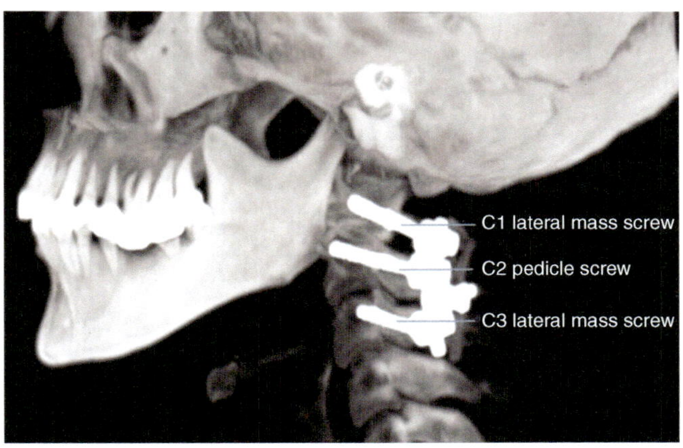

Fig. 1.41 Location of internal fixation (*lateral view*)

References

1. Gallie WE. Skeletal traction in the treatment of fractures and dislocations of the cervical spine. Ann Surg. 1937;106(4):770–6.
2. Brooks AL, Jenkins EB. Atlanto-axial arthrodesis by the wedge compression method. J Bone Joint Surg Am. 1978;60(3):279–84.
3. Dickman CA, et al. The interspinous method of posterior atlanto-axial arthrodesis. J Neurosurg. 1991;74(2):190–8.
4. Holness RO, et al. Posterior stabilization with an interlaminar clamp in cervical injuries: technical note and review of the long term experience with the method. Neurosurgery. 1984;14(3):318–22.
5. Jeanneret B, Magerl F. Primary posterior fusion C1/2 in odontoid fractures: indications, technique, and results of transarticular screw fixation. J Spinal Disord. 1992;5(4):464–75.
6. Goel A, Laheri V. Plate and screw fixation for atlanto-axial subluxation. Acta Neurochir. 1994;129(1–2):47–53.
7. Harms J, Melcher RP. Posterior C1-C2 fusion with polyaxial screw and rod fixation. Spine (Phila Pa 1976). 2001;26(22):2467–71.
8. Tan M, et al. Morphometric evaluation of screw fixation in atlas via posterior arch and lateral mass. Spine (Phila Pa 1976). 2003;28(9):888–95.
9. Christensen DM, et al. C1 anatomy and dimensions relative to lateral mass screw placement. Spine (Phila Pa 1976). 2007;32(8):844–8.

C2 Internal Fixation Techniques and Their Applications

2

Junxiong Ma, Liangbi Xiang, and Wei Lei

Abstract

There are four types of axis fixation: axis pedicle screw, axis pars screw, axis transarticular screw, and axis laminar screw. Each of those techniques has its advantages and disadvantages. Although pedicle screw is the most commonly used technique, the others are also applied as alternative in some cases.

The entry point of pedicle screw is located 2 mm superomedial to the center of the C2 lateral mass. The entry angle is 30° medially and 20° in the cephalad direction. The screw length is usually 24–28 mm.

When placing C2 pedicle screw, the surgeon should be cautious about the potential injury to the vertebral artery. Anatomic variations of the vertebral artery are frequent, which are often accompanied by C2 pedicle maldevelopment. So preoperative CTA is mandatory. For example, high riding deformity of the vertebral artery is a contraindication for C2 pedicle screw placement. Then other internal fixation techniques should be employed.

Keywords

Axis · Screw · Pedicle · Pars screw · Transarticular
Translaminar

2.1 Axis Internal Fixation: A Historical Perspective

The techniques of atlas and axis internal fixation coevolved, and atlas and axis fixation and fusion are often undertaken simultaneously because of requirements of an illness. There are four types of axis fixation: axis pedicle screw, axis pars screw, axis transarticular screw, and axis laminar screw.

Goel developed the C2 pedicle screw technique in 1994 [1] (Fig. 2.1). In the same year, he also invented the C2 pars screw (Fig. 2.2). In 1992, Jeanneret and Magerl developed the C1–C2 transarticular screw technique [2] (Fig. 2.3). In 2004, Wright developed translaminar screw fixation tech-

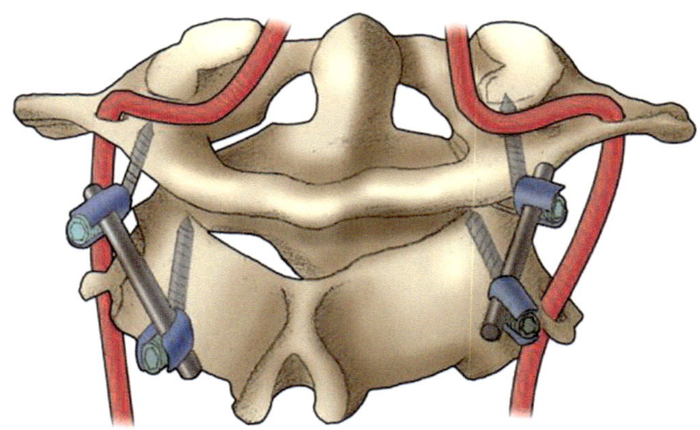

Fig. 2.1 C2 pedicle screw

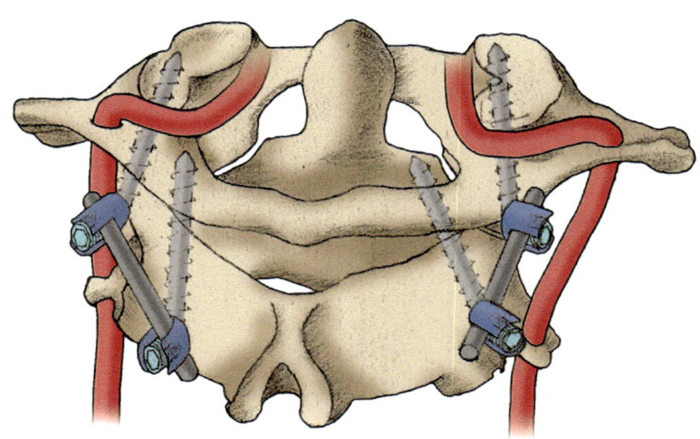

Fig. 2.2 The C2 pars screw

J. Ma · L. Xiang
Department of Orthopedics, General Hospital of Northern Theater Command, Shenyang, China

W. Lei (✉)
Department of Orthopedics, Xijing Hospital, Air Force Medical University, Xi'an, Shaanxi, China
e-mail: leiwei@fmmu.edu.cn

W. Lei, Y. Yan (eds.), *Internal Fixation of the Spine*, https://doi.org/10.1007/978-981-16-1562-7_2

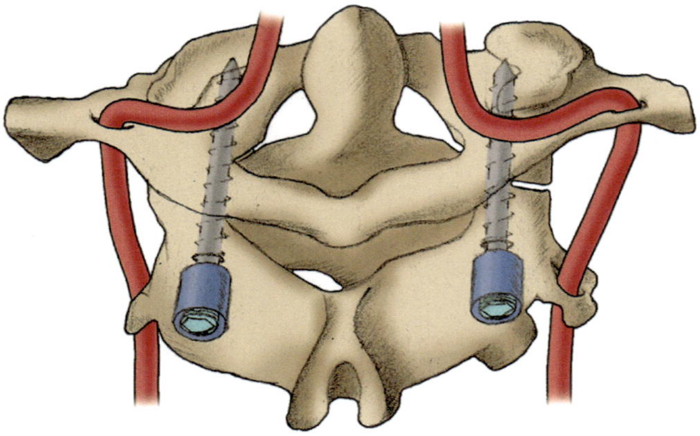

Fig. 2.3 The C1–C2 transarticular screw

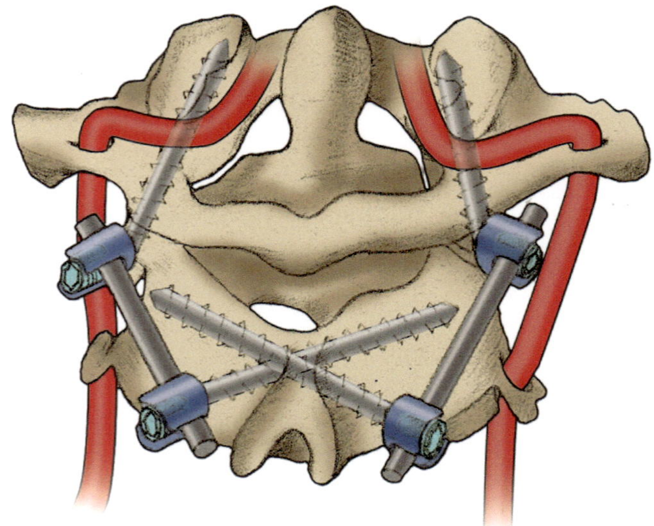

Fig. 2.4 The C2 translaminar screw

Table 2.1 Comparison of techniques of axis screw fixation

	Pedicle screw	Short pars screw	Transarticular screw	Translaminar screw
Technical difficulty	High	Low	High	Low
C2 anatomic requirement	Normal development of the vertebral artery and pedicle	No	Normal development of the vertebral artery and pedicle	Normal development of laminar thickness
C1/C2reduction requirement	No	No	Yes	No
Spine requirement	No	No	Not suitable thoracic kyphosis deformity patients	No
Functional reduction	Yes	Yes	No	Yes
Screw length	24–28 mm	14–20 mm (not extending the posterior wall of the transverse foramen)	32–34 mm (not disrupting the anterior cortex)	24–26 mm, no more than 28 mm (to avoid vertebral artery injury)
Internal fixation strength	High	Moderate	High	High
Risk with screw insertion	Potential injury to the vertebral artery or spinal cord	Small	Potential injury to the vertebral artery or spinal cord	Potential injury to the spinal cord;, less likely to injure the vertebral artery
Recommended technique	Preferred	Second choice	Others	Second choice

nique [3] (Fig. 2.4). The comparison of techniques of axis screw fixation was shown in Table 2.1.

2.2 Anatomy of the Axis

2.2.1 The Gross Anatomy of C2 Was Shown Below (Figs. 2.5, 2.6, 2.7, 2.8, and 2.9)

2.2.2 The Vertebral Artery in Relation to the Axis

Under normal circumstances, the vertebral artery enters the skull through the transverse foramen of the axis and the atlas. The intra-axial vertebral artery, the vertebral artery segment that passes through the transverse foramen of C2, often exhibits anatomic variations. Lee et al. [5] showed that the

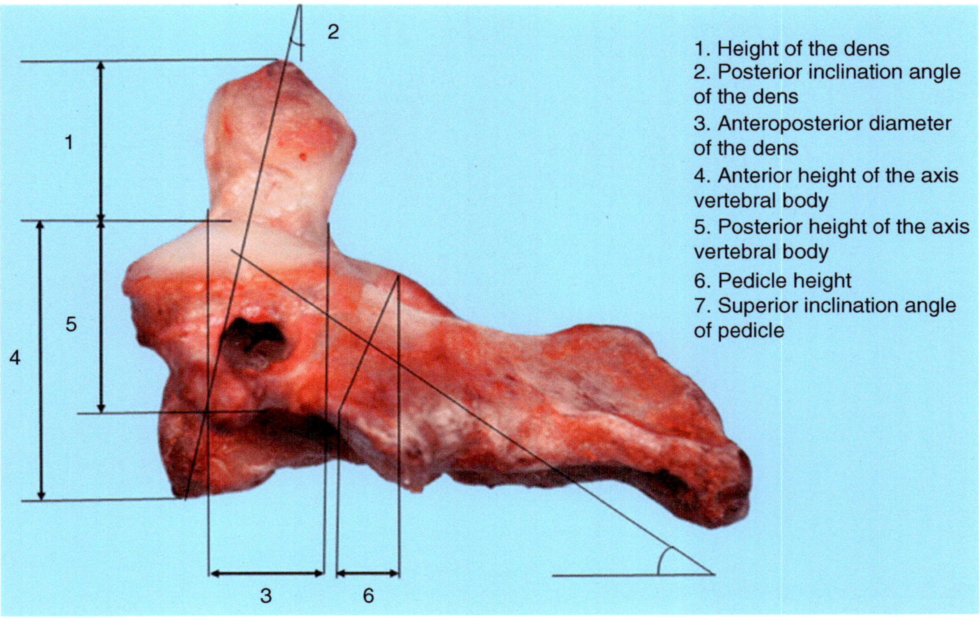

Fig. 2.5 The lateral view of the axis. The height of the dens is 14.7 ± 1.9 mm. The posterior inclination angle of the dens is 10.3° ± 3.5°. The anteroposterior diameter of the dens is 10.5 ± 1.1 mm. The anterior height of the axis vertebral body is 22.8 ± 1.1 mm. The posterior height of the axis vertebral body is 19.5 ± 0.9 mm. The pedicle height is 8.5 ± 0.7 mm. The superior inclination angle of pedicle is 42.3° ± 5.4° [4]

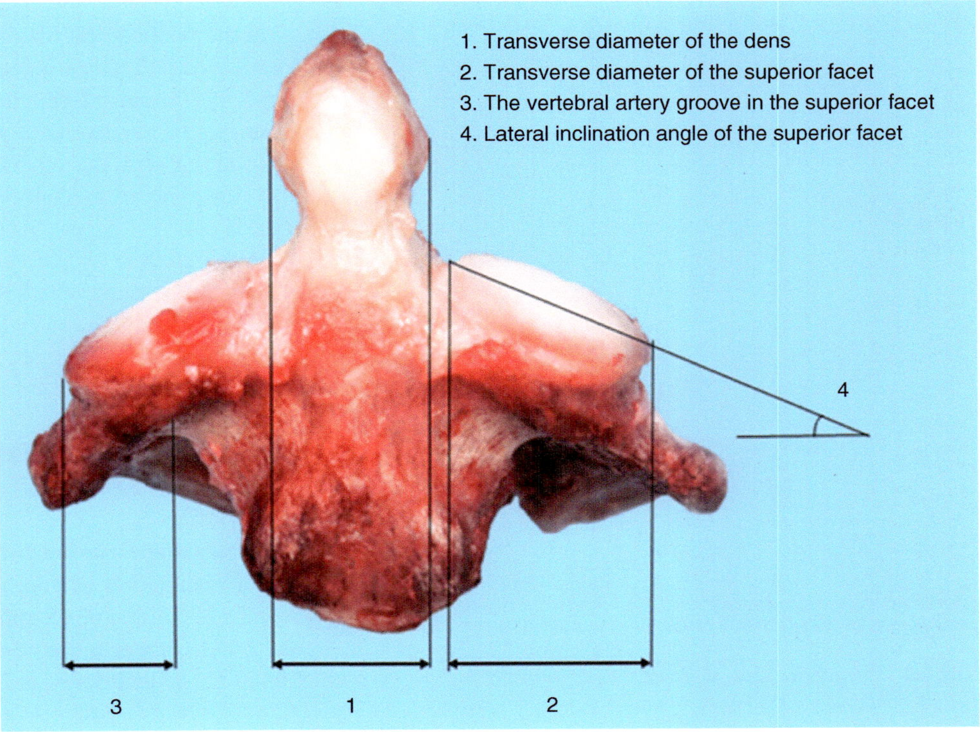

Fig. 2.6 The anterior view of the axis

intra-axial vertebral artery may exhibit medial shifting and high riding. Medial shifting was seen in 25.5% and high riding in 24% of 200 intra-axial vertebral artery segments on three-dimensional, vascular-enhanced computed tomographic scans. Medial shifting positively correlated with high riding (Fig. 2.10).

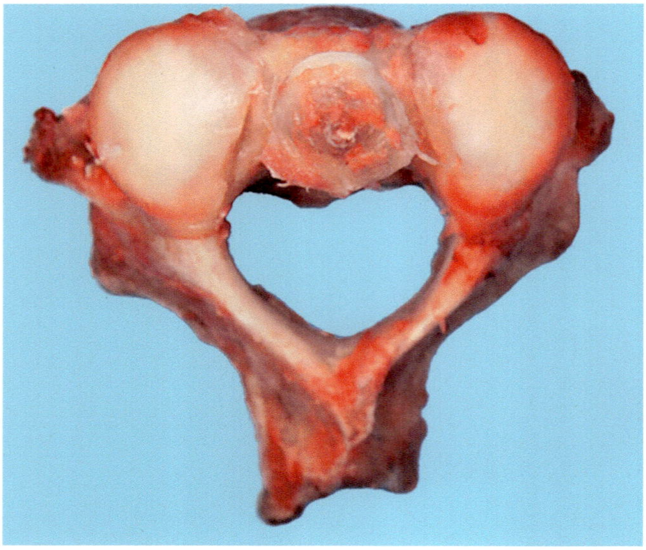

Fig. 2.7 The superior view of the axis

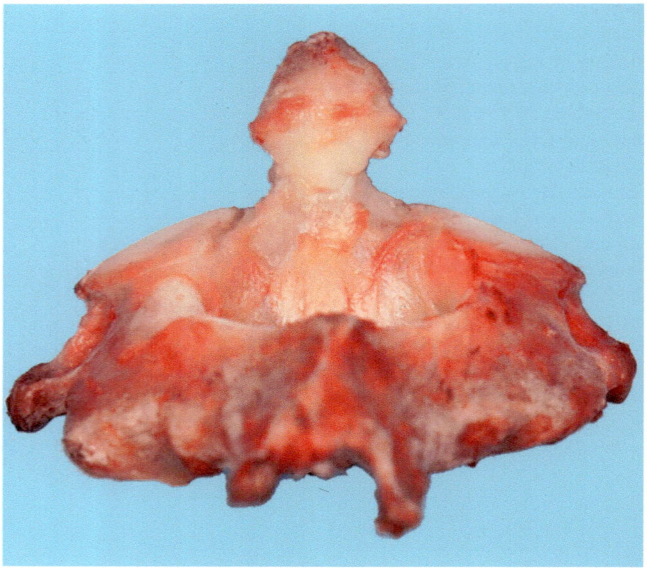

Fig. 2.8 The posterior view of the axis

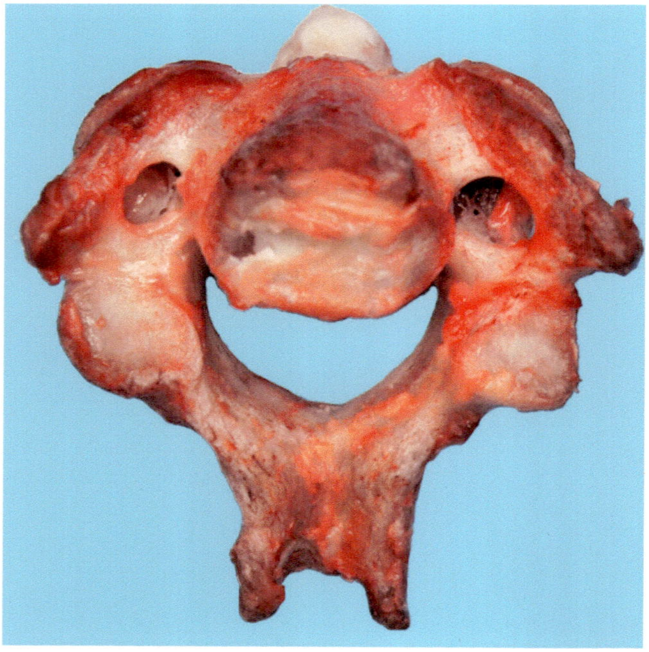

Fig. 2.9 The inferior view of the axis

2.3 Key Points of Axis Pedicle Screw Techniques

2.3.1 Determining Entry Points of C2 Pedicle Screws

Many methods are available for entry of a C2 pedicle screw. The most reliable method is pedicle screw insertion under direct vision.

In the method described by Xu et al. [6], the entry point for a C2 pedicle screw is located at the junction of the transverse line 5 mm inferior to the superior margin of the C2 lamina and 7 mm lateral to the medial border of the vertebral canal in line with the superior margin of the C2 lamina. The drill is angled 30° medially and 20° in the cephalad direction (Fig. 2.11).

In the method by the current authors, the entry point is located 2 mm superomedial to the center of the C2 lateral mass (Fig. 2.12). The entry angle is the same as described by Xu et al.

2.3.2 Entry Angle of the Pedicle Screw of the Axis

The entry angles in the two methods are identical, with a medial inclination of approximately 30° (Fig. 2.13) and a cephalad inclination of approximately 20° [7] (Figs. 2.14 and 2.15). Chin et al. showed that the optimal medial inclination of C2 pedicle screw is 29.2° [8].

2.3.3 Depth of the Pedicle Screw of the Axis

Based on our experience and intraoperative measurements, the screw is inserted for an approximate depth of 24–28 mm using the aforementioned entry points and angles.

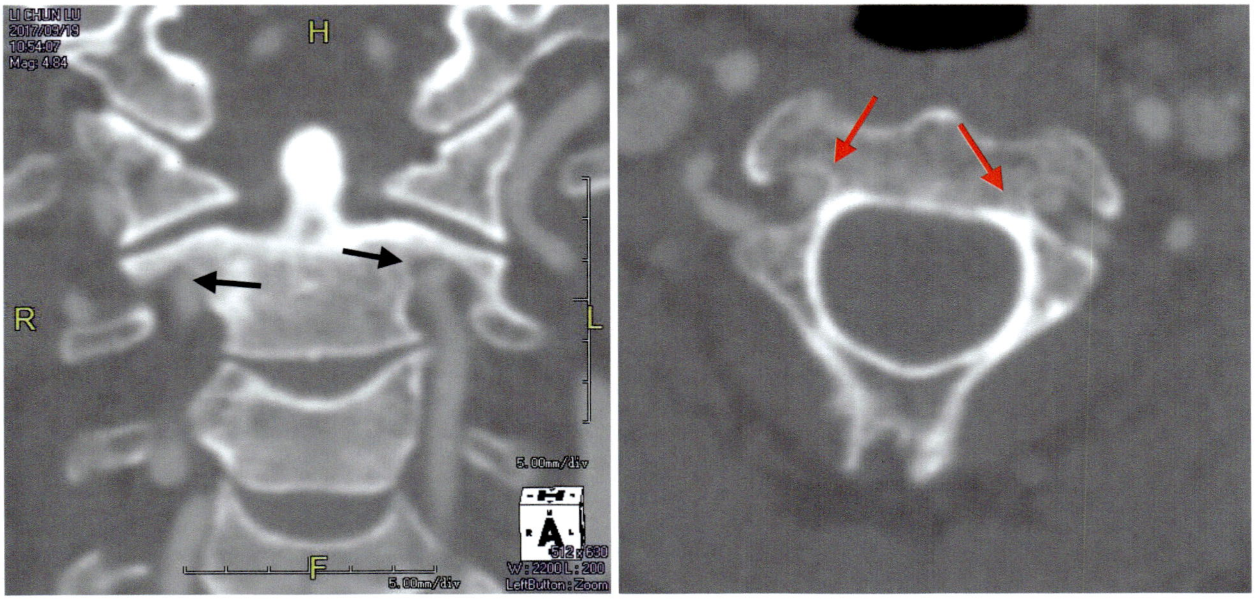

Fig. 2.10 Variations of the vertebral artery. *Black arrows* (*left*) indicate tortuosity, medial shifting, and high riding of bilateral vertebral arteries. *Red arrows* (*right*) show medial shifting of the vertebral artery and underdevelopment of bilateral pedicles

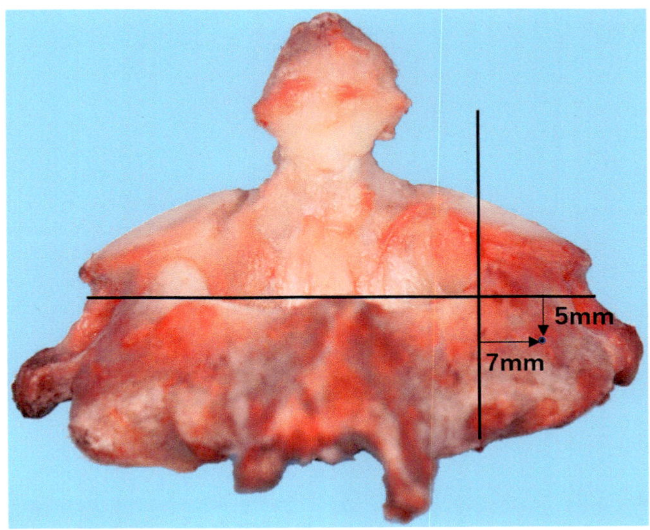

Fig. 2.11 Determining the entry point of the pedicle screw of the axis according to Xu et al. The posterior view is shown in C2. The *transverse line* and the *vertical line* define the superior margin of the C2 lamina and the lateral margin of the vertebral canal, respectively. The entry point for a C2 pedicle screw is located 7 mm lateral to the vertical line and 5 mm caudal to the transverse line

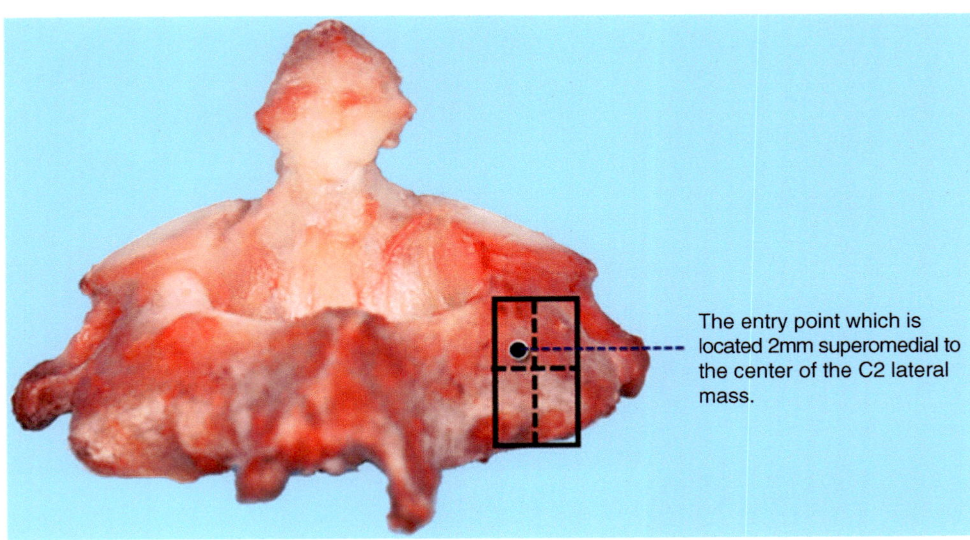

Fig. 2.12 Determining the entry point of the pedicle screw of the axis according to the current authors

Fig. 2.13 Angle between the screw path and the sagittal plane

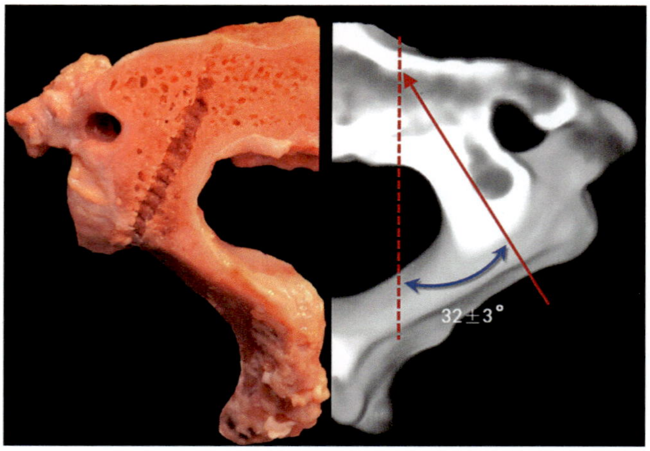

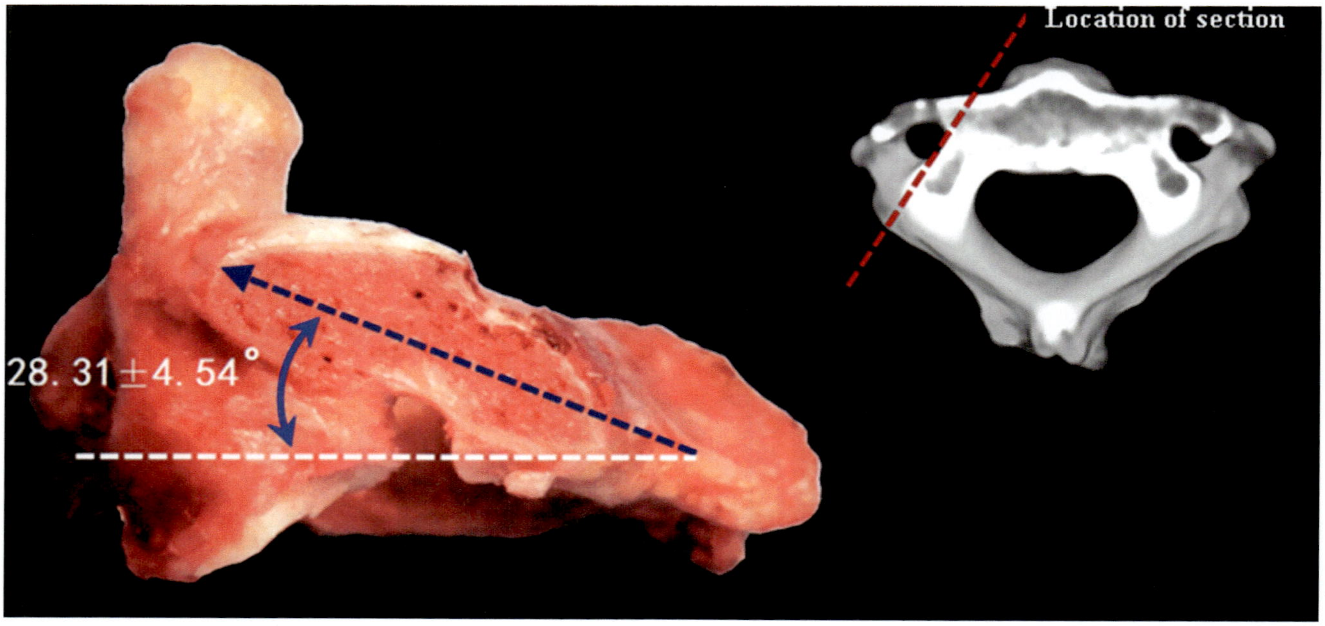

Fig. 2.14 Angle between the screw path and the horizontal plane

Fig. 2.15 An illustrative drawing showing the angle between the screw path and the horizontal plane

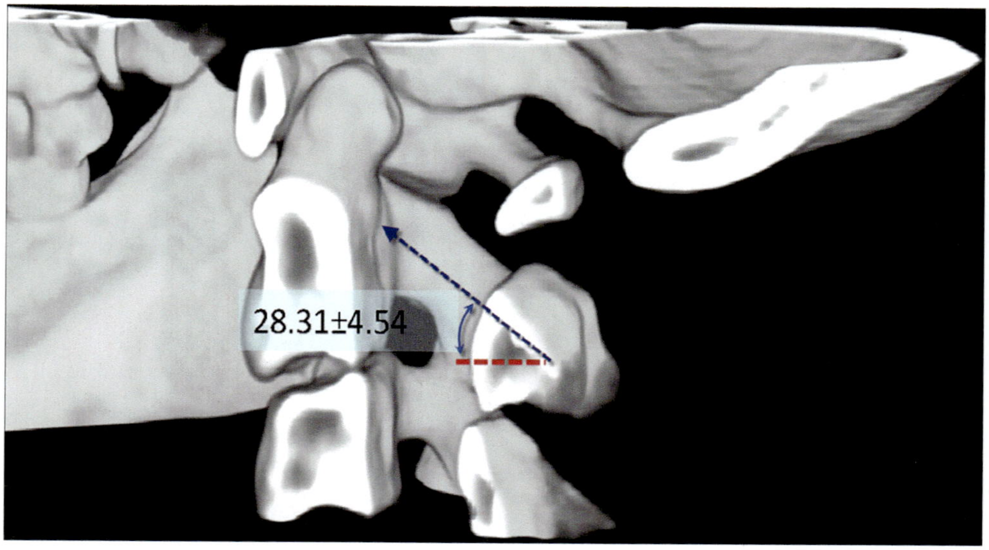

2.3.4 Surgical Steps

1. The entry point is determined (Fig. 2.16).
2. The screw hole is drilled using a drill bit (Fig. 2.17).
3. Drill depth is increased using a 3.5-mm drill bit with drill guide (Fig. 2.18).
4. The screw is implanted after the screw path is processed (Fig. 2.19).
5. The contralateral screw path is handled (Fig. 2.20).
6. Screw implantation is completed (Fig. 2.21).
7. The sectional view of the screw path (Figs. 2.22 and 2.23).

2.4 Imaging Features of Standard Pedicle Screws of the Axis (Figs. 2.24, 2.25, 2.26, 2.27, 2.28, and 2.29)

Case 1 Patient: A 48-year-old male complained of a sore neck and numbness of extremities with difficulty in walking for 3 years.

Diagnosis: Congenital malformation of the odontoid process.

Surgery: Atlas reduction, VERTEX internal fixation with cervico-occipital bone graft and fusion (Figs. 2.30, 2.31, 2.32, 2.33, 2.34, and 2.35).

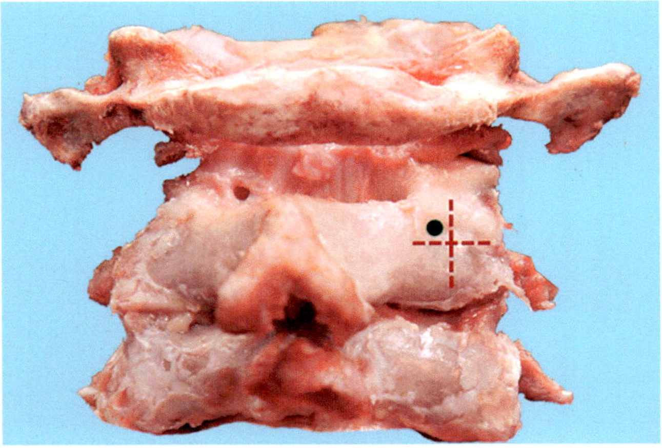

Fig. 2.16 Choosing the screw entry site

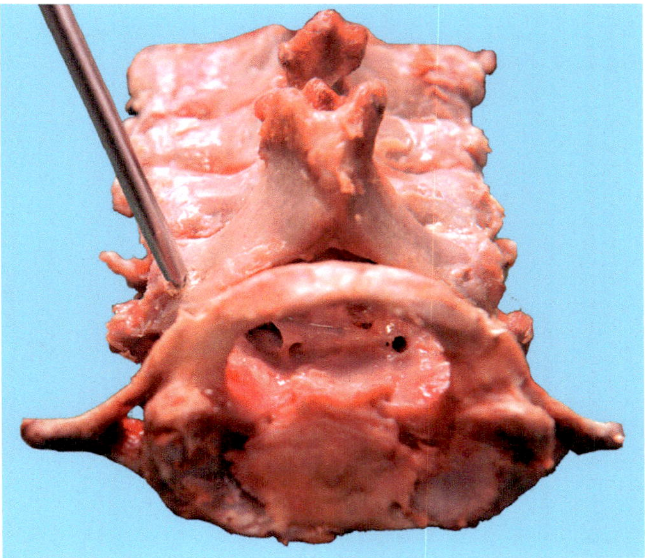

Fig. 2.17 A screw hole is drilled

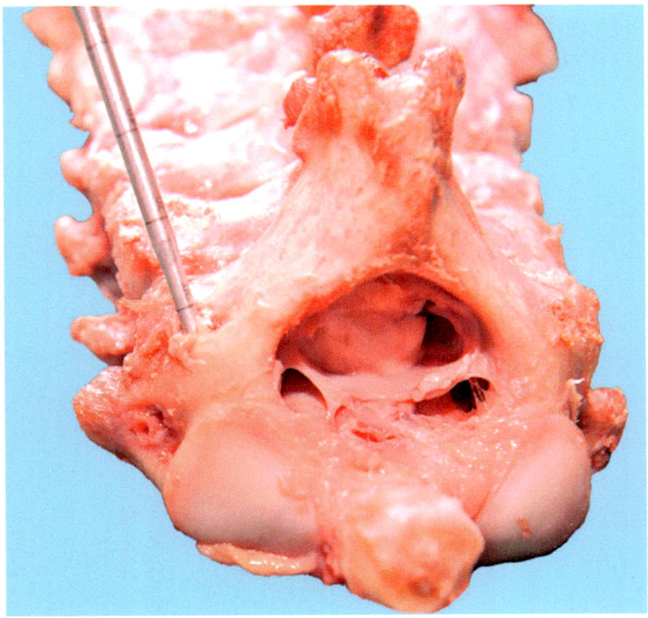

Fig. 2.18 Lengthening the screw path

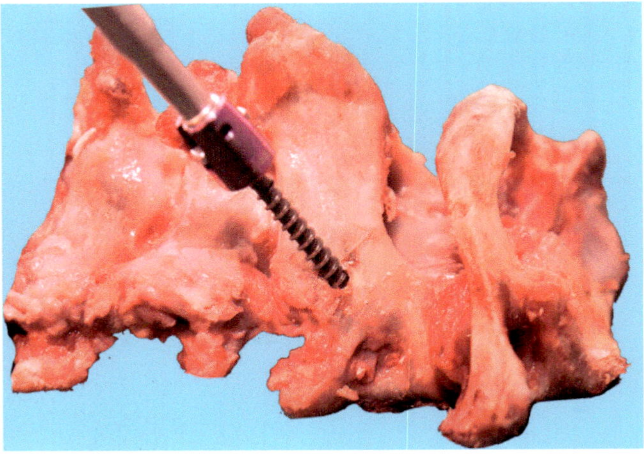

Fig. 2.19 Implanting the screw

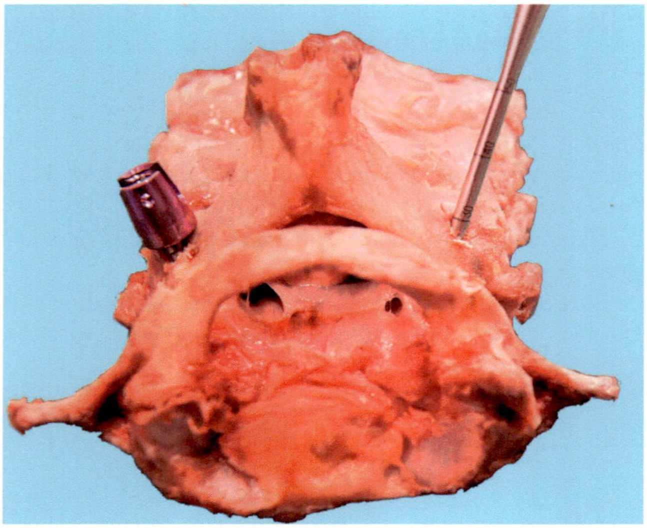

Fig. 2.20 Processing the contralateral screw path

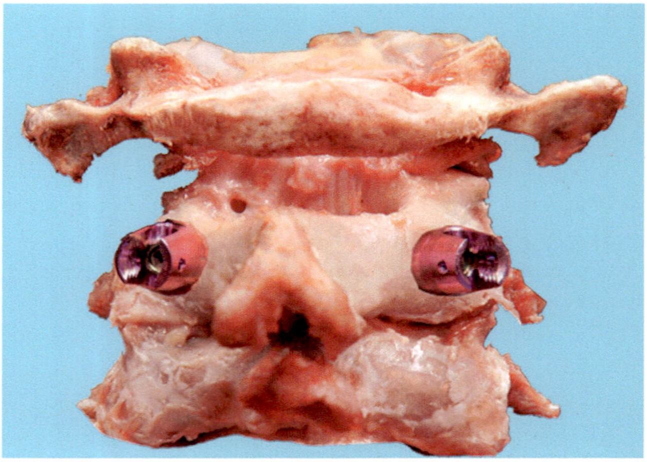

Fig. 2.21 The screw is implanted

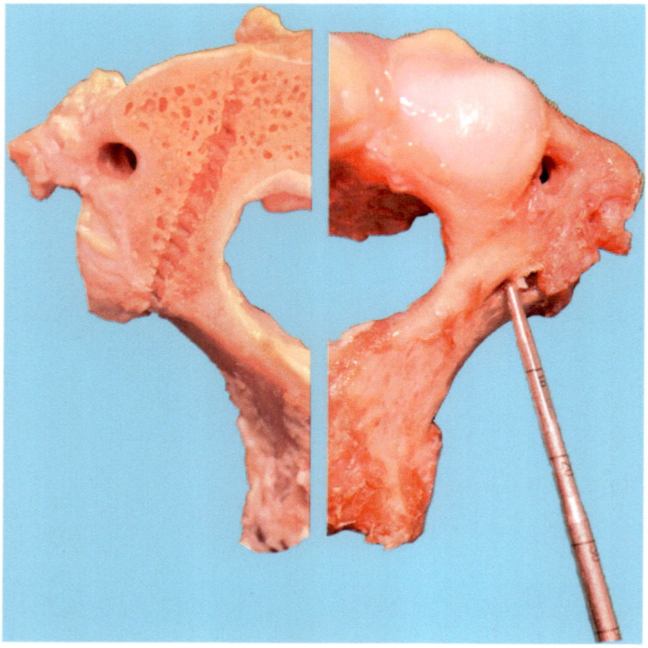

Fig. 2.22 Sectional view of the screw path

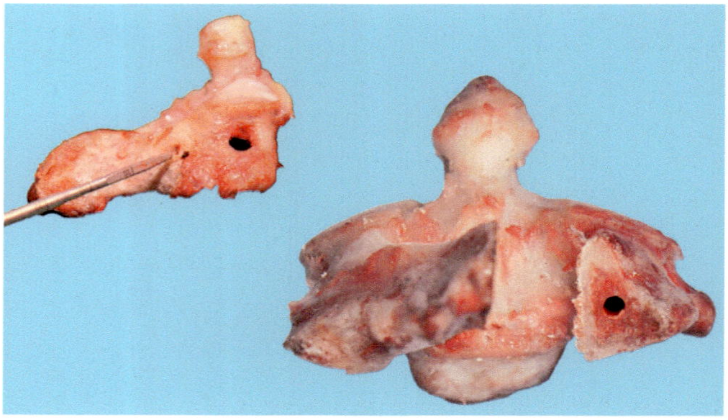

Fig. 2.23 Sectional view of the screw path

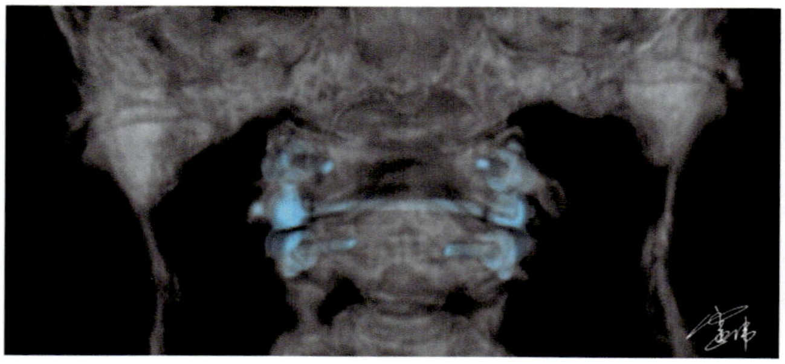

Fig. 2.24 Anterior view of C2 pedicle screw

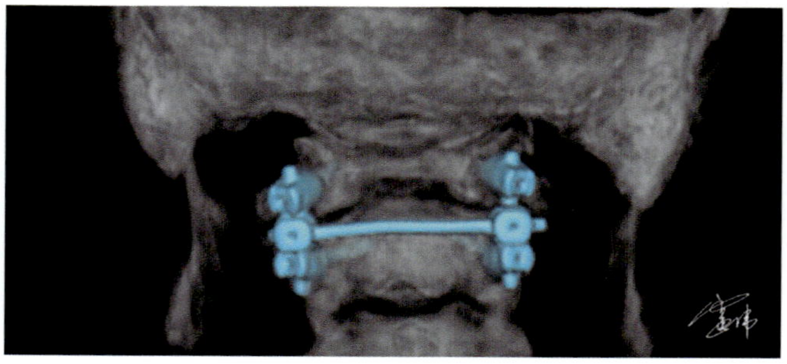

Fig. 2.25 Posterior view of C2 pedicle screw

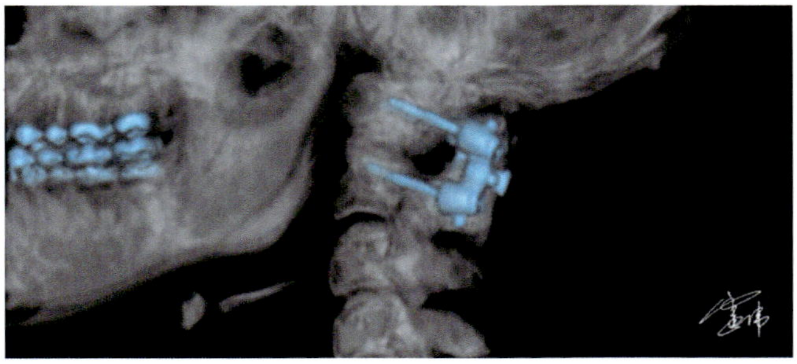

Fig. 2.26 Lateral view of C2 pedicle screw

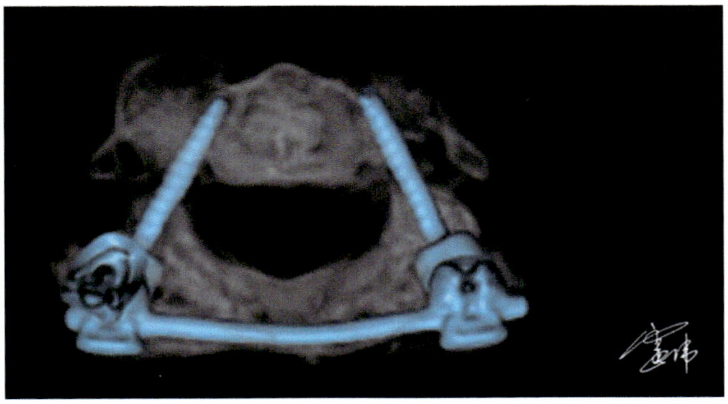

Fig. 2.27 Superior view of C2 pedicle screw

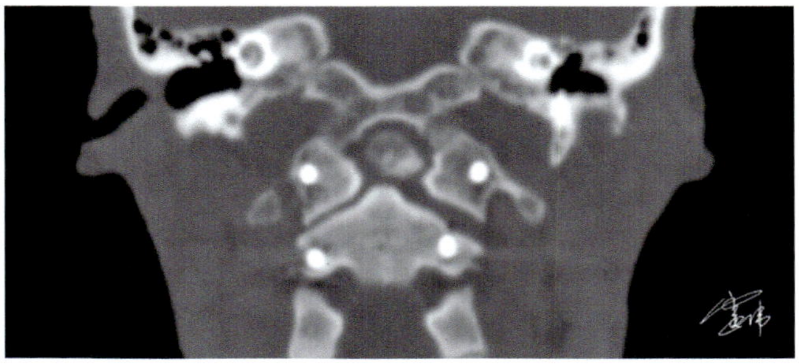

Fig. 2.28 Coronal section of C2 pedicle screw

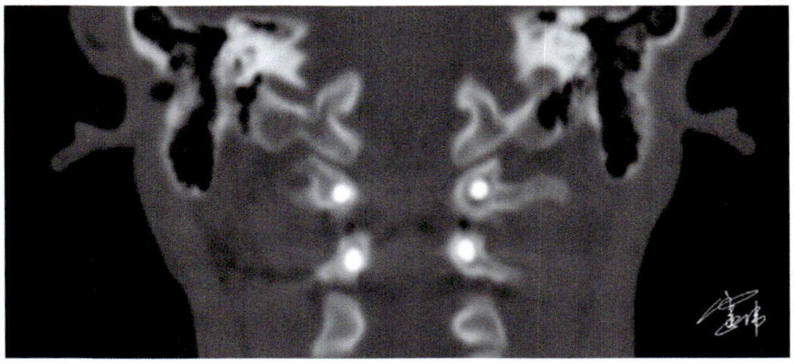

Fig. 2.29 Coronal section of C2 pedicle screw

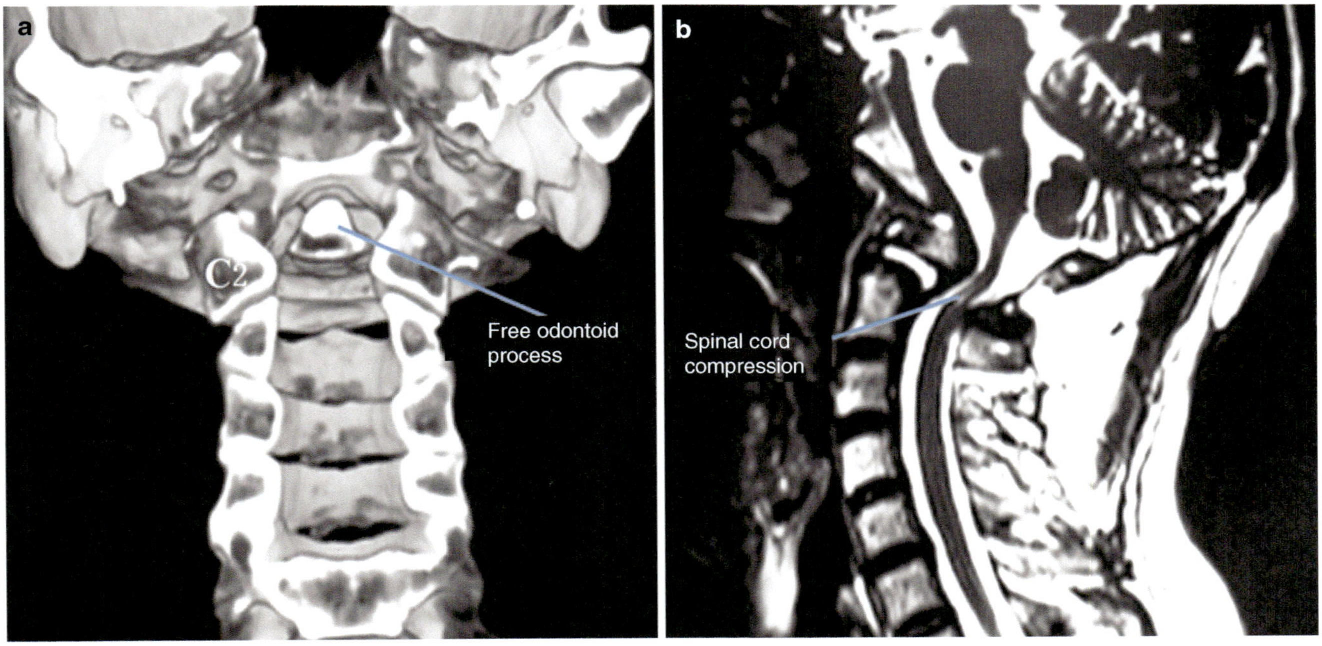

Fig. 2.30 Preoperative images. (**a**) Split coronal image of the spinal canal (*posterior view*); (**b**) MRI (*lateral view*); (**c**) Cervico-occipital reconstruction (*sagittal view*)

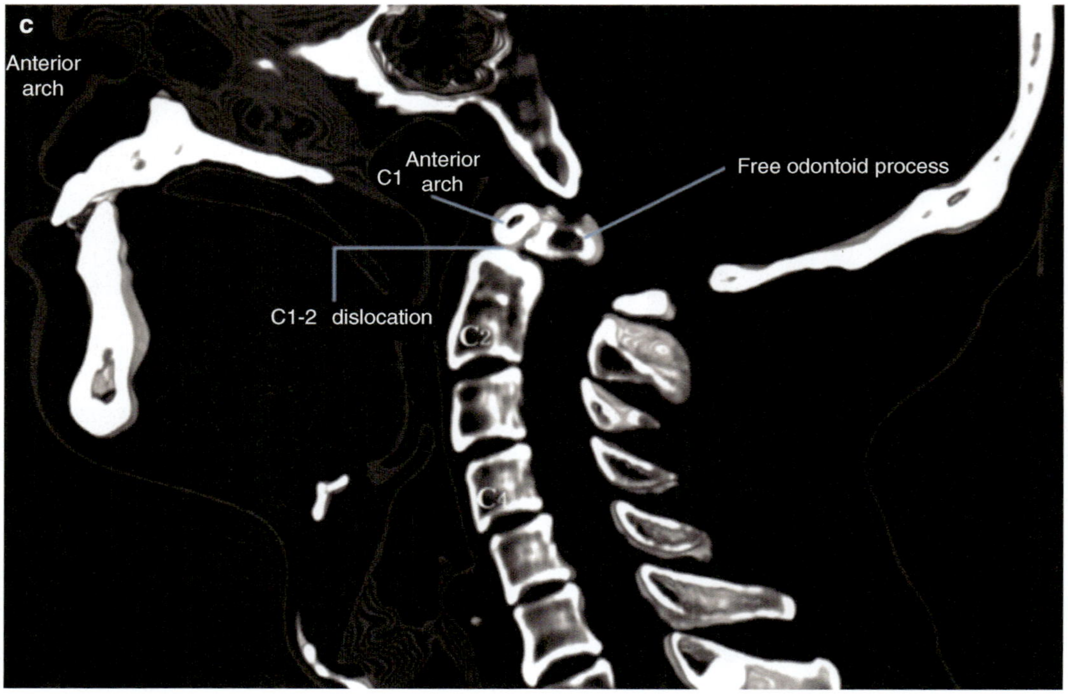

Fig. 2.30 (continued)

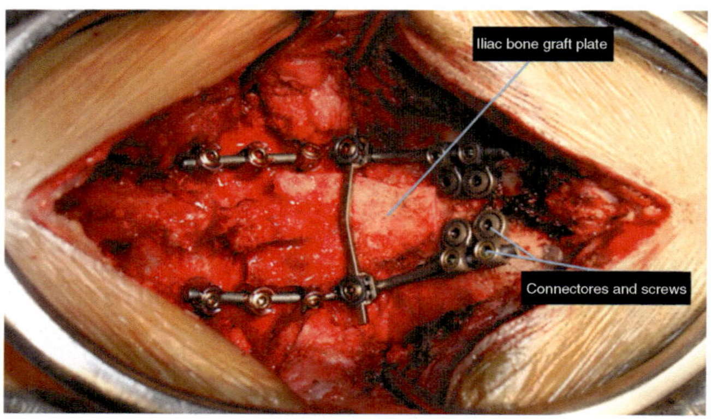

Fig. 2.31 Intraoperative internal fixation

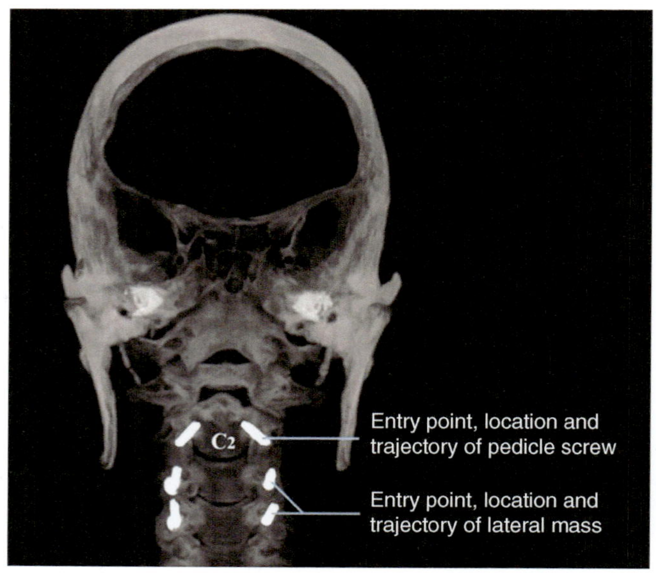

Fig. 2.33 The spinal canal is split in the coronal section (*posterior view*)

Case 2

Patient: A 69-year-old female complained of numbness of four extremities with weakness in walking for 3 years and worsening for 1 year.

Diagnosis: Ossification of the posterior longitudinal ligament of the cervical spine and cervical spinal stenosis.

Surgery: Decompression by laminectomy via a posterior approach, vertex internal fixation, bone graft and fusion (C2–C6) (Figs. 2.36, 2.37, and 2.38).

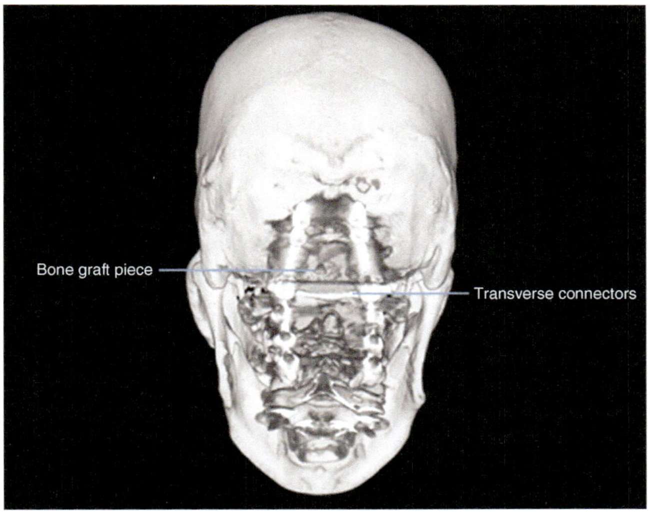

Fig. 2.32 Position of internal fixation (flexion, *posterior view*)

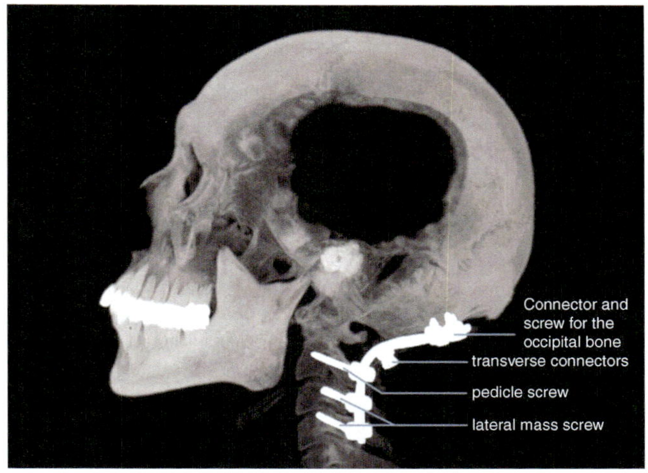

Fig. 2.34 Position of internal fixation (*lateral view*)

Fig. 2.35 Location of internal fixation (*posterior view*). Caution: The patient only has C1–C2 instability, which requires decompression by partial bone removal of the foramen magnum and C1 posterior arch removal. Stabilization should be limited to the occipital bone, C1 and C2. If C1 cannot be stabilized, or if the surgeon cannot carry out internal fixation with confidence, stabilization can be extended to C3. In the current patient, C4 is stabilized; though fixation is well positioned, it goes beyond the set limit of stabilization. The space between C4 and C5 is the largest space for cervical mobility; C4 fixation may accelerate degenerative changes of the intervertebral space

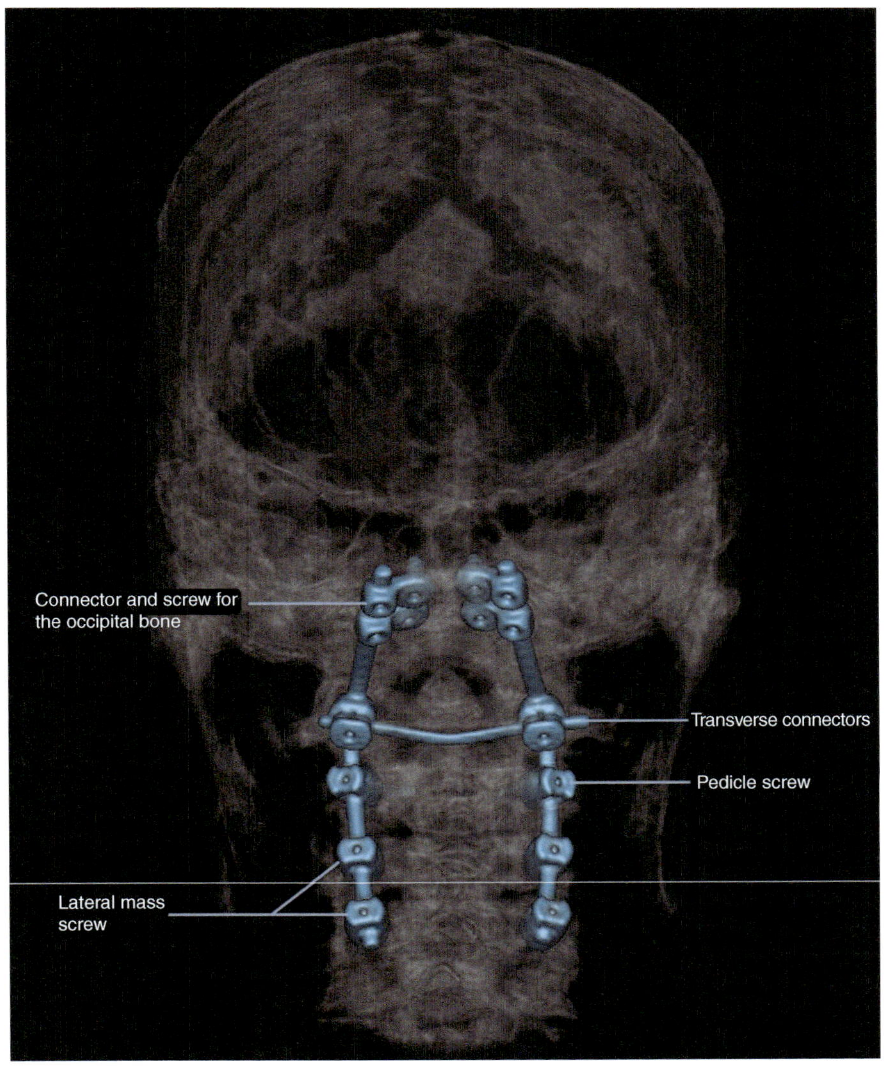

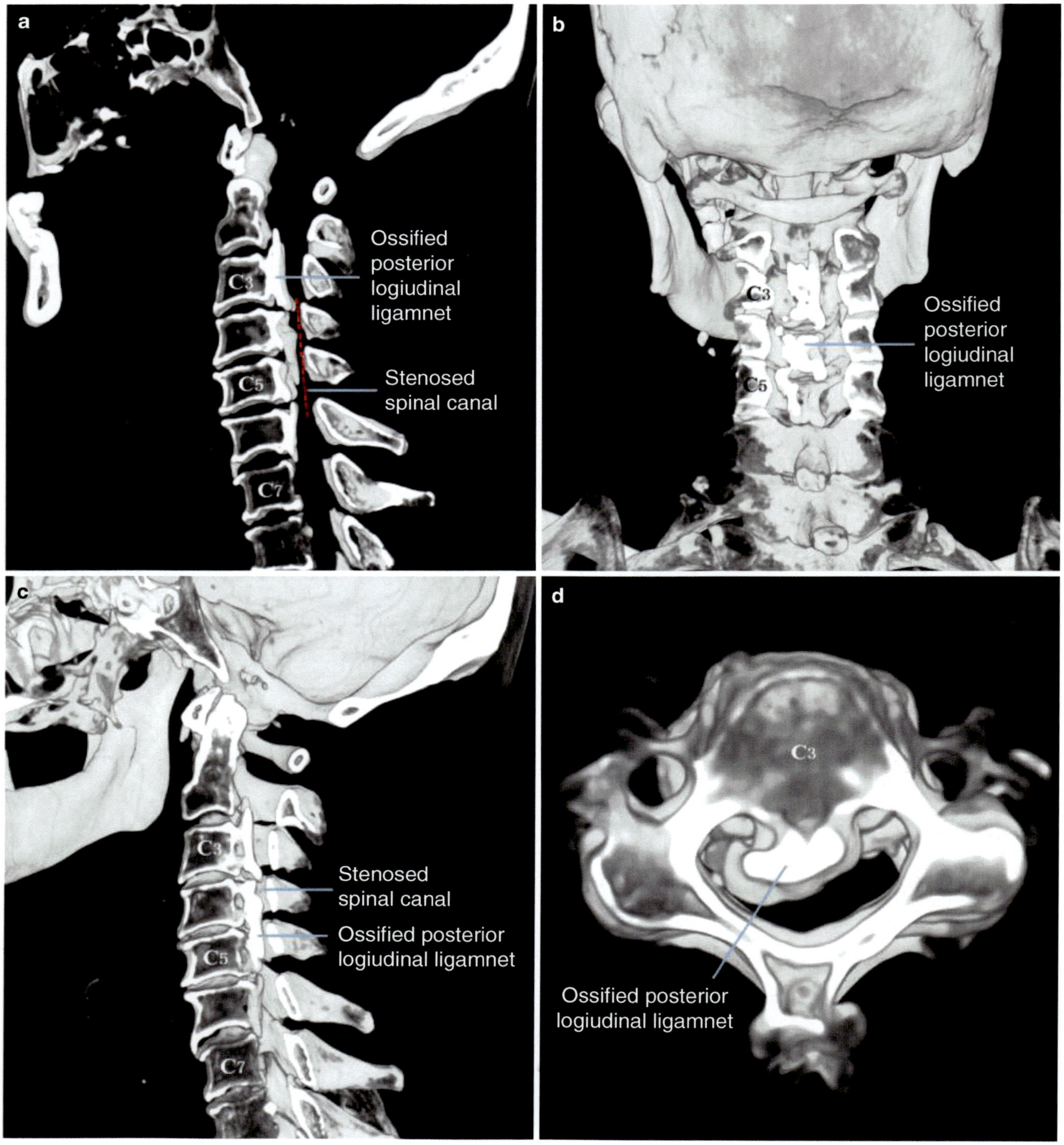

Fig. 2.36 Preoperative 3D CT reconstruction. (**a**) Spinal canal reconstruction (*sagittal view*); (**b**) The spinal canal is split in the coronal section (posterior view); (**c**) The spinal canal is split in the longitudinal section (*sagittal view*); (**d**) Reconstruction of the spinal canal at C3–C6 (*the overlooking view*)

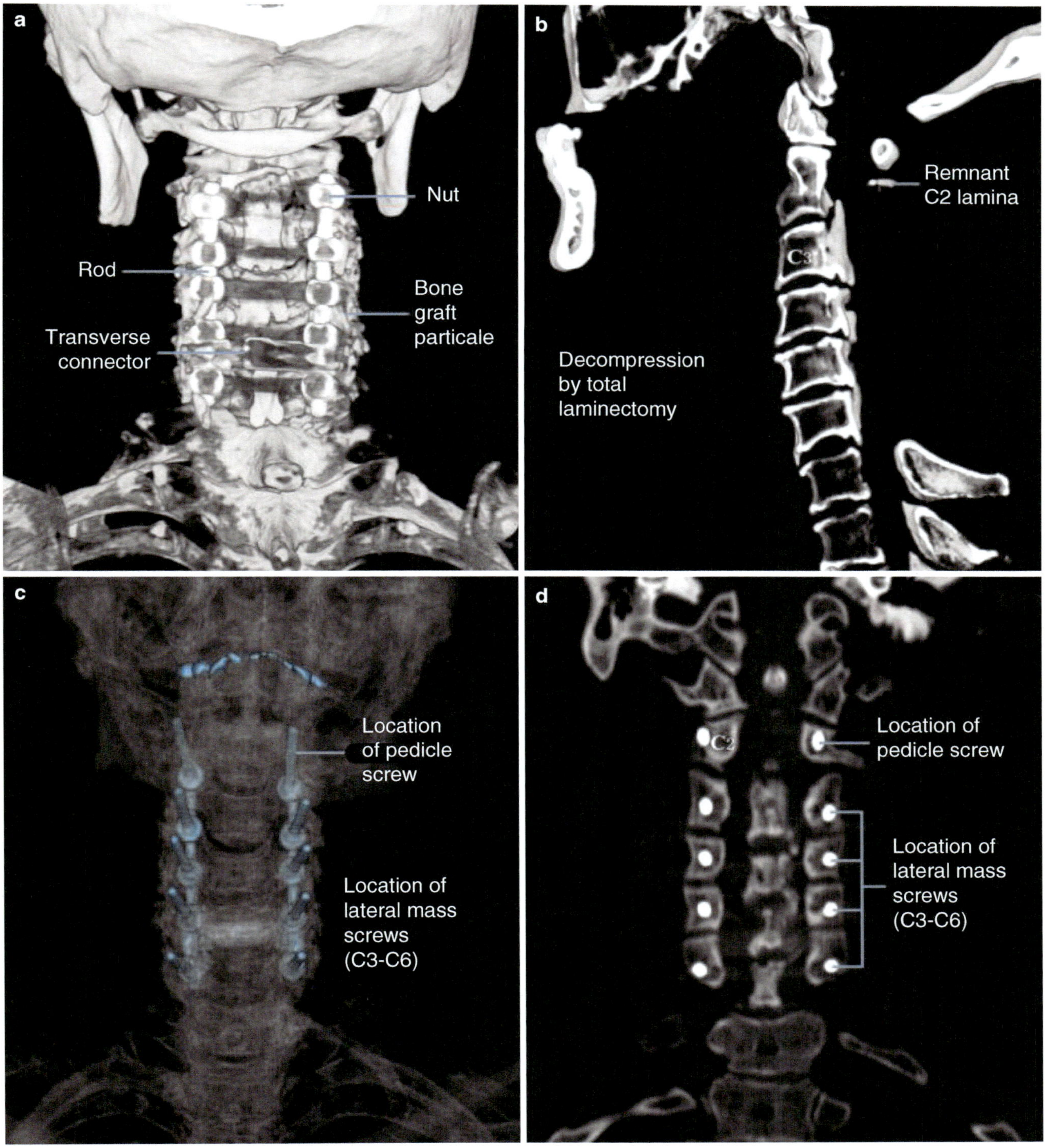

Fig. 2.37 Postoperative 3D CT reconstruction. (**a**) Location of internal fixation (*posterior view*); (**b**) Spinal canal reconstruction (*sagittal view*); (**c**) Location of internal fixation (*anterior view*); (**d**) The spinal canal is split in the coronal section (*posterior view*)

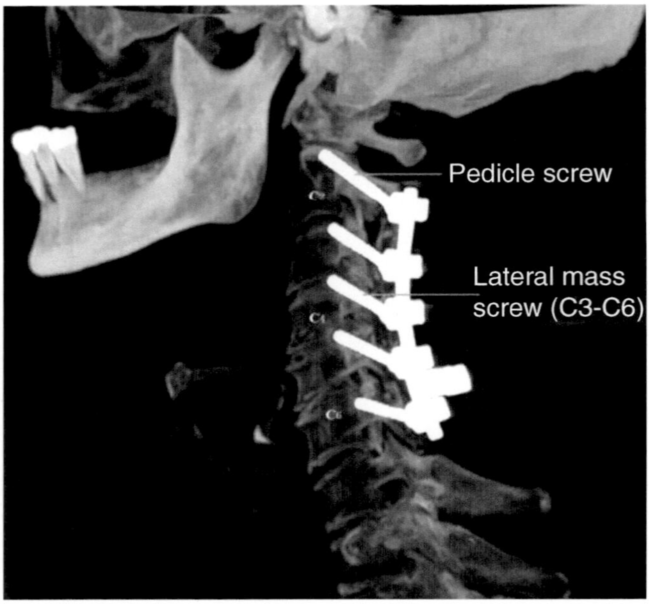

Fig. 2.38 Location of internal fixation (*lateral view*)

2.5 Pearls and Pitfalls

1. The axis has an intimate relation with the vertebral artery. Great caution is advised against causing inadvertent vertebral artery injury when axis pedicle screw techniques are undertaken. Preoperative CTA is mandatory.
2. Anatomic variations of the vertebral artery are frequent, which are often accompanied by C2 pedicle maldevelopment. For example, high riding deformity of the vertebral artery is a contraindication for C2 pedicle screw placement; other internal fixation techniques should be employed.

References

1. Goel A, Laheri V. Plate and screw fixation for atlanto-axial subluxation. Acta Neurochir. 1994;129(1–2):47–53.
2. Jeanneret B, Magerl F. Primary posterior fusion C1/2 in odontoid fractures: indications, technique, and results of transarticular screw fixation. J Spinal Disord. 1992;5(4):464–75.
3. Wright NM. Posterior C2 fixation using bilateral, crossing C2 laminar screws: case series and technical note. J Spinal Disord Tech. 2004;17(2):158–62.
4. Chao Z. Z.S., and Xu C, *An illustrative figure showing measurements of the axis*. Chin J Clin Anat. 2000;18(2):299–301.
5. Lee SH, et al. Analysis of 3-dimensional course of the intra-axial vertebral artery for C2 pedicle screw trajectory: a computed tomographic study. Spine (Phila Pa 1976). 2014;39(17):E1010–4.
6. Ebraheim N, et al. Anatomic consideration of C2 pedicle screw placement. Spine (Phila Pa 1976). 1996;21(6):691–5.
7. Benzel EC. Anatomic consideration of C2 pedicle screw placement. Spine (Phila Pa 1976). 1996;21(19):2301–2.
8. Chin KR, et al. Ideal starting point and trajectory for C2 pedicle screw placement: a 3D computed tomography analysis using perioperative measurements. Spine J. 2014;14(4):615–8.

Lateral Mass Screw Fixation Techniques for the Lower Cervical Spine

3

Lei Shi, Yabo Yan, and Wei Lei

Abstract

Lateral mass screws combined with rods are widely used in treating cervical spine diseases, such as ossification of the posterior longitudinal ligament, spinal stenosis, trauma, tumor, etc. Although lateral mass screw fixation is not as strong as lateral pedicle screw fixation, surgeons prefer to use it due to its safety and convenience. Several lateral mass screw fixation techniques have been described, among which the most used are Roy-Camille, Magerl, Anderson, and An. In this chapter, we introduce surgical anatomy of the lateral mass and carefully describe how to use the lateral mass screws in lower cervical spine based on Magerl techniques. The entry point, entry angle, and entry depth of lateral mass screws are clearly showed. At the end of the chapter, one clinical case was performed. The patient was diagnosed to have ossification of the posterior longitudinal ligament of the cervical spine and cervical spinal stenosis. Decompression and lateral mass screw fixation were done, and after the surgery, the patient got good function.

Keywords

Lateral mass screws · Fixation · Lower cervical spine Spinal stenosis

3.1 Lateral Mass Screws for the Lower Cervical Spine: A Historical Perspective

Roy-Camille et al. developed lateral mass screw techniques in 1980 [1]. Magerl subsequently improved the entry method for lateral mass screws [2], which has become the most frequently used entry method for lateral mass screws currently (Fig. 3.1).

3.2 Surgical Anatomy of the Lateral Mass of the Lower Cervical Spine

The lateral masses, one on each side, lie posterolateral to the cervical vertebra and connect the superior and inferior articular facets. The lateral mass is divided from the laminar via the medial line of the articular facets and connects the vertebral body via the pedicle (Figs. 3.2, 3.3, 3.4, and 3.5).

3.2.1 Defining the Lateral Mass Boundaries

The margins of the lateral masses are defined superiorly by the lowest point of the superior articular facet and inferiorly by the most distal point of the inferior articular facet and medially by the junction of the lamina and the articular process and laterally by the bony border (Fig. 3.6). The distance between the centers of adjacent lateral masses is 13 mm on average.

3.2.2 Important Neurovascular Structures in Relation to the Lateral Masses

The anteromedial border of the lateral mass is the lateral border of the cervical spinal cord. The medial two quadrants are the projection of the vertebral artery anteriorly, and the inferior two quadrants are the projection of cervical nerves anteriorly. The superolateral quadrant, under which vital neurovascular structures do not lie, is considered a safe zone (Figs. 3.7 and 3.8).

L. Shi · Y. Yan · W. Lei (✉)
Department of Orthopedics, Xijing Hospital, Air Force Medical University, Xi'an, Shaanxi, China
e-mail: leiwei@fmmu.edu.cn

W. Lei, Y. Yan (eds.), *Internal Fixation of the Spine*, https://doi.org/10.1007/978-981-16-1562-7_3

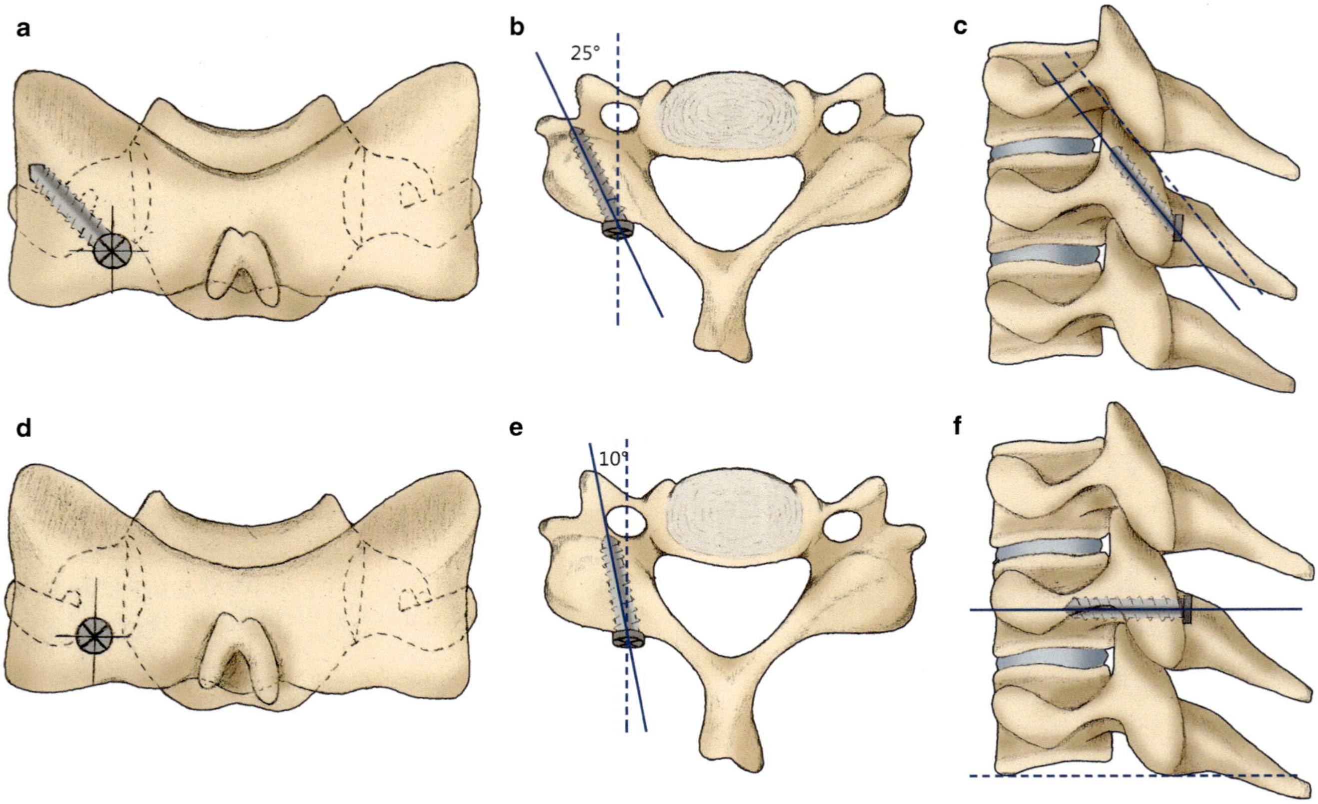

Fig. 3.1 The Magerl technique (**a**–**c**) versus the Roy-Camille technique (**d**–**f**)

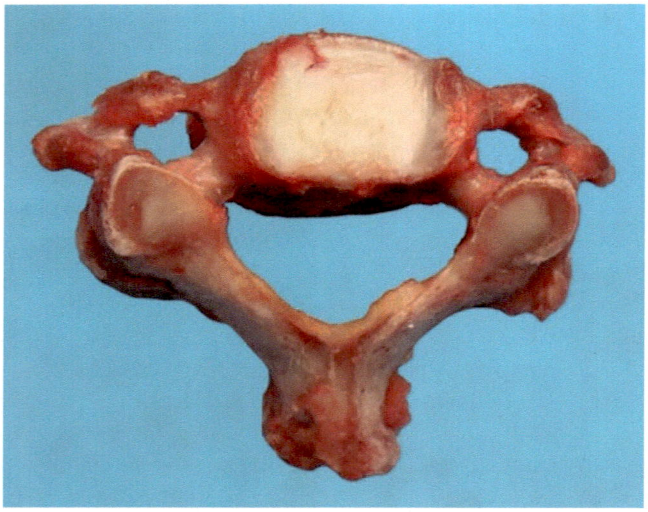

Fig. 3.2 The superior view of C5

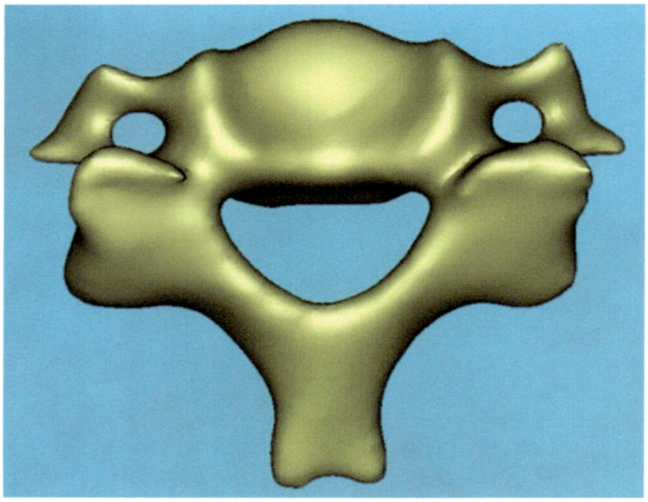

Fig. 3.3 The inferior view of C5

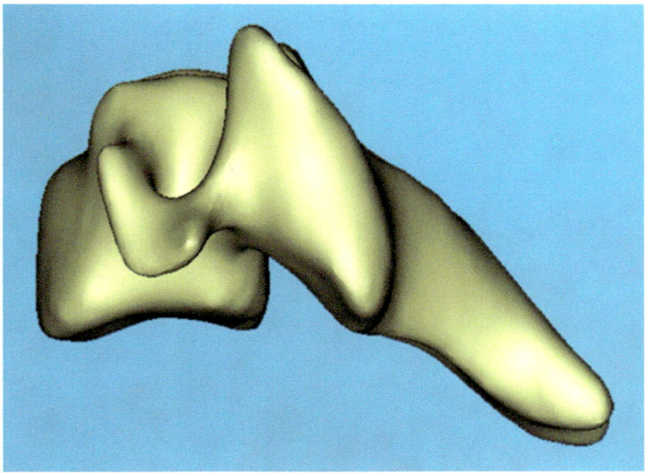

Fig. 3.4 The lateral view of C5

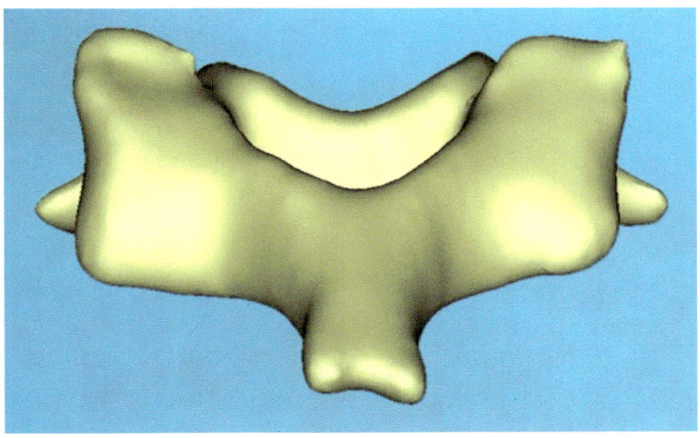

Fig. 3.5 The lateral view of C5

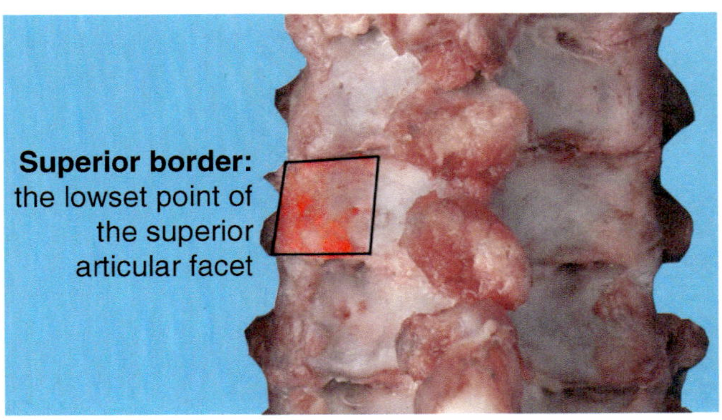

Fig. 3.6 The borders of the lateral mass

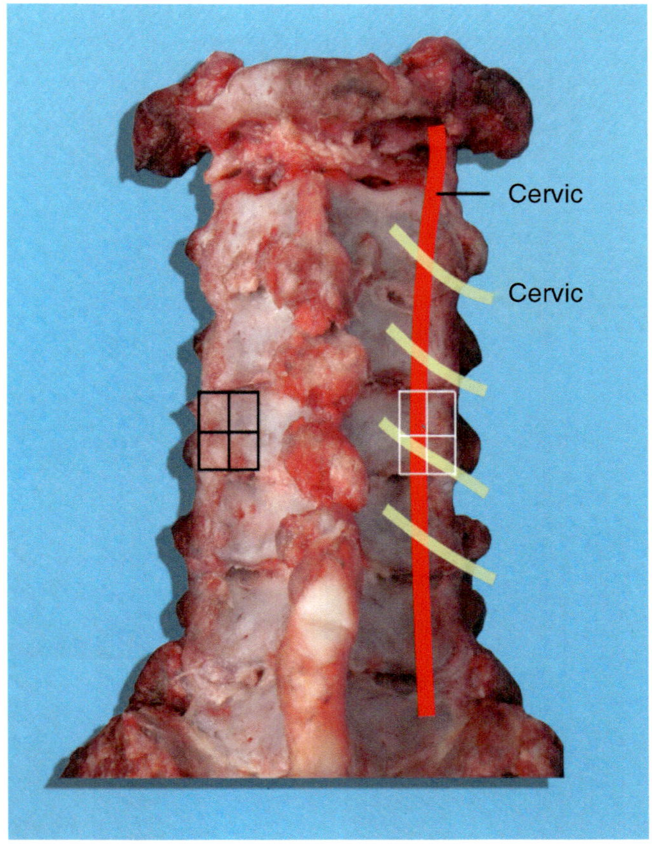

Fig. 3.7 The relations between the lateral mass and important neurovascular structures

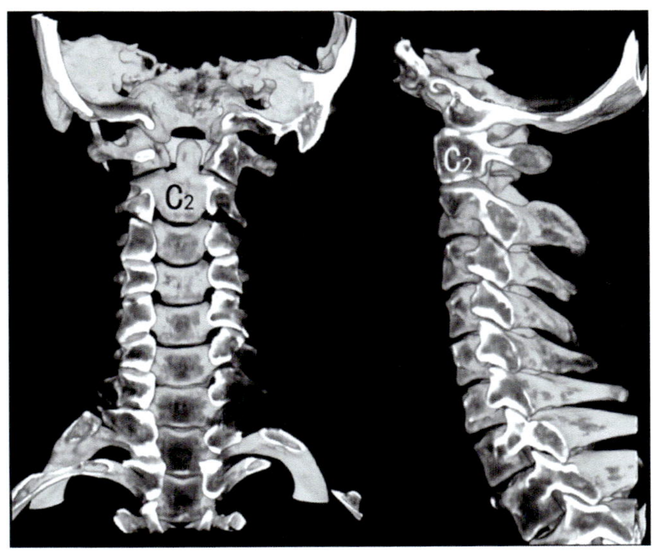

Fig. 3.8 The sectional view of the lateral mass. *Left*: the coronal section; *Right*: the sagittal section

3.2.3 Measured Dimensions of the Lateral Mass of the Cervical Spine (Figs. 3.9 and 3.10; Table 3.1)

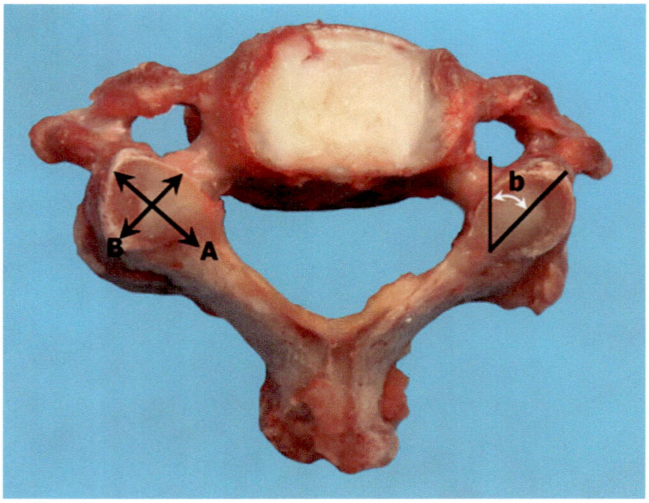

Fig. 3.10 The superior view of the lateral mass [3]. (*A*) the left to right diameter of the lateral mass, (*B*) the anteroposterior diameter of the lateral mass, (*b*) angle in the sagittal plane

3.3 Lateral Mass Screw Techniques for the Lower Cervical Spine

3.3.1 Determining the Screw Entry Points in the Lateral Mass of the Cervical Spine

The Magerl technique is the most common method (Fig. 3.11).

1. The entry point is located 2–3 mm cephalic and medial to the midpoint of the lateral mass.
2. The entry angle is 45° in the cephalad direction relative to the sagittal plane and is parallel to the small joint facet and laterally 25° relative to the transverse plane.

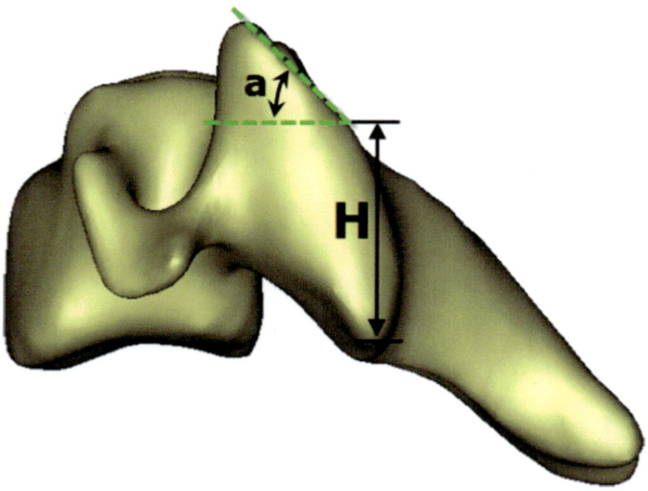

Fig. 3.9 The lateral view of the lateral mass [3]. (*a*) the inclinations of the surface of the superior articular surface. (*H*) the height of the later mass

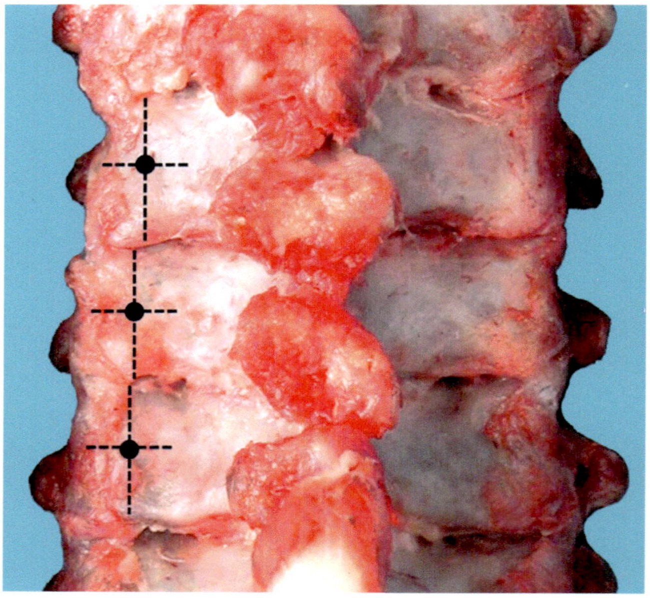

Fig. 3.11 Entry points of the lateral mass screws

Table 3.1 Measured dimensions of the lateral mass

Cervical vertebra	A (mm)	B (mm)	H (mm)	a (°)	b (°)
C3	10.7 ± 1.0	8.1 ± 1.2	12.3 ± 1.8	48.4 ± 8.3	49.8 ± 5.0
C4	11.2 ± 1.2	8.0 ± 1.0	13.2 ± 1.9	49.9 ± 5.5	49.5 ± 4.5
C5	11.4 ± 1.0	8.0 ± 1.2	14.5 ± 2.2	48.5 ± 7.1	50.0 ± 3.7
C6	11.7 ± 1.6	8.2 ± 1.7	14.6 ± 2.2	53.2 ± 5.9	49.0 ± 4.7
C7	12.0 ± 1.2	7.0 ± 1.2	15.7 ± 2.0	62.7 ± 5.4	48.8 ± 4.6

Data is expressed as mean ± SD

3.3.2 Entry Angles of Lateral Mass Screws of the Cervical Spine (Figs. 3.12 and 3.13)

3.3.3 Entry Depth of Lateral Mass Screws

In general, the screw is inserted for 12–16 mm into the lateral mass of the cervical spine. The most commonly used screw has a diameter of 3.5 mm.

3.3.4 Surgical Steps

For detailed description of the surgical procedures, please refer to Surgical Techniques for Pedicle Screw Fixation of the Cervical Spine. Implanted screws are shown in Fig. 3.14.

3.3.5 Imaging Features of Standard Lateral Mass Screws of the Cervical Spine (Figs. 3.15, 3.16, 3.17, and 3.18)

Case Patient: A 69-year-old female complained of numbness of four extremities with weakness in walking for 3 years and worsening for 1 year.

Diagnosis: Ossification of the posterior longitudinal ligament of the cervical spine and cervical spinal stenosis.

Surgery: Decompression by laminectomy via a posterior approach, vertex internal fixation, bone graft and fusion (C2–C6) (Figs. 3.19, 3.20, and 3.21).

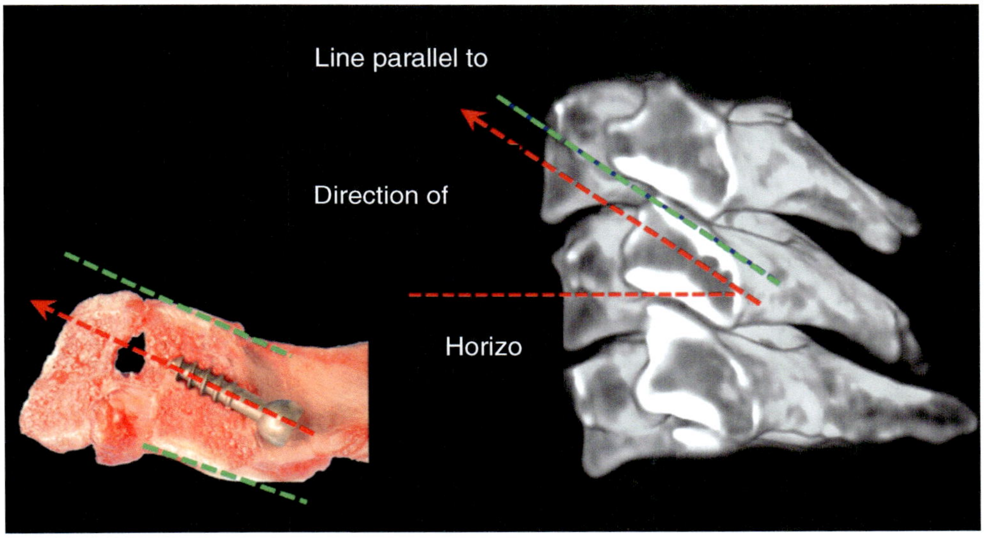

Fig. 3.12 Entry angles of lateral mass screws of the cervical spine. The angle along the articular facet in the sagittal plane is shown. Injury of the articular facet should be avoided

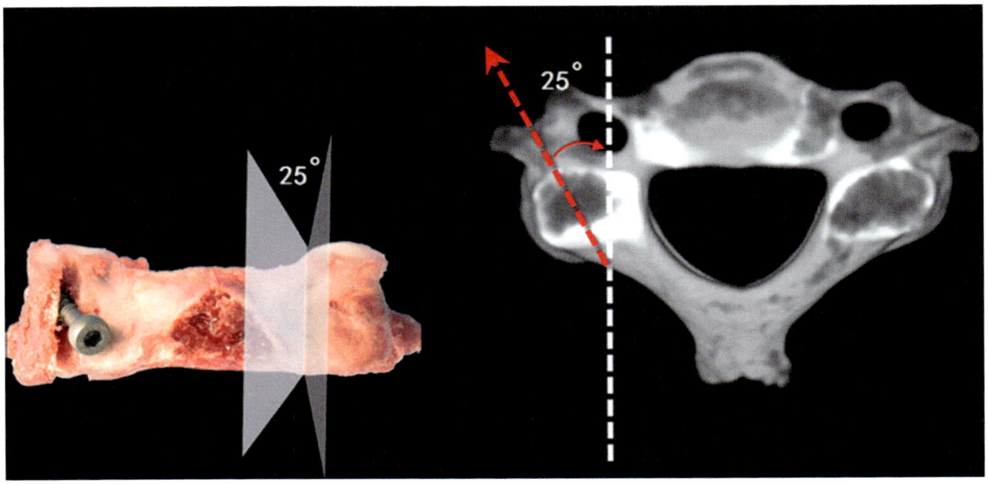

Fig. 3.13 Entry angles of lateral mass screws of the cervical spine. The horizontal plane forms a 25° angle with the sagittal plane, and the entry angle points to the root of the transverse process

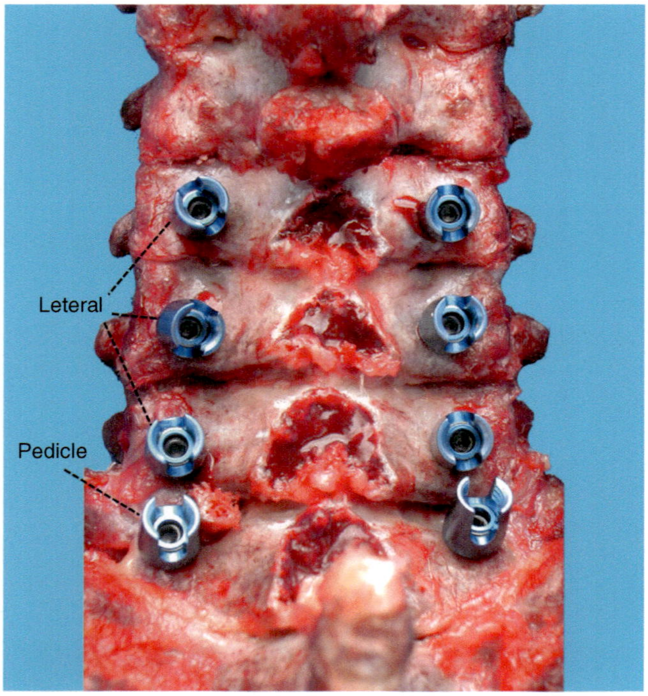

Fig. 3.14 Implanted lateral mass screws and pedicle screws

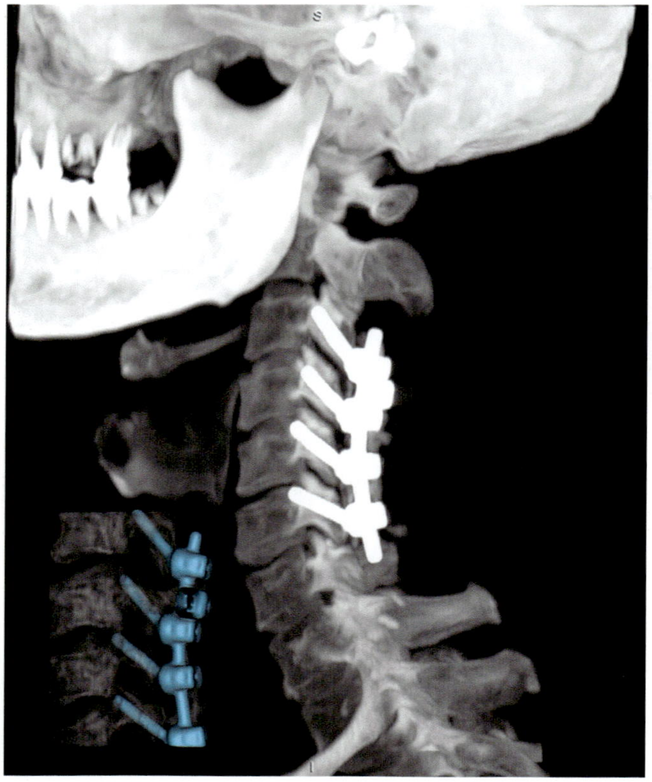

Fig. 3.15 The lateral view of implanted lateral mass screws

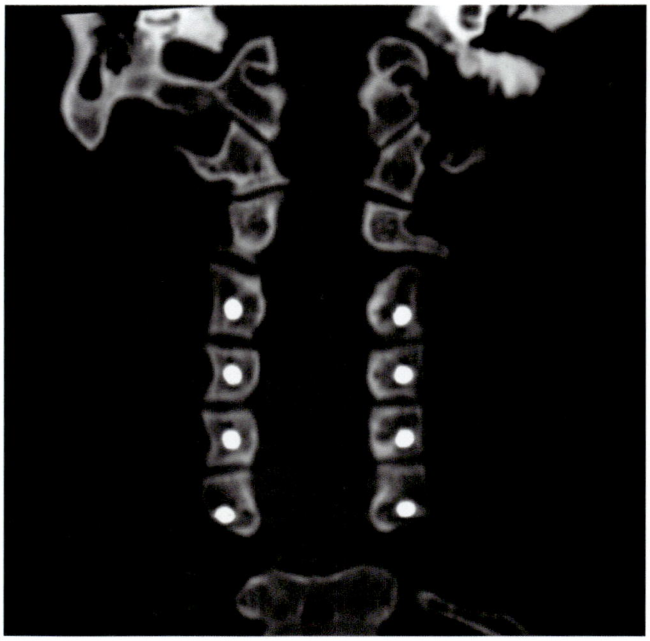

Fig. 3.16 The coronal sectional view of lateral mass screws

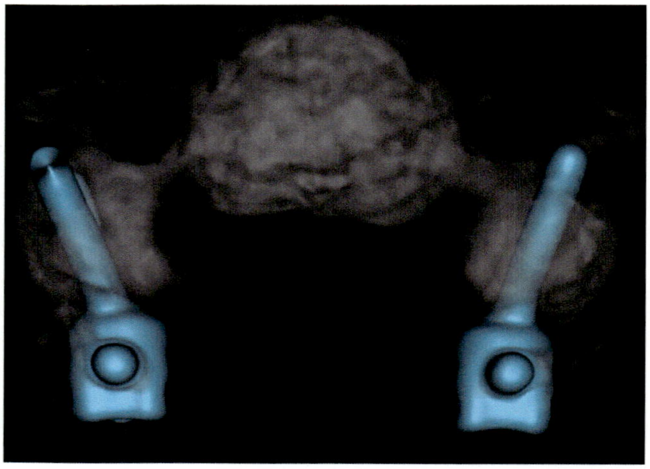

Fig. 3.17 The horizontal sectional view of C3 lateral mass screws

3.3.6 Pearls and Pitfalls

1. The surgeon should be familiar with the anatomical features of lateral masses of the cervical spine and screw entry methods in order to avoid lateral mass fracture and injuries to the vertebral artery and cervical spinal cord.
2. The lateral mass for fixation should be normal.
3. Fixation should be performed before decompression by laminectomy. If decompression is performed before fixation, the vertebral canal is open and the cervical spinal cord may be injured if surgical procedures are not properly performed.
4. If lateral mass screw fixation fails, pedicle screw fixation can be done instead.

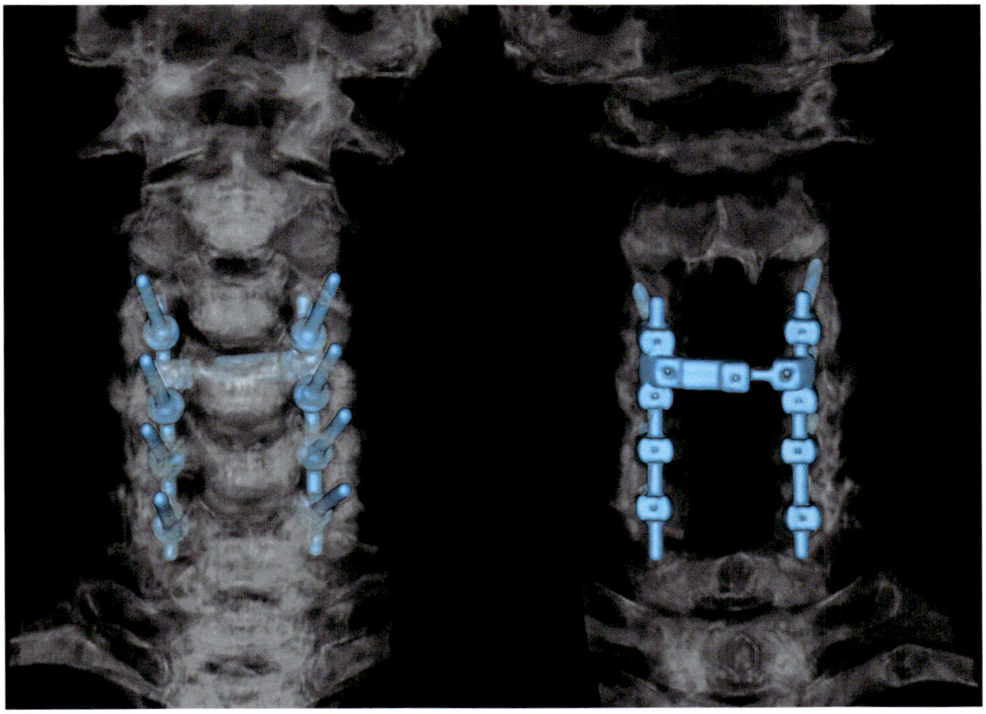

Fig. 3.18 Implanted lateral mass screws. *Left*: the anterior view; *Right*: the posterior view

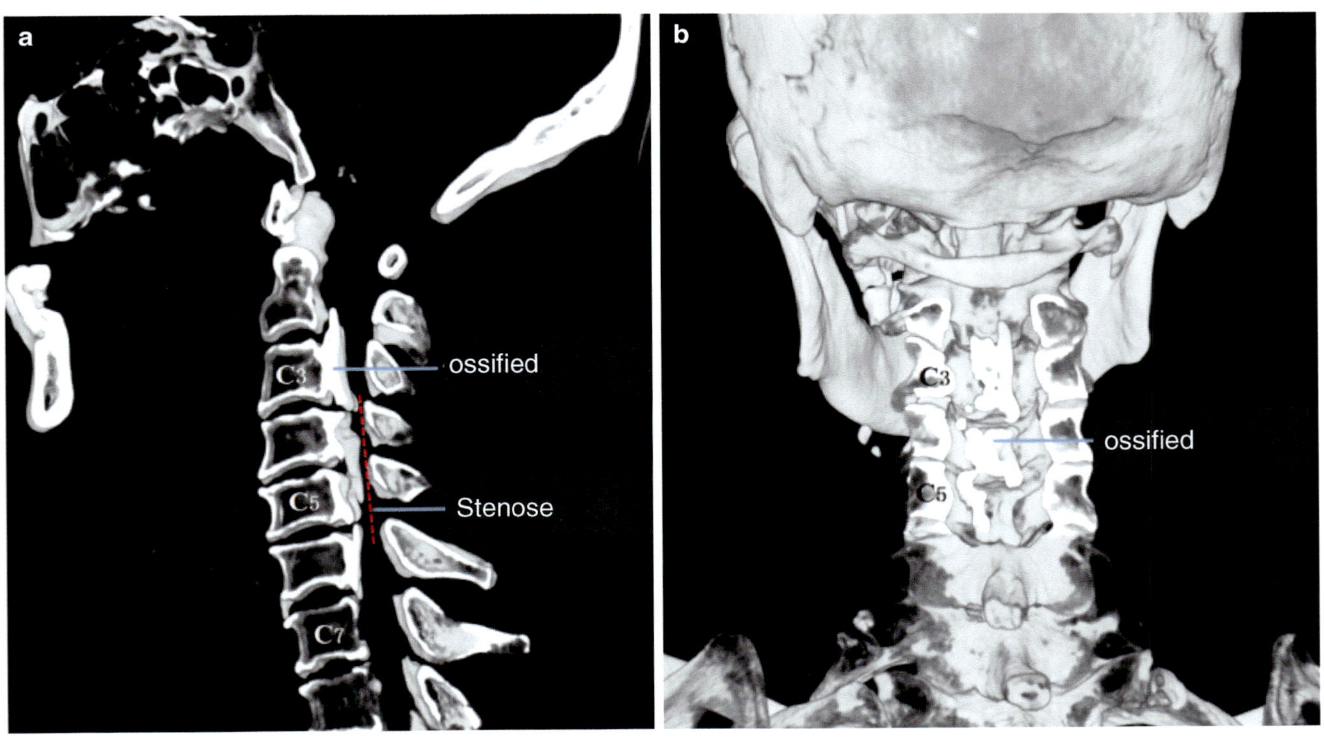

Fig. 3.19 Preoperative 3D CT reconstruction. (**a**) Spinal canal reconstruction (*sagittal view*); (**b**) The spinal canal is split in the coronal section (*posterior view*); (**c**) The spinal canal is split in the longitudinal section (*sagittal view*); (**d**) Reconstruction of the spinal canal at C3–C6 (*the overlooking view*)

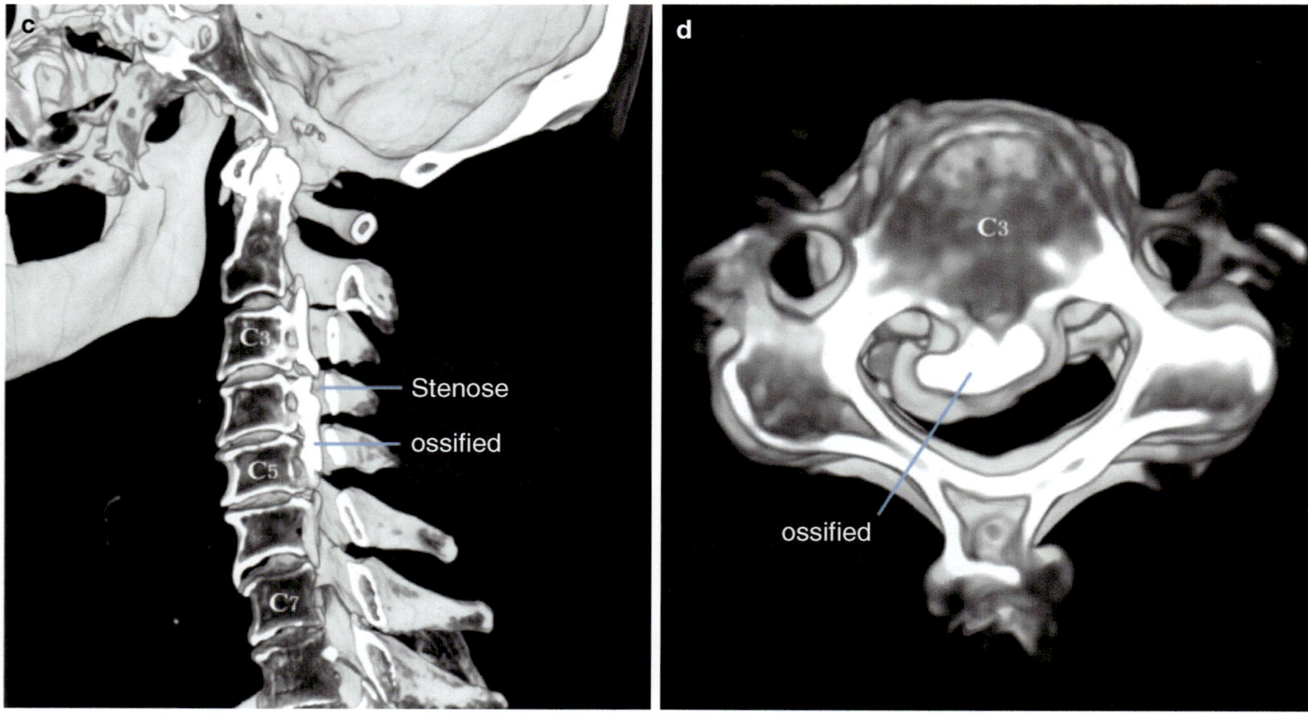

Fig. 3.19 (continued)

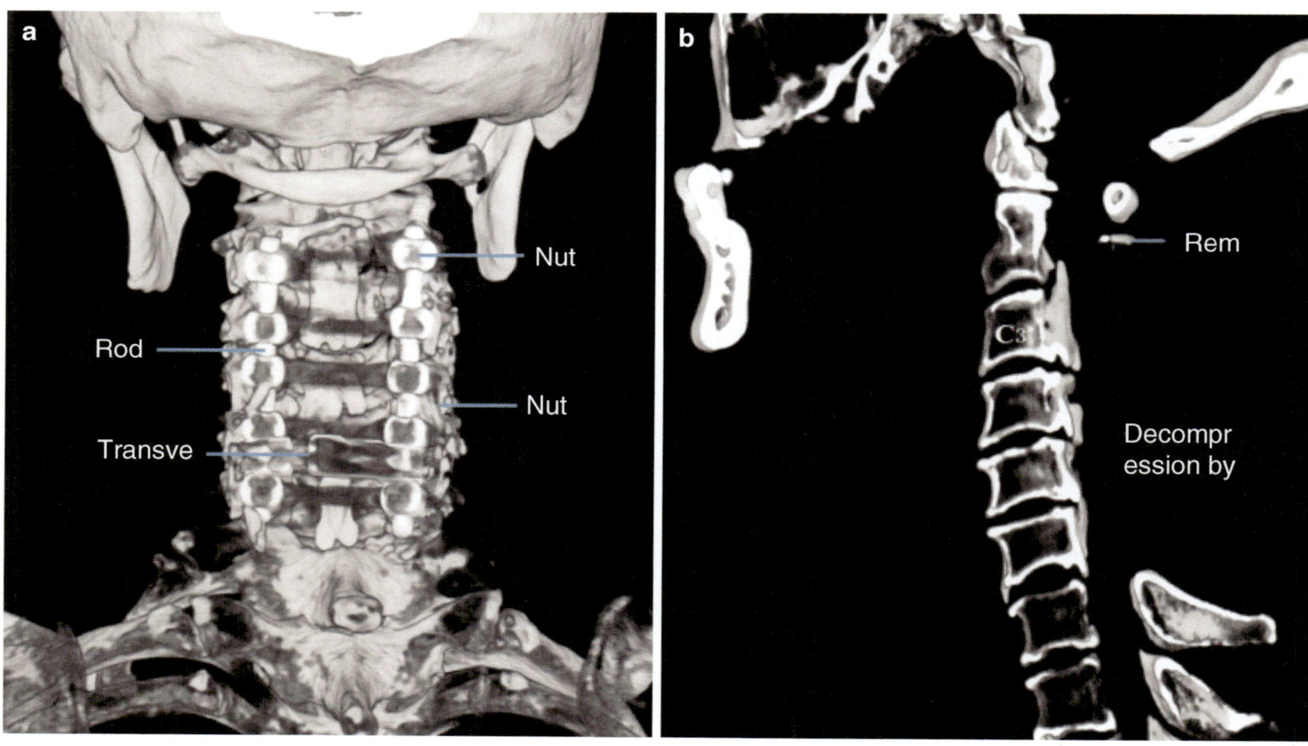

Fig. 3.20 Postoperative 3D CT reconstruction. (**a**) Location of internal fixation (*posterior view*); (**b**) Spinal canal reconstruction (*sagittal view*); (**c**) Location of internal fixation (*anterior view*); (**d**) The spinal canal is split in the coronal section (*posterior view*)

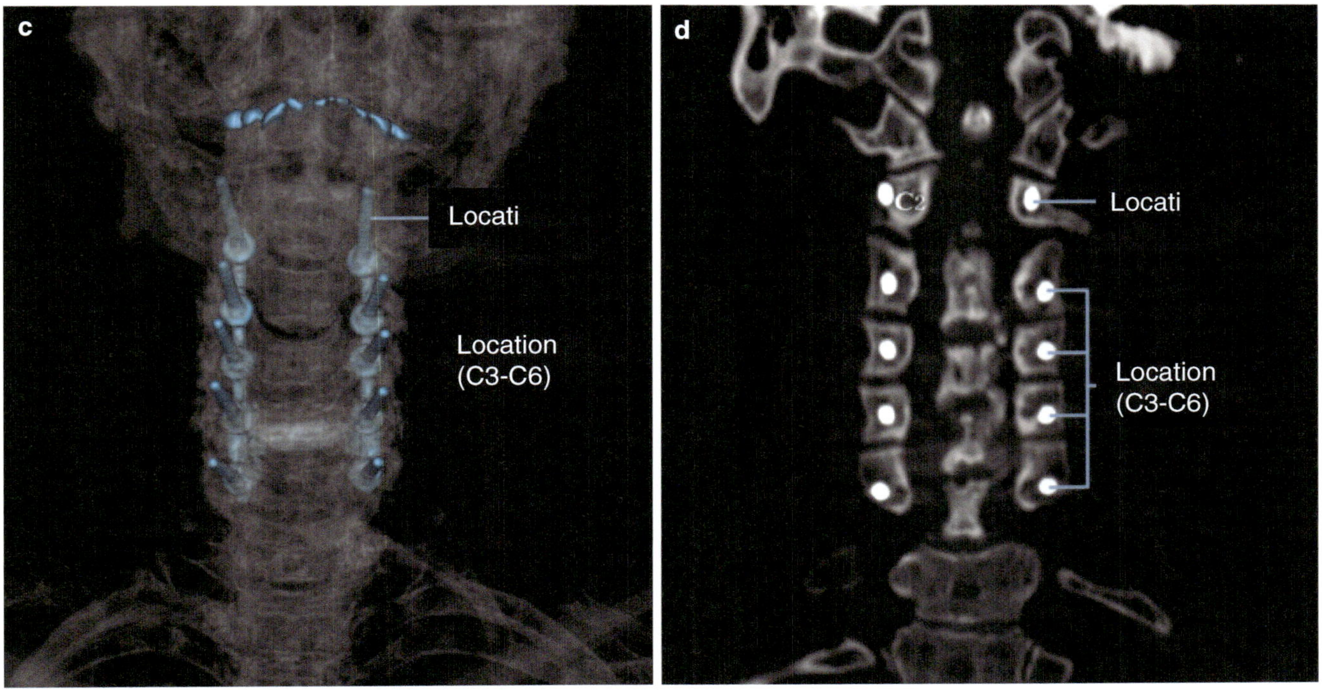

Fig. 3.20 (continued)

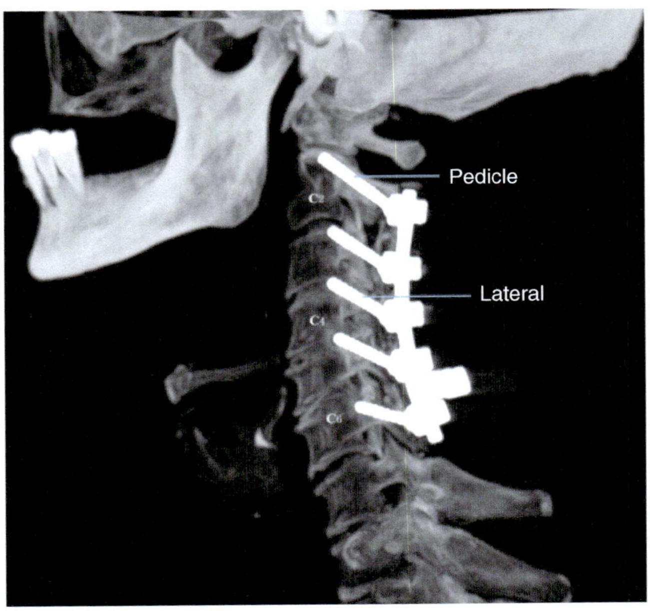

Fig. 3.21 Location of internal fixation (*lateral view*). Pedicle screw; lateral mass screws (C3–C6)

References

1. Roy-Camille RSG, Berteaus D, Serge MA. Early management of spinal injuries. Recent Adv Orthopae. 1979;1979(17):57–87.
2. Grob D, Magerl F. Dorsal spondylodesis of the cervical spine using a hooked plate. Orthopade. 1987;16(1):55–61.
3. Ji LCZ, Fan F. Anatomical measurements of the lateral masses for safe screw fixation lower cervical spine. Chin J Spine Spinal Cord. 2008;2008(18):286–9.

Surgical Techniques for Pedicle Screw Fixation of the Cervical Spine and Their Applications

4

Hailong Yu, Yi Huan, and Wei Lei

Abstract

Pedicle screw fixation of the cervical spine allows superior, simultaneous stabilization of all three columns of the cervical spine. However, pedicle screw fixation has the risk of neurovascular injury from penetration of the small cervical pedicle. The chapter introduces the anatomic parameters of the cervical pedicle and describes screw entry points, angles, and depth in details. At the same time, the procedure of inserting C4 pedicle screw in the cadaver is shown as a step-by-step example. Pearls and pitfalls of cervical pedicle screw fixation are summarized at the end of the chapter.

Keywords

Cervical spine · Pedicle screw fixation · Anatomy

4.1 Pedicle Screw Fixation Technique for the Cervical Spine: A Historical Perspective

The development of pedicle screw techniques for fixation of the cervical spine is highlighted below:

In 1994, Abumi et al. invented the pedicle screw fixation technique [1] (Fig. 4.1). In the same year, Jeanneret et al. modified the Abumi technique by increasing the medial inclination of pedicle screw [2] (Fig. 4.2). In 1996, Miller proposed laminectomy with exploration under direct X-ray or fluoroscopic guidance [3] (Fig. 4.3). In 2001, Karaikovic et al. proposed the funnel technique [4] (Fig. 4.4).

4.2 Surgical Anatomy of the Pedicles of the Cervical Spine

4.2.1 Gross Anatomy (Figs. 4.5, 4.6, 4.7, and 4.8)

4.3 Data in Relation to the Pedicles of the Cervical Spine

Morphological studies of the cervical spine have demonstrated that the pedicle of C2 and C7 has a larger diameter, while the diameter of C3 is the smallest (Table 4.1). In general, the diameter of pedicles of the cervical spine is more than 4 mm. Pedicle screw fixation of C2 and C7 is relatively safe because the vertebral artery is located anatomically in the anterolateral quadrant of the C2 lateral mass. In addition, because the C7 lateral mass is thin and has a peculiar shape, effective length of a C7 lateral mass screw is very short; as a result, fixation is insecure and may put the nerves at risk. Therefore, lateral mass screw fixation of C3 to C6 is an ideal choice (Figs. 4.9 and 4.10).

4.4 Key Points of Pedicle Screw Techniques for Fixation of the Cervical Spine

4.4.1 Determining Pedicle Screw Entry Points in the Cervical Spine (Fig. 4.11)

The Abumi method is the most commonly used pedicle screw technique for fixation of the cervical spine [1]. The entry point for C3 to C6 pedicle screws lies at the junction of

H. Yu
General Hospital of Northern Theater Command, Shenyang, China

Y. Huan
Department of Radiology, Xijing Hospital, Air Force Military Medical University, Xi'an, China

W. Lei (✉)
Department of Orthopedics, Xijing Hospital, Air Force Medical University, Xi'an, Shaanxi, China
e-mail: leiwei@fmmu.edu.cn

W. Lei, Y. Yan (eds.), *Internal Fixation of the Spine*, https://doi.org/10.1007/978-981-16-1562-7_4

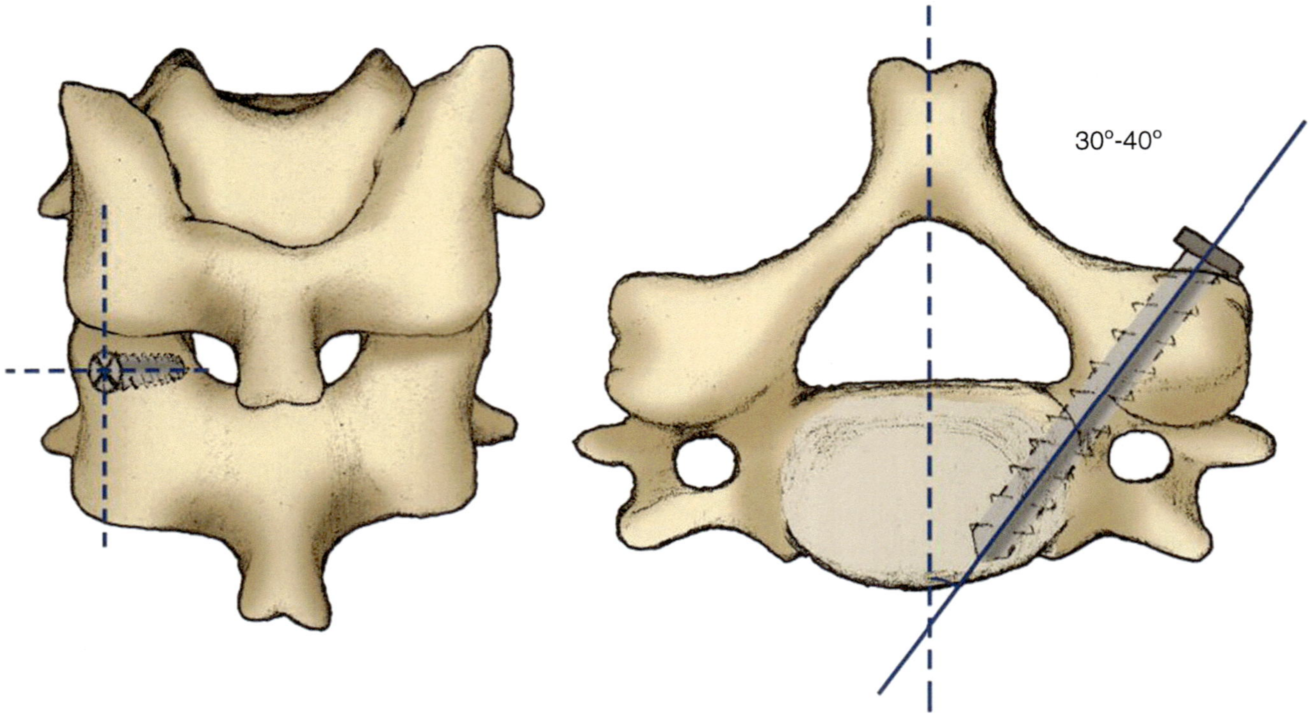

Fig. 4.1 The Abumi technique for cervical pedicle screw fixation

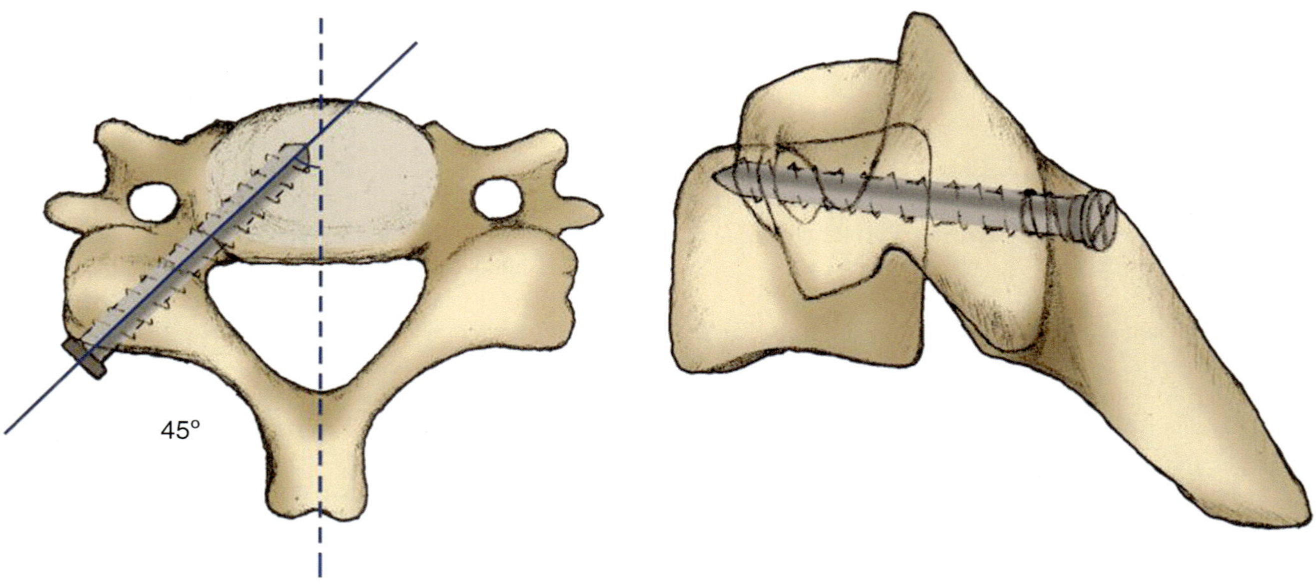

Fig. 4.2 Jeanneret technique

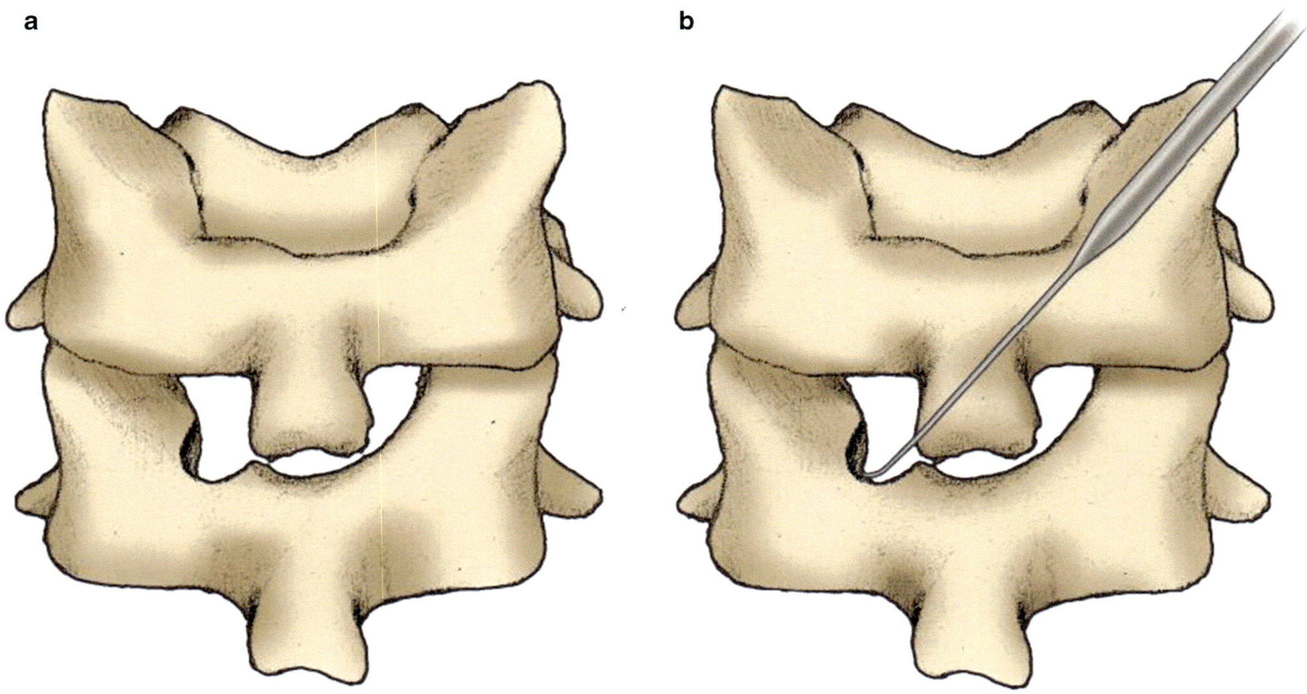

Fig. 4.3 Miller technique. (**a**) Laminectomy; (**b**) Exploration of the interior wall of the pedicle

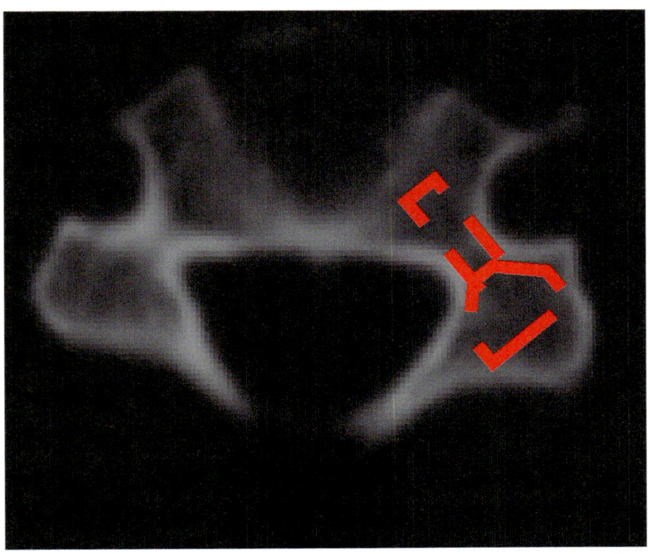

Fig. 4.4 The funnel technique

the transverse line and the vertical line crossing the center of the superolateral quadrant at the posterior surface of the lateral mass. The entry point for C7 pedicle screw lies superior to the junction of the mid-vertical line of the lateral mass and the transverse line crossing the centers of the superolateral and superomedial quadrant.

In our clinical practice, we choose the entry point for C3 to C6 pedicle screws at the junction of the transverse line and the vertical line crossing the center of the superolateral quadrant at the posterior surface of the lateral mass. The entry point for C7 pedicle screw lies slightly superior.

4.4.2 Pedicle Screw Entry Angles in the Cervical Spine (Fig. 4.12)

The C2 pedicle screw entry angle is 30° medial to the midline in the transverse plane and 20° in the cephalad direction. The C3 to C6 pedicle screw entry angle is 40° to 45° from the sagittal plane (Fig. 4.12), and the transverse plane is parallel to the superior and inferior endplate. The C7 pedicle screw entry angle is 30° to 40° from the sagittal plane, and the transverse plane is parallel to the superior and inferior endplate.

4.4.3 Entry Depths of Pedicle Screws in the Cervical Spine

In general, the trajectory depth of pedicle screws is 18–20 mm. When the fixation depth reaches 80% of the trajectory depth (from the start of the entry point to the anterior

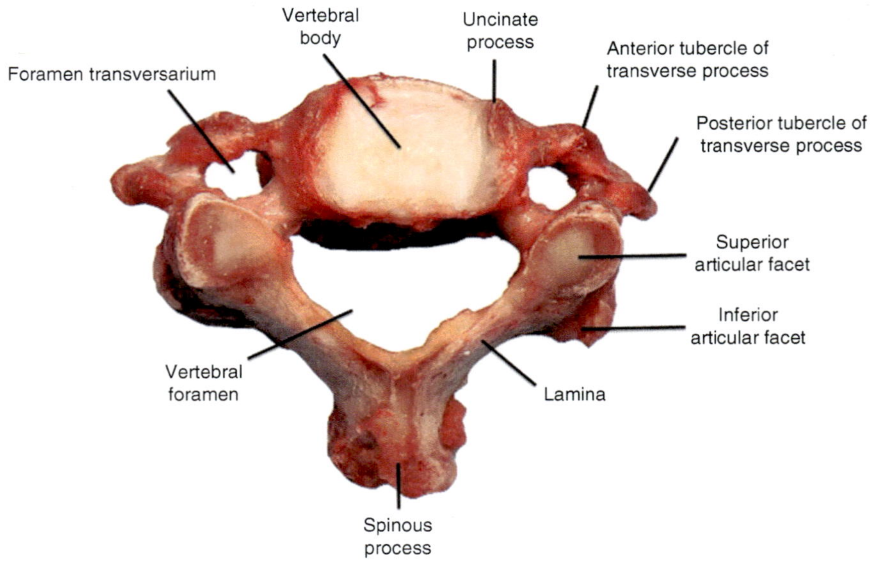

Fig. 4.5 The superior view of C5

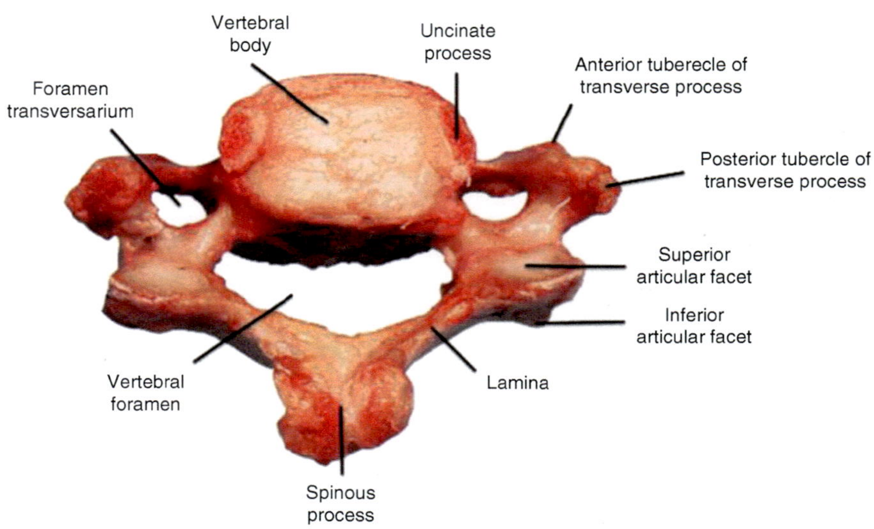

Fig. 4.6 The inferior view of C5

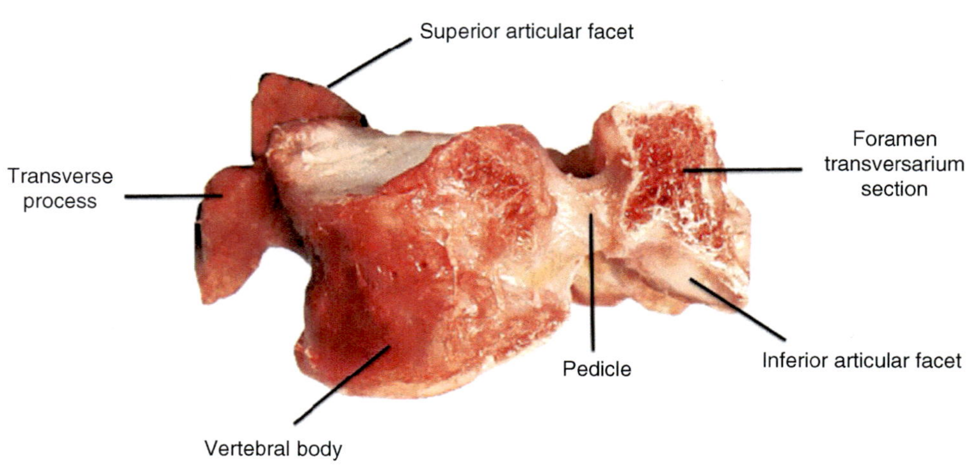

Fig. 4.7 The lateral view of C5

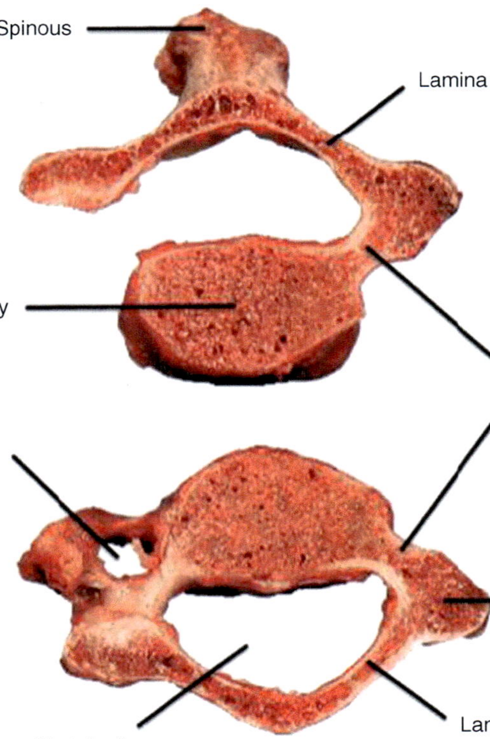

Fig. 4.8 The sectional view of C5

Table 4.1 Anatomic parameters of the pedicles of the cervical spine

	Panjabi et al. [5]		Tan et al. [6]	
	Width (mm)	Height (mm)	Width (mm)	Height (mm)
C3	5.6 ± 0.5	7.4 ± 0.4	4.5 ± 0.2	6.7 ± 0.2
C4	5.4 ± 0.5	7.4 ± 0.5	4.6 ± 0.2	6.6 ± 0.2
C5	5.6 ± 0.4	7.0 ± 0.4	4.7 ± 0.1	6.3 ± 0.3
C6	6.0 ± 0.4	7.3 ± 0.4	5.1 ± 0.2	6.0 ± 0.3
C7	6.0 ± 0.4	7.5 ± 0.3	5.6 ± 0.2	6.5 ± 0.2

Data is expressed as mean ± SD

border of the vertebral body along the pedicle axis), the fixation strength of the screw is sufficient. Further increase of entry depth does not lead to significant increase in fixation strength while increasing surgical risks. The diameter of the most commonly used pedicle screws is 3.5 mm.

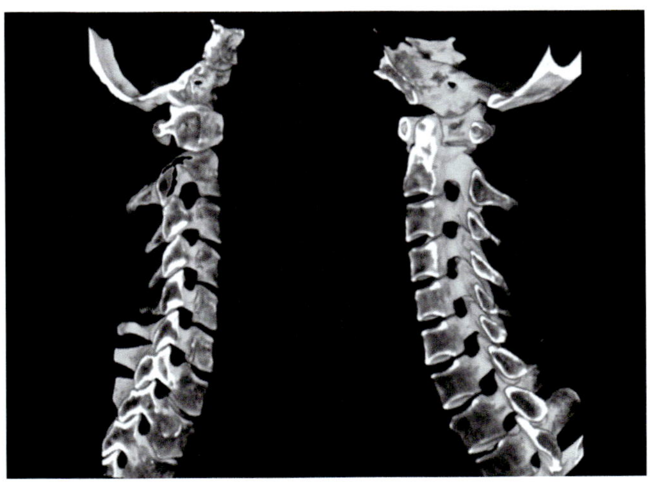

Fig. 4.9 The pedicles of the cervical spine (3D CT reconstruction). *Left*: lateral view; *Right*: medial view

4.4.4 Surgical Steps (Insertion of C4 Pedicle Screw Is Used as an Example)

1. Determining the pedicle screw entry point (see Fig. 4.11 for the location of the entry point of pedicle screw for the cervical spine).
2. Removing the cortical bone: A mill or burr is used to disrupt the cortical bone at the screw entry point (Fig. 4.13).
3. Drilling the screw hole: A screw hole is gradually drilled in the cancellous bone of the pedicle and vertebral body using a drill bit with drill guide. During drilling, the surgeon should have an obvious manual feedback of having entered into the cancellous bone. If resistance is encountered, the surgeon should consider whether the entry point or entry angle is correct. If the surgeon continuously feels

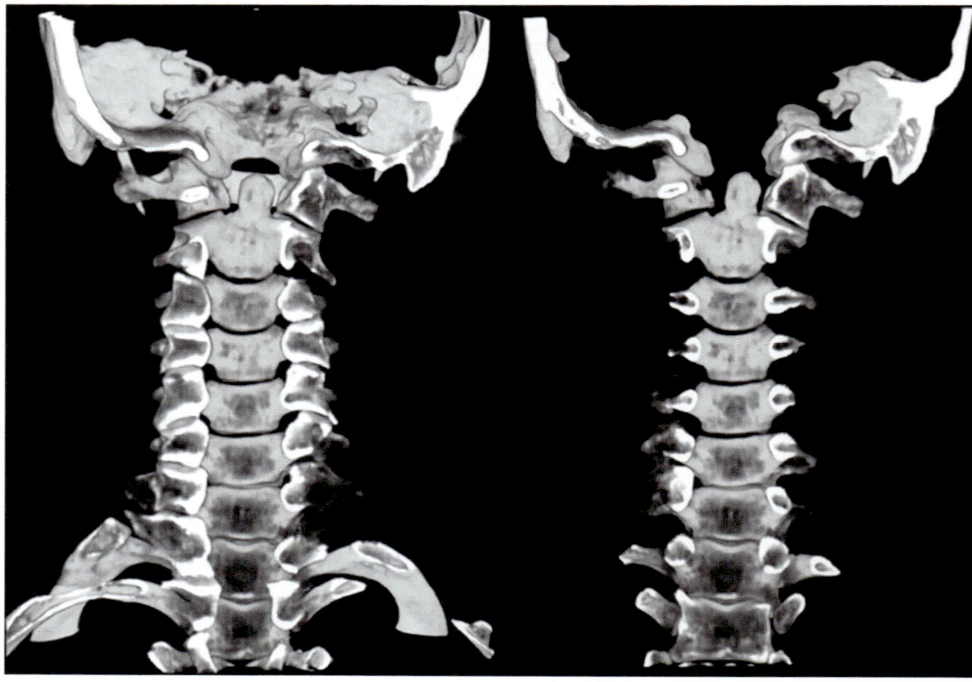

Fig. 4.10 The coronal section of the pedicles of the cervical spine (3D CT reconstruction). *Left*: the proximal pedicle; *Right*: the distal pedicle

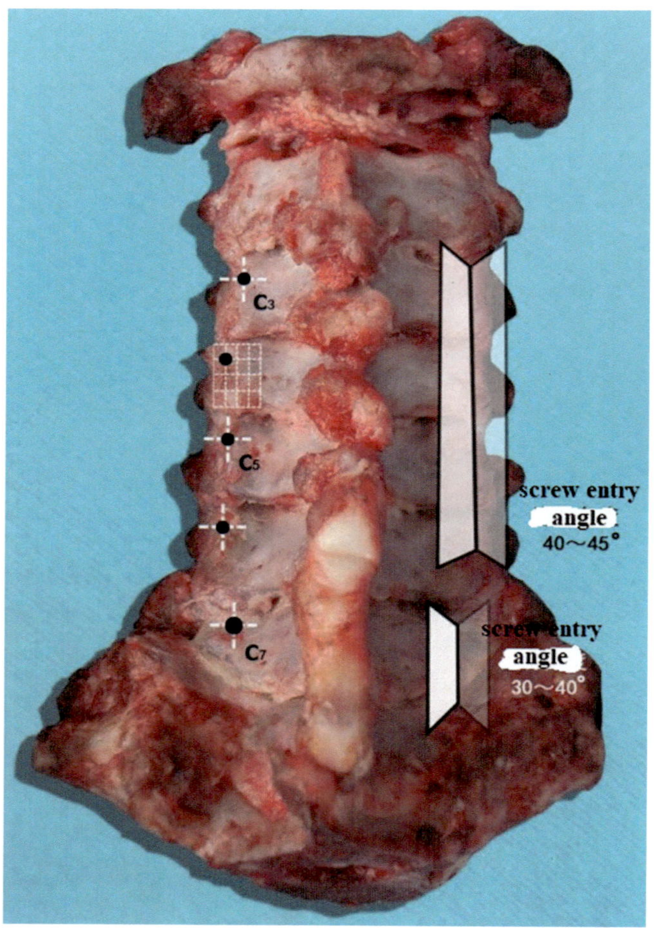

Fig. 4.11 Pedicle screw entry points in the cervical spine

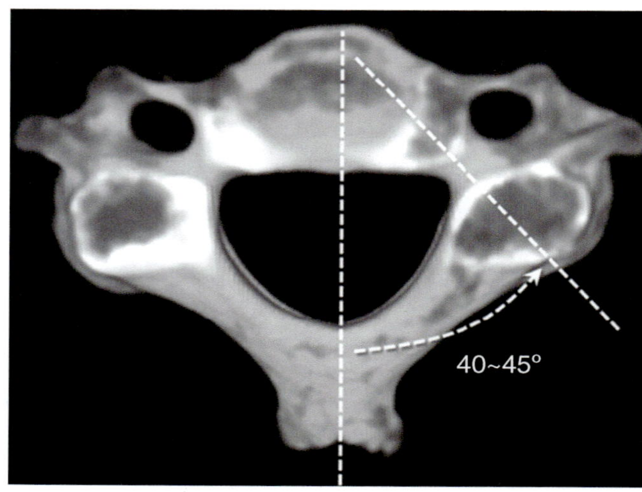

Fig. 4.12 The pedicle screw entry angle in the cervical spine

resistance or changes in bone density during insertion, the surgeon should determine by X-ray whether the burr has disrupted the lateral wall of the pedicle (Fig. 4.14).

4. Probing insertion depth: A blunt pedicle probe is advanced into the vertebral body via the pedicle screw path. When the walls of the screw path are probed, the surgeon should have the manual feedback of probing the cancellous bone and make sure that the integrity of the walls is not violated. If resistance or discontinuity is encountered during probing, the surgeon should consider whether the entry

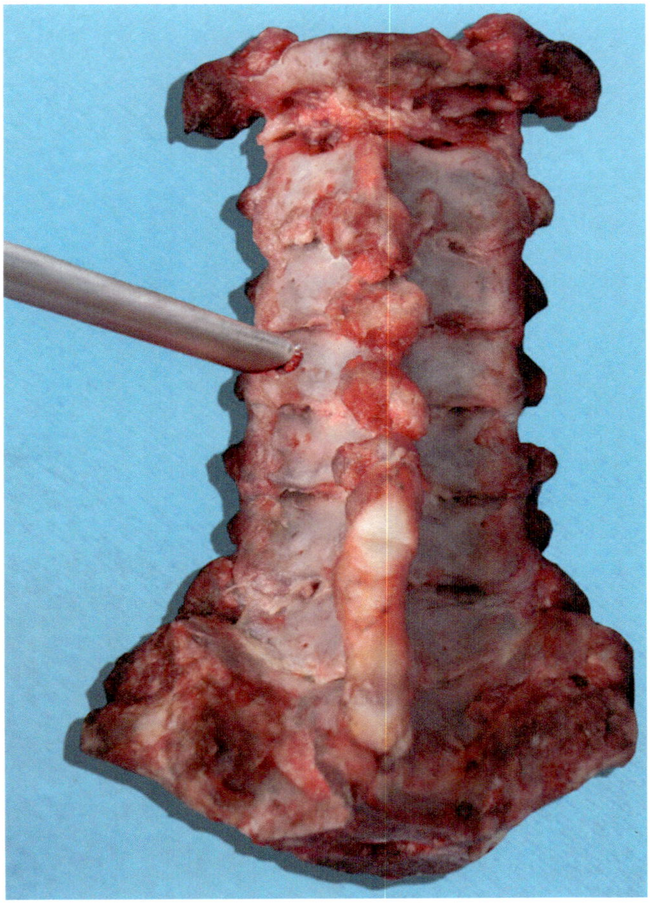

Fig. 4.13 Removing the cortical bone

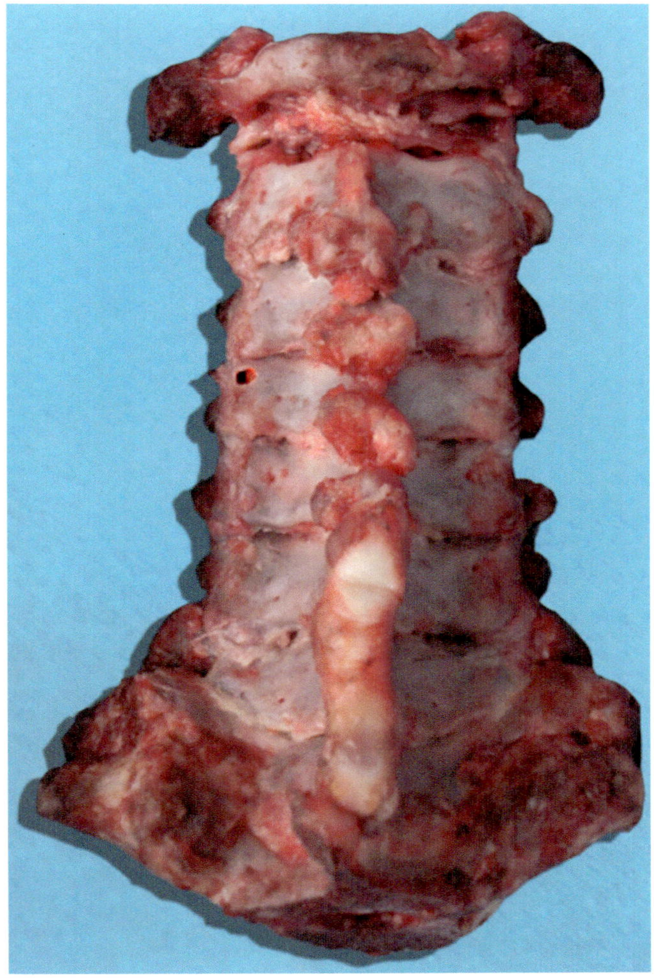

Fig. 4.14 Drilling the screw hole

angle is correct and verify by X-ray that the probe is within the pedicle under fluoroscopic guidance (Fig. 4.15).

5. Determining the location: After the hole is drilled, a metal probe is put in the screw hole and located under fluoroscopic guidance. Adjustment is made until satisfaction is achieved under fluoroscopic guidance (Fig. 4.16).
6. Screw insertion: Appropriate screws are selected based on the screw trajectory and intraoperative need for correction. Suitable screws are inserted into the prepared screw path using a screwdriver. Screws should be completely inserted and enter 80% of the vertebral body; the screw path should be parallel to the endplates (Fig. 4.17).

4.5 Imaging Features of Standard Pedicle Screws of the Cervical Spine (Figs. 4.18, 4.19, and 4.20)

Case 1

Patient: A 67-year-old male complained of numbness of four extremities with weakness in walking for 2 years.

Diagnosis: Cervical spondylosis and ossification of the posterior longitudinal ligament of the cervical spine

Surgery: Decompression by laminectomy via a posterior approach, vertex internal fixation, bone graft and fusion (C3–C7) (Figs. 4.21, 4.22, and 4.23).

Case 2

Patient: A 52-year-old female complained of numbness of both hands with instability in walking for 1 year.

Diagnosis: Cervical spondylosis and ossification of the posterior longitudinal ligament of the cervical spine.

Surgery: Decompression by laminectomy via a posterior approach, vertex internal fixation, bone graft and fusion (C3–C7) (Figs. 4.24 and 4.25).

Case 3

Patient: A 45-year-old male complained of neck and shoulder pain due to a fall with weakness of bilateral upper extremities for 19 days.

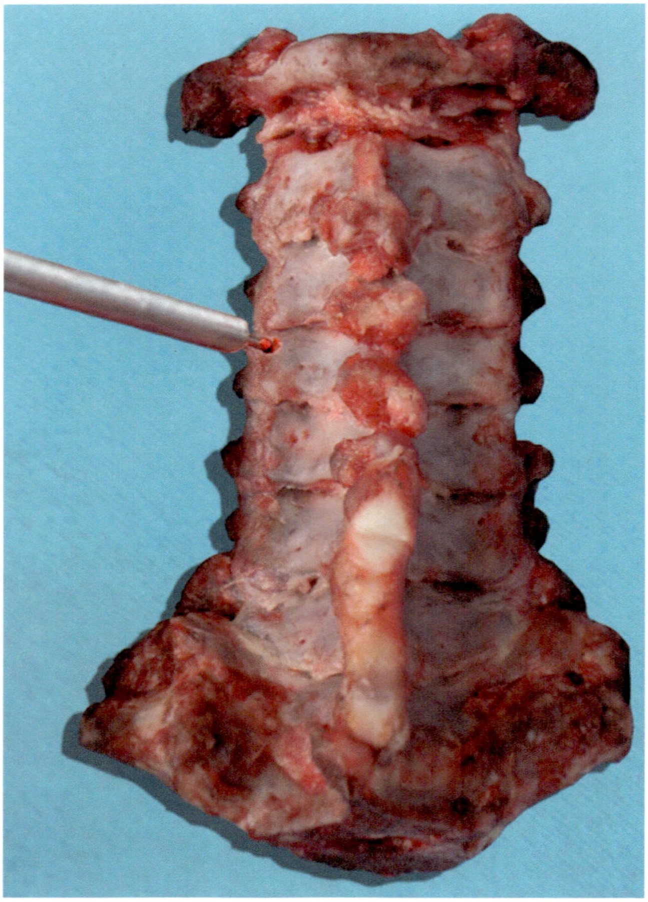

Fig. 4.15 Probing the screw path

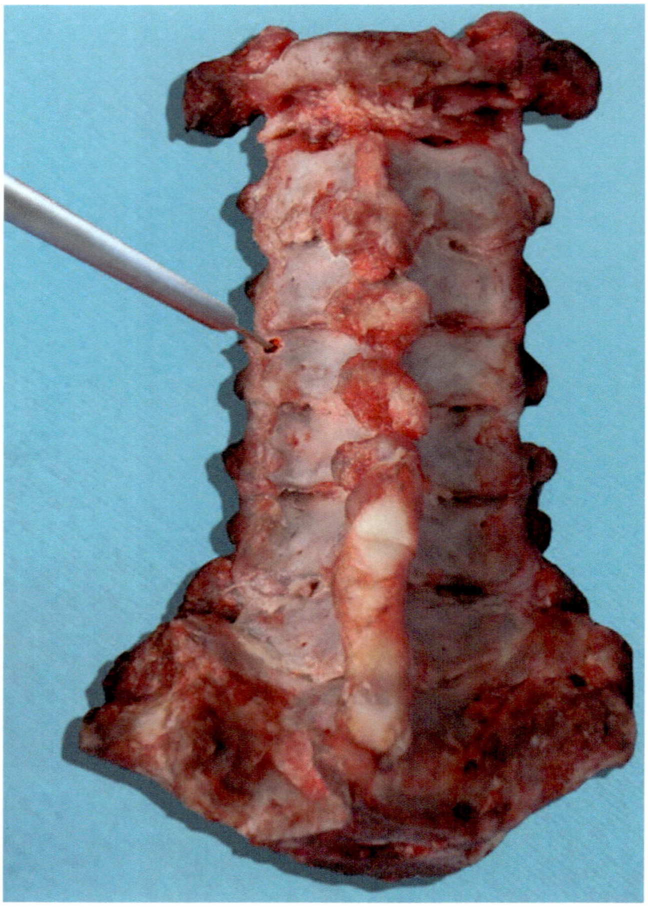

Fig. 4.16 Determining the location

Diagnosis: Fracture of the cervical spine: hangman's fracture, C7 compression fracture, C3–C6 fracture of the lamina.

Surgery: **C2–T1** bone graft and fusion and internal fixation via a posterior approach (Figs. 4.26 and 4.27).

4.6 Pearls and Pitfalls

1. Currently, there are three pedicle screw insertion methods, including anatomic pedicle screw insertion, laminectomy with exploration, and computer-assisted pedicle screw insertion. The first two methods are both associated with a certain rate of screw failures; even pedicle insertion under direct vision is associated with a certain rate of perforations. Therefore, caution should be exercised during pedicle screw insertion. Computer-assisted navigation allows the surgeon to evaluate the site and direction of pedicle screw insertion, thus greatly increasing safety and accuracy of screw placement and reducing risk of neurovascular injury. However, navigation equipment is expensive and the procedure is complicated; besides, the operative time is long and sterilization is inconvenient. A surgeon should carefully choose an insertion method based on the surgeon's familiarity with cervical spine anatomy and the surgeon's mastery of a pedicle screw fixation technique [1, 2].
2. Preoperative accurate measurement should be made of imaging data to assist development of an individualized

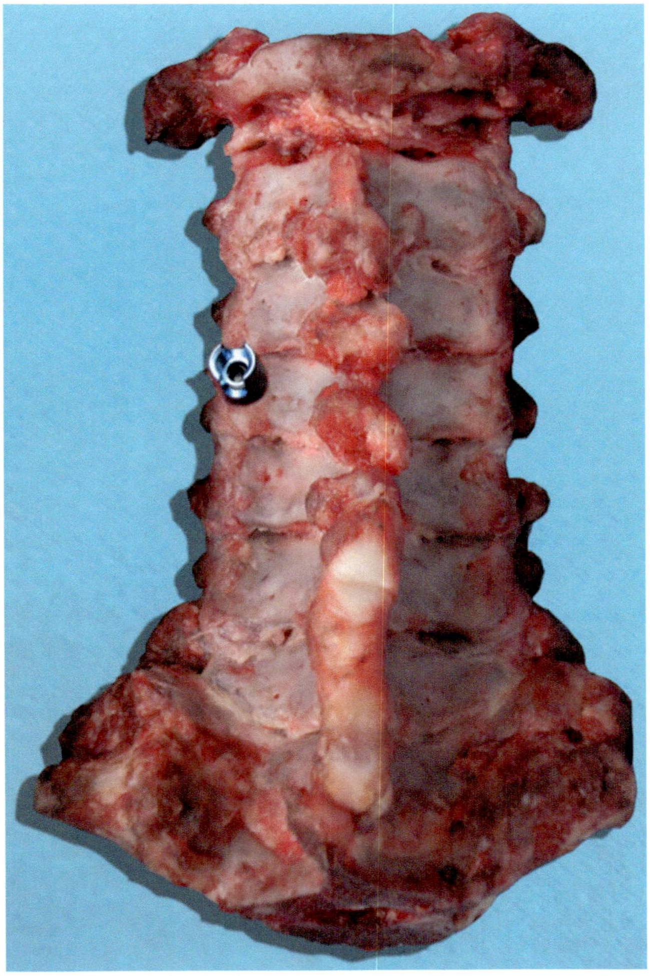

Fig. 4.17 An implanted screw

screw placement protocol for determination of direction and position of pedicle screws for each cervical segment. Particular attention should be paid to the pedicle that is too small, has no medullary cavity, and has presence of pedicle injury, which preclude pedicle screw fixation [3, 4].

3. The surgical incision should be adequately exposed, and surgical procedures should be meticulously carried out. For patients requiring vertebral decompression, pedicle screw placement before decompression may lessen the risk of nerve injuries.
4. Lateral mass screw fixation of C3 to C6 is safer and easier than pedicle screw fixation.
5. The lateral wall of the pedicle should not be violated by a surgical instrument; otherwise, it will incur injuries to adjacent nerves and vessels [5].
6. Screw entry angles should be adjusted according to changes in pedicle angles.
7. Caution should be taken to avoid penetration of the cortical bone of the anterior vertebral body [6].
8. Intraoperative fluoroscopy allows accurately locating the vertebral body and intervertebral spaces and accurate screw insertion and helps avoid violation of the intervertebral spaces and vertebral canal.

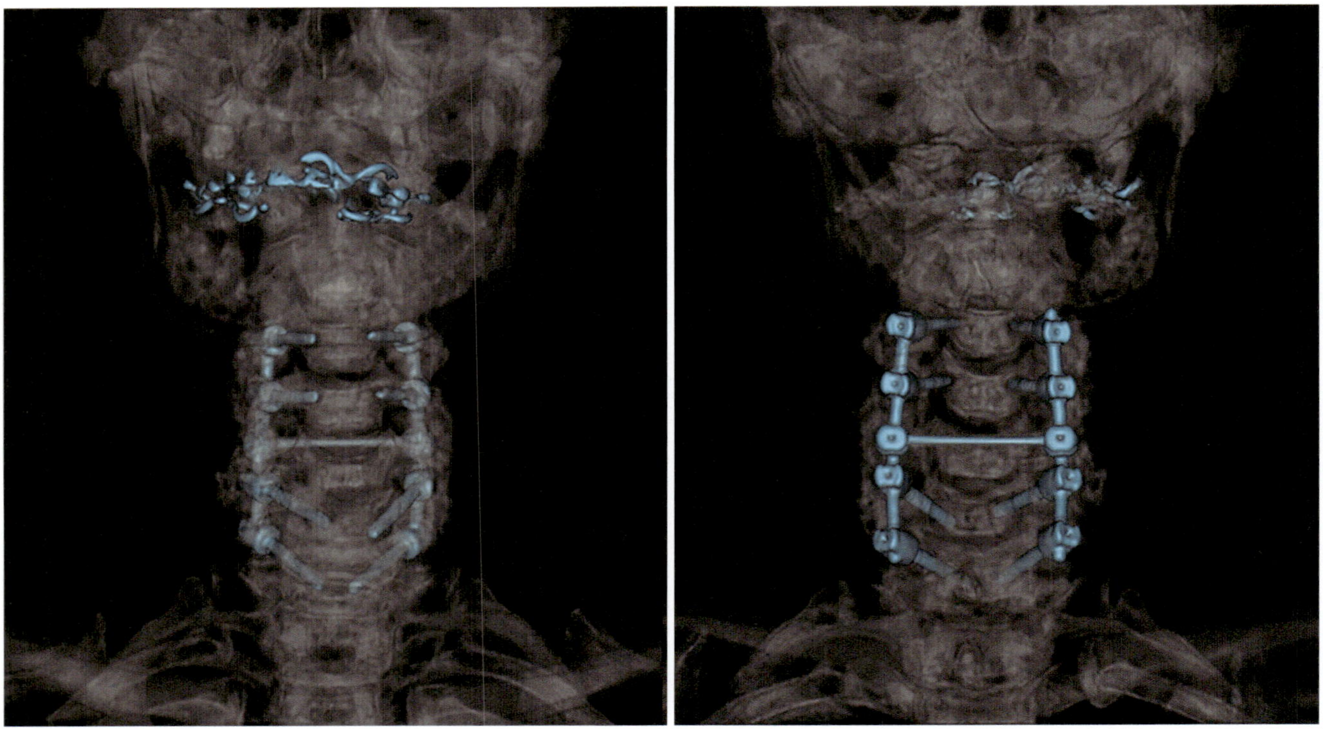

Fig. 4.18 Implanted C3–C7 pedicle screws. *Left*: anterior view; *Right*: posterior view

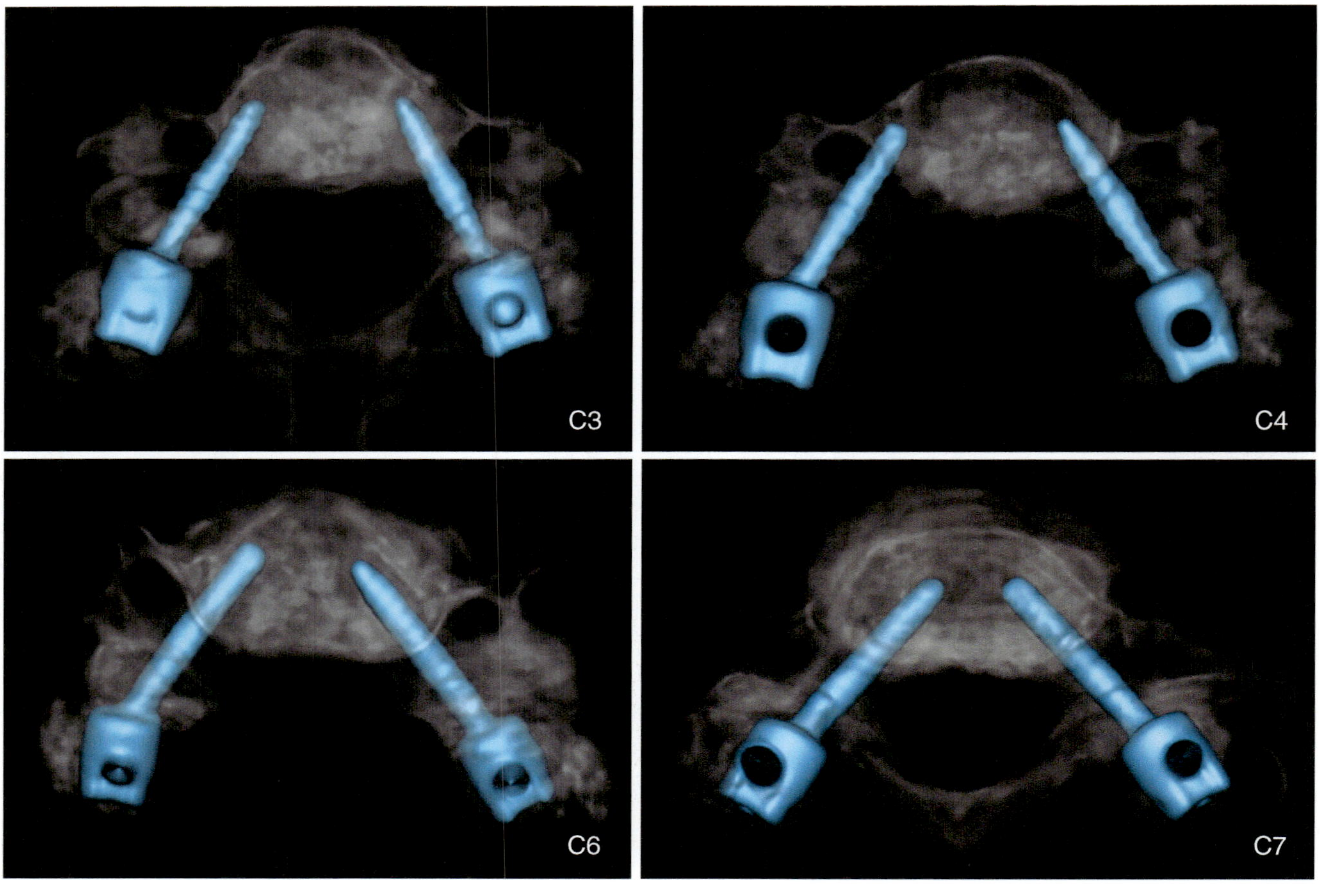

Fig. 4.19 Cervical pedicle screws

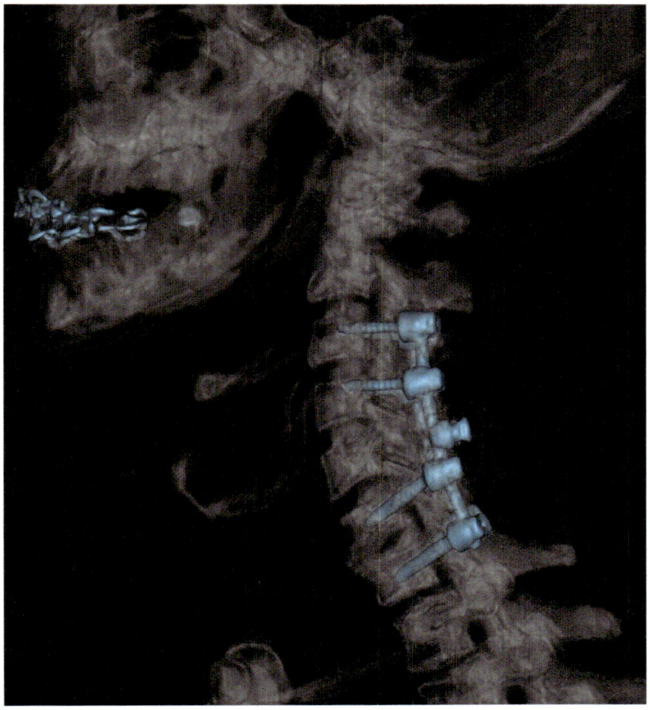

Fig. 4.20 The lateral view of C3–C7 pedicle screws

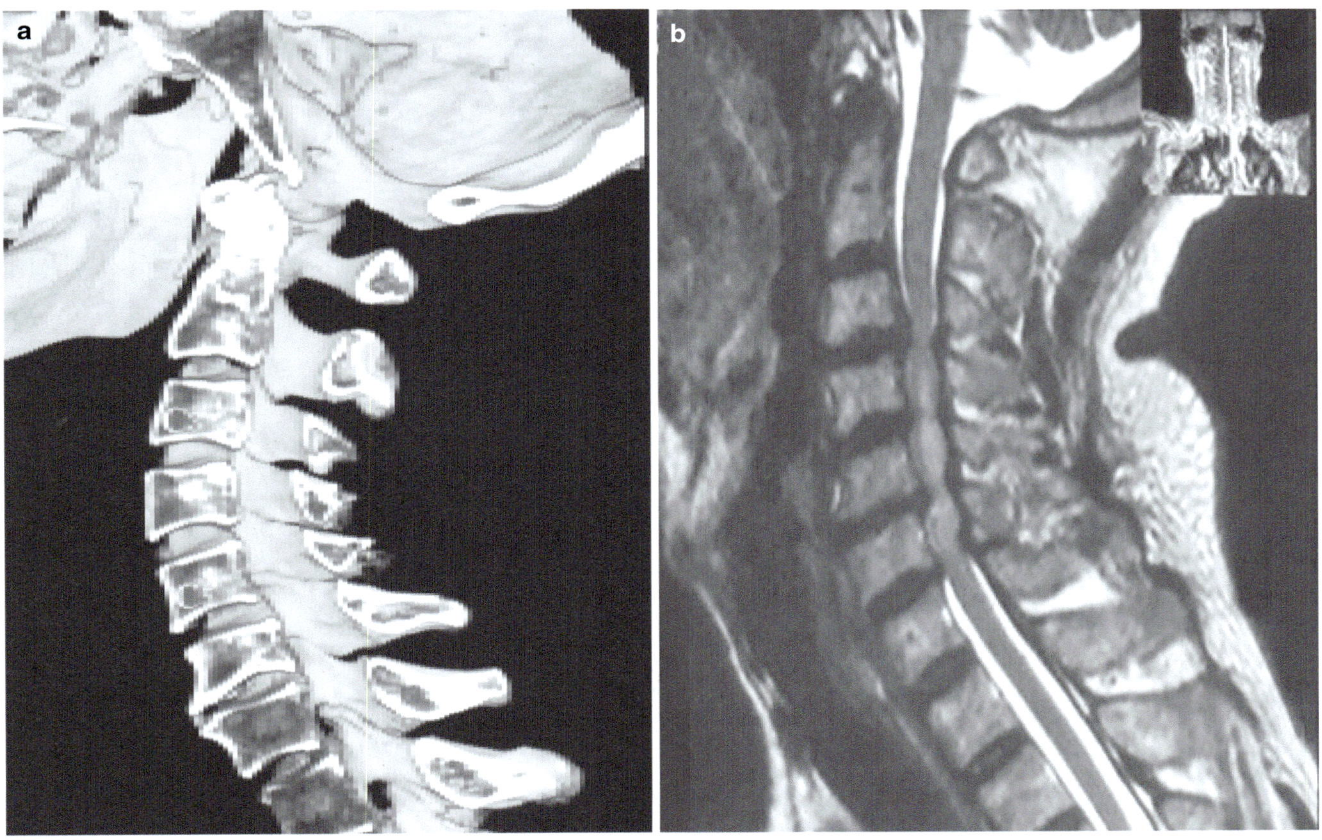

Fig. 4.21 Preoperative images. (**a**) 3D CT reconstruction. The spinal canal is split in the longitudinal section (*sagittal view*); (**b**) MRI (*sagittal view*)

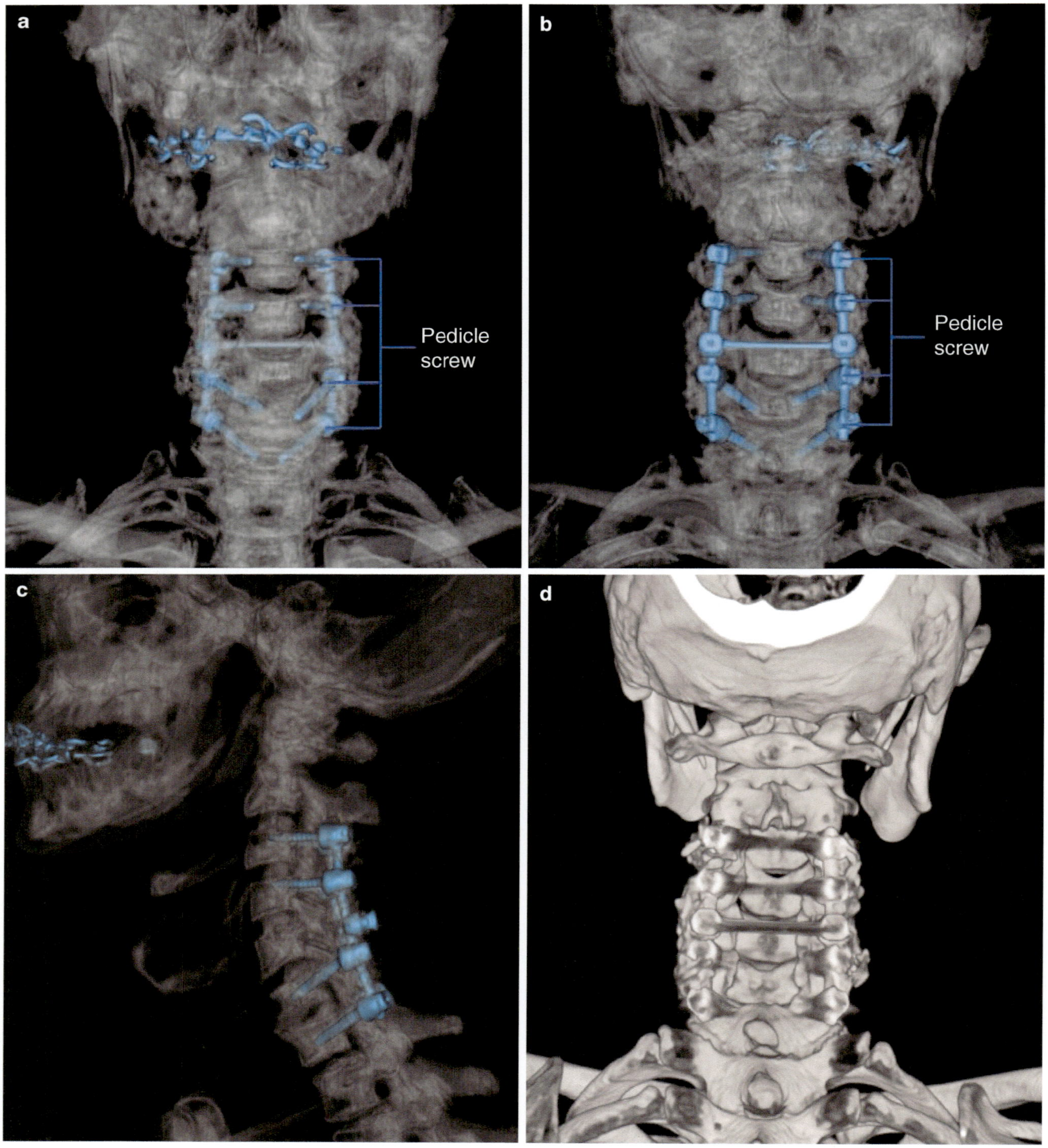

Fig. 4.22 Preoperative 3D CT reconstruction. (**a**) Location of internal fixation (*anterior view*); (**b**) Location of internal fixation (*posterior view*); (**c**) Location of internal fixation (*lateral view*); (**d**) Decompression and location of fixation (*posterior view*)

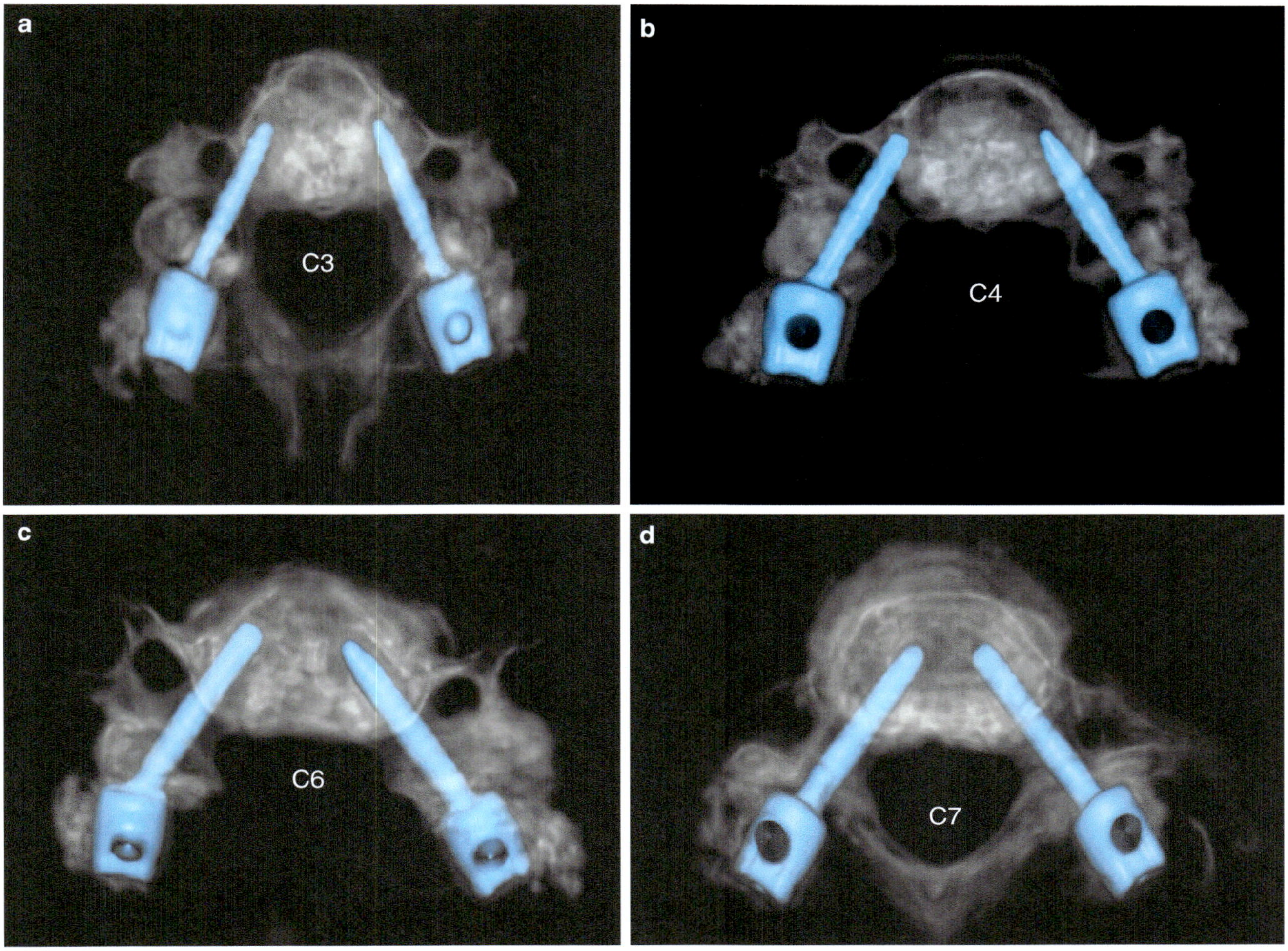

Fig. 4.23 Entry sites and angles of C3, C4, C6, and C7 screws (*horizontal view*). (**a**) C3; (**b**) C4; (**c**) C5; (**d**) C6

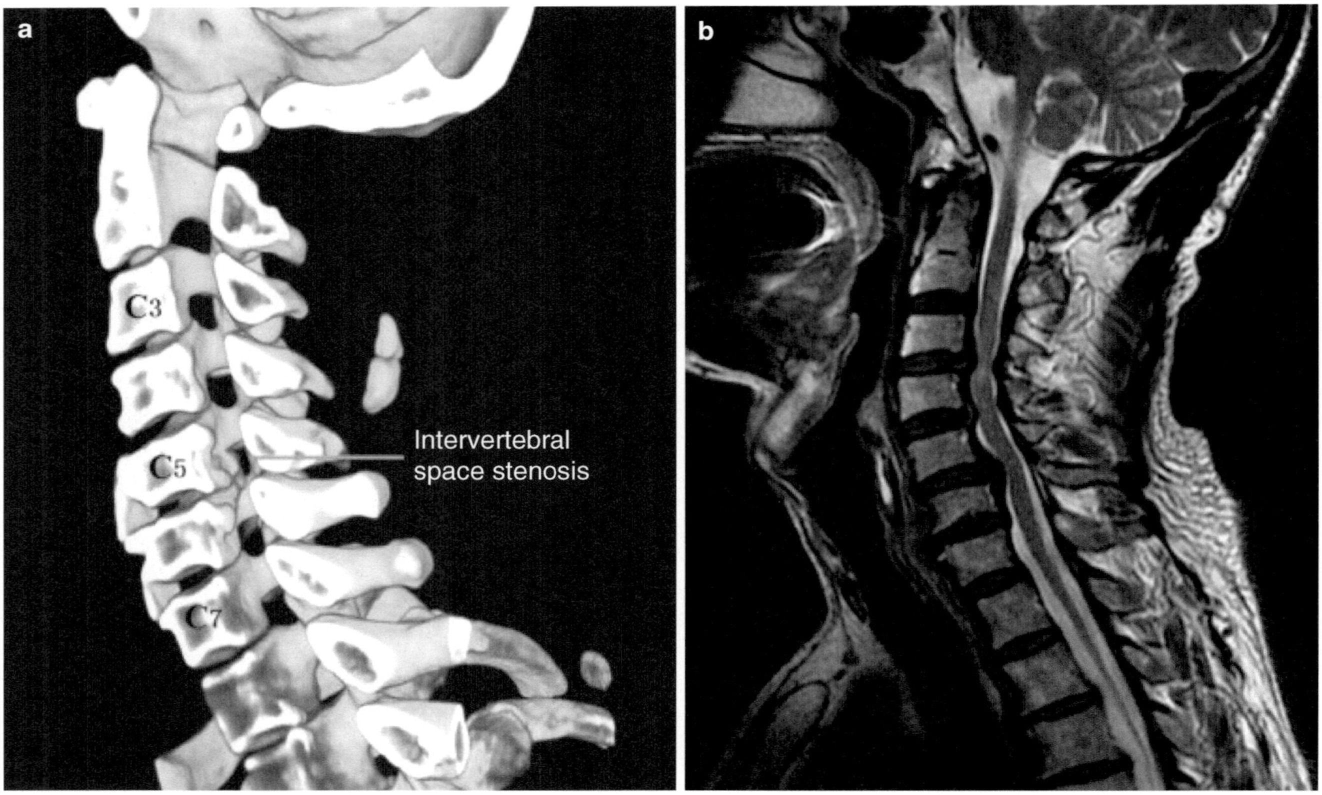

Fig. 4.24 Preoperative imaging data. (**a**) 3D CT reconstruction. The spinal canal is split in the longitudinal section (*sagittal view*); (**b**) MRI (*sagittal view*)

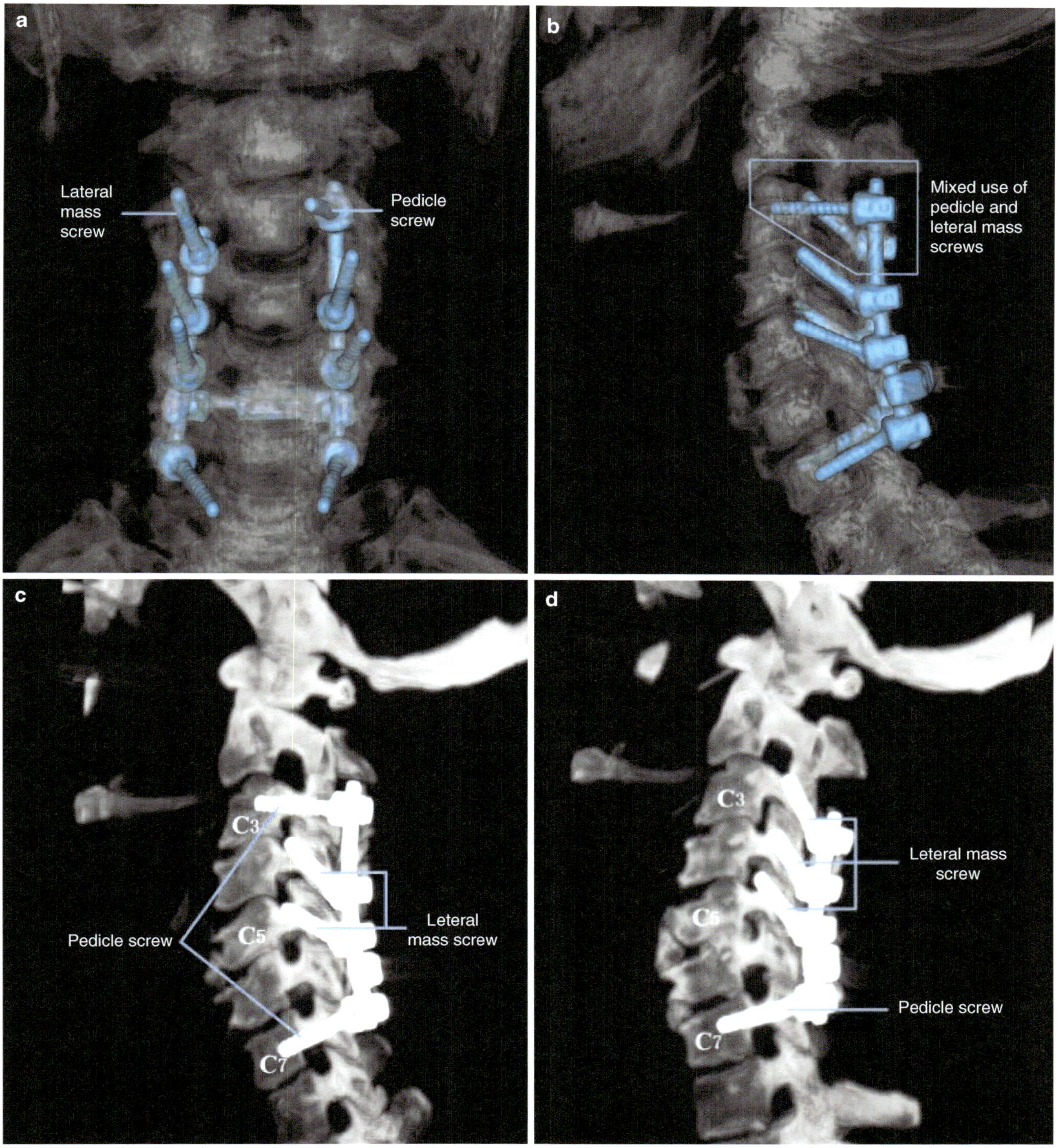

Fig. 4.25 Postoperative location of internal fixation. (**a**) Location of internal fixation (*anterior view*); (**b**) Location of internal fixation (*lateral view*); (**c**) Placement sites of screws on the left (*left view*); (**d**) Placement sites of screws on the right (*right view*)

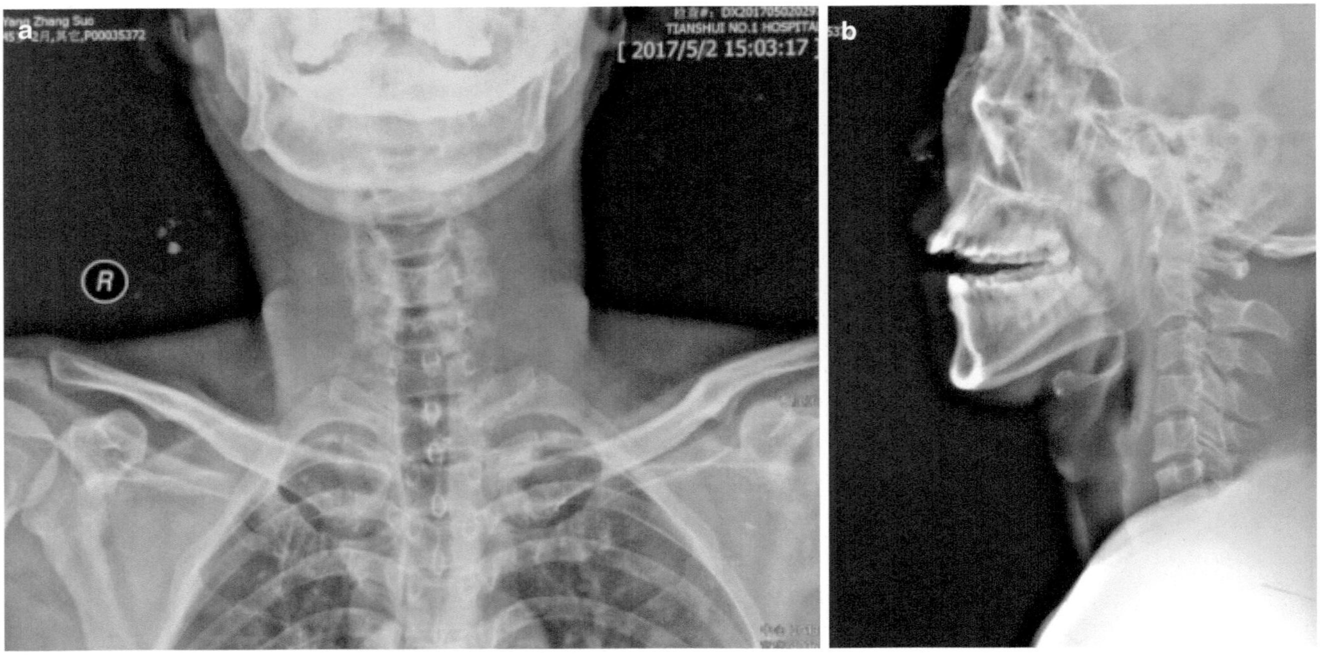

Fig. 4.26 Preoperative radiographs. (**a**) Anteroposterior view; (**b**) Lateral view

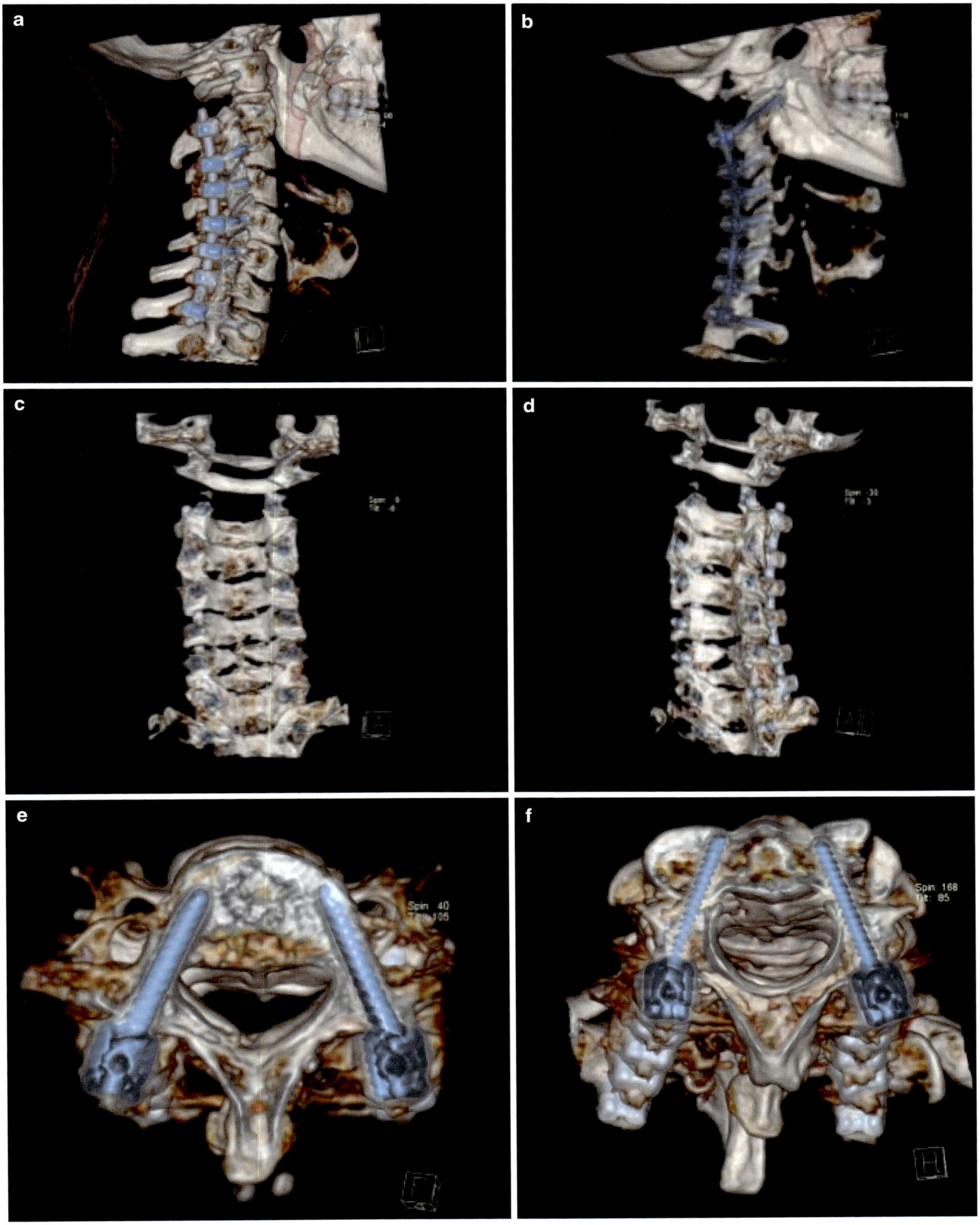

Fig. 4.27 Postoperative 3D CT reconstruction images. (**a**) Lateral view; (**b**) Lateral view (*split*); (**c**) Anteroposterior view (*split*); (**d**) Oblique view (*split*); (**e**) Horizontal section; (**f**) Horizontal section

References

1. Abumi K, et al. Transpedicular screw fixation for traumatic lesions of the middle and lower cervical spine: description of the techniques and preliminary report. J Spinal Disord. 1994;7(1):19–28.
2. Jeanneret B, Gebhard JS, Magerl F. Transpedicular screw fixation of articular mass fracture-separation: results of an anatomical study and operative technique. J Spinal Disord. 1994;7(3):222–9.
3. Miller RM, et al. Anatomic consideration of transpedicular screw placement in the cervical spine. An analysis of two approaches. Spine (Phila Pa 1976). 1996;21(20):2317–22.
4. Karaikovic EE, Yingsakmongkol W, Gaines RW. Jr., *Accuracy of cervical pedicle screw placement using the funnel technique*. Spine (Phila Pa 1976). 2001;26(22):2456–62.
5. Panjabi MM, et al. Cervical human vertebrae. Quantitative three-dimensional anatomy of the middle and lower regions. Spine (Phila Pa 1976). 1991;16(8):861–9.
6. Tan SH, Teo EC, Chua HC. Quantitative three-dimensional anatomy of lumbar vertebrae in Singaporean Asians. Eur Spine J. 2002;11(2):152–8.

5 Anterior Cervical Plate Techniques and Their Applications

Tianqing Li, Yabo Yan, and Wei Lei

Abstract

Surgery is the most direct and effective treatment for cervical spondylosis and cervical traumas. Anterior cervical surgery effectively relieves compression against the anterior spinal cord and restores cervical stability and physiological curvature by means of bone graft fusion plate fixation. With the evolution of treatment concepts and technologies, new surgical equipment and various surgical improvement methods have emerged one after another. This paper summarizes the development of this surgery and the characteristics of various surgical methods and mainly introduces the commonly used anterior cervical plate and technology.

Keywords

Cervical spine · Cervical plate · ACDF · ACCF

5.1 A Historical Review and Anatomic Parameters

5.1.1 A Historical Review of Anterior Cervical Plate Techniques

In 1955, Cloward et al. proposed autologous iliac bone graft for anterior cervical discectomy (Fig. 5.1). In 1967, Bohler put forward plate internal fixation following anterior bone graft fusion, i.e., anterior cervical discectomy and fusion (ACDF) and anterior cervical corpectomy and fusion (ACCF) (Fig. 5.2). In 1986, Morscher et al. designed the cervical spine locking plate for anterior cervical fusion (Fig. 5.3).

5.1.2 Anatomic Parameters Related to Cervical Anterior Plates

1. The superior view of the vertebral body (Fig. 5.4) [1]
2. The superior view of the vertebral body (Fig. 5.5)
3. The anterior view of the vertebral body (Fig. 5.6) [2]
4. The lateral view of the vertebral body (Fig. 5.7)

5.2 Internal Fixation with the ATLANTIS Anterior Cervical Plate System

5.2.1 Surgical Indications and Contraindications

1. Indications

The anterior cervical plate system is suitable for anterior fixation of C2 to T1 segments.

A. Trauma (Fig. 5.8)
   a. Instabilities of traumatic cervical spine injuries or intervertebral disc herniation
   b. Subluxation of the vertebral body without locked facet joint
   c. Vertebral body fracture or vertebral body fracture with compression of the spinal cord
   d. Anterior stabilization of severe traumatic cervical spine injuries requiring both anterior and posterior stabilization
B. Degenerative changes (Fig. 5.9)
   a. Single- or multilevel cervical disc herniation
   b. Single- or multilevel instability or spondylolisthesis
   c. Ossified posterior longitudinal ligament with fewer than two to three surgically resectable segments
   d. Cervical spondylotic myelopathy or cervical spondylotic radiculopathy
   e. Cervical kyphosis or swan neck deformity post posterior laminectomy
C. Tumors

T. Li · Y. Yan · W. Lei (✉)
Department of Orthopedics, Xijing Hospital, Air Force Medical University, Xi'an, Shaanxi, China
e-mail: leiwei@fmmu.edu.cn

W. Lei, Y. Yan (eds.), *Internal Fixation of the Spine*, https://doi.org/10.1007/978-981-16-1562-7_5

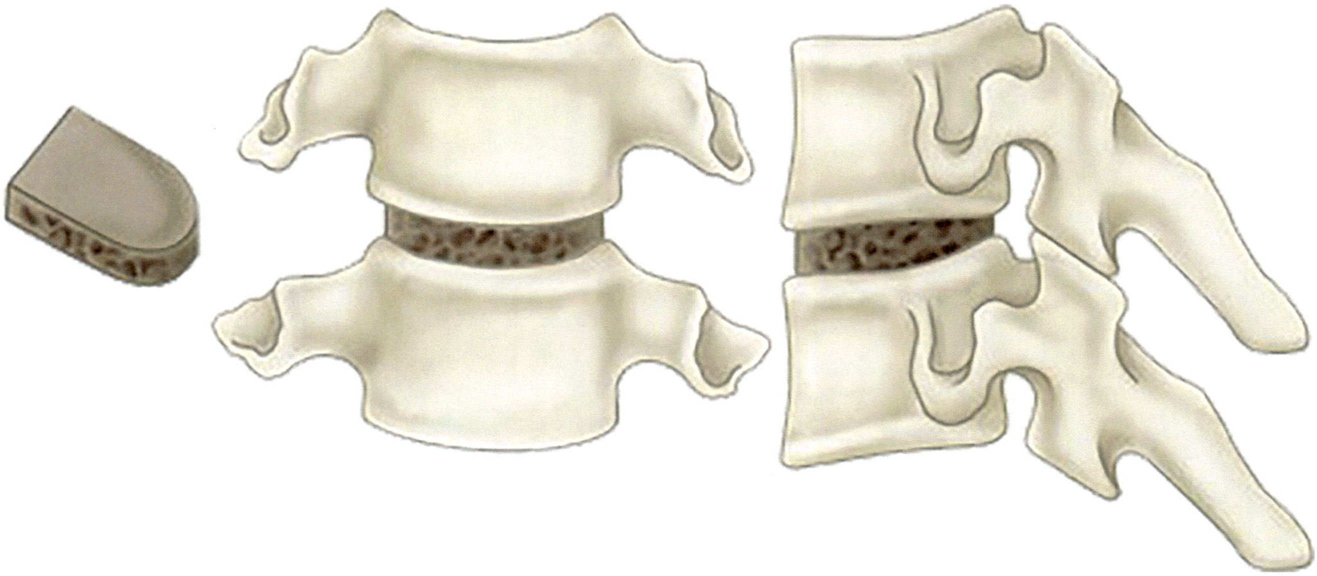

Fig. 5.1 Autologous iliac bone graft for anterior cervical discectomy

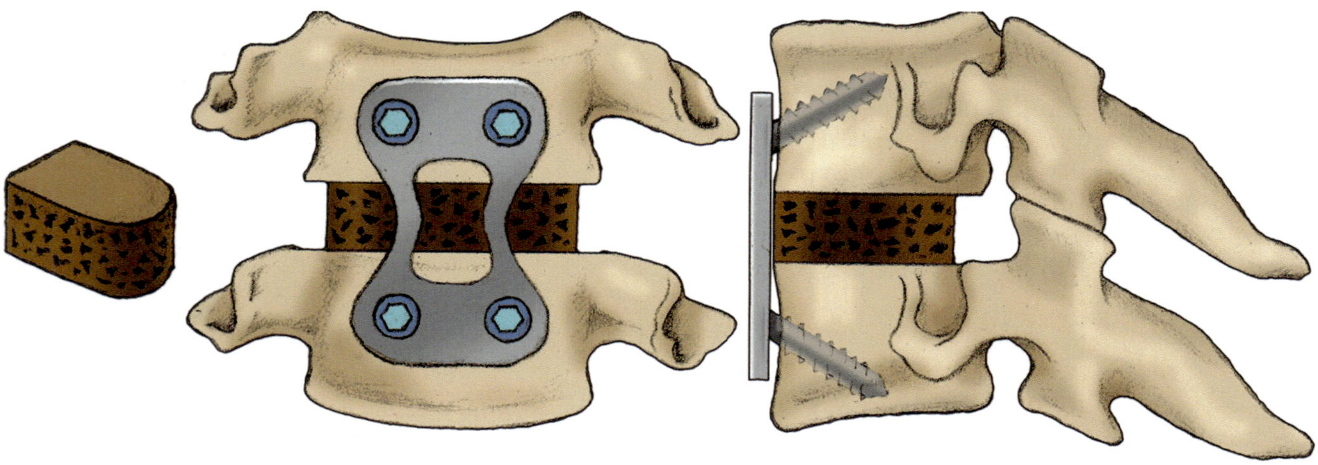

Fig. 5.2 Anterior cervical discectomy and fusion

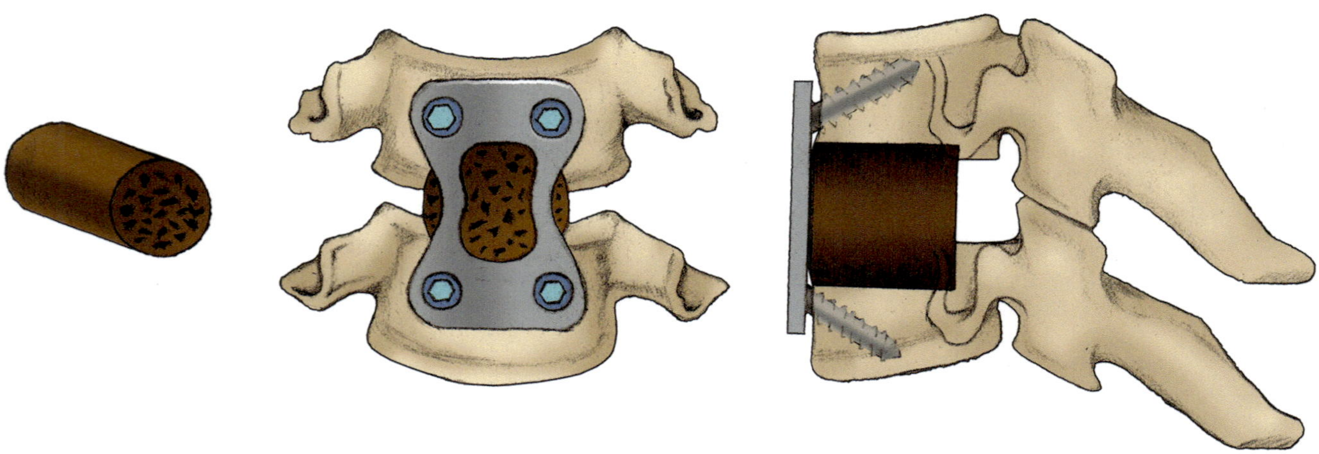

Fig. 5.3 Anterior cervical corpectomy and fusion

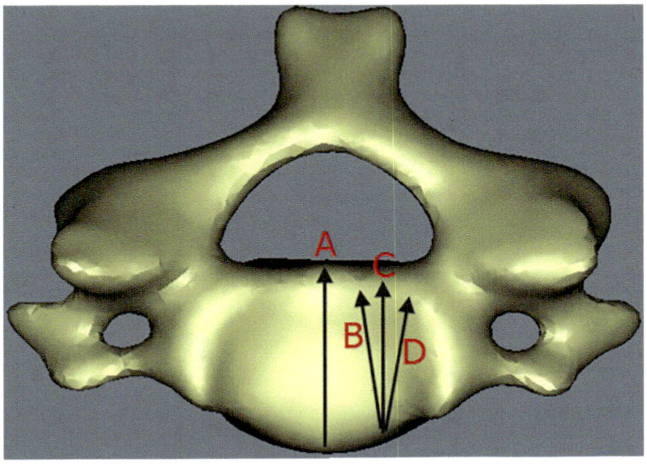

Fig. 5.4 Dimensions of the superior endplate. The screw entry depth from the middle sagittal plane (Depth *A*) ranged from 14.7 to 15.5 mm in the lower cervical spine. The screw entry depth in the 5-mm lateral and 10° medial inclination to Depth A (Depth *B*) ranged from 13.6 to 15.4 mm in the lower cervical spine. The screw entry depth in the 5 mm lateral and parallel to Depth A (Depth *C*) ranged from 13.2 to 15.4 mm in the lower cervical spine. The screw entry depth in the 5-mm lateral and 10° lateral inclination to Depth A (Depth *D*) ranged from 13.3 to 15.9 mm in the lower cervical spine

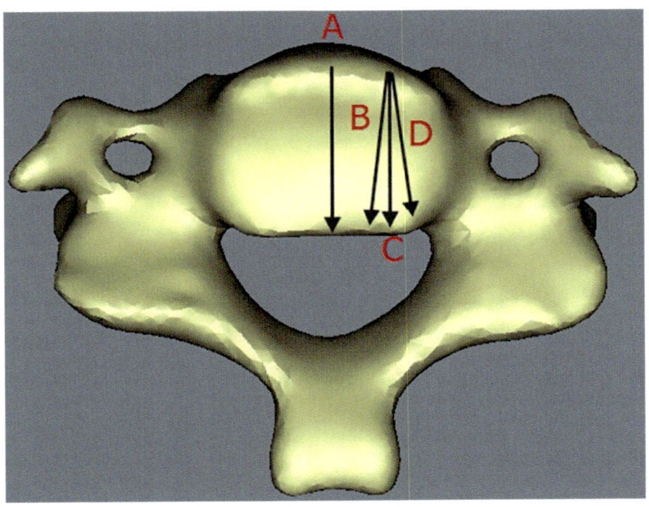

Fig. 5.5 Dimensions of the inferior endplate. The screw entry depth from the middle sagittal plane (Depth *A*) ranged from 15.1 to 14.8 mm in the lower cervical spine. The screw entry depth in the 5-mm lateral and 10° medial inclination to Depth A (Depth *B*) ranged from 14.5 to 14.9 mm in the lower cervical spine. The screw entry depth in the 5 mm lateral and parallel to Depth A (Depth *C*) ranged from 14.3 to 15.2 mm in the lower cervical spine. The screw entry depth in the 5-mm lateral and 10° lateral inclination to Depth A (Depth *D*) ranged from 13.7 to 15.4 mm in the lower cervical spine

Spine stability reconstruction post surgical resection of benign or metastatic tumors of the spine

D. Tuberculosis

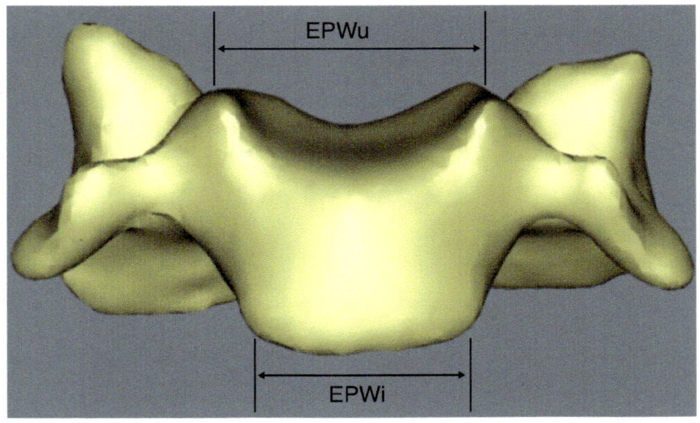

Fig. 5.6 The anterior view of the vertebral body. EPWu, width of the upper endplate; EPWi, width of the inferior endplate. The superior endplate width of the lower cervical spine ranged from 15.8 to 21.8 mm. The inferior endplate width of the lower cervical spine ranged from 17.0 to 23.4 mm

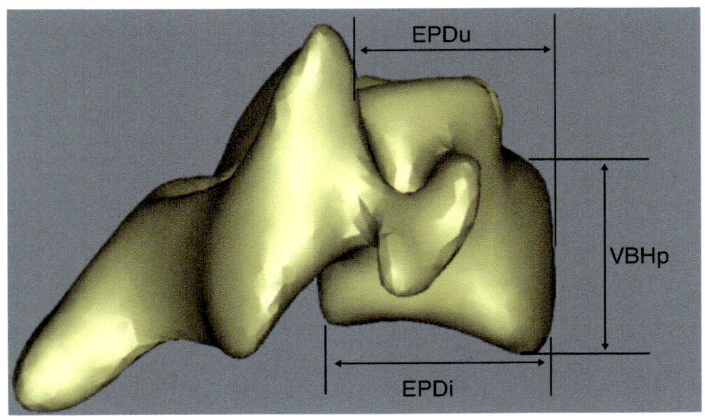

Fig. 5.7 The lateral view of the vertebral body. EPDu, upper endplate depth; EPDi, inferior endplate depth; VBHp, vertebral body height. The superior endplate depth of the lower cervical spine ranged from 15 to 18.1 mm. The inferior endplate depth of the lower cervical spine ranged from 15.6 to 16.8 mm. The height of the vertebral body in the lower cervical spine ranged from 11.6 to 12.8 mm

Segmental stability reconstruction following focal tuberculosis debridement

E. Congenital deformities

Cervical spine instability or cervical kyphosis due to congenital malformations

Contraindications

1. Suppurative infection of the surgical site
2. Fever of unknown cause or elevation of leukocyte count or increased erythrocyte sedimentation rate (ESR)
3. Morbid obesity
4. Mental disease
5. Suspected or confirmed metal allergy or intolerance

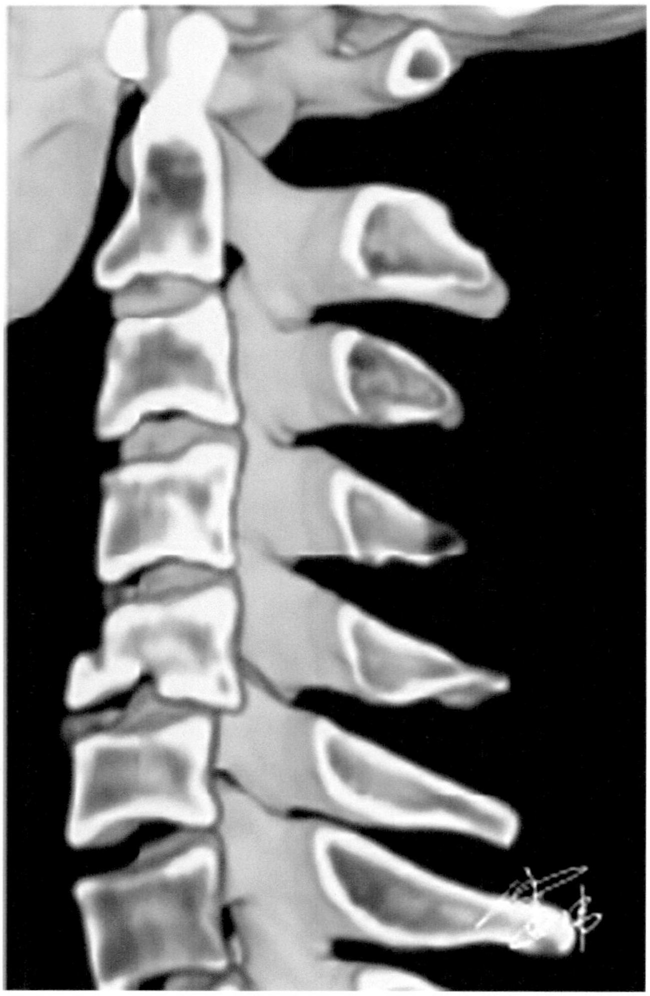

Fig. 5.8 Fracture of the cervical spine

Relative contraindications
1. Severe bone absorption
2. Severe osteoporosis
3. Osteomalacia

5.2.2 Surgical Steps

1. Patient position and incision

The patient is placed in the supine position with the head slightly extended. The posterior cervical spine is supported to establish and maintain normal cervical lordosis. A right or left approach to the cervical vertebral column must be chosen by the surgeon then (Fig. 5.10a). Typically, a transverse skin incision is made, and an avascular dissection plane is developed between the trachea/esophagus medially and the sternocleidomastoid/carotid sheath laterally. Handheld retractors are utilized to provide initial exposure of the anterior vertebral column and the adjacent longus colli muscles (Fig. 5.10b).

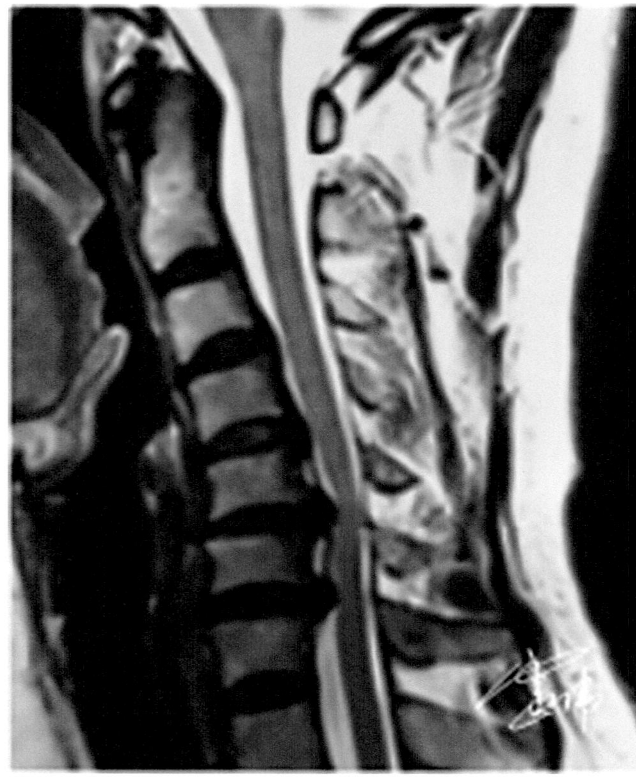

Fig. 5.9 Cervical disc herniation

2. Exposure of the cervical vertebral column

After the cervical vertebral column has been exposed, the medial border of the longus colli muscles is dissociated. Then, the self-retaining retractor blades are securely positioned, and the longitudinal self-retaining retractor is placed to provide optimal visualization (Fig. 5.11a, b). A vertebral body distractor may be used. The distraction pins are positioned midline in the vertebral bodies adjacent to the corpectomized vertebral body (Fig. 5.11c). The distractor is placed over the pins and appropriate distraction is applied.

3. Discectomy and corpectomy

Discectomies are completed at each level. To expose the posterior longitudinal ligament, pituitaries, curettes, and kerrisons may be used to remove the disc material and cartilage (Fig. 5.12a, b). To further decompress the spine, a corpectomy or partial corpectomy may be performed after removal of the discs. A portion of the vertebrae may be removed with a rongeur and the remaining portion of the vertebrae with a high-speed drill with a large bore bur (Fig. 5.12c). The posterior longitudinal ligament and osteophytes are then carefully removed.

4. Graft preparation and placement

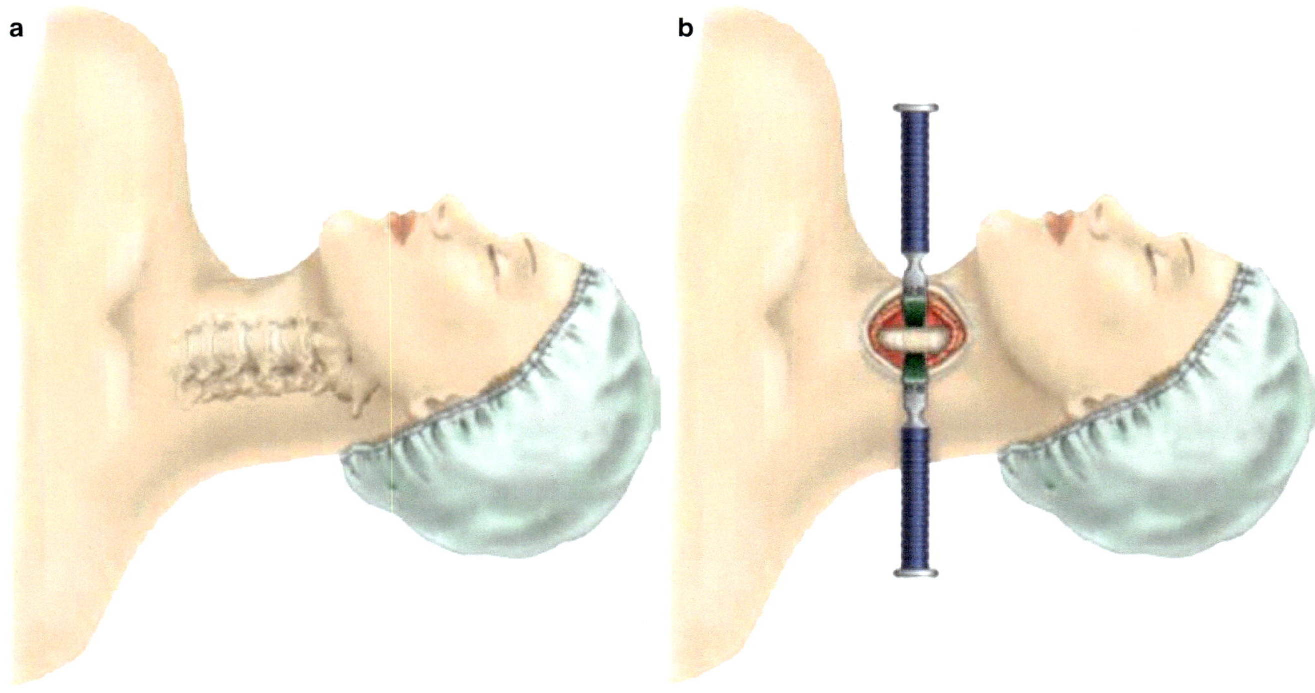

Fig. 5.10 Position of the patient and incision. (**a**) The patient is placed in the supine position with the head in slight extension. (**b**) A transverse skin incision is made

Following completion of decompression, the endplate is milled with a high-speed bur into a mortise that is precisely matched with the bone graft (Fig. 5.13a).

Either autograft or allograft may be utilized. The dimensions of the corpectomy site are precisely measured, and the bone graft is shaped and then held with a bone graft holder and tapped into place in the bone groove with a mallet (Fig. 5.13b, c).

5. Selecting appropriate plate length

Soft tissue and anterior osteophytes are removed from the adjacent vertebral bodies so that the plate sits evenly on the anterior cortex. The plate is positioned to allow the superior and inferior screw holes to locate at approximately the mid-portion of the vertebral body (Fig. 5.14a). This assures that fixed or variable bone screws are placed in the center of the vertebrae. The plate edge should not interfere with the adjacent unfused disc spaces (Fig. 5.14b). The plate may be further contoured using the plate bender to fit the lordotic curvature of the anterior cervical spine.

6. Plate contouring

The ATLANTIS VISION ELITE cervical plate has a pre-machined cervical lordotic curve (Fig. 5.15a). When required, the plate may be contoured using the plate bender to increase (Fig. 5.15b) or decrease the amount of lordotic curvature (Fig. 5.15c). Abrupt changes in curvature should be avoided by gradually bending the plate.

7. Use of the plate holder

The plate holder in ATLANTIS VISION ELITE anterior cervical plate system may be used for any screw holes. It has a sharp tip that prevents plate migration while positioning. The tip of the plate holder retracts when pressure is applied to the locking sleeve cap (Fig. 5.16a). The retracted tip is inserted into the appropriate screw hole. After the locking sleeve cap is released, the plate holder becomes securely engaged with the plate.

8. Positioning the plate

The plate that is of appropriate length is selected by carefully observing the anatomic landmarks of the cervical vertebra and is centered medially on the anterior surface of the cervical spine. The plate can also be temporarily affixed to the vertebral bodies by inserting Plate Holding Pins in the midline of the plate through the locking cap (Fig. 5.17a). Use caution not to turn the locking cap when seating the Holding Pin. This could preclude the screws from being inserted. These pins are threaded for increased hold strength in the vertebral body. The instrument set includes a Plate Holding Pin Driver to facilitate pin insertion. Drive the sharp tip of the pin into the bone until the dorsal portion of the pin is

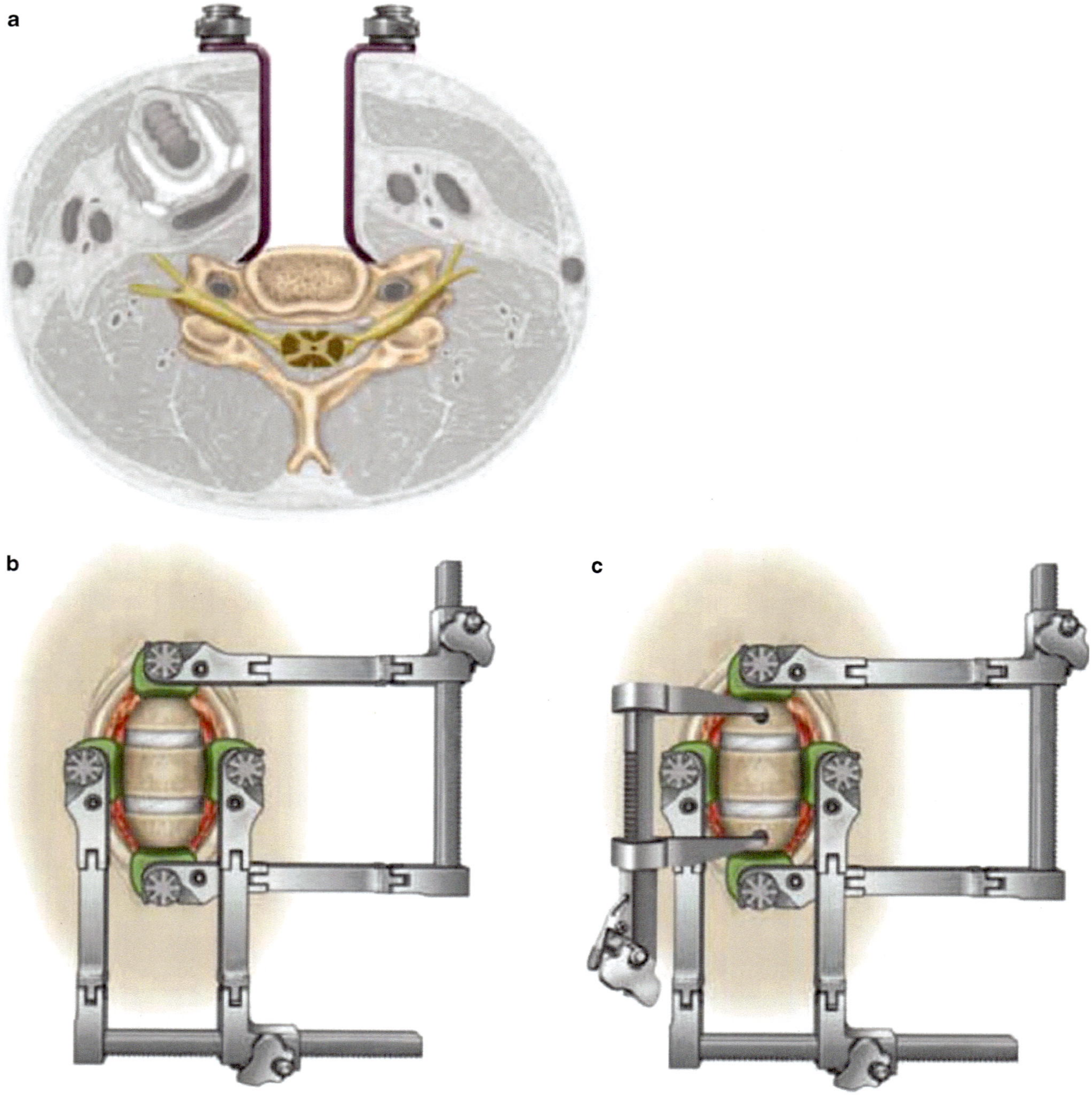

Fig. 5.11 Exposure of the cervical vertebral column. (**a**) The target vertebral body is exposed. (**b**) The retractor is placed. (**c**) The vertebral body distractor is placed

flush with the plate (Fig. 5.17b). To release a Plate Holding Pin from the Pin Driver, place upward pressure on the locking sleeve collar.

9. Optional Bone Screw Hole Preparation

An awl can be used to break through the cortex of the vertebral body. The instrument set includes a Fixed Angle Awl (Fig. 5.18a) and a Universal Awl to provide multiple options for screw hole preparation.

Use the Variable or Fixed Drill Guide. Snap the tri-flat end of the Universal Awl shaft into the Universal Handle. Ensure that the selected guide is securely seated in the aperture of the bone screw hole on the plate. Insert the Universal Awl into the guide. Place downward pressure on the awl to puncture the cortex of the bone (Fig. 5.18b).

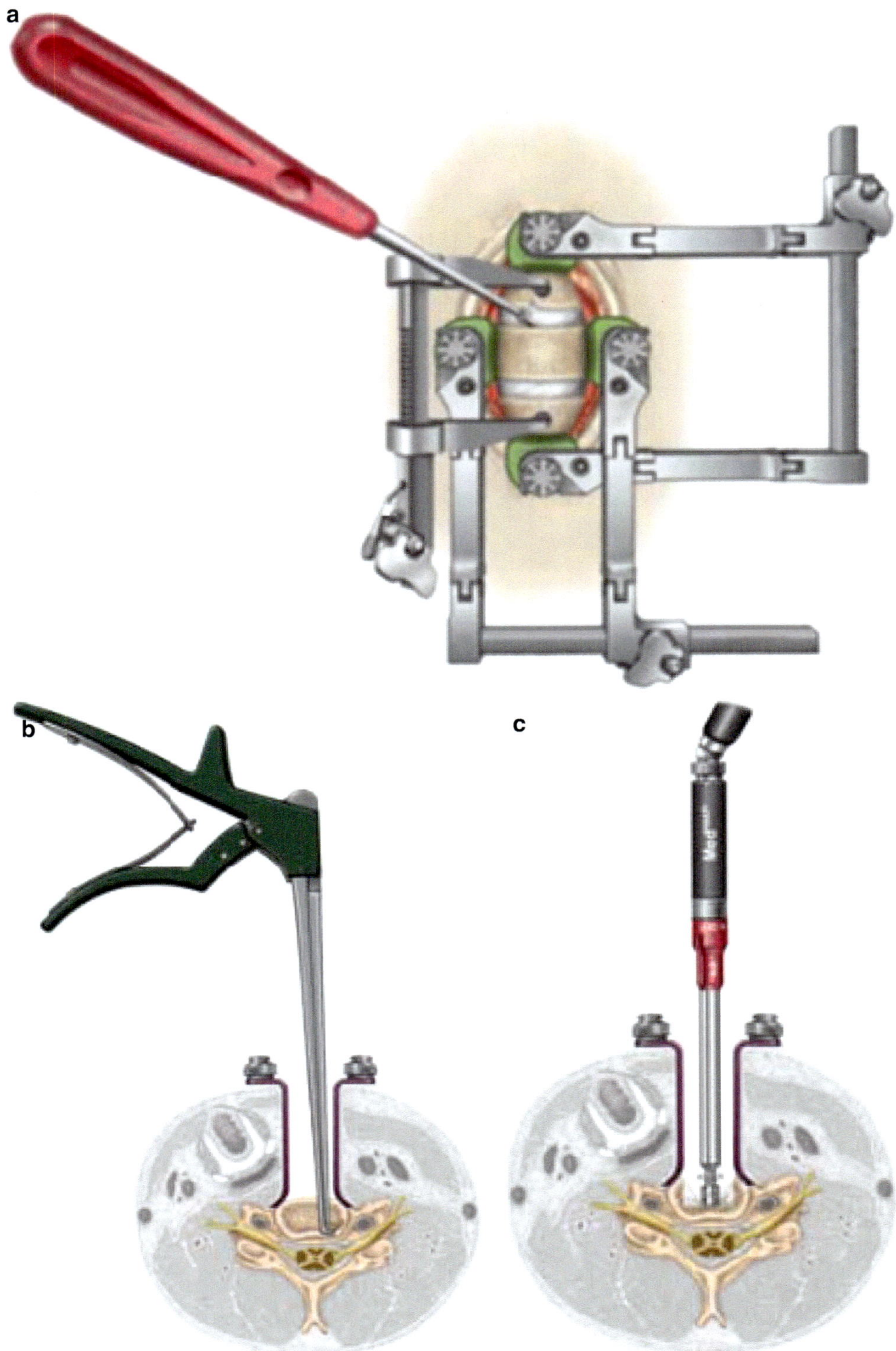

Fig. 5.12 Discectomy and corpectomy. (**a**) Discectomy is done. (**b**) The intervertebral disc is excised. (**c**) The vertebral body is removed

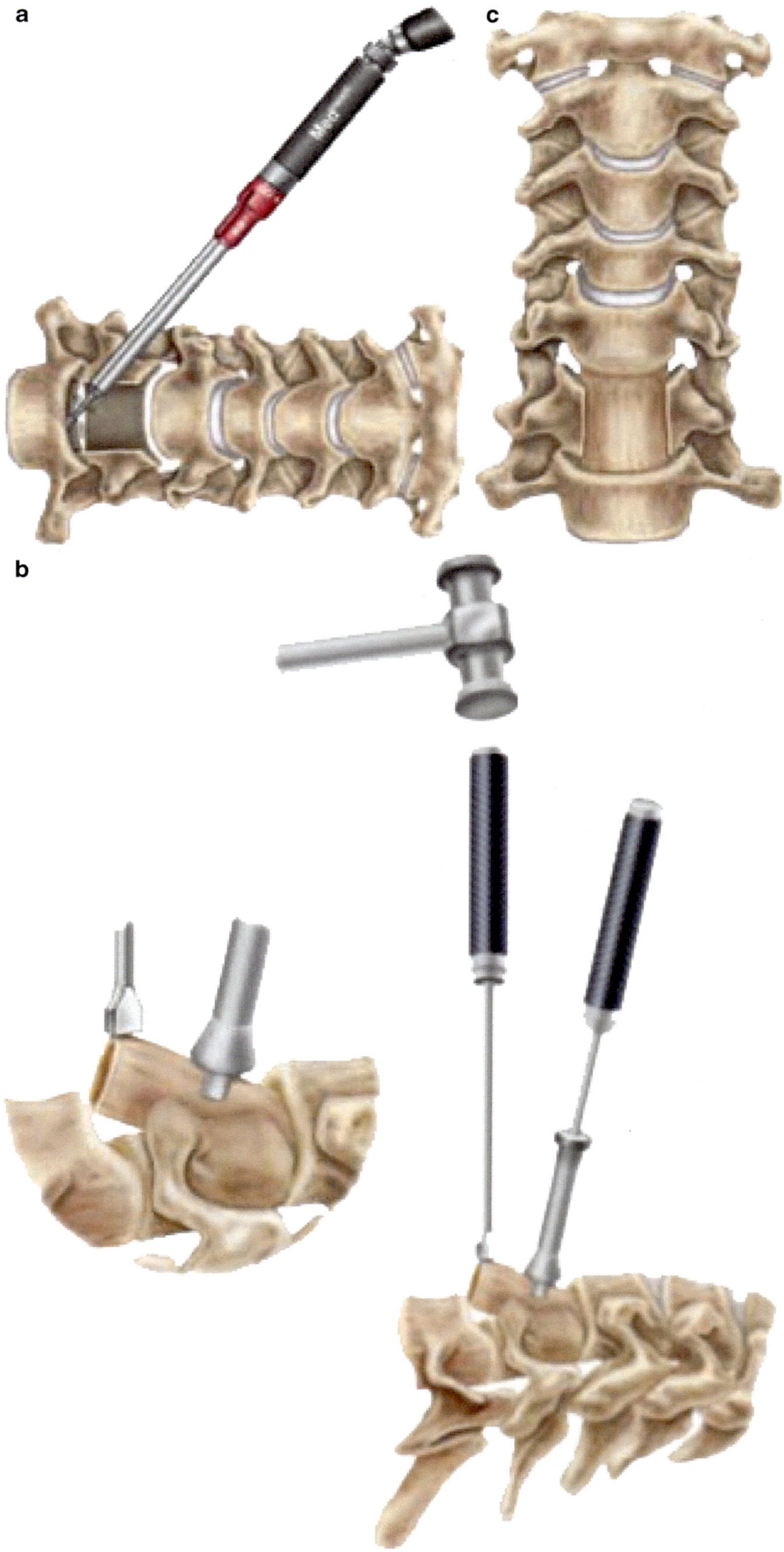

Fig. 5.13 Preparation and placement of bone graft. (**a**) Milling the endplate; (**b**) Bone graft placement; (**c**) Completion of bone graft implantation

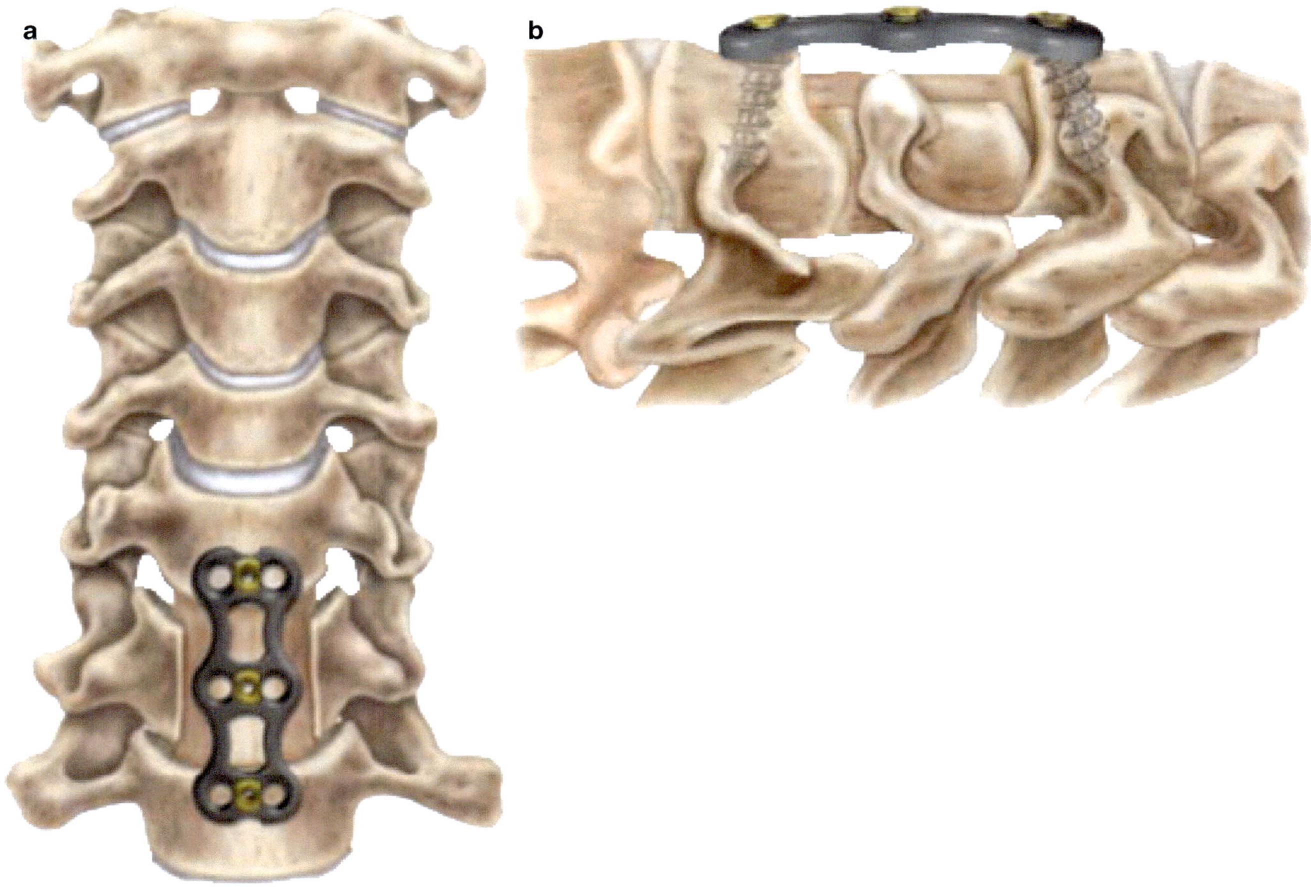

Fig. 5.14 Selecting the appropriate plate length. (**a**) Determining the plate position; (**b**) Attention should be paid to positioning of the plate edge

10. Selection of constructs

The ATLANTIS VISION ELITE cervical anterior plate system offers the surgeon the versatility of mastery of intra-operative dynamics of the construct. Color-coded fixed or variable angle bone screws are used to configure fixed, variable, or hybrid angle constructs.

11. Screw positioning

a. Screw positioning method

The positioning method for fixed angle screws: The fixed angle drill guide is seated within the bone screw hole of the plate, and the handle is pressed lightly downward (Fig. 5.19a, b), making sure to align the drill guide in the correct 12°cephalad or 12°caudad and 6° medial convergent angle (Fig. 5.19c).

The positioning method for variable screws: The variable angle drill guide is secured within the bone screw hole of the plate. The variable angle drill guide can be aligned with the proper screw entry path (Fig. 5.19a). When 4-mm variable angle screw is selected, any angle within the following angles can be chosen: 22° distant angle, −2° proximal angle, 17° medial convergent angle, and 4° lateral divergent angle (Fig. 5.19b, c).

The positioning method hybrid screws: The variable or fixed angle drill guide is secured within the bone screw hole of the plate and can be aligned with the proper screw entry path.

b. Angle range

The range for fixed angle: The handle of the fixed angle drill guide is pressed lightly downward (Fig. 5.19b, c) and is securely screwed into the plate in the 12° cephalad or 12° caudal and 6° medial convergent angle (Fig. 5.20a). The drill guide handle has a color band that facilitates selection of same color screws.

The range for variable angle: The variable angle drill guide (Fig. 5.20a, b) can restrict the screw path within the angle range of 4-mm variable screws, i.e., 22° distant angle and −2° proximal angle (Fig. 5.20b) and 17° medial convergent angle and 4° lateral divergent angle (Fig. 5.20c).

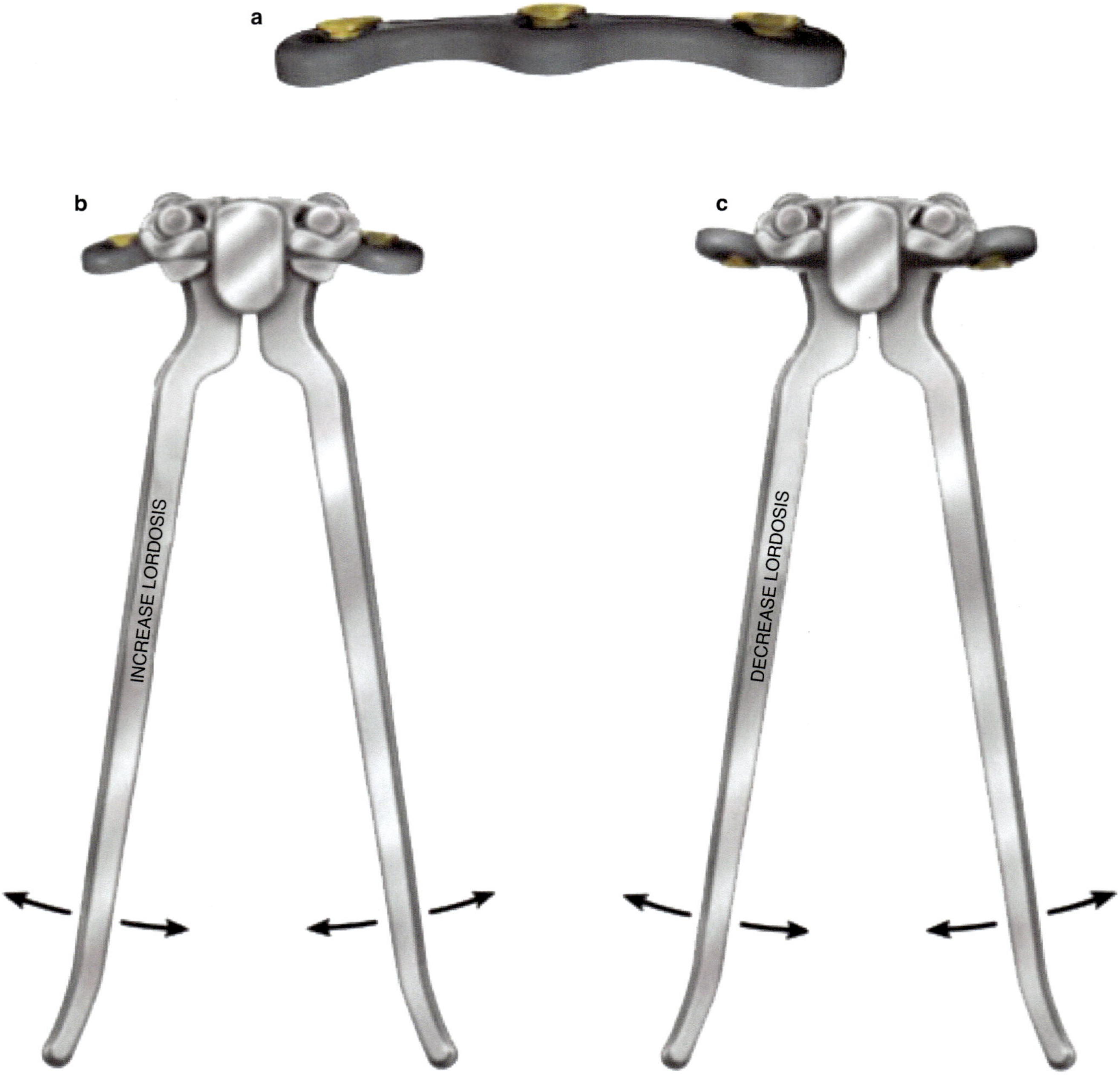

Fig. 5.15 Plate contouring. (**a**) Pre-machined lordotic curvature of the plate; (**b**) Increasing the plate curvature; (**c**) Decreasing the plate curvature

12. Bone screw implantation

The appropriate length screw can be verified using the screw gauge located in the fixed or variable angle bone screw block (Fig. 5.21a). The appropriate length bone screw is inserted through the plate, using the screwdriver with tapered, self-holding tip and preliminarily tightening the bone screw (Fig. 5.21b) (not final tightening).

Note: Place the initial screws deep enough so that the head of the screw "slips past" the gold washer. This allows the washer to move freely, thus providing space for the contralateral screw drilling.

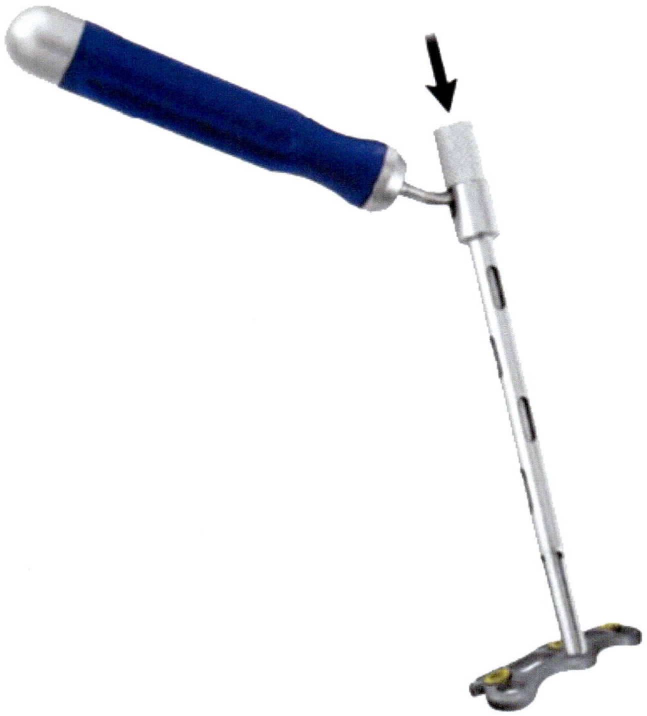

Fig. 5.16 Holding the plate. Pressure is applied to the locking sleeve cap

The following are recommended steps for screw implantation:

- Drill, tap, and place one bone screw securely through the plate (not final tightening).
- Drill, tap, and place the second bone screw securely on the opposite end of the plate, diagonally from the first screw position.
- If necessary, the plate holder can be removed with a pin driver.
- The remaining two bone screw implant sites are then drilled and tapped with the bone screws securely inserted.

13. Final tightening of screws

The screw is finally tightened so that the plate is evenly and firmly applied to the anterior cortical surface of the spine

14. Tightening of the attached lock mechanism

The ATLANTIS VISION ELITE anterior cervical plate system includes an attached locking cap mechanism. The lock detail has a positive stop that prevents the cap from turning more than 90° clockwise. Avoid turning the locking cap counterclockwise as this will detach the cap from the plate.

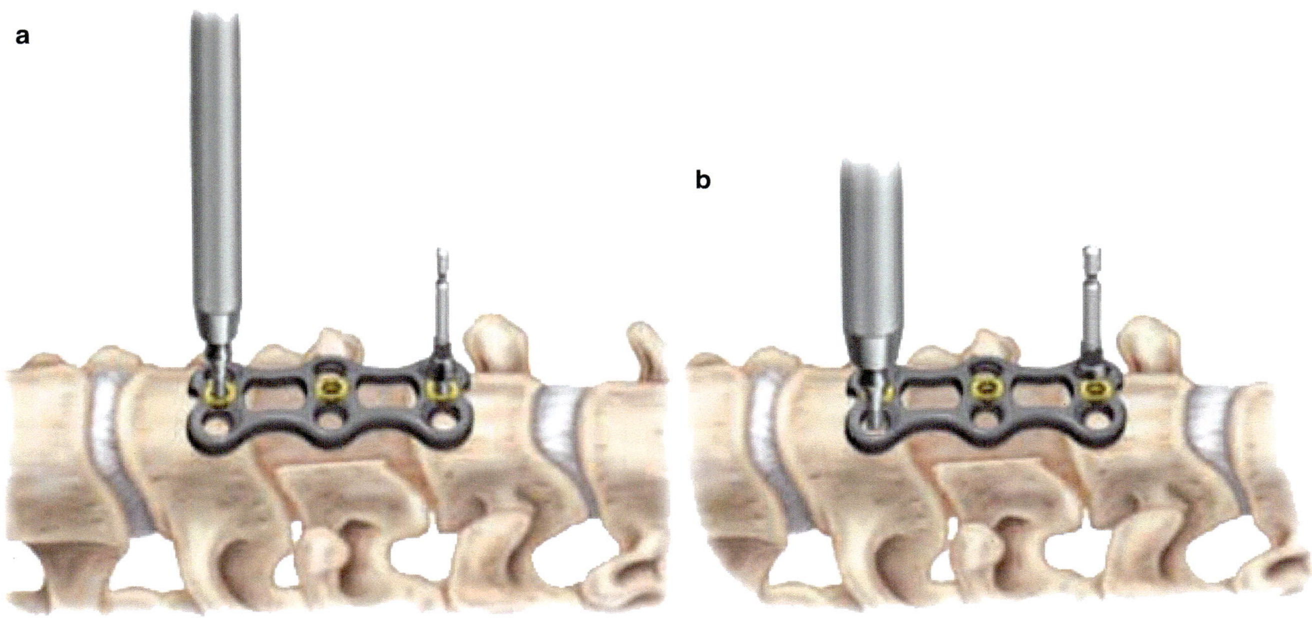

Fig. 5.17 Positioning the plate. (**a**) Inserting Plate Holding Pins the locking cap; (**b**) Inserting the Plate Pin Driver

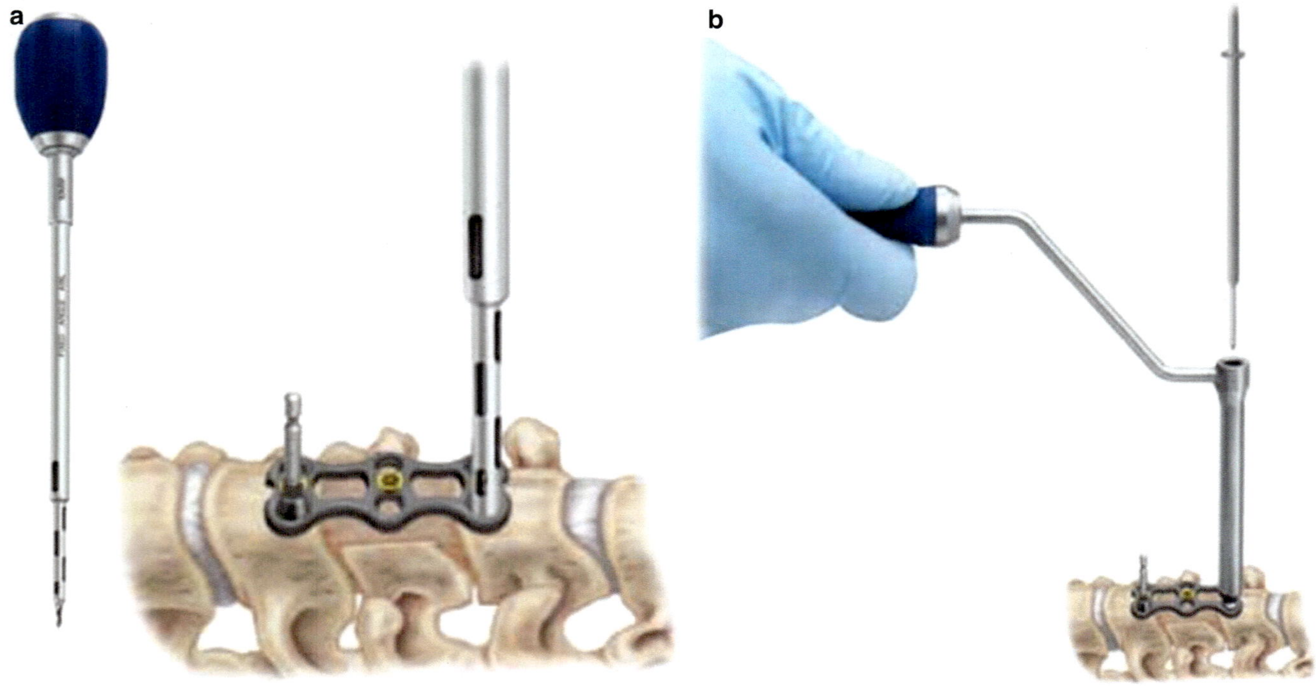

Fig. 5.18 Optional bone screw hole preparation. (**a**) 10 mm of bone penetration at a trajectory of 12° cephalad or 6° caudal. (**b**) 22° to −2° cephalad or caudal and 17°–4° medially convergent with the Variable Drill Guide. 12° cephalad or 6° caudal and 4° medially convergent with the Fixed Drill Guide

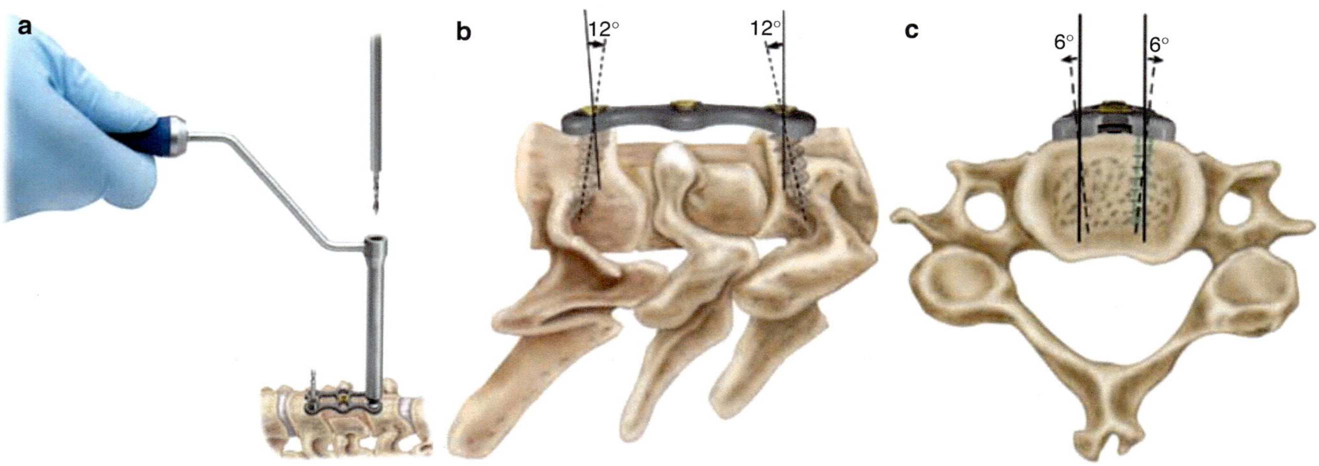

Fig. 5.19 Positioning of fixed screws. (**a**) The fixed angle drill guide is seated. (Note: (**b**) The drill guide is aligned in the correct 12°cephalad or 12°caudad and (**c**) 6° medial convergent angle)

The same standard 2.5-mm Hex Screwdriver used for screw insertion can be used to engage the locking cap mechanism. Insert the 2.5-mm Hex Screwdriver into the head of the locking cap and rotate it 90° until the cap covers both screw heads and a positive stop is felt. The stop provides tactile feedback that the cap is fully engaged and covering both screw heads (Fig. 5.22a). A Ball Tip Lock Driver is also included in the instrument set to allow the locking cap to be engaged from an angle (Fig. 5.22b). If the locking cap does not rotate and cover both screw heads, check to make sure that the screws are fully seated. If bone screws are not fully seated, locking it could cause pressure on the skin from component parts in patients with inadequate tissue coverage over the implant, possibly causing skin penetration, irritation, and/or pain.

15. Construct removal

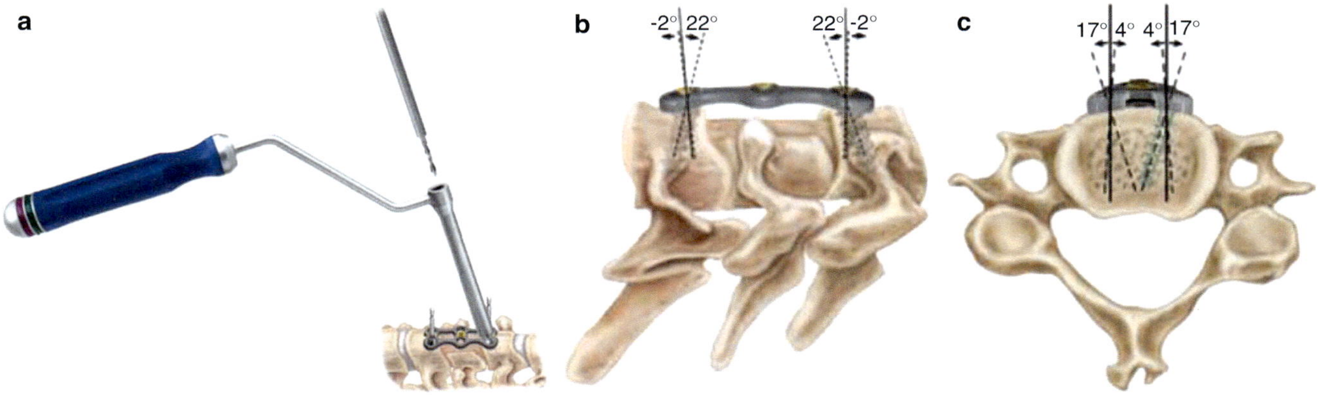

Fig. 5.20 Positioning of hybrid angle screws. (**a**) The cephalad drill guide is assembled. (**b**) 22° distant angle, −2° proximal angle (**c**), 17° medial convergent angle and 4° lateral convergent angle

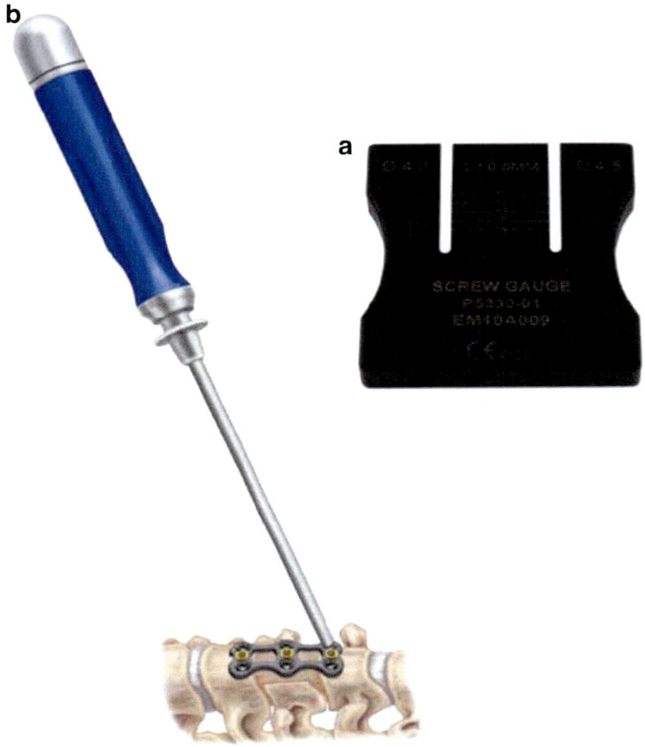

Fig. 5.21 Screw implantation. (**a**) The screw length is measured. (**b**) The screw is inserted

If removal of the construct is necessary, the lock screwdriver is first used to loosen the lock screw. The tip of the lock screwdriver is placed into the lock screw, and the tip is completely inserted and does not strip the screw head. The lock screwdriver is turned 90° counterclockwise to loosen the lock screw from the plate. Then, the 2.5-mm hex driver can be used for removal of the bone screws. The tip of the 2.5-mm hex driver is properly placed into the head of the screw by avoiding stripping of the screw head. The 2.5-mm hex driver is turned counterclockwise until the screw backs out completely from the plate. This is repeated for all screws within the construct.

5.3 Clinical Cases

Case 1

Patient: A 32-year-old female complained of traumatic neck pain with limited mobility for 8 h.

Diagnosis: Hangman's fracture.

Surgery: C2–C3 discectomy, CONERSTONE fusion, and internal fixation with the ATLANTIS system.

Imaging data: Preoperative imaging study is shown in Fig. 5.23, and postoperative imaging study is shown in Fig. 5.24.

Case 2

Patient: A 32-year-old male complained of sensorimotor impairment of bilateral upper and lower extremities after trauma for 1 day.

Diagnosis: Cervical cord injury with incomplete paralysis.

Surgery: C3 to C4 and C4 to C5 disc decompression surgery, CONERSTONE fusion, and internal fixation with the ATLANTIS system.

Imaging data: Preoperative imaging study is shown in Fig. 5.25, and postoperative imaging study is shown in Fig. 5.26.

Case 3

Patient: A 46-year-old female complained of numbness in both upper and lower extremities and weakness in walking for 2 years.

Diagnosis: Cervical spondylosis and ossified posterior longitudinal ligament of the cervical spine.

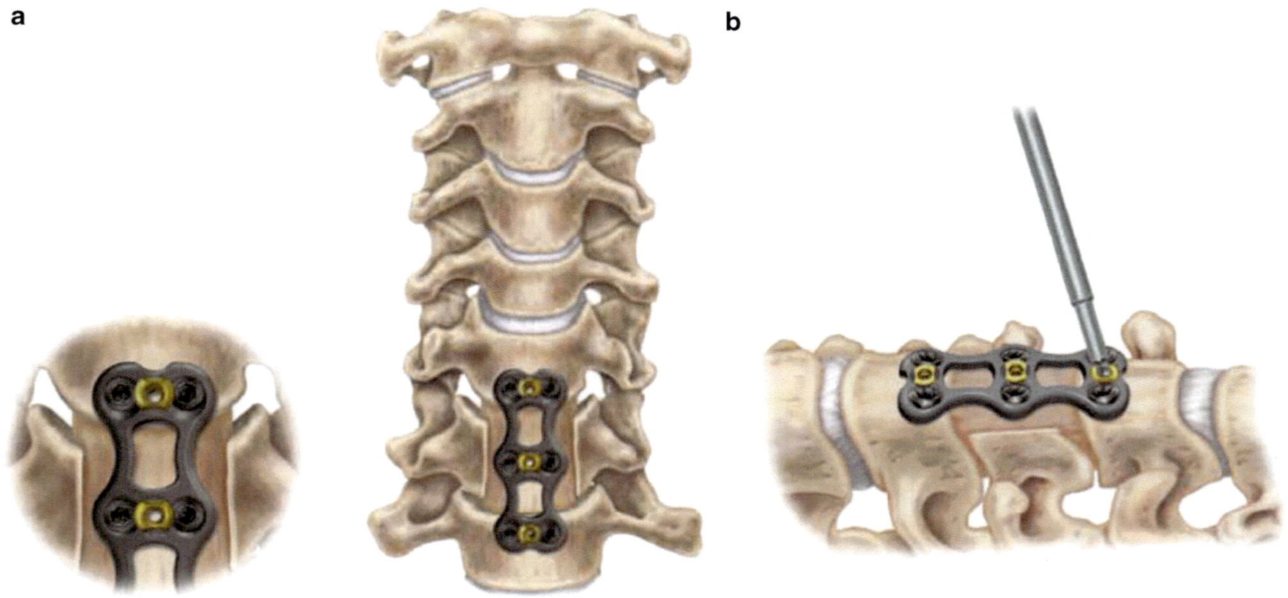

Fig. 5.22 Tightening the screw. (**a**) The lock screw is tightened. (**b**) Ball Tip Lock Driver allows the locking cap to be engaged from an angle

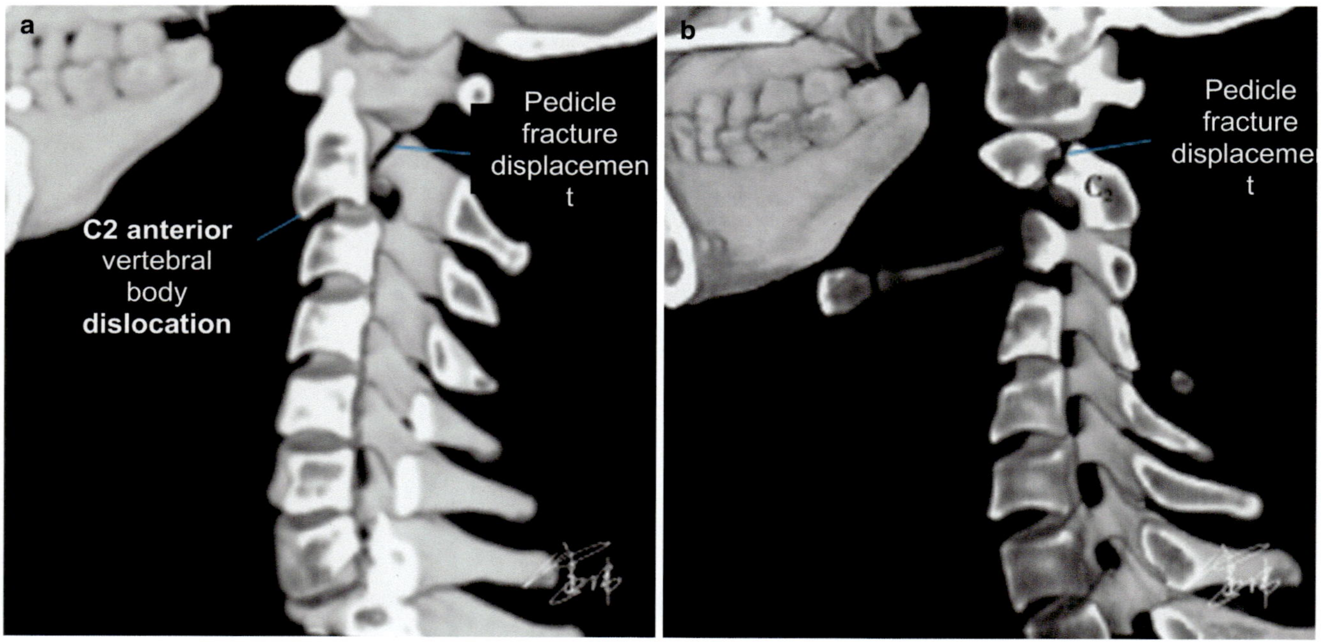

Fig. 5.23 Preoperative imaging study. Split sagittal (**a**) and 3D CT reconstruction image of the spinal canal (**b**)

Surgery: C4 to C5 discectomy and decompression surgery, CONERSTONE fusion, C6 corpectomy, PYRAMESH fusion, and internal fixation with the ATLANTIS system.

Imaging data: Preoperative imaging study is shown in Fig. 5.27, and postoperative imaging study is shown in Fig. 5.28.

Case 4

Patient: A 40-year-old male complained of sensorimotor impairment of bilateral upper and lower extremities after trauma for 20 h.

Diagnosis: C6 fracture and dislocation with paraplegia.

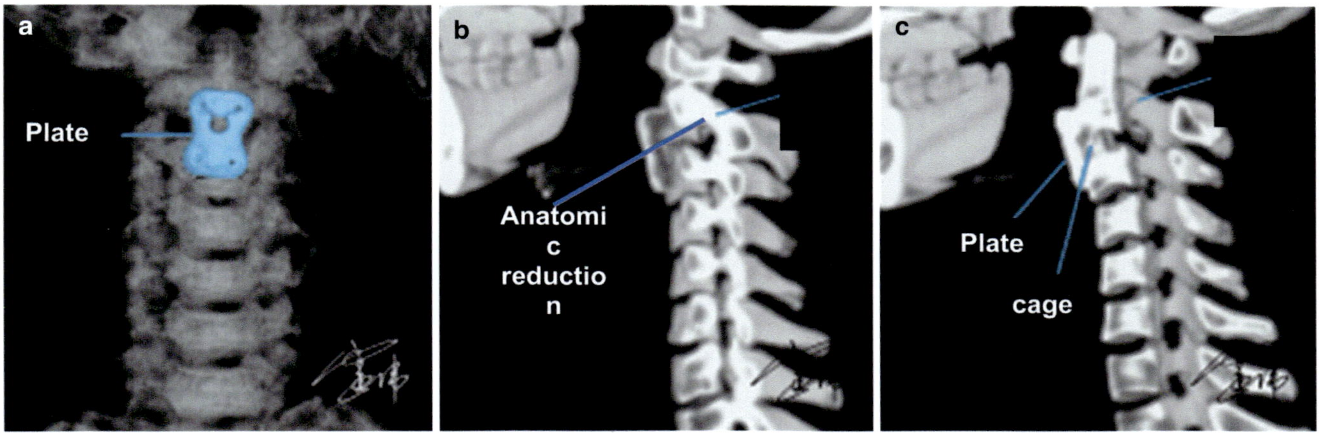

Fig. 5.24 Postoperative imaging study. (**a**) Three-dimensional CT reconstruction (anterior view). Split sagittal (**b**) and coronal (**c**) 3D CT reconstruction image of the spinal canal

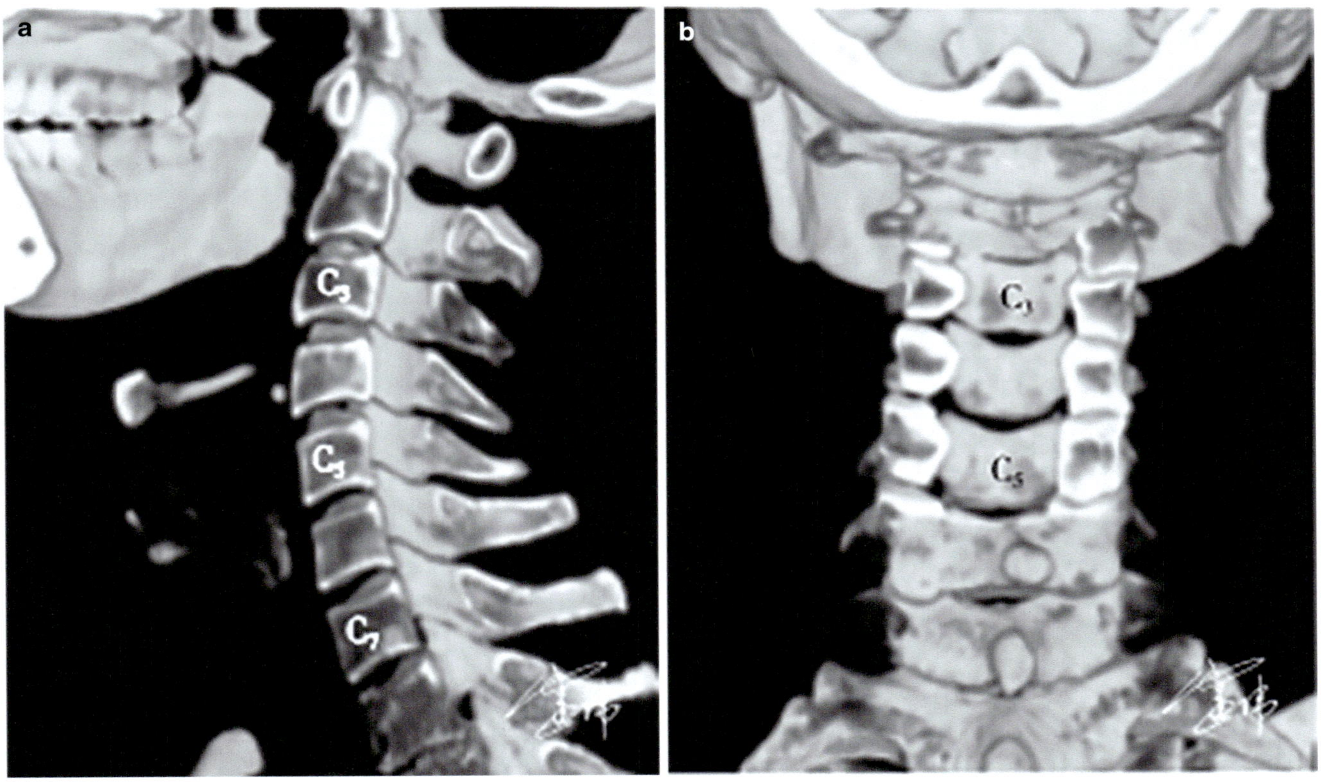

Fig. 5.25 Preoperative imaging study. Split sagittal (**a**) and coronal (**b**) 3D CT reconstruction image of the spinal canal

Surgery: C6 corpectomy, iliac graft fusion and ATLANTIS VISION internal fixation, and posterior C5 to C7 screw and rod internal fixation.

Imaging data: Preoperative imaging study is shown in Fig. 5.29, and postoperative imaging study is shown in Fig. 5.30.

Case 5

Patient: A 68-year-old female complained of neck pain for 15 months with weakness of bilateral lower extremities for 14 months and worsening for 20 days.

Diagnosis: Cervical spondylotic myelopathy

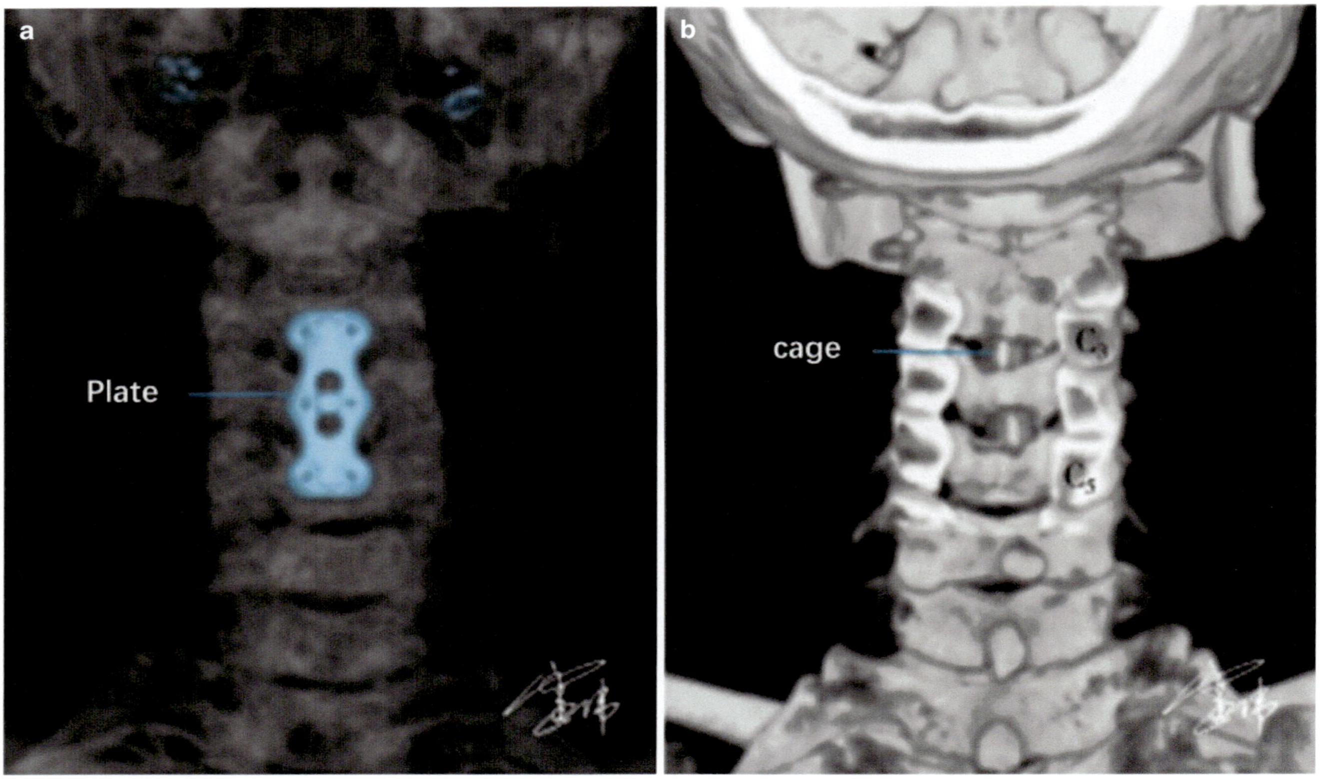

Fig. 5.26 Postoperative imaging study. (**a**) Three-dimensional CT reconstruction (*anterior view*). (**b**) Anteroposterior split 3D CT reconstruction image of the spinal canal

Surgery: C4/C5 and C5/C6 discectomy via an anterior approach, C5 vertebral subtotal resection, bone graft and fusion and internal fixation

Imaging data: Preoperative imaging study is shown in Fig. 5.31, and postoperative imaging study is shown in Figs. 5.32, 5.33, 5.34, and 5.35.

5.4 Pearls and Pitfalls

1. Plate selection

The correct length of the plate is selected according to bone groove length and height of the upper and lower vertebral body to ensure that the screw is implanted into the middle of the vertebral body, thereby enhancing internal fixation stability. A plate that is unduly long affects the function of adjacent vertebral segments, and a plate that is unduly short impacts on spine stability.

2. Plate bending

The plate has predesigned curvature in both horizontal and vertical directions. When required, the plate may be contoured using the plate bender to increase or decrease the amount of lordotic curvature. The plate should not be bent excessively; otherwise, the lock mechanism in the plate may be jeopardized.

3. Plate placement

Osteophytes in the anterior vertebral body that are to undergo internal fixation are removed so that the plate is evenly and firmly applied to the anterior cortical surface of the spine according to the physiological curvature of the cervical spine. The plate should be placed in the center of the vertebral body, preferably in the midpoint of the upper and lower vertebral body. The bilateral longus colli muscles can be used as landmarks for plate placement, and palpation of the suprasternal notch facilitates plate placement in the center of the cervical vertebra. If a surgeon cannot determine the superior and inferior border of the vertebral bodies during surgery, he or she can temporarily affix the plate to the cortex of the vertebral body and then determine the position and length of the plate by X-ray. This prevents the use of inappropriately sized plate and avoids implantation of the screw into the intervertebral space. The final position of the plate should be confirmed by intraoperative X-ray.

4. Advantages of multi-segment plate fixation

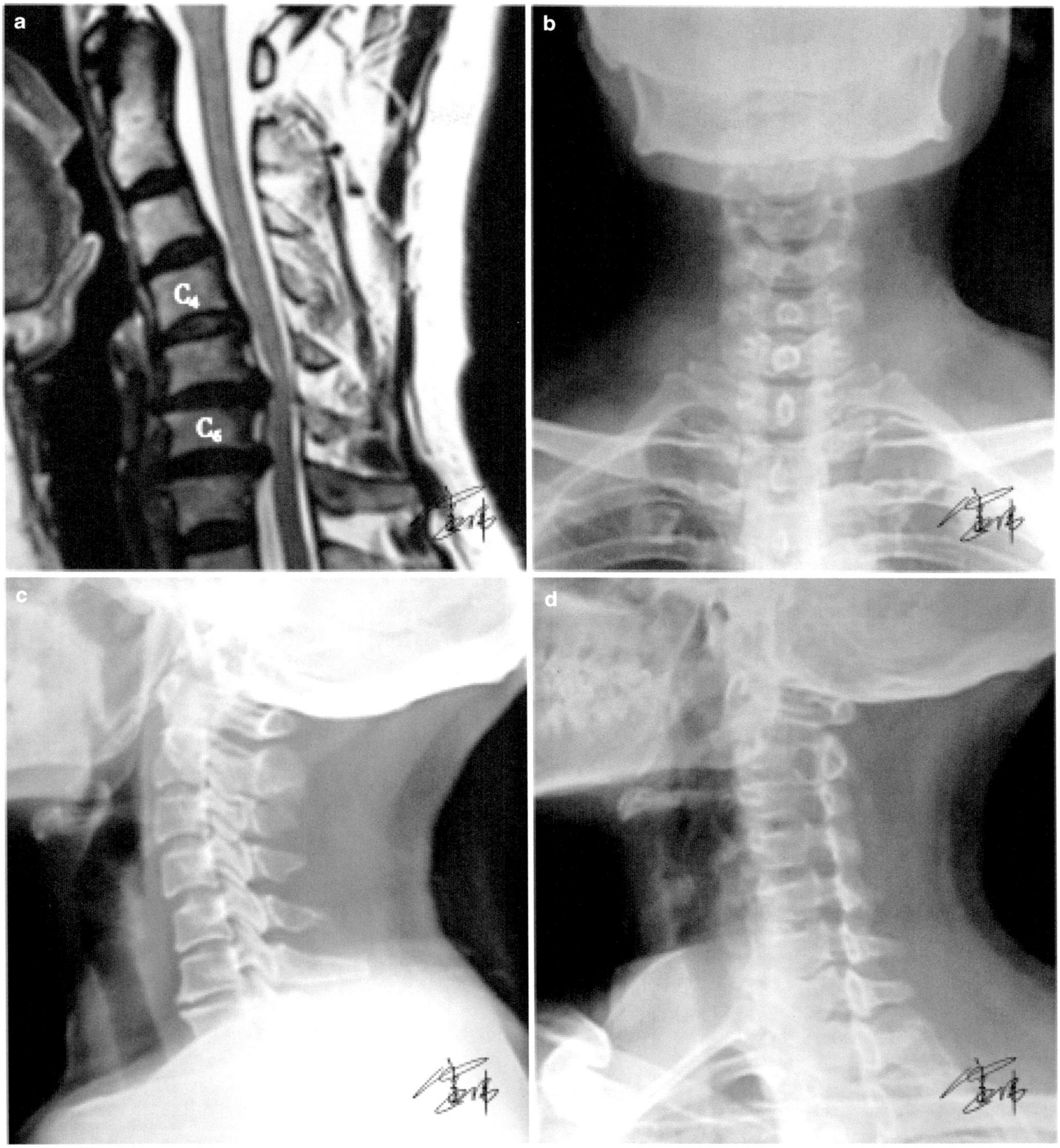

Fig. 5.27 Preoperative imaging study. (**a**) MRI (*sagittal*); (**b**) X-ray (*anterior*); (**c**) X-ray (*lateral*) (**d**) X-ray (*left lateral*)

For patients with multi-segment cervical spondylotic myelopathy (up to four segments) for decompression and autologous bone fusion, anterior plate fixation offers great advantages. The approach provides excellent postoperative stability at the junction; therefore, osteophytes may be radically removed during surgery to achieve extensive and effective decompression. Meanwhile, there will be no risk of bone and vertebral collapse, non-fusion, instability, and formation of kyphotic angles.

5. Requirements for drilling holes

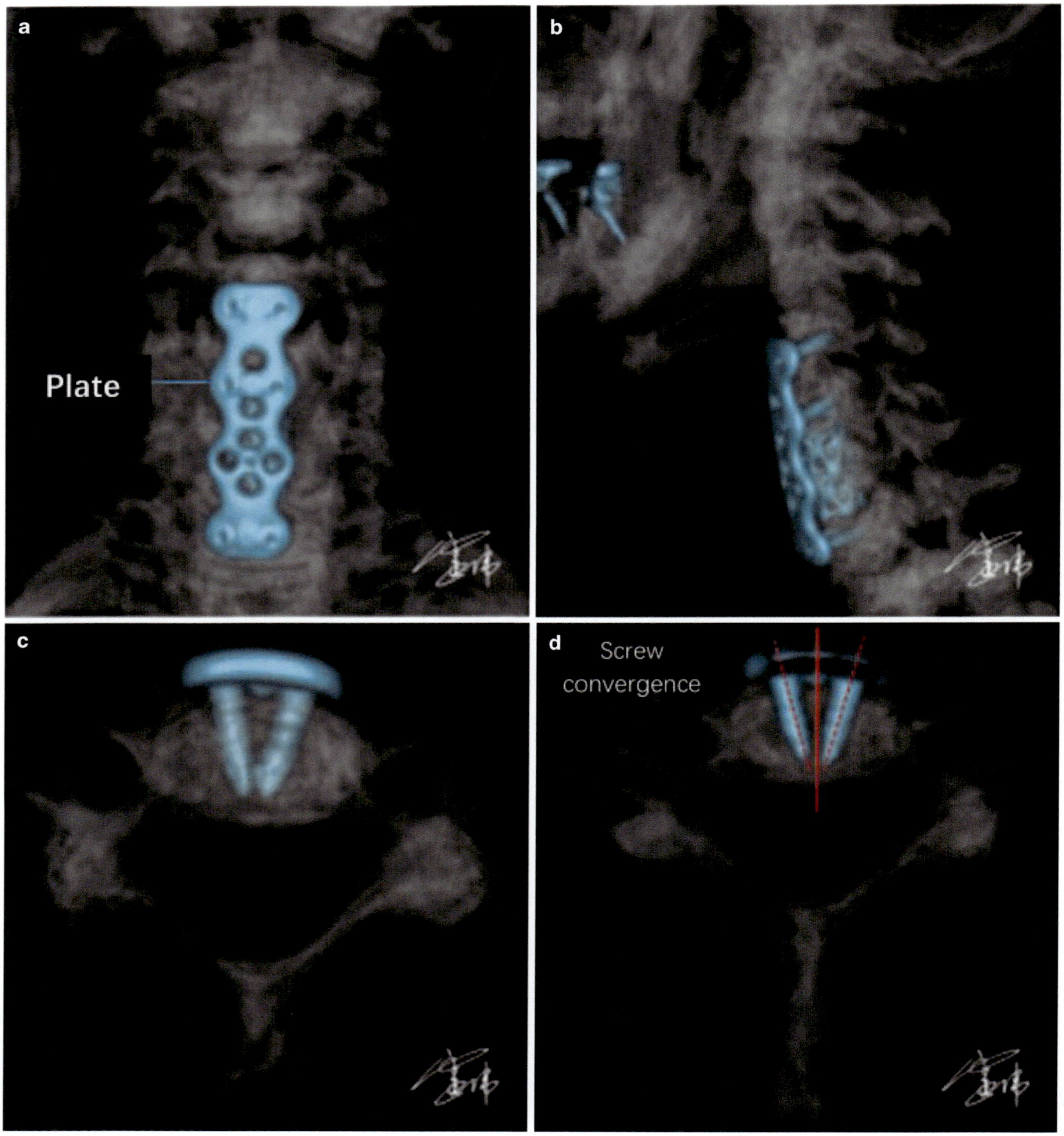

Fig. 5.28 Postoperative imaging study. (**a**) Three-dimensional CT reconstruction (*anterior view*) and (**b**) three-dimensional CT reconstruction (*lateral view*). (**c**) C4 screw depth (*horizontal plane*). (**d**) C7 screw depth (*horizontal plane*)

The drill sleeve should be used when drilling holes in order to control penetration depth and avoid inadvertent injury due to entry of the drill bit into the vertebral canal. The use of sleeve also assures accurate and error-proof screw implantation. In addition, drilling holes multiple times could cause diminished bone purchase, leading to loosening of screws and plates. If the above scenario occurs during surgery, 4-mm correction screws should replace 3.5-mm s standard crews for plate fixation.

6. Screw usage

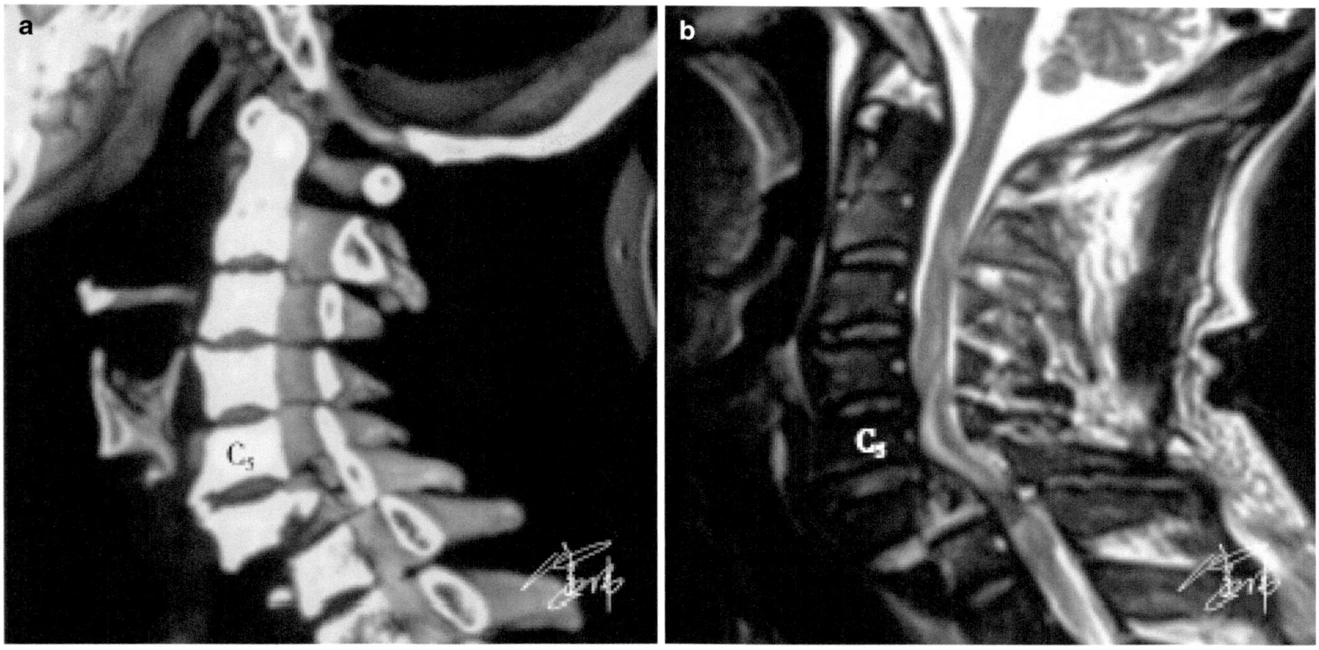

Fig. 5.29 Preoperative imaging study. (**a**) Split sagittal 3D CT reconstruction image of the spinal canal. (**b**) MRI (*sagittal*)

Caution must be taken not to use standard 3.5-mm screw in the middle holes of the plate for graft fixation. The standard screws do not have anti-pullout function, while the 4-mm correction screws possess such function.

7. Correct preparation of the graft recipient area

Regions anterior and posterior to the intervertebral disc, including the anterior and posterior 1/3 of the endplate of the upper vertebral segment and half of the endplate of the lower vertebral segment, should be partially removed for preparation of the rectangular recipient bed. This avoids the creation of a slope, which is critical for Smith-Robison method. For corpectomy, the posterior portions of the upper and lower vertebral segments of the bone graft are not excised as long as the sides of the anterior bed are parallel, which helps prevent the bone block from slipping into the vertebral canal. The bone graft should be parallel to and tightly applied to the recipient bed, with no intervening gap between the two, which minimizes the risk of pseudoarthrosis and graft necrosis. In addition, the inferior border of the upper vertebral body and the superior border of the lower vertebral body should not be excised excessively, which impacts on the stability of implanted screws.

8. Securing bone graft or titanium mesh

The size and length of bone graft or titanium mesh should be based on the size of the bone groove in the appropriately distracted intervertebral body so that the graft or mesh is tightly applied to the bone groove and secured after implantation. If the contact of the bone graft and titanium mesh with the upper and lower vertebral body is not secured or the contact surface is too small, bone graft stability and quality of bone graft fusion may be jeopardized. The height of the graft should be 2–4 mm lower than the measured height of the groove so that there is an approximately 3-mm safety distance in the deep surface after implantation, which prevents compression against the dural sac. Meanwhile, graft length should be approximately 2 mm longer than the measured length of the bone groove so that when the distractor is released, the graft sits on the upper and lower vertebral endplates, forming a support and locking mechanism. This prevents anterior or posterior displacement of bone graft and promotes bony fusion (pressure bone healing). If the bone graft is higher than the cortex of adjacent vertebral segments, it readily produces shear force in the anterior cortical bone and partially in the adjacent cancellous bone. Arch-shaped bone grafting technique should be avoided as it easily leads to displacement and fracture of bone graft in the intervertebral space. Bone graft can only be safely secured after accurate measurement and thorough preparation of the recipient bed. Figure 5.34 shows loosening of the plate due to incorrect titanium mesh placement.

9. Use of the lock mechanism

The lock mechanism should be used to prevent postoperative screw breaking off, which may injure the esophagus. After plate placement, make sure that the plate and all lock

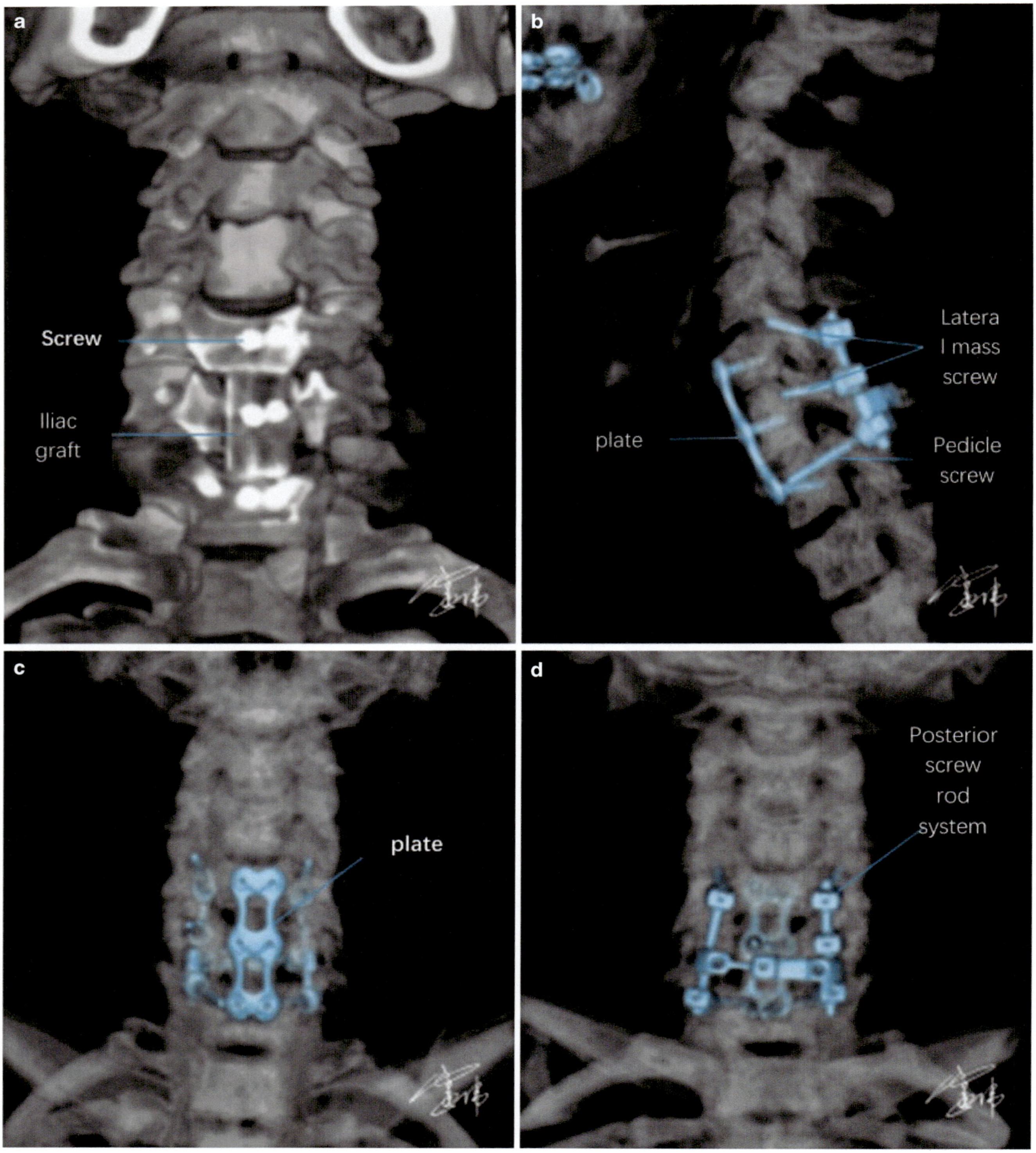

Fig. 5.30 Postoperative imaging study. (**a**) Three-dimensional CT reconstruction (*anterior view*) and (**b**) three-dimensional CT reconstruction (*lateral view*). (**c**) Three-dimensional CT reconstruction (*anterior view*) and (**d**) three-dimensional CT reconstruction (*posterior view*)

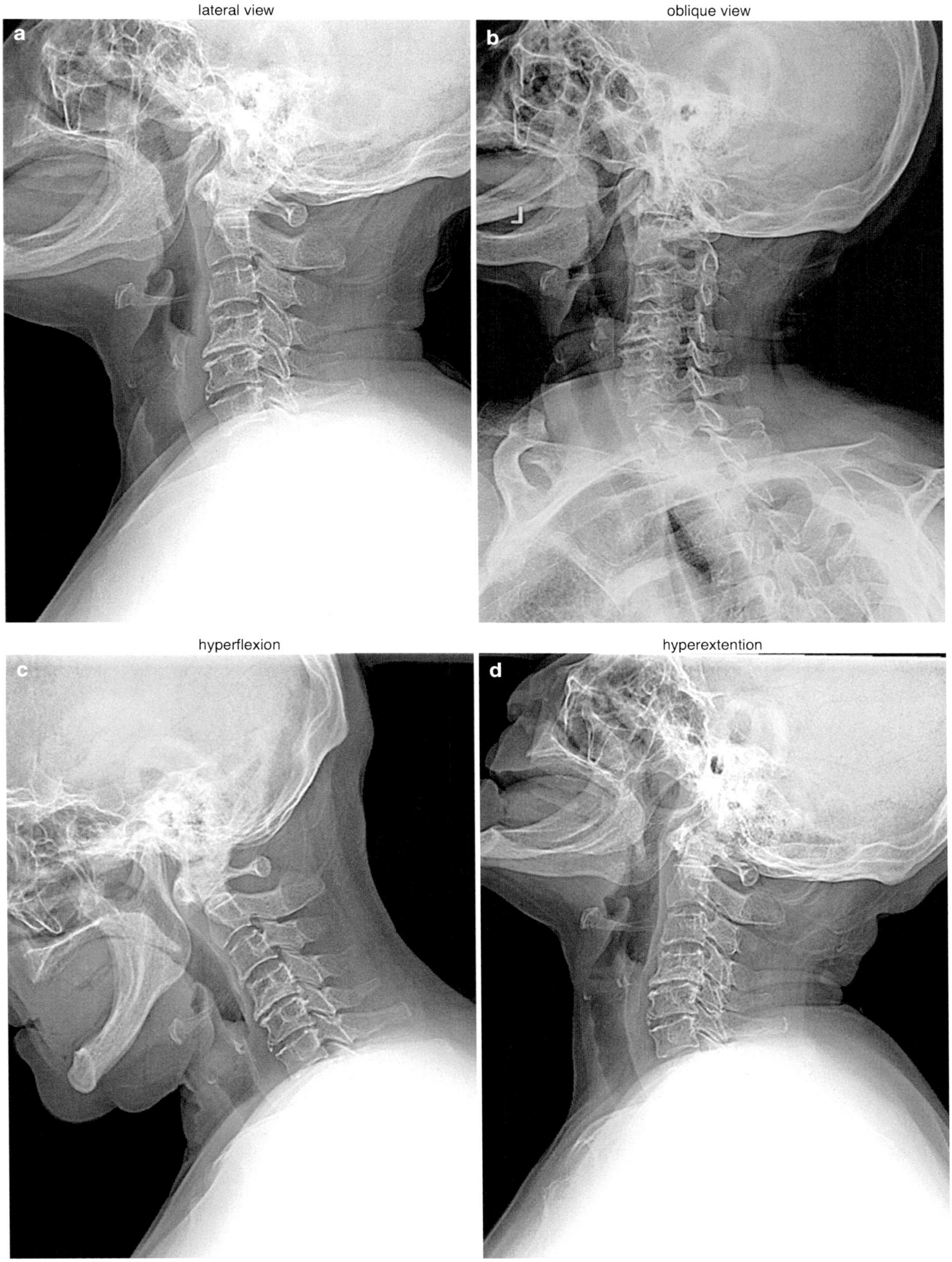

Fig. 5.31 Preoperative imaging. (**a**) Lateral view; (**b**) Oblique view. Preoperative radiograph

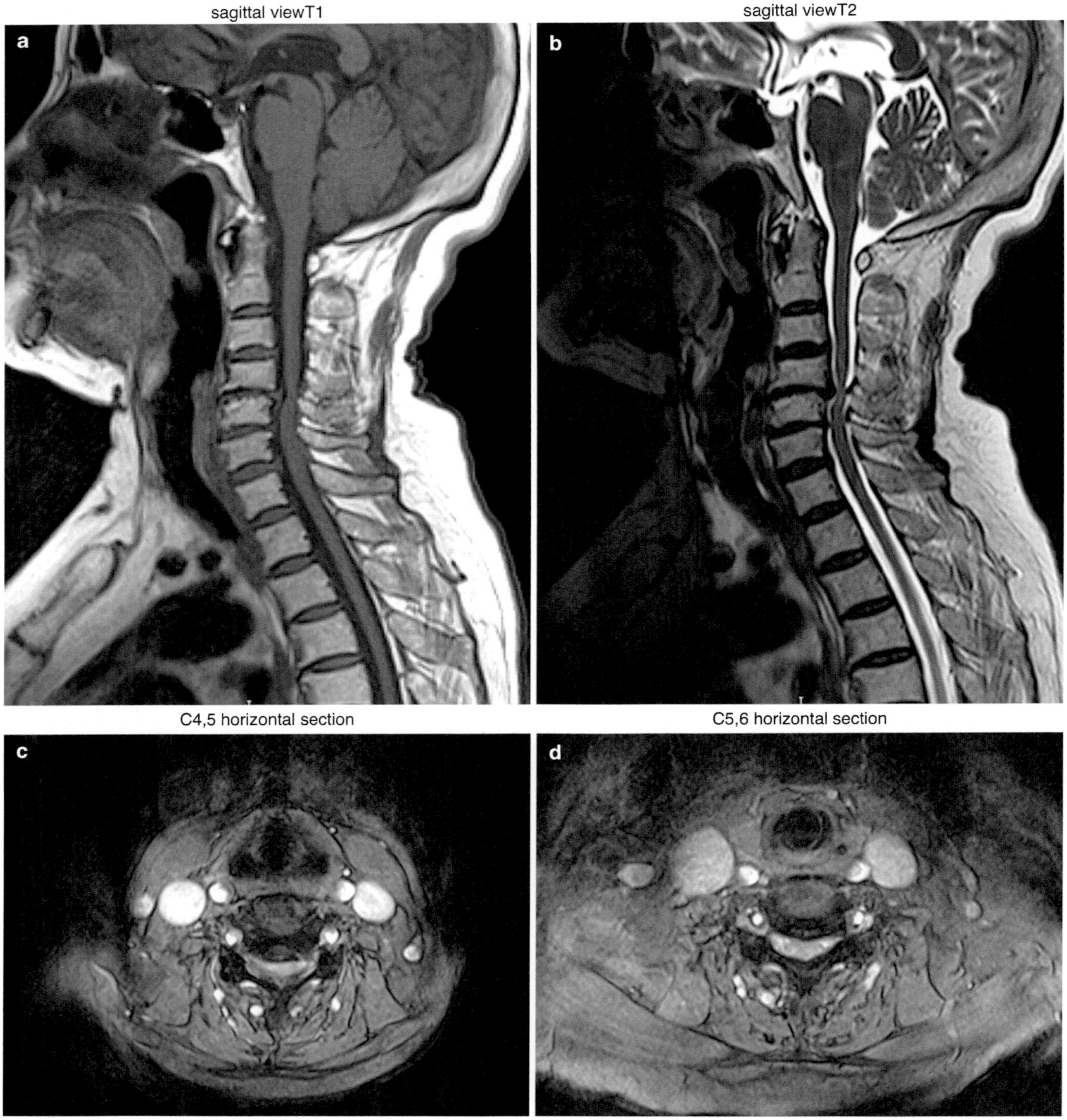

Fig. 5.32 Preoperative imaging study. (**a**) Sagittal view T1 MRI; (**b**) Sagittal view T2 MRI; (**c**) C4 and C5 horizontal section MRI; (**d**) C5 and C6 horizontal section MRI

screws within the plate must be fully engaged and tightened as confirmed by intraoperative fluoroscopy before the lock procedure is complete. Figure 5.35a and b shows that a screw breaks off because the screw is not fully tightened.

10. Selecting position of screw placement

Plate screws should not be affixed to diseased vertebrae. Severely osteoporotic patients should avoid anterior plate fixation alone because the interface between osteoporotic bone tissues and bone screws is unstable, which may lead to breaking off of both plate and screws.

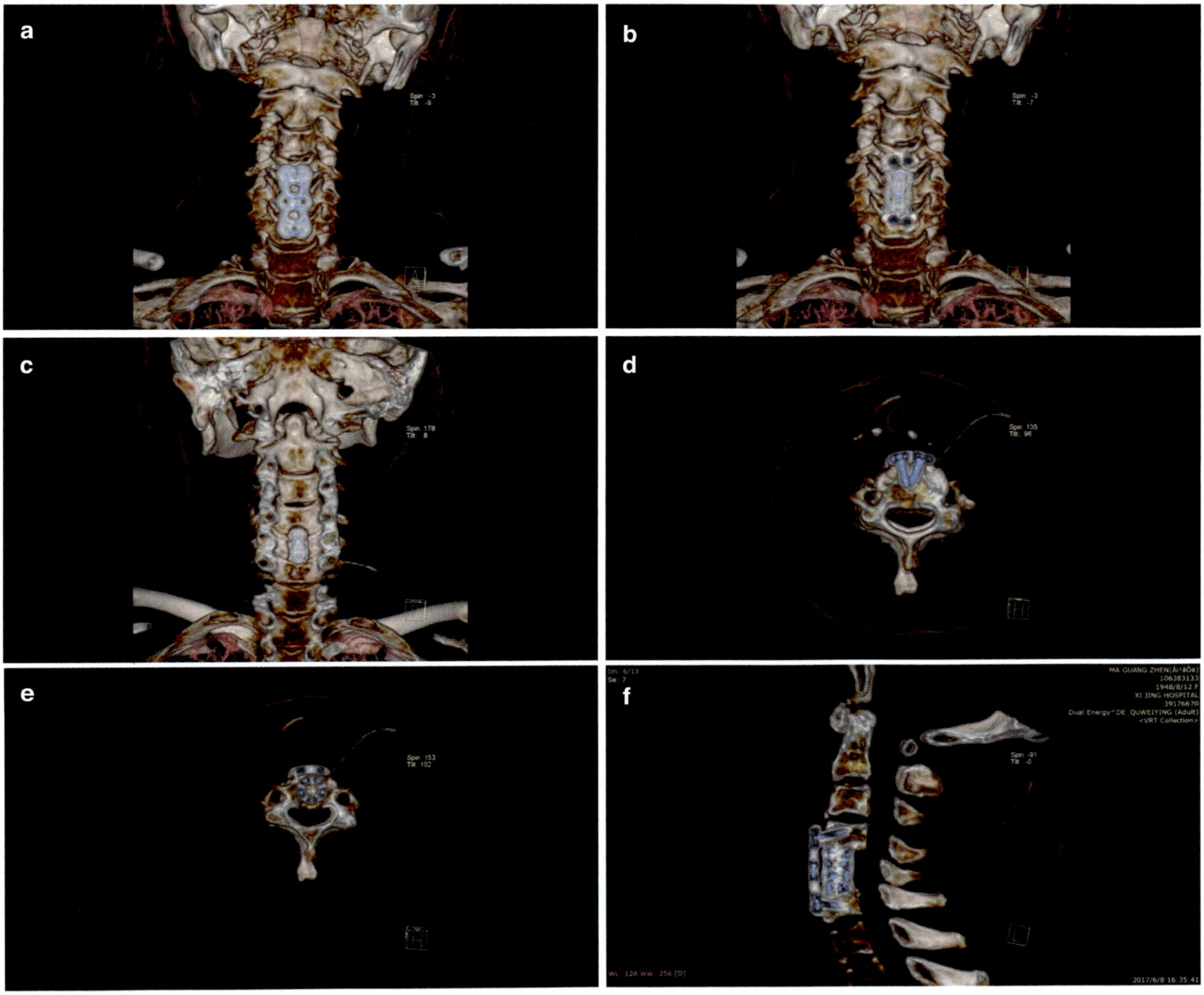

Fig. 5.33 Postoperative imaging study. (**a**, **b**, **c**, **d**, **e**, **f**, **g**) three-dimensional CT reconstruction

11 Causes of screw and plate loosening
   a. Drilling holes multiple times increases the diameter of screw holes, leading to reduced bone purchase.
   b. The selected screw is too short.
   c. Excessive force is used when the screw is inserted, destroying the interface between the screw and bone tissues.
   d. Erroneous screw placement includes inadequate screw implantation depth, implantation in the intervertebral space, or implantation in the gap between the bone graft and endplate. Figure 5.36 shows breaking-off of the titanium mesh and plate due to screw implantation in the gap between the titanium mesh and the endplates.
   e. The quality of bone in the screw fixation area is poor such as due to osteoporosis or diseased vertebral bodies.
   f. The plate is not tightly applied to the cortical bone and is not placed evenly, leading to uneven tension (e.g., osteophytes are not removed or inadequately removed from the bone surface).
   g. Improper use of the lock mechanism.
   h. Poor preparation of graft and titanium mesh or graft recipient bed leads to instability in the early phase and pseudoarthrosis later on.
   i. Inadequate postoperative activities.
   j. Infection.

12 Advantages of intraoperative fluoroscopy

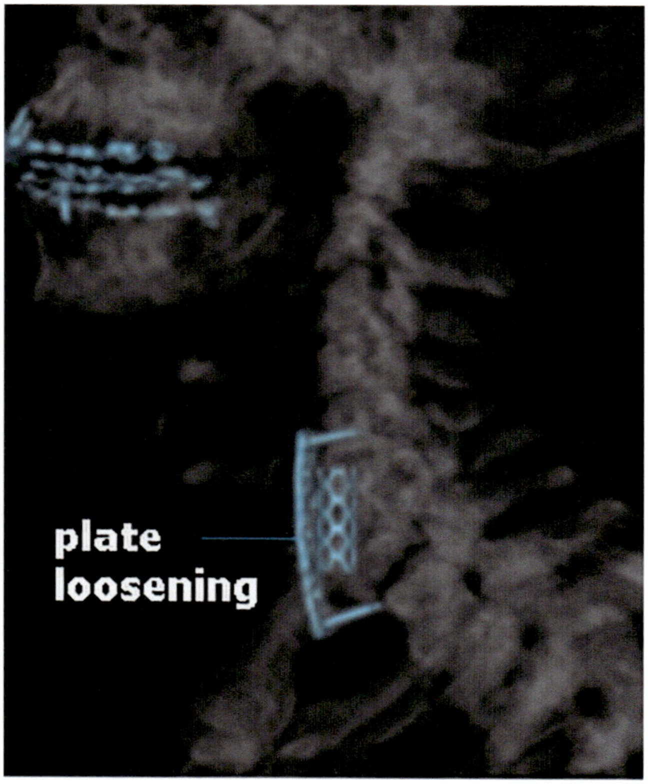

Fig. 5.34 Loosening of the plate due to incorrect titanium mesh placement

a. Accurate determination of location of the vertebral body and intervertebral space.
b. It offers better guidance for the circular drill to excise the degenerative intervertebral disc in parallel to the endplate.
c. It helps to achieve a more intimate contact between the bone graft and fusion device with the endplates.
d. It helps to achieve normal physiologic curvature of the cervical spine during reduction, bone grafting, and plate fixation.
e. It helps accurate screw implantation and prevention of screw implantation in the intervertebral space.
f. It helps plate placement in the center of the vertebral body.

13 Issues to consider by surgeons before surgery
  a. Is the cervical spine or fracture stable? Are there any risks in transport, change of body positions, or anesthesia of the patient?
  b. Is the anterior or the posterior approach or the combined approach optimal for decompression and restoration of spine stability?
  c. What is the range of decompression? How many segments should be fixed or fused?
  d. Which internal fixation equipment should a surgeon choose?

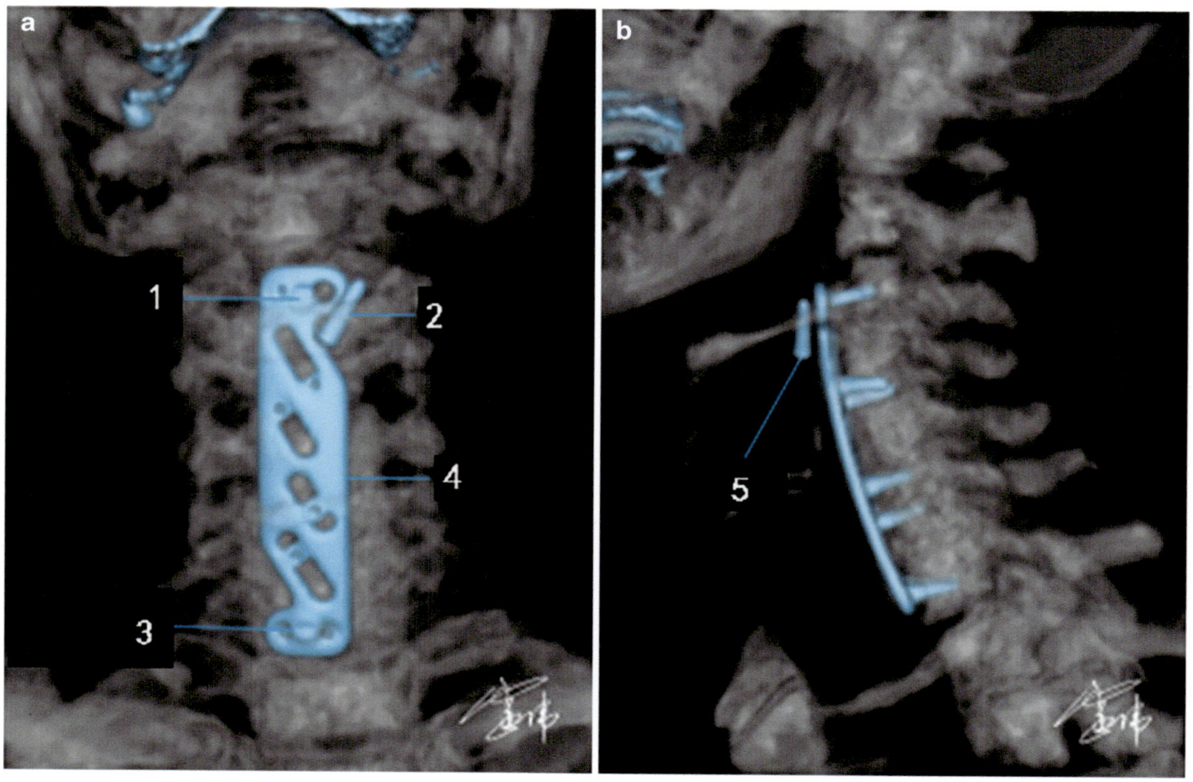

Fig. 5.35 Screw breaking-off. (**a**) Three-dimensional CT reconstruction (*anterior view*). (**b**) Three-dimensional CT reconstruction (*lateral view*). (*1*) Screw is not fully tightened before the lock mechanism is triggered. (*2*) Screw has broken off. (*3*) Properly tightened screw. (*4*) Plate. (*5*) Screw has broken off

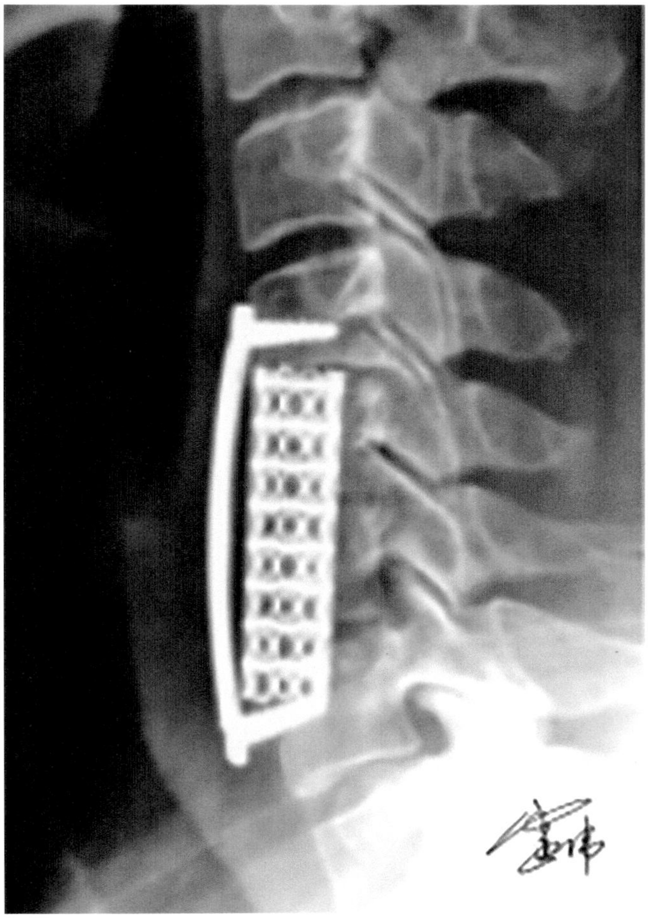

Fig. 5.36 Erroneous screw placement

e. Which type of anesthesia and which mode of spinal cord monitoring should a surgeon use (SSEP, wake-up test)?
f. What is to be used for intraoperative determination of screw and plate position (C arm or bedside fluoroscopy)?
g. What are the nursing and monitoring conditions post surgery?
h. Have the supplies for operation and orthosis post surgery been ordered?
i. Has the surgeon well communicated with the patient before surgery in a professional manner?

5.5 Postoperative Management

1. Temporary postoperative external fixation of the cervical spine

Neck brace is used for cervical external fixation. The support is worn for 1–3 months depending on the condition of the patient such as age, bone quality, type of injury and reliability of support, and quality of fusion. X-ray examination is done at 1 week, 3 months, and 6 months postoperatively to learn about the condition of plate fixation and bone fusion, and then the time to remove the neck brace is determined.

2. Postoperative activities

In general, the head of the bed can be adjusted to the 30° semi-recumbent position 6 h postoperatively, and the angle can be gradually increased to prepare the patient for ambulation. The patient can start ambulation 3 days postoperatively depending on the condition of the patient. During ambulation, the patient wears neck brace, which prevents excessive activities, especially for young patients. Neck brace is typically worn for 6–8 weeks. Longer use of neck brace can cause neck muscle degeneration and atrophy, leading to re-emergence of neck symptoms.

3. Fate of the plate

The plate can remain in the body for a long period of time, but can be removed after 1 year if required by the patient because bone fusion has been completed at that time. In fact, bone fusion has been achieved in 2–4 months in most patients. The quality of bone fusion and the integrity of bone graft are better in patients undergoing plate fixation than those simply receiving bone graft. The former approach provides solid fixation and promotes recovery of nerve roots and spinal cord injury by eliminating fine movements and stimulation.

The application of the anterior plate internal fixation system effectively reduces the incidence of postoperative complications, reduces patients' physical suffering and psychological disorders, and significantly improves the postoperative quality of life of patients.

References

1. Ebraheim NA, et al. The vertebral body depths of the cervical spine and its relation to anterior plate-screw fixation. Spine (Phila Pa 1976). 1998;23(21):2299–302.
2. Panjabi MM, et al. Cervical human vertebrae. Quantitative three-dimensional anatomy of the middle and lower regions. Spine (Phila Pa 1976). 1991;16(8):861–9.

Artificial Cervical Disc Techniques and Their Applications

6

Mingxuan Gao and Wei Lei

Abstract

Cervical disc replacement has undergone a dramatic evolution of prosthesis and techniques since the first device was invented and tested in the 1960s. This chapter presents the history of prosthesis development, anatomy of cervical intervertebral discs, and the standard surgical procedures of one currently developed device, including some successful and failed cases. According to some recent clinical trials, the early outcomes of such techniques are encouraging though its viability needs to be confirmed by more long-term studies.

Keywords

Artificial cervical disc · Cervical disc replacement · Cervical arthroplasty · Surgical techniques · Evolution of prosthesis

6.1 A Historical Review of Artificial Cervical Disc Techniques

The history of the development of artificial cervical disc techniques is marked by the ever improvement and renovation of prosthesis. The designs and technical features of representative prostheses are described below:

In 1966, Fernstrom invented artificial cervical intervertebral discs (Fig. 6.1) [1]. In 1991, Cummins invented the Bristol prosthesis [2], which was modified in 2002 and became the Frenchay prosthesis (Fig. 6.2) [3]. The prosthesis was renamed as the PRESTIGE prosthesis in 2007 and has been ever since widely used clinically (Figs. 6.3 and 6.4) [4]. Currently, the fifth-generation PRESTIGE LP artificial cervical disc is made of titanium alloy and ceramics, and the bone interface is applied with titanium plasma spray coating to promote bone ingrowth (Fig. 6.5). The ProDisc-C prosthesis by Synthes Spine was used clinically in 2007 (Fig. 6.6). In 2002, Bryan designed the Bryan prosthesis (Fig. 6.7) [5]. Other types of prostheses soon followed and were subsequently used widely, including Secure-C prosthesis by Globus Medical Co., PCM prosthesis by NuVasive, Mobi-C prosthesis by LDR Spine USA, and CerviCore prosthesis by Stryker Spine (Fig. 6.8).

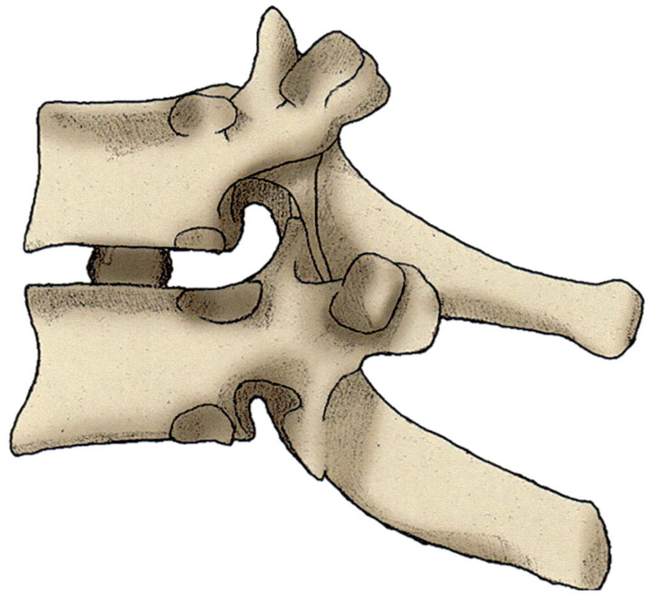

Fig. 6.1 Fernstrom technique: this implant is widely considered to be the first disc implant and has a simple ball bearing adapted from use in the cervical intervertebral discs

M. Gao · W. Lei (✉)
Department of Orthopedics, Xijing Hospital, Air Force Medical University, Xi'an, Shaanxi, China
e-mail: leiwei@fmmu.edu.cn

W. Lei, Y. Yan (eds.), *Internal Fixation of the Spine*, https://doi.org/10.1007/978-981-16-1562-7_6

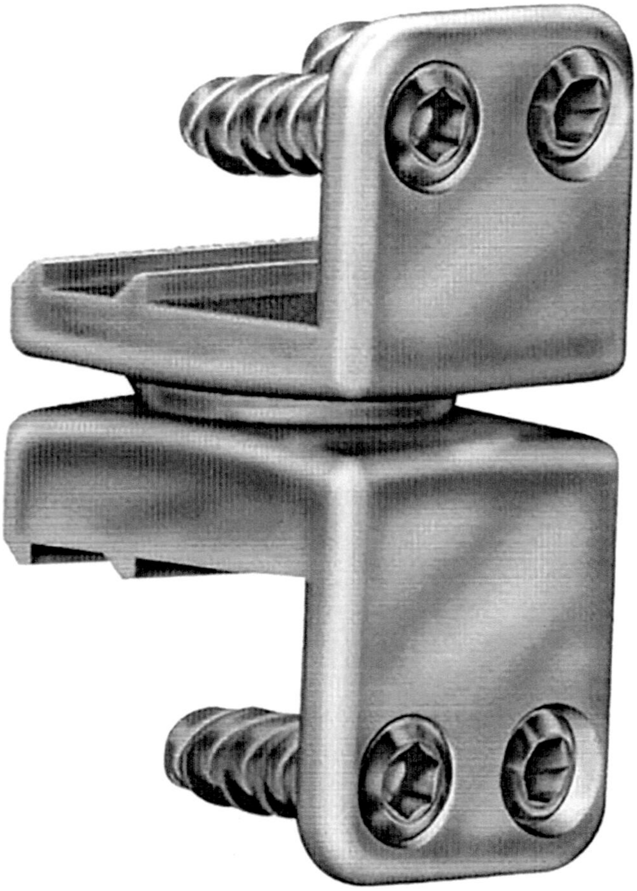

Fig. 6.2 The Cummins/Bristol prosthesis is considered the prototype of the PRESTIGE prosthesis

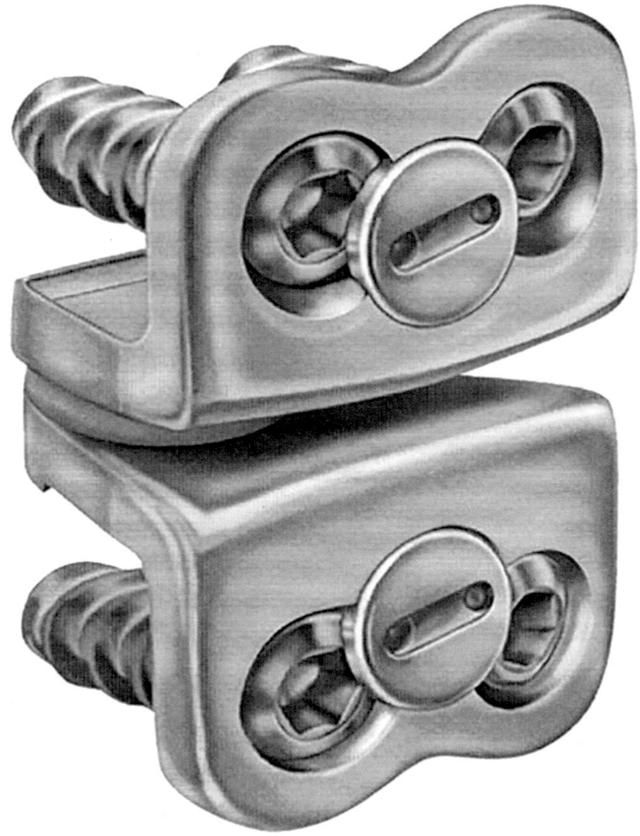

Fig. 6.3 The Frenchay prosthesis was subsequently renamed as the PRESTIGE prosthesis

6.2 Anatomy of Cervical Intervertebral Discs

The morphometric characteristics of human cervical spine are related to ethnicity, gender, age, and other factors. Mahto and Omar [6] measured the anteroposterior and transverse diameter as well as the height of 240 adult cervical vertebrae with 60 specimens for each vertebral segment from C3 to C6. They found that C6 has the largest and C3 has the smallest anteroposterior diameter (Fig. 6.9a). C5 has the largest and C3 has the smallest transverse diameter (Fig. 6.9b). In addition, C6 has the largest height, while C4 has the smallest height (Fig. 6.9c).

6.3 Artificial Cervical Intervertebral Disc Replacement Technique

6.3.1 Standard Location of Artificial Cervical Intervertebral Disc Replacement

1. Determination of the location of artificial cervical intervertebral disc replacement should take into consideration of the center of rotation and insertional torque.
2. The location of replacement should not disturb horizontal, coronal, and sagittal mechanical balance.
3. The posterior border of the prosthesis should be ideally parallel to the posterior border of the adjacent upper and lower vertebral bodies. The posterior cortical bone provides support for and prevents the prosthesis from caving in.

6.3.2 Preoperative Planning for Artificial Cervical Intervertebral Disc Replacement and Key Operative Techniques

1. The anteroposterior diameter and height of the intervertebral disc should be accurately determined before surgery so that the appropriately sized prosthesis is selected.
2. The surgical position of the patient should maintain the cervical curvature to be consistent with the cervical spine angle in the neutral position. Neck position should mirror the position in the preoperative standing neutral lateral X-rays.
3. The posterior border of the corresponding segment should be clearly visualized under fluoroscopy. Otherwise, replacement surgery should be converted to fusion surgery.

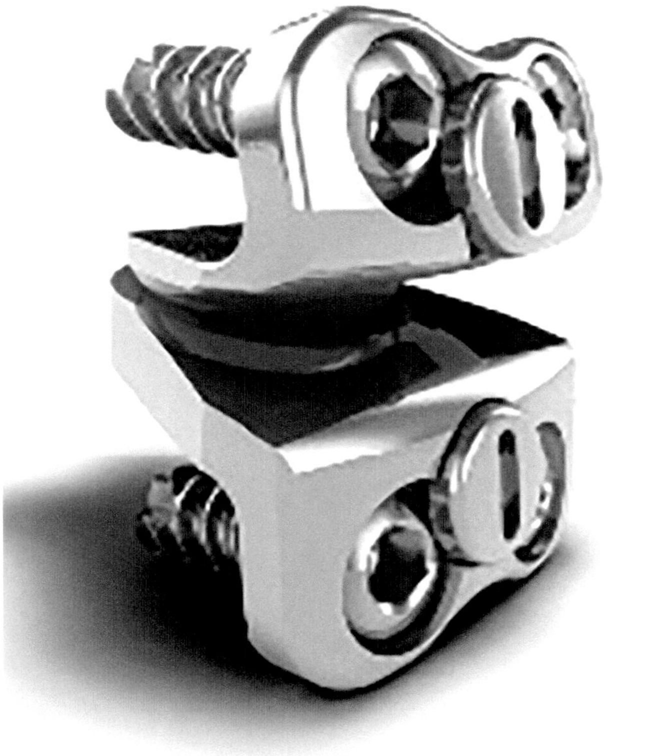

Fig. 6.4 PRESTIGE ST is the first artificial intervertebral disc prosthesis approved by the US FDA

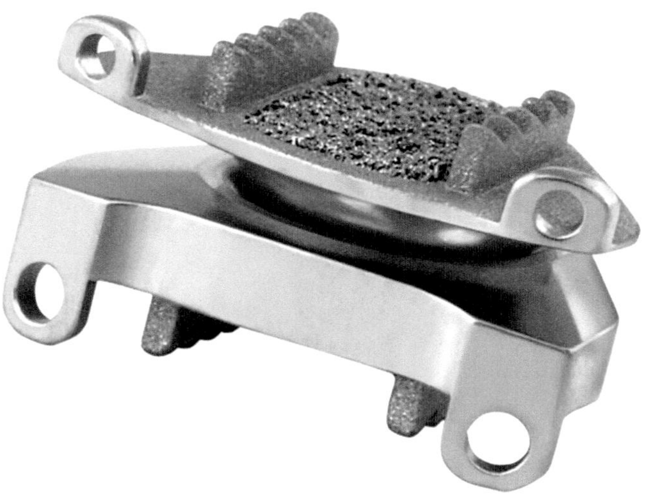

Fig. 6.5 Titanium alloy and ceramics are used in the fifth-generation PRESTIGE LP artificial cervical discs

4. Bilateral nerve root decompression should be undertaken even though only unilateral nerve root compression symptoms are present preoperatively.
5. The cortical bone should be preserved as much as possible when the upper and lower endplates are prepared.

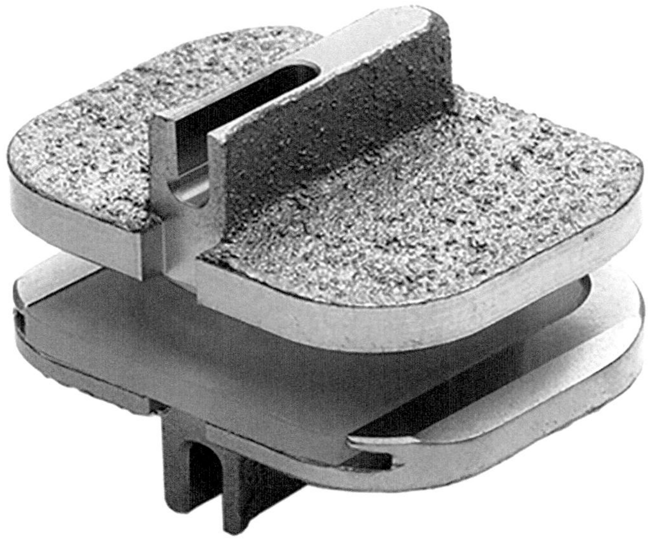

Fig. 6.6 ProDisc-C prosthesis

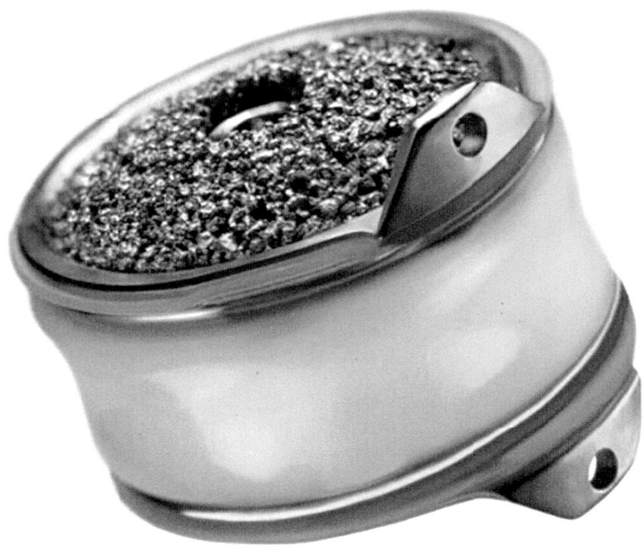

Fig. 6.7 Bryan prosthesis was approved by the US FDA in 2009

6. For preparation of rail for prosthesis, it is critical that the guide be centered on the midline of the vertebral bodies.
7. The appropriately sized prosthesis should be selected, and the posterior border of the prosthesis should reach the posterior cortical bone of the vertebral body as much as possible.

6.4 Personalized Surgical Plan

A personalized surgical plan for artificial cervical intervertebral disc replacement or artificial cervical intervertebral disc replacement in combination with cervical spine fusion

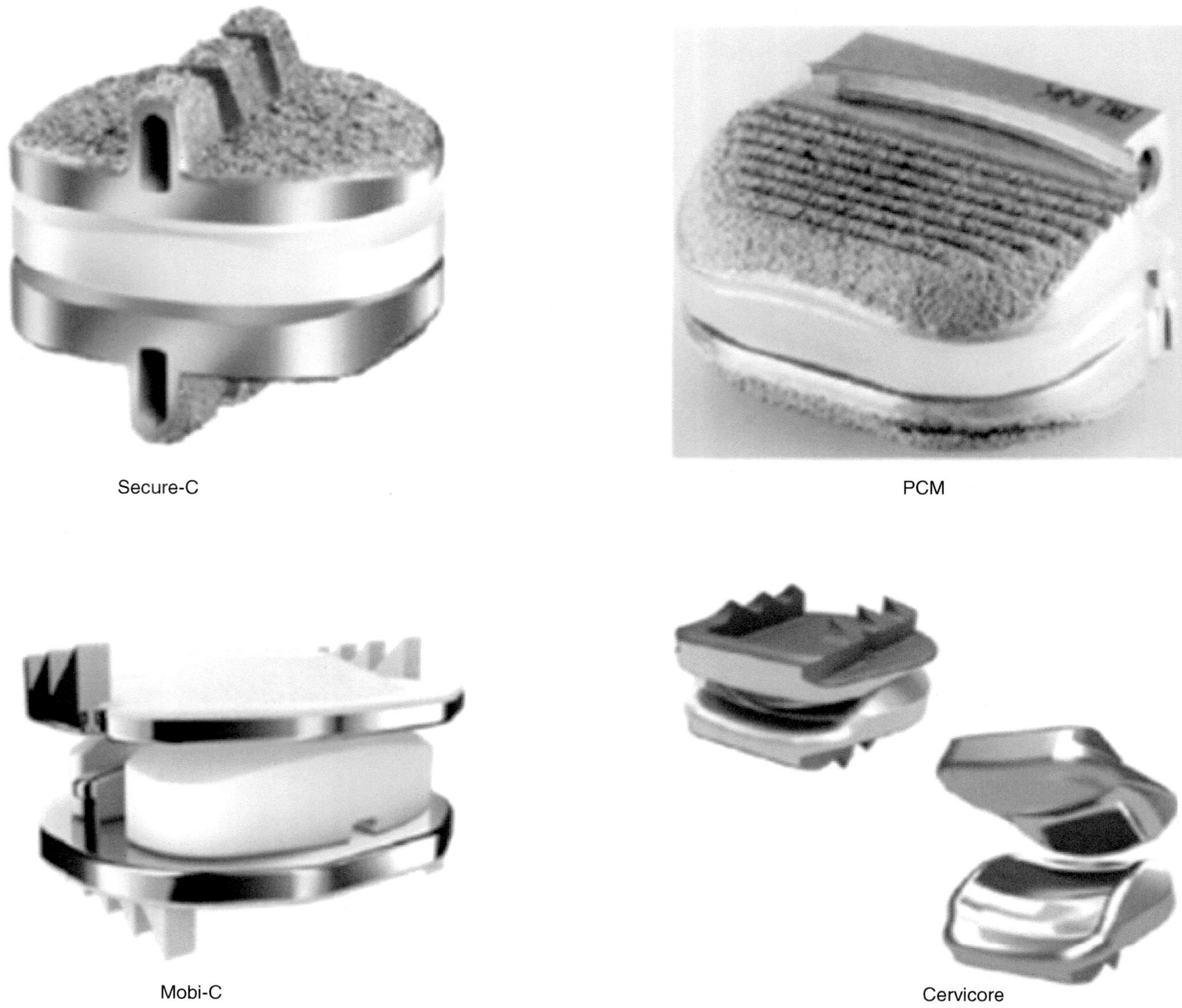

Fig. 6.8 Secure-C prosthesis, PCM prosthesis, Mobi-C prosthesis, and CerviCore prosthesis

surgery at one level, multilevel contiguous, or noncontiguous may be designed based on individual patient characteristics.

6.4.1 Surgical Indications and Contraindications

6.4.1.1 Indications

Artificial cervical intervertebral disc replacement is generally indicated for intervertebral disc replacement at any level from C3 to C7 in adults aged above 21 years. It is suitable for use at a single intervertebral disc space or two adjacent intervertebral disc spaces.

1. Prolapse cervical intervertebral disc
2. Cervical myelopathy or cervical spondylotic radiculopathy

6.4.1.2 Contraindications

1. A history of previous cervical spine surgery
2. Active infection
3. Metabolic bone disease such as osteoporosis
4. Cervical spine instability or articulate process disorder

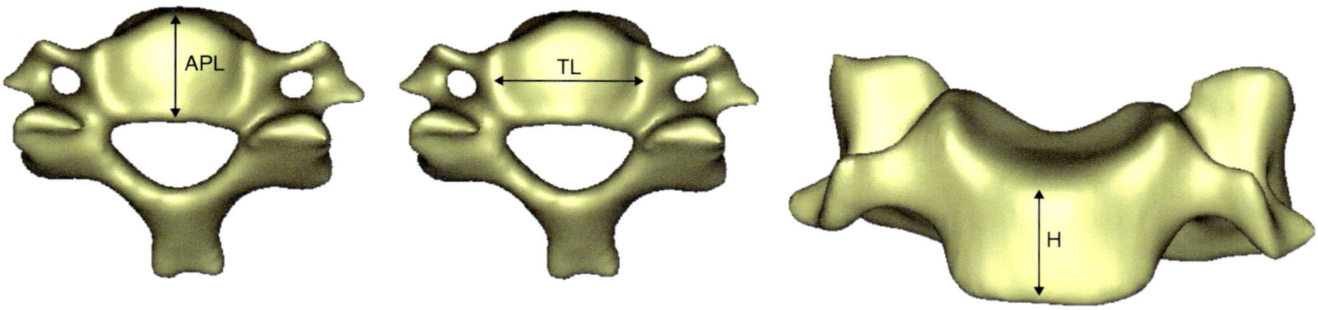

Fig. 6.9 (a) Measuring the anteroposterior length (APL), (b) the transverse length (TL), and (c) the height of the cervical vertebral body (H). The APL ranged from 13.6 ± 0.18 to 15.8 ± 0.19 mm in the lower cervical spine. The TL ranged from 22.8 ± 0.21 to 25.2 ± 0.23 mm. The height of the vertebral in the lower cervical spine ranged from 8.9 ± 0.11 to 11.3 ± 0.16 mm

5. Loss of mobility of the target cervical intervertebral disc or occurrence of vertebral body fusion

6.5 Surgical Steps

The surgical steps differ by types of prostheses. The following descriptions use the PRESTIGE prosthesis as an illustrative example.

6.5.1 Preoperative Measurement

Magnetic resonance imaging (MRI) or preferably CT scan should be performed before surgery. The slices are parallel to the vertebral body endplates, and the smaller endplate in the adjacent upper and lower vertebral bodies at the target disc space is selected. Spurs or ridges are not included in determining endplate size as they will be removed in subsequent burring/decompression process. The magnification factor of the image is determined using the PRESTIGE LP cervical disc template set (Fig. 6.10a), the prosthesis template corresponding to the measured magnification factor is chosen, and the prosthesis size is selected based on the instructions on the template (Fig. 6.10b). This process determines the appropriate footprint, but not the height, of the implant (Fig. 6.10c, d).

Cautionary notes: Templating provides only approximate sizing. This initial assessment may vary because of magnification factors inherent in CT or MRI images. The final selection of the implant size should be based on clinical judgment, disc space preparation, and trialing.

6.5.2 Patient Positioning

With the head and neck in the neutral position, the patient is placed in the supine position (Fig. 6.11). The posterior cervical spine should be supported to establish and maintain this position. A standard right- or left-sided approach may be adopted. Neck position should mirror that in the preoperative standing neutral lateral X-rays and remain fixed throughout the procedure. Failure to reproduce preoperative neutral neck position may lead to improper implant position or improper sagittal balance of the cervical spine at the operative level. For better visualization of the lower cervical spine during fluoroscopy, both shoulders may be pulled down and secured if necessary. A fusion procedure will be required if visualization of the target disc space does not allow for an optimal lateral view.

6.5.3 Exposure

A transverse skin incision is typically made. An avascular dissection plane is developed between the trachea and the esophagus medially, and the carotid sheath laterally. To provide exposure of the anterior vertebral column and the adjacent longus colli muscles, handheld retractors are utilized (Fig. 6.12)

Cautionary notes: The presence of anatomical abnormalities and/or deformities may reduce the ability to ensure proper placement of the instrumentation and/or prosthesis. Under such circumstances, a fusion procedure is recommended (Fig. 6.12).

6.5.4 Decompression

Discectomy is performed at the target disc space level. Pituitaries, curettes, and kerrisons may be used to remove disc and cartilage and to expose the posterior longitudinal ligament. A vertebral body or halter distractor may be used for a complete and thorough decompression. Vertebral body distraction pins are positioned midline in the vertebral bodies adjacent to the discectomy. The distractor is placed over the pins and the appropriate amount of distraction needs to be applied. To remove the posterior disc and osteophytes, a

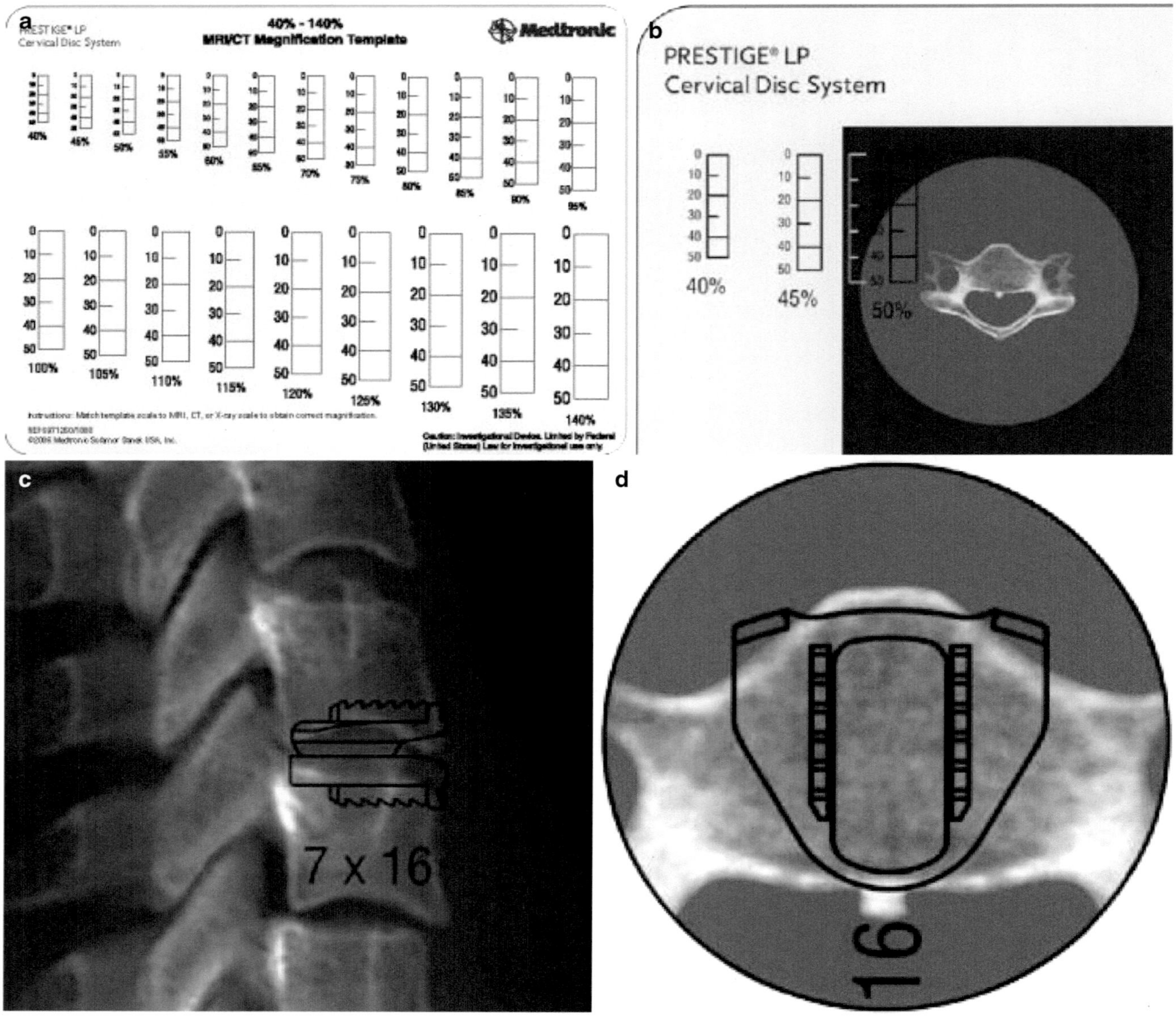

Fig. 6.10 Preoperative measurement. (**a**) Magnification template. (**b**) Template magnification factor. (**c**) Comparing implant. (**d**) Determining implant size

high-speed drill with a burr (match tip/round) may be utilized. If necessary, the posterior longitudinal ligament is carefully removed. Osteocytes on the anterior surface of the vertebral bodies are also removed to create a flat surface. Excessive anterior bone removal should be avoided (Fig. 6.13).

6.5.5 Endplate Preparation

After completion of discectomy and decompression, the exterior distraction devices are relaxed and removed. The endplates are prepared using a burr and rendered flat and parallel to the upper and lower endplates (Fig. 6.14a). The cortical bone should be preserved as much as possible. It is also important to complete endplate preparation of the posterior aspects of the vertebral bodies to ensure maximum implant/endplate interface (Fig. 6.14b). After removal of the distractor, the vertebral body height may be lost. When this occurs, a shim distractor may be used to facilitate surgery (Fig. 6.14c).

The appropriately sized rasp is selected to maximize contact surface for the endplate. This step can also be completed in conjunction with a burr so that the positive stop in the rasp is positioned superiorly. The rasp can be moved up and down in the disc space, with slight medial/lateral rocking (Fig. 6.15a). Rasping helps remove any protrusions remaining after parallel burring. The size dimensions of the rasp

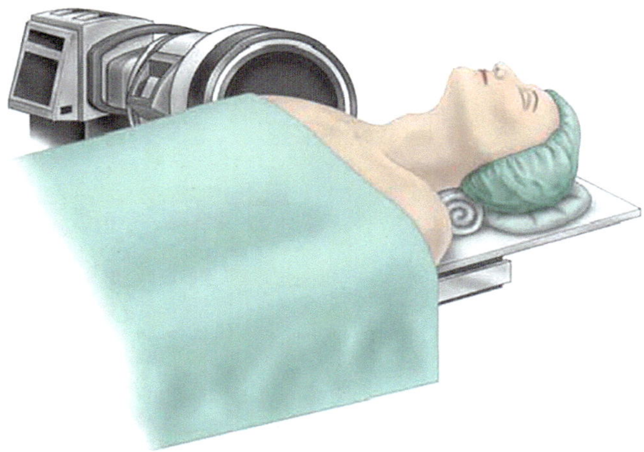

Fig. 6.11 Patient position

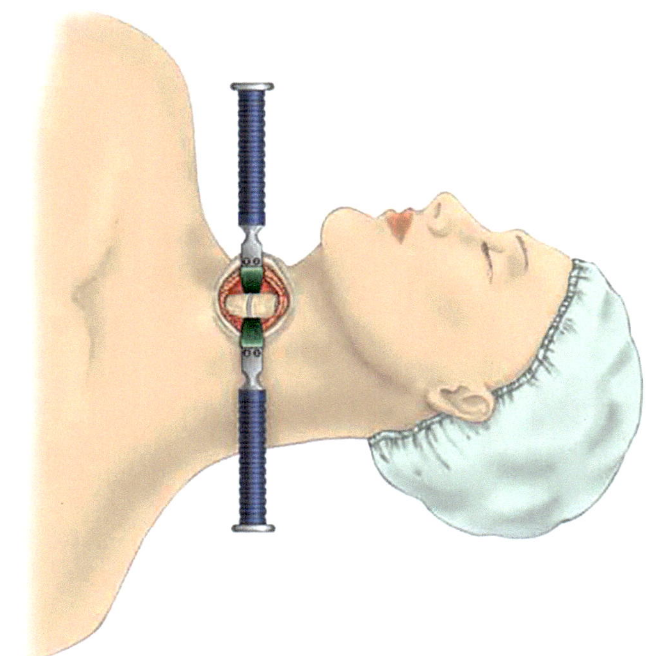

Fig. 6.12 Exposure

head should precisely match the endplate interfacing dimensions of the implant, ensuring adequate endplate preparation. The handle extension can be used to remove the rasp if necessary (Fig. 6.15b).

6.5.6 Selection of Appropriate Implant Sizes

Once the endplates are prepared in a flat, parallel fashion, the appropriately sized implant trial is used to confirm the size of the prepared disc space. The size dimensions of the implant trial head should also precisely match the endplate interfacing dimensions of the implant. The implant trial, which measures disc space height, depth, and width, should fit snugly without distracting the disc space. If more than gentle tapping is required to insert the implant trial into the disc space, a smaller implant trial should be considered, or additional endplate preparation should be done. Selection of the size of the implant trial can be assisted with fluoroscopy. The four anterior tabs in the implant trial match the anterior tabs of the prosthesis. The anterior vertebral body surfaces are double-checked to ensure that no protruding bone interferes with the placement of the implant trial tabs flush with the anterior surface.

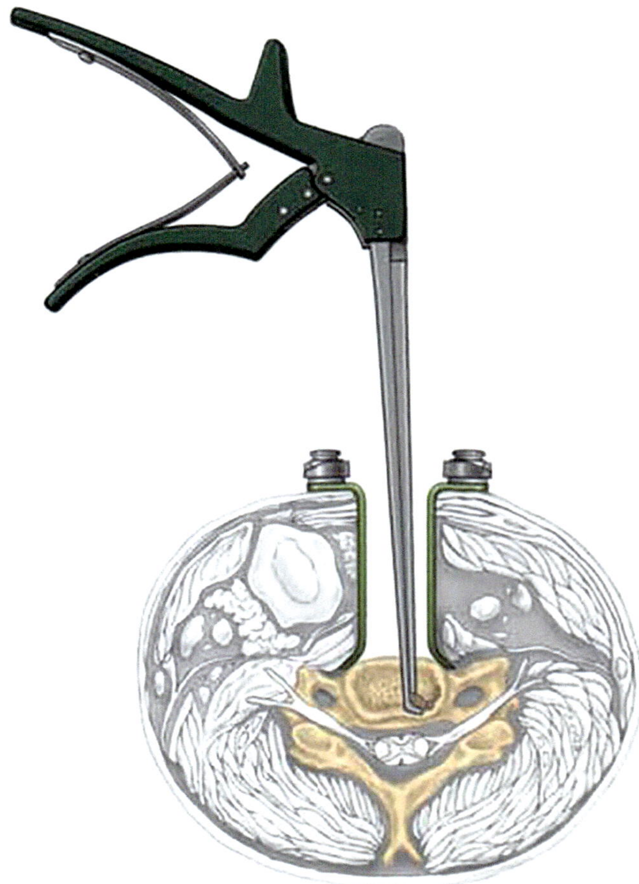

Fig. 6.13 Decompression. A complete and thorough discectomy and bilateral decompression are essential

*Cautionary notes: It is important that the prepared endplates be in complete contact with the flat portions of the implant trial and that the posterior tip of the implant trial reaches the posterior aspects of the disc space (*Fig. 6.16*).*

6.5.7 Rail Preparation

Once the appropriate implant size is determined, the corresponding guide may be selected to prepare the implant fixation channels in the endplates. The guide is gently impacted

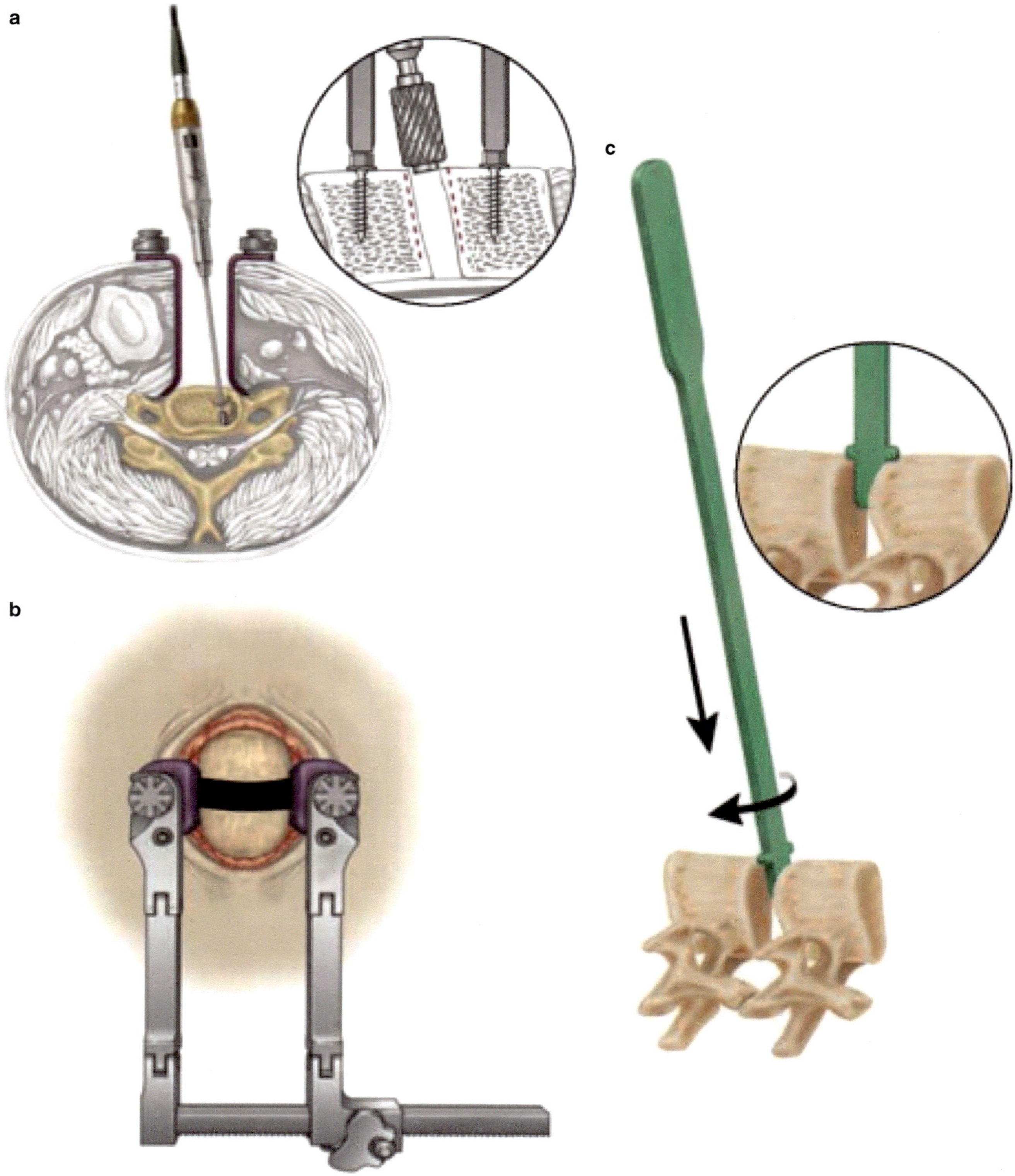

Fig. 6.14 Endplate preparation. (*a*) The endplate is rendered parallel to the adjacent upper and lower endplates. (*b*) The inferior aspect of the endplate is processed. (*c*) A shim distractor is used

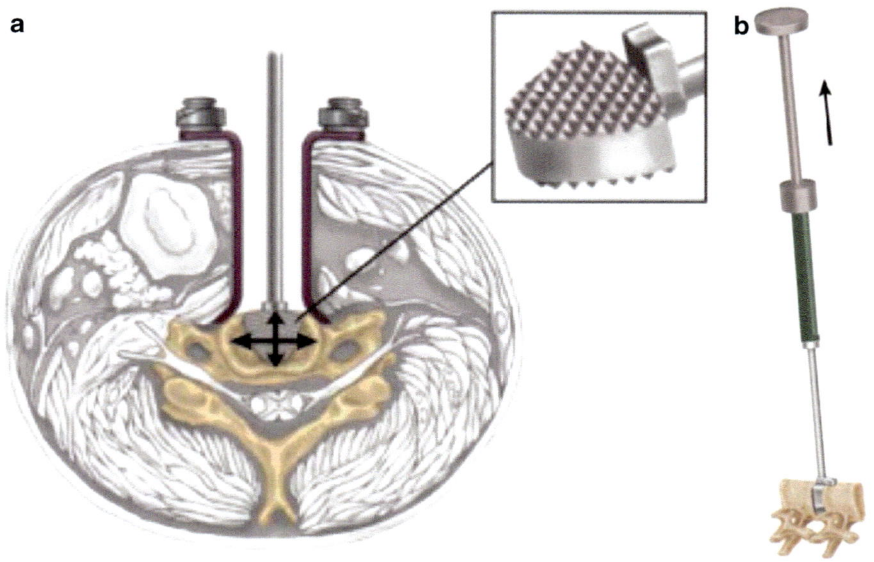

Fig. 6.15 Endplate preparation. (*a*) Direction of rasp movement. (*b*) Removing the rasp

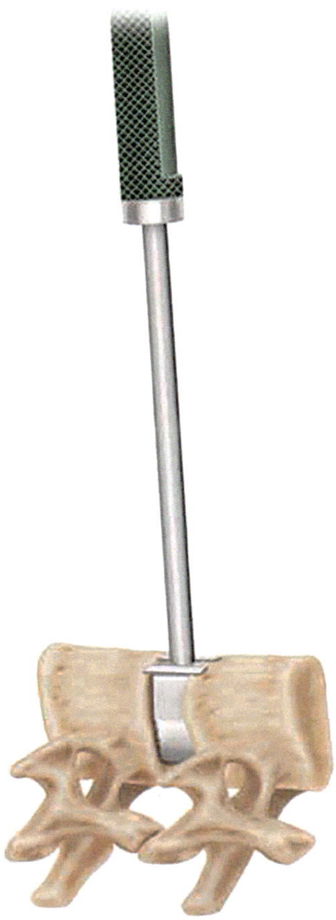

Fig. 6.16 Position of the implant trial

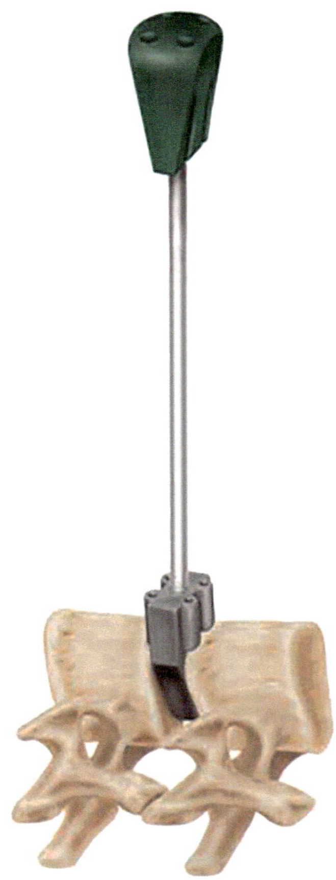

Fig. 6.17 Position of the guide

into the prepared disc space. It is critical that the guide be centered on the midline of the vertebral bodies.

*Cautionary note: The four drill guide ports on the head of the guide should touch the anterior surface of the spine (*Fig. 6.17*).*

After the bit is attached to the handle, it is inserted into one port on the guide. The first fixation channel is drilled in the endplate. While the guide is held firmly in place, the bit is removed, and a temporary fixation pin is placed in the channel. A second channel is drilled in the contralateral port

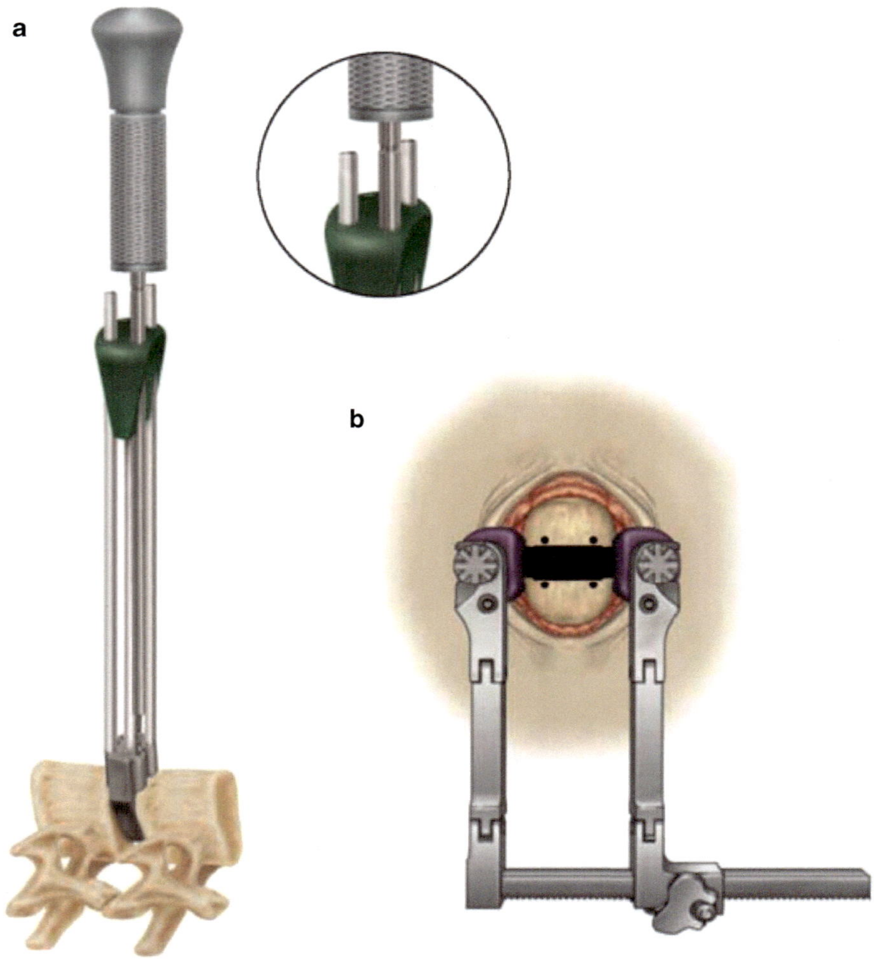

Fig. 6.18 Rail preparation. (*a*) A rail is prepared. (*b*) The rail is completed

and another fixation pin is placed. Similarly, the third and fourth channel is drilled (Fig. 6.18a). Then, the fixation pins and the guide are removed. Each properly prepared endplate should have two parallel channels as shown in Fig. 6.18b. If this is not the case, the endplates are double-checked to see if they are properly paralleled, and if not, this step should be repeated.

6.5.8 Rail Cutting

The four cutting blades of the rail punch are aligned into the four pilot holes made by the guide (Fig. 6.19a), and the rail punch is gently tapped into the disc space until depth stops contact the anterior surface of the spine (Fig. 6.19b). The handle extension may be used to remove the rail punch (Fig. 6.19c). This should complete the preparation of the four channels into the endplates (Fig. 6.19d).

6.5.9 Implantation

The appropriately sized implant is placed in the corresponding slot of the loading block (Fig. 6.20a). The four inserter prongs are placed into the ports on the anterior disc tabs (Fig. 6.20b). Then, the outer sheath is advanced toward the disc and rotated clockwise to lock in position (Fig. 6.20c).

Cautionary note: The ball portion of the implant should be superior.

The ball portion of the prosthesis is positioned superiorly, and the PRESTIGE LP disc rails are aligned with the channels on the endplates and inserted into the prepared disc space. The prosthesis is gently tapped into place with a mallet until the anterior tabs come into contact with the anterior surface of the vertebral bodies by exerting gentle pressure in a direction perpendicular to the anterior surface of the device to avoid the possibility of breaking an anterior disc tab. It is acceptable that a slight gap may remain between the tabs and

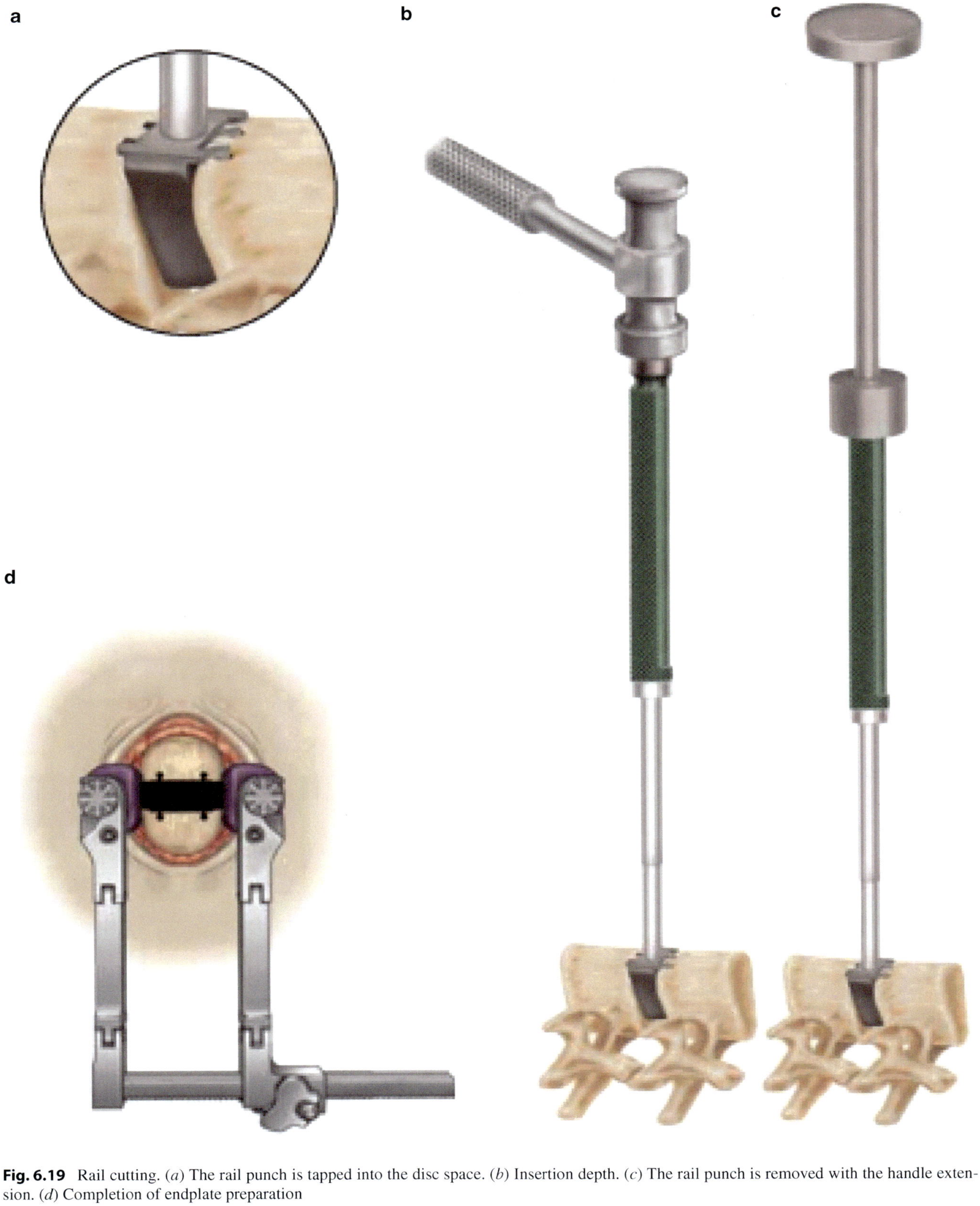

Fig. 6.19 Rail cutting. (*a*) The rail punch is tapped into the disc space. (*b*) Insertion depth. (*c*) The rail punch is removed with the handle extension. (*d*) Completion of endplate preparation

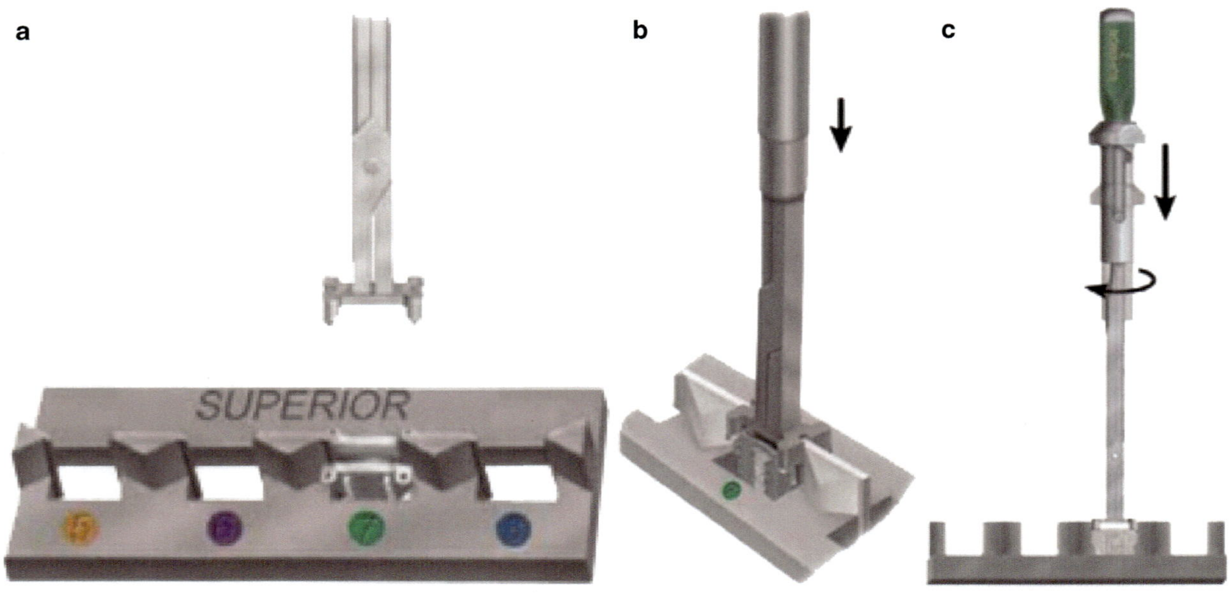

Fig. 6.20 Inserting the prosthesis. (*a*) The prosthesis is placed. (*b*) The rail punch is inserted. (*c*) The prosthesis is locked into place

the anterior surface on either the inferior or superior body if the anterior surfaces are not exactly level. The prosthesis is released by rotating the sheath counterclockwise (Fig. 6.21a) and the outer sheath is slid back, and the inserter is gently removed (Fig. 6.21b).

Cautionary notes: If necessary, the final impactor may be used to fully seat the implant by aligning it with the anterior aspects of the implant and gently tapping with a mallet (Fig. 6.21c).

6.5.10 Placement Verification

Following implantation, lateral and anteroposterior radiographs should be taken to verify proper placement (Fig. 6.22).

Cautionary notes: If explantation of the implant is required, separation of the implant from the endplate can be achieved by utilizing standard surgical instruments.

If removal is required after the implant has bonded with the endplates, a small osteotome may be used, along with an angled curette and forceps to separate the fixation surface from the bone.

6.5.11 Bi-level Implantation

For treatment of multilevel cervical diseases with the PRESTIGE prosthesis, the bi-level surgical technique can be used for implantation at two adjacent levels. The bi-level implantation procedure can follow the initial steps of the single-level surgical technique for PRESTIGE prosthesis implantation (Fig. 6.23). The following should be considered during your preoperative planning:

1. The two affected disc spaces should be adequately exposed.
2. When the first implant is placed, special attention should be paid to achieve normal sagittal balance and select appropriate implant height by using the implant trials.

The baseline of the intervertebral disc space is determined assisted by the use of a protractor and a level measuring device. The sagittal wedge locator and bi-rail punch guide are placed, and examination is undertaken by fluoroscopy to verify whether they are in intimate contact with the anterior border of the superior and inferior vertebral bodies.

6.6 Standard Imaging Features

The postoperative imaging features of ideal PRESTIGE artificial cervical disc replacement surgery include the following:

1. The prosthesis is centered on the midline of the vertebral bodies and appropriately sized.
2. The opening is appropriate, and mobility is normal.
3. The prosthesis is parallel to the intervertebral disc space, and the physiologic curvature of the cervical spine is maintained.

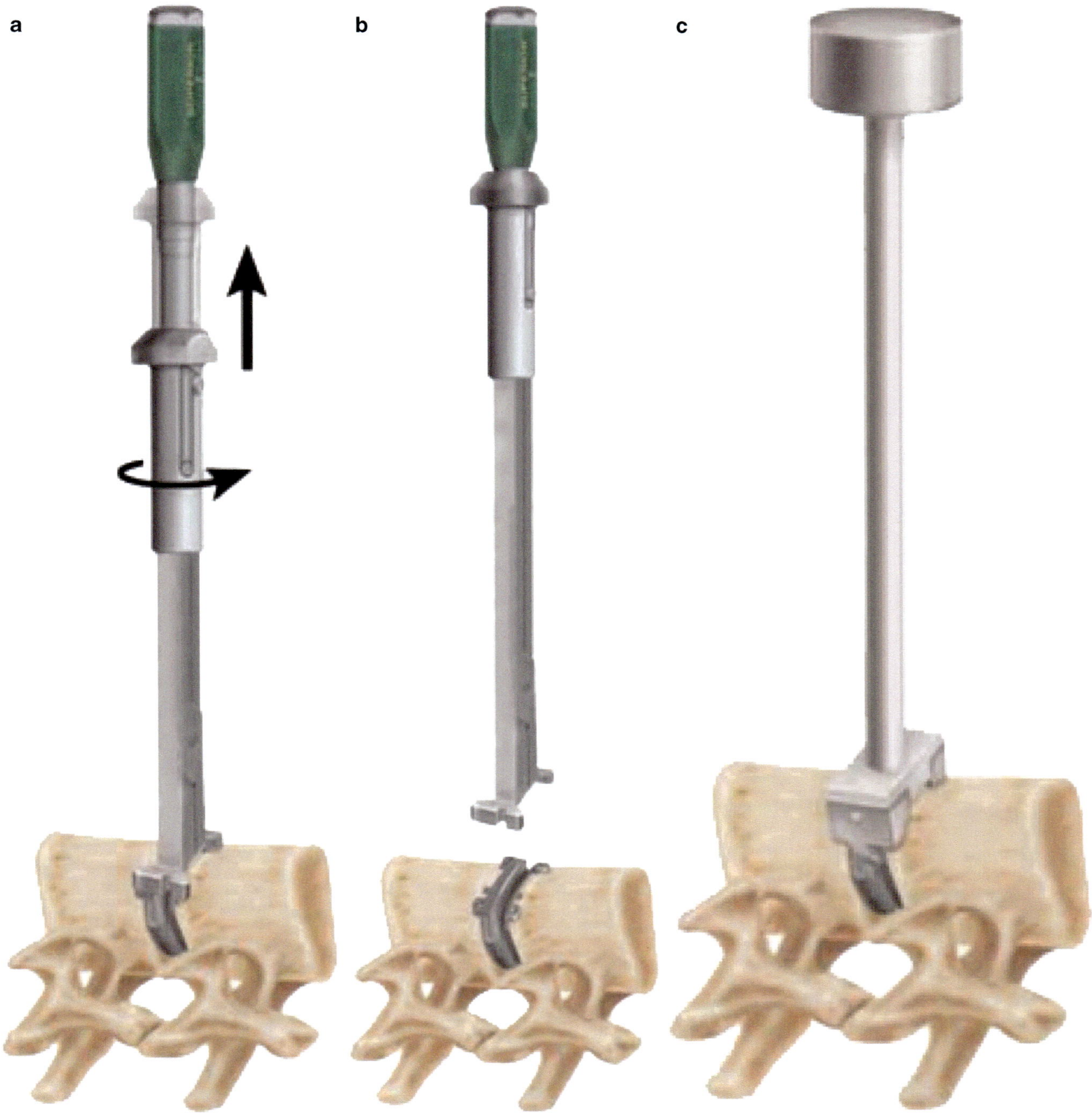

Fig. 6.21 Implanting the prosthesis. (*a*) Loosening the prosthesis. (*b*) Removing the rail punch. (*c*) Tapping the prosthesis into place

6.7 Clinical Cases

Case 1

Patient: A 47-year-old woman with neck pain and numbness of the right hand for 1 year

Diagnosis: Cervical disease (radiculopathy).

Surgery: C4–C5 PRESTIGE artificial cervical disc replacement.

Imaging data: Figure 6.24 shows preoperative findings. Figure 6.25 shows radiological findings at postoperative day 3, and Fig. 6.26 shows radiological findings 1 month post the operation.

Case 2

Patient: A 48-year-old woman with neck pain and numbness and pain of the right hand for 1 year.

Diagnosis: Cervical disease (myelopathy).

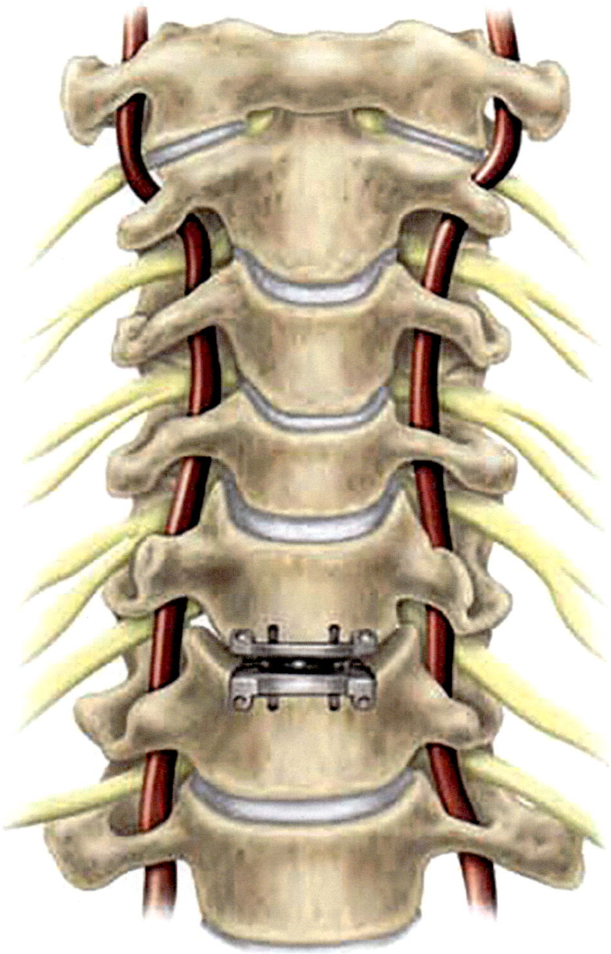

Fig. 6.22 Placement verification

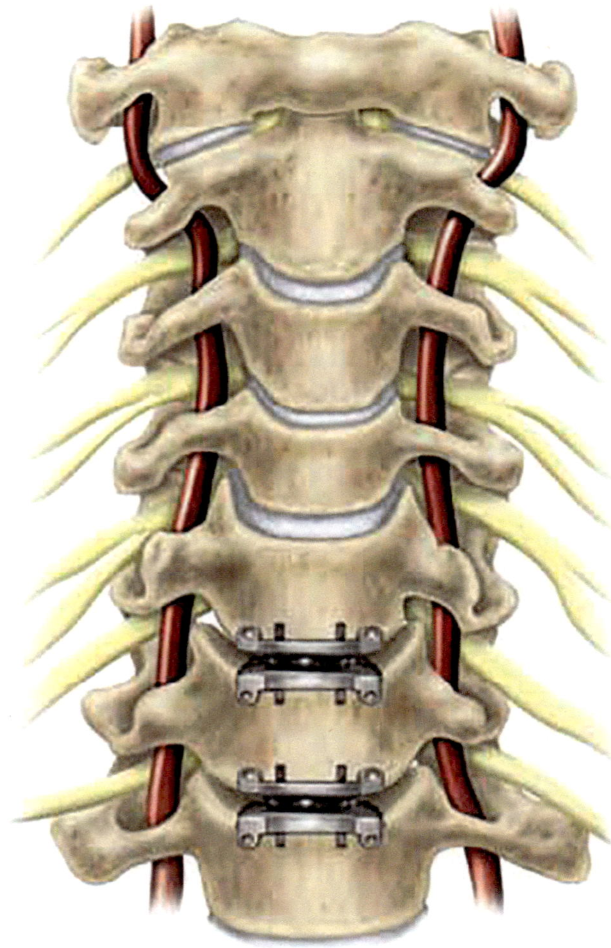

Fig. 6.23 Bi-level implantation

Surgery: C4–C5 and C5–C6 PRESTIGE artificial cervical disc replacement.

Imaging data: Figure 6.27 shows preoperative radiological findings. Figure 6.28 shows postoperative radiological findings.

6.8 Pearls and Pitfalls

6.8.1 The Imaging Features of Undesirable PRESTIGE Artificial Disc Replacement

1. Poor dilation of the disc space.

With excessive excision of the posterior edge of the vertebral body or inadequate excision of the anterior edge of the vertebral body, the upper and lower endplates of the intervertebral space are not in a parallel fashion with each other, causing cervical kyphosis and poor dilation of the disc space (Fig. 6.29, C5–C6 artificial disc replacement).

The posterior edge of the superior and inferior vertebral body shows severe hyperplasia. When the posterior edge of the vertebral body is excised for the purpose of intraoperative decompression, it may easily lead to cervical kyphosis with poor dilation of the disc space (Fig. 6.30, C5–C6 artificial disc replacement). In this scenario, interbody fusion surgery is recommended.

2. Loss of balance because the implant is not centrally positioned (Fig. 6.31).
3. The size of the implant is too large or too small (Fig. 6.32).

Comparison of the PRESTIGE and BRYAN artificial disc systems:

1. The PRESTIGE system is easier to use but has poorer bioconic properties than the BRYAN system.
2. The PRESTIGE system requires that the surgeons be more clinically experienced, but the system has poorer objectivity and precision.
3. The PRESTIGE system is more prone to regional cervical kyphosis or poor dilation of the disc space.

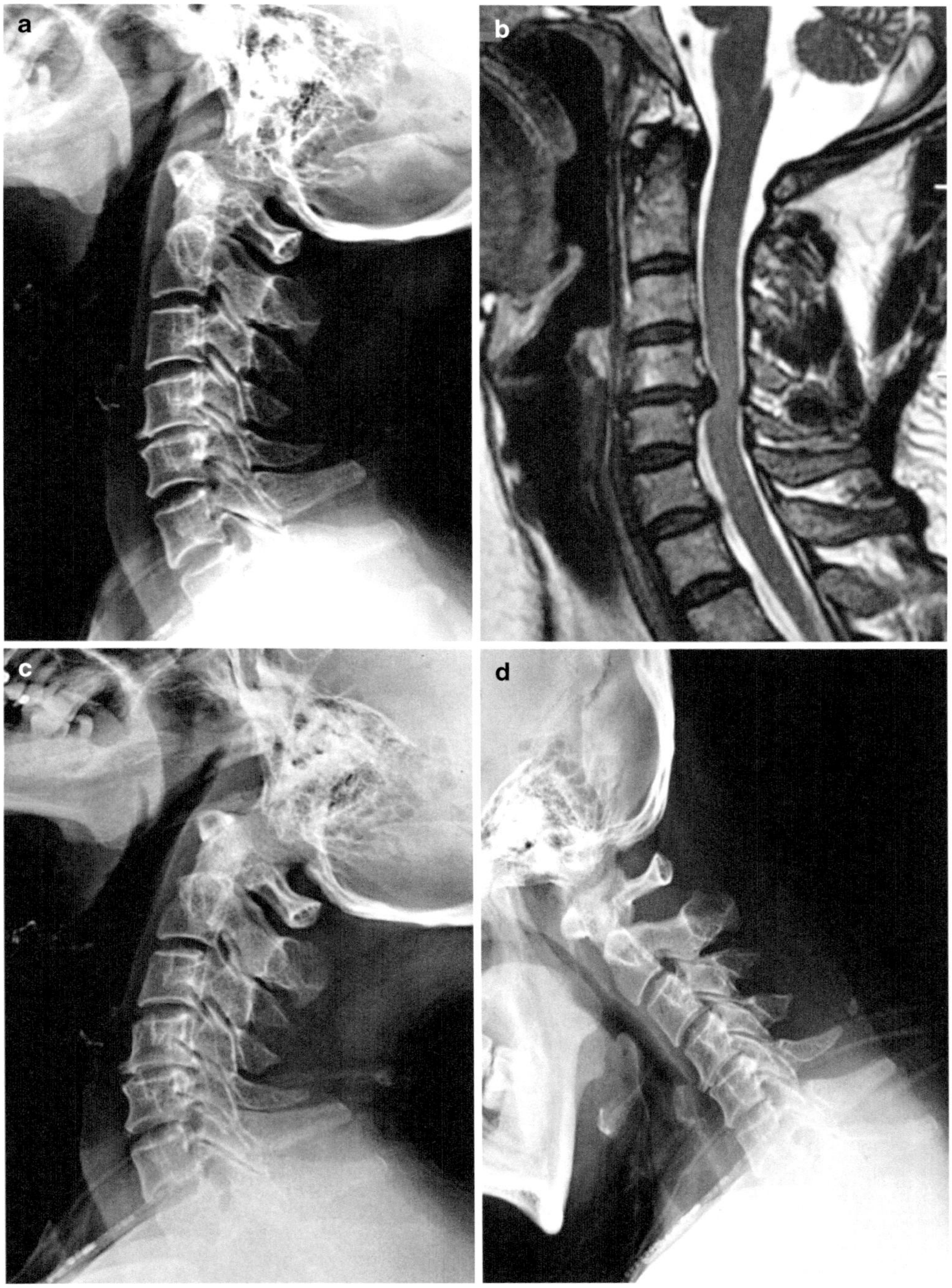

Fig. 6.24 Preoperative radiological findings. (**a**) Anteroposterior radiograph. (**b**) MRI, sagittal view. (**c**) Radiograph, overextension. (**d**) Radiograph, overflexion

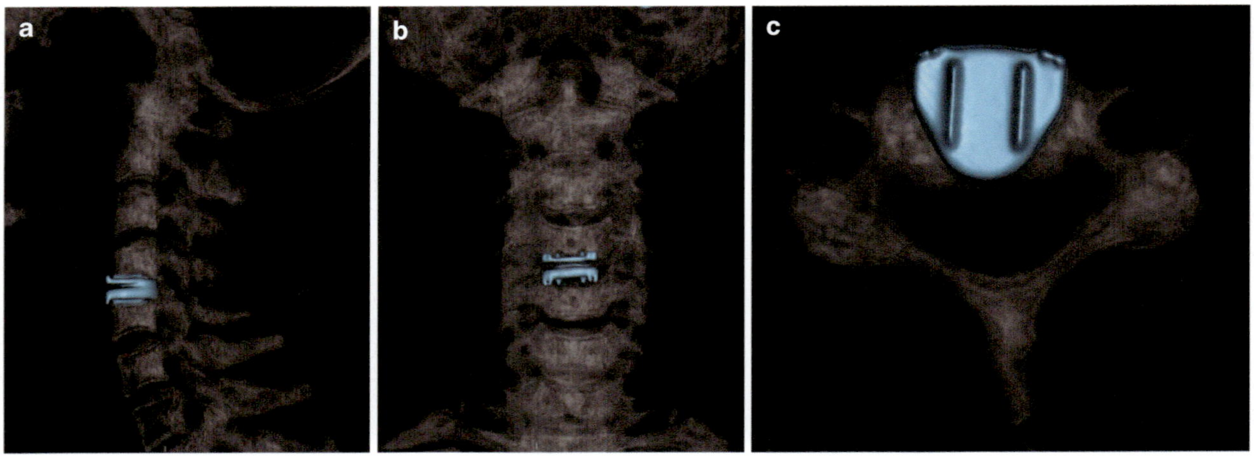

Fig. 6.25 Radiological findings at postoperative day 3. (**a**) CT 3D reconstruction, sagittal view. (**b**) CT 3D reconstruction, coronal view. (**c**) CT 3D reconstruction, horizontal view

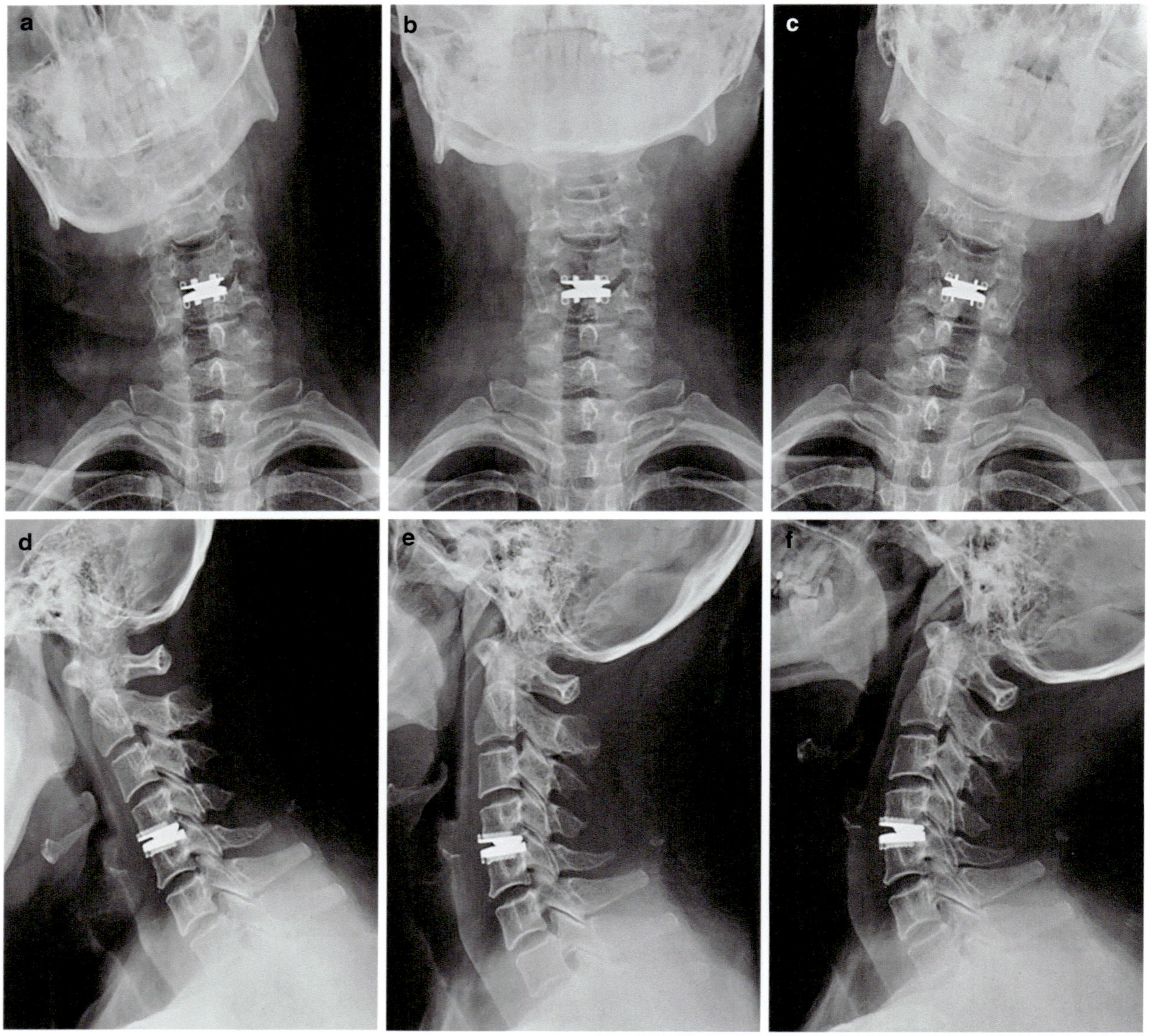

Fig. 6.26 Postoperative radiological findings at 1 month. (**a**) Radiograph, right flexion. (**b**) Anteroposterior radiograph. (**c**) Radiograph, left flexion. (**d**) Radiograph, overextension. (**e**) Lateral radiograph. (**f**) Radiograph, overflexion

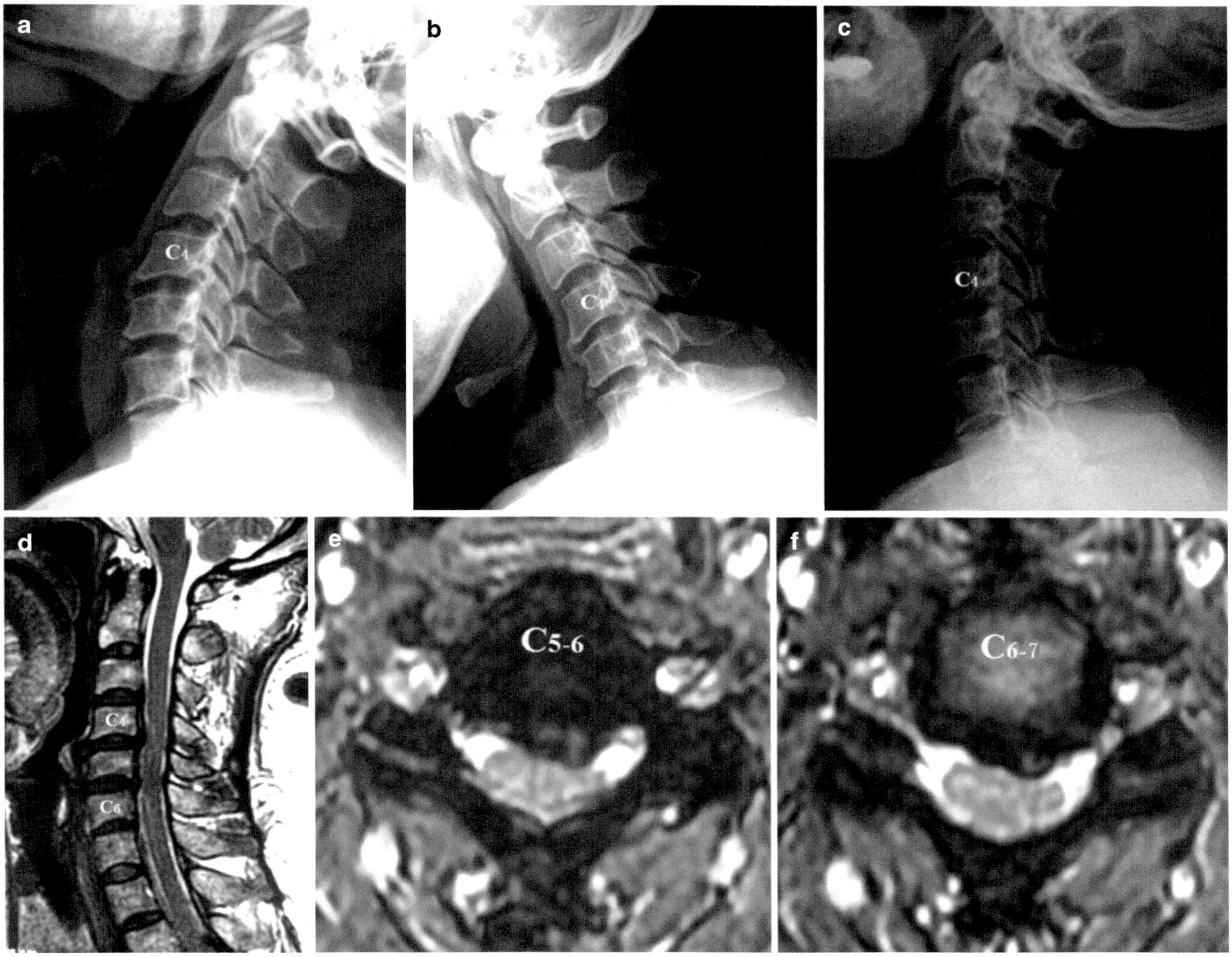

Fig. 6.27 Preoperative radiological findings. (**a**) Radiograph, overextension. (**b**) Radiograph, overflexion. (**c**) Lateral radiograph. (**d**) MRI, sagittal view. (**e**) MRI, C5–C6 intervertebral disc. (**f**) MRI, C6–C7 intervertebral disc

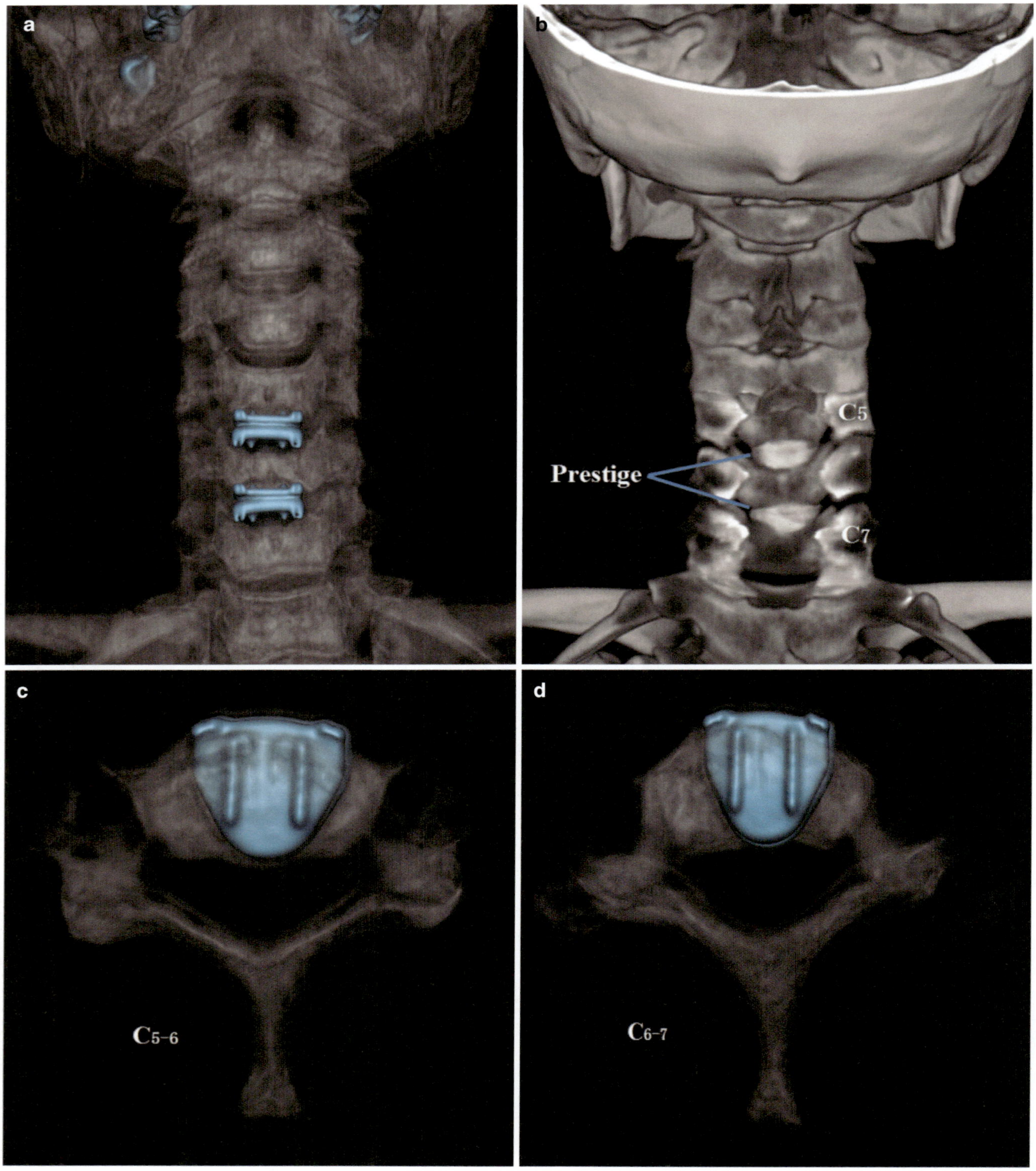

Fig. 6.28 Postoperative radiological findings. (**a**) CT 3D reconstruction, anterior view. (**b**) CT 3D reconstruction, posterior view. (**c**) CT 3D reconstruction, C5–C6 intervertebral disc. (**d**) CT 3D reconstruction, C6–C7 intervertebral disc

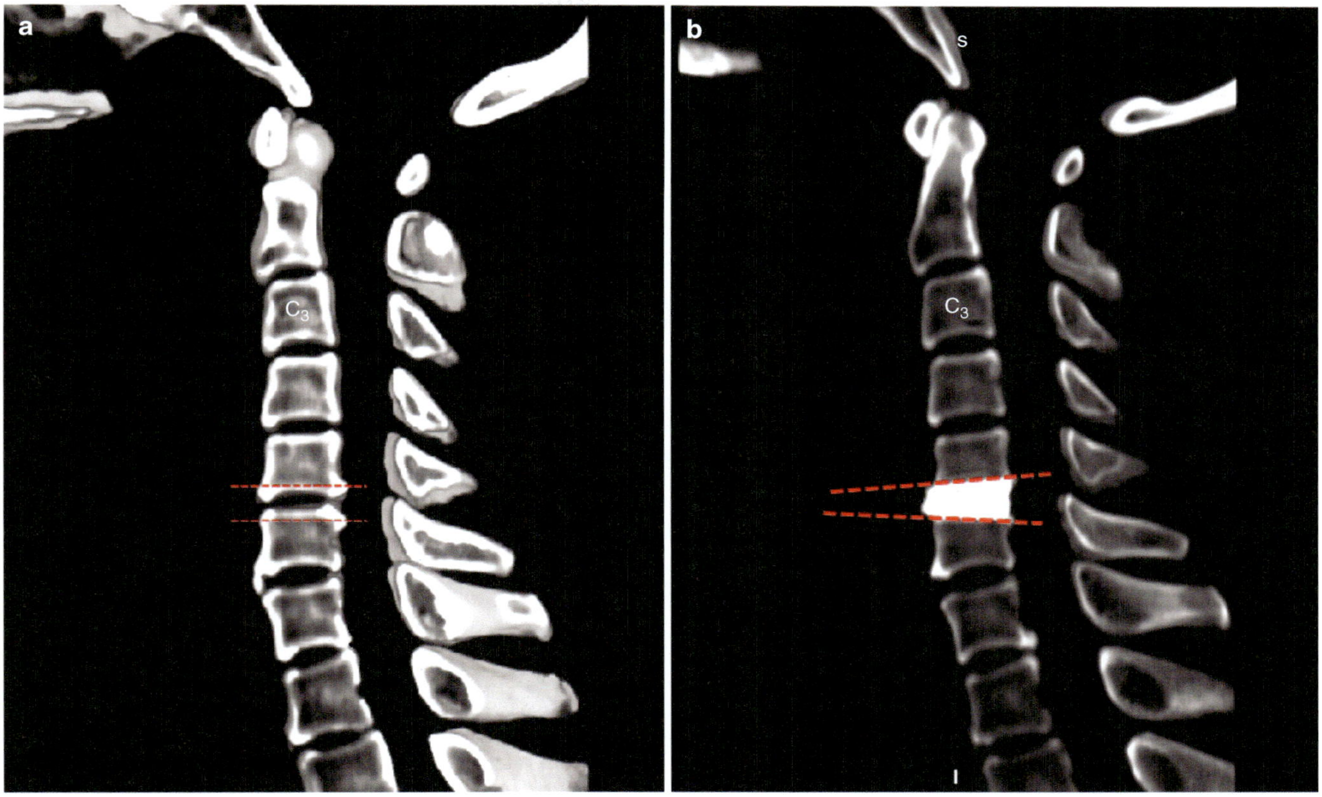

Fig. 6.29 Poor dilation of disc space. (**a**) CT 3D reconstruction, prior to surgery. (**b**) CT 3D reconstruction, post surgery

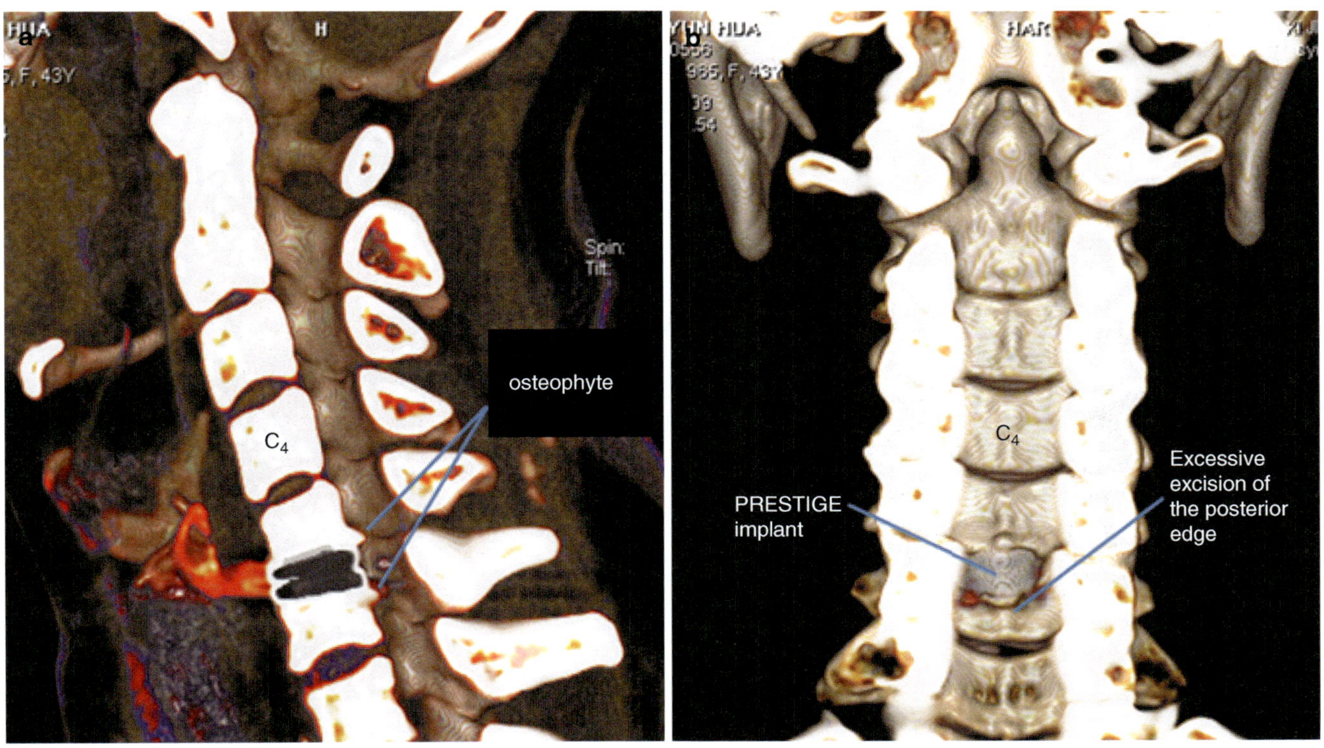

Fig. 6.30 Poor dilation of disc space. (**a**) CT 3D reconstruction, sagittal view; osteophyte at the posterior edge is too large and excision is inadequate. (**b**) CT 3D reconstruction, coronal view, PRESTIGE implant, excessive excision of the posterior edge of C_6

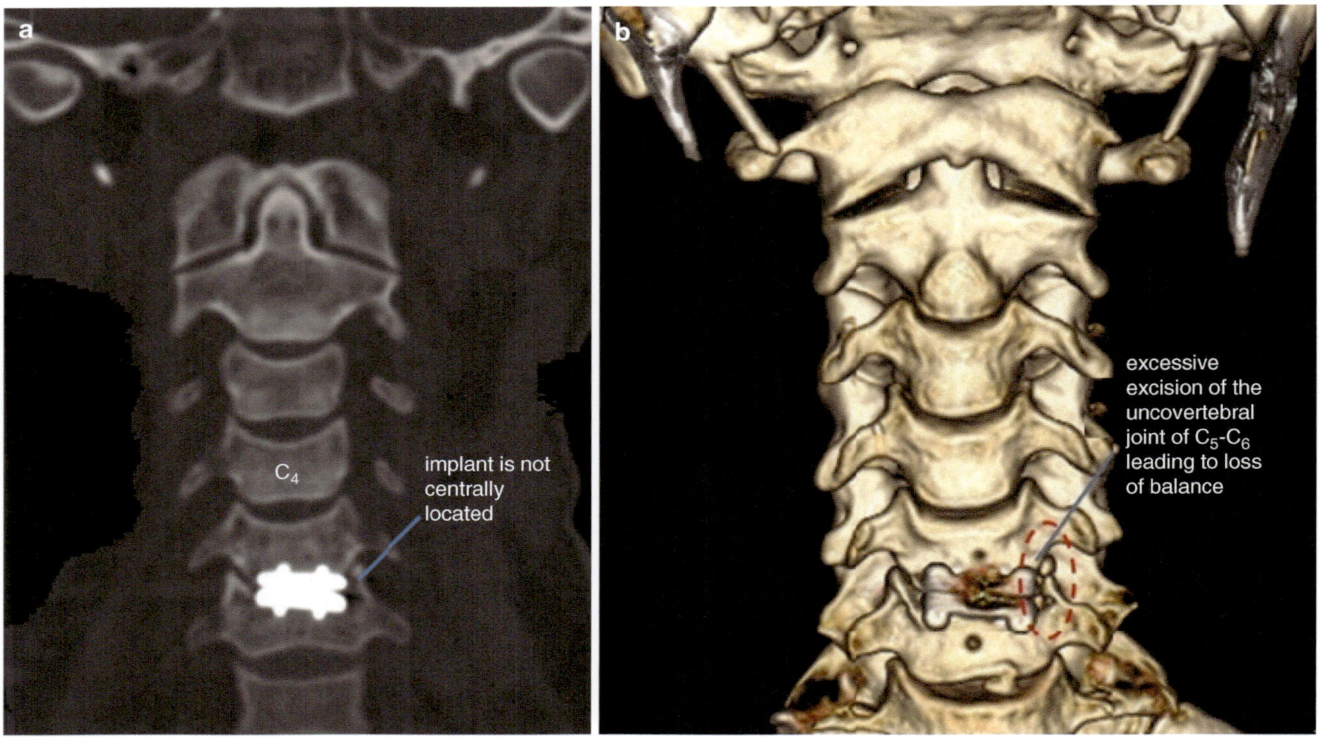

Fig. 6.31 Poor dilation of disc space. (**a**) CT 3D reconstruction, coronal view; implant is not centrally located leading to loss of balance. (**b**) CT 3D reconstruction, excessive excision of the uncovertebral joint of C5–C6 leading to loss of balance

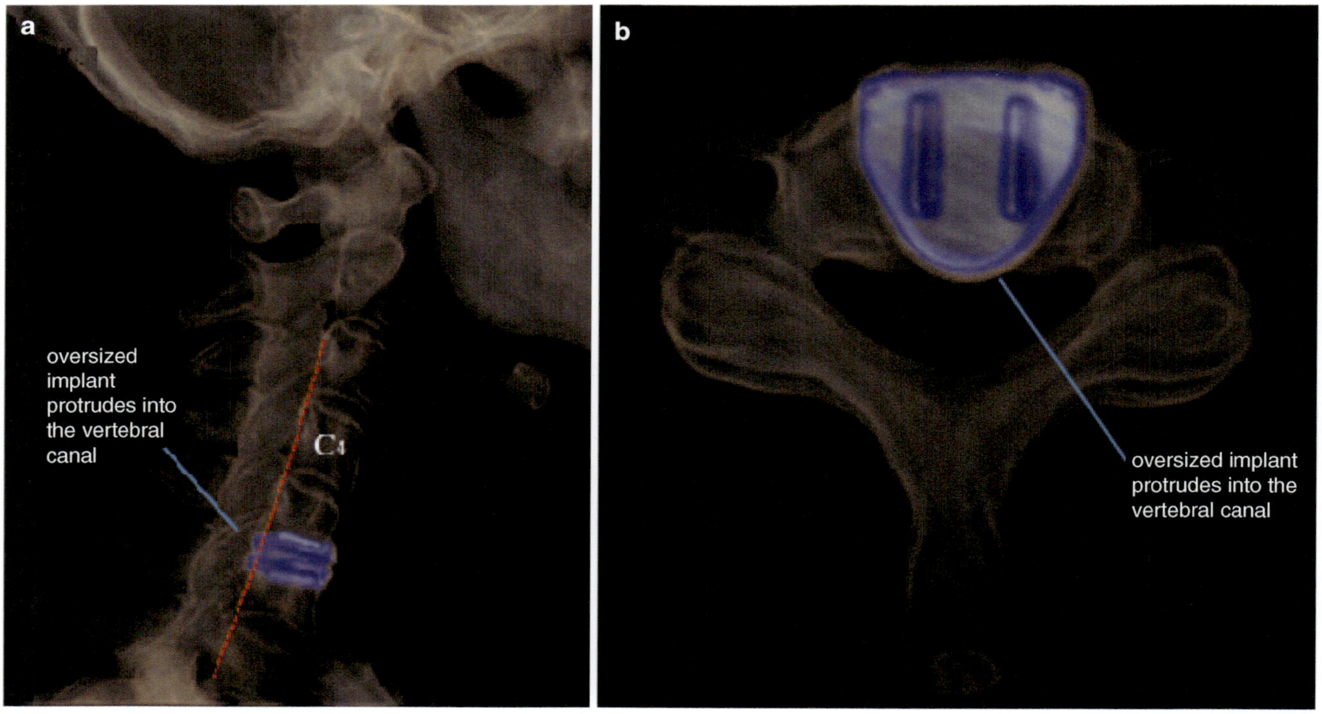

Fig. 6.32 Oversized implant. (**a**) CT 3D reconstruction, sagittal view; oversized implant protrudes into the vertebral canal. (**b**) CT 3D reconstruction, horizontal view; oversized implant protrudes into the vertebral canal

References

1. Fernstrom U. Arthroplasty with intercorporal endoprothesis in herniated disc and in painful disc. Acta Chir Scand Suppl. 1966;357:154–9.
2. Cummins BH, Robertson JT, Gill SS. Surgical experience with an implanted artificial cervical joint. J Neurosurg. 1998;88(6):943–8.
3. Wigfield CC, et al. The new Frenchay artificial cervical joint: results from a two-year pilot study. Spine (Phila Pa 1976). 2002;27(22):2446–52.
4. Mummaneni PV, et al. Clinical and radiographic analysis of cervical disc arthroplasty compared with allograft fusion: a randomized controlled clinical trial. J Neurosurg Spine. 2007;6(3):198–209.
5. Goffin J, et al. Preliminary clinical experience with the Bryan cervical disc prosthesis. Neurosurgery. 2002;51(3):840–5; discussion 845–7
6. Mahto AK, Omar S. Clinico-anatomical approach for instrumentation of the cervical spine: a morphometric study on typical cervical vertebrae. Int J Sci Study. 2015;3(4):143–5.

The CENTERPIECE™ Posterior Cervical Laminoplasty and Internal Fixation System

7

Yang Zhang and Wei Lei

Abstract

The technique of posterior cervical laminoplasty was developed to decompress the spinal canal in patients with multilevel compression caused by ossification of the posterior longitudinal ligament or cervical spondylosis. Several studies have confirmed its superiority to laminectomy with regard to neurological outcome, preserving spinal stability, and preventing post-laminectomy kyphosis. This chapter introduces the CENTERPIECE™, one of the most commonly used plate fixation systems for cervical laminoplasty. Meanwhile, the detailed steps and surgical precautions are explained with specific illustrative cases.

Keywords

Cervical spine · Laminoplasty · Miniplates

7.1 Posterior Cervical Laminoplasty: A Historical Perspective

Posterior cervical laminoplasty evolved from cervical laminectomy and is mainly used for treatment of cervical spinal stenosis, posterior longitudinal cervical ligament ossification, and multilevel cervical spondylosis [1, 2].

In 1973, Oyama et al. proposed expansive Z-laminoplasty (Fig. 7.1a–d).

In 1982, Kurokawa first put forward double-door laminoplasty, which is also called "French-window," "French-door," or "Kurokawa" laminoplasty (Fig. 7.2a–d).

In 1983, Hirabayashi first proposed single-door expansive laminoplasty, which is currently the most commonly used form of expansive laminoplasty (Fig. 7.3a–d).

Many scholars subsequently put forward new laminoplasties, which are all modified techniques based on the classic single-door or double-door laminoplasty [3, 4], including the following:

- Implant-secured Hirabayashi laminoplasty, in which lamina stabilization is done with a titanium alloy microplate on the basis of single-door laminoplasty.
- Implant-secured Kurokawa expansive laminoplasty, which is based on double-door laminoplasty, and the space between the spinous processes is filled with allograft or hydroxyapatite blocks.
- Muscle-preserving Hirabayashi expansive laminoplasty, in which the integrity of the interspinous ligament and C7 spinous process should be preserved. The muscle dissection technique is employed, or the spinous process is temporarily cut and retracts into the contralateral lamina trough. This could protect the attached muscle tissues on one side, and the muscles attached to C2 spinous process should be preserved.
- Muscle-preserving Kurokawa expansive laminoplasty, in which the rhomboid and trapezius which are attached to C7 should be preserved. In addition, dissection of the muscles attached to C2 spinous process should be best avoided if possible. Therefore, the surgical technique is also called minimally invasive expansive laminoplasty.

The above surgical approaches of expansive laminoplasties are shown in the figure below [5, 6] (Fig. 7.4):

7.2 Implants

1. Open-door plate

The "kickstand" design of the plate helps to secure the plate when it is placed on the lateral mass (Fig. 7.5).

2. Graft plate

Y. Zhang · W. Lei (✉)
Department of Orthopedics, Xijing Hospital, Air Force Medical University, Xi'an, Shaanxi, China
e-mail: zhangyang@fmmu.edu.cn; leiwei@fmmu.edu.cn

W. Lei, Y. Yan (eds.), *Internal Fixation of the Spine*, https://doi.org/10.1007/978-981-16-1562-7_7

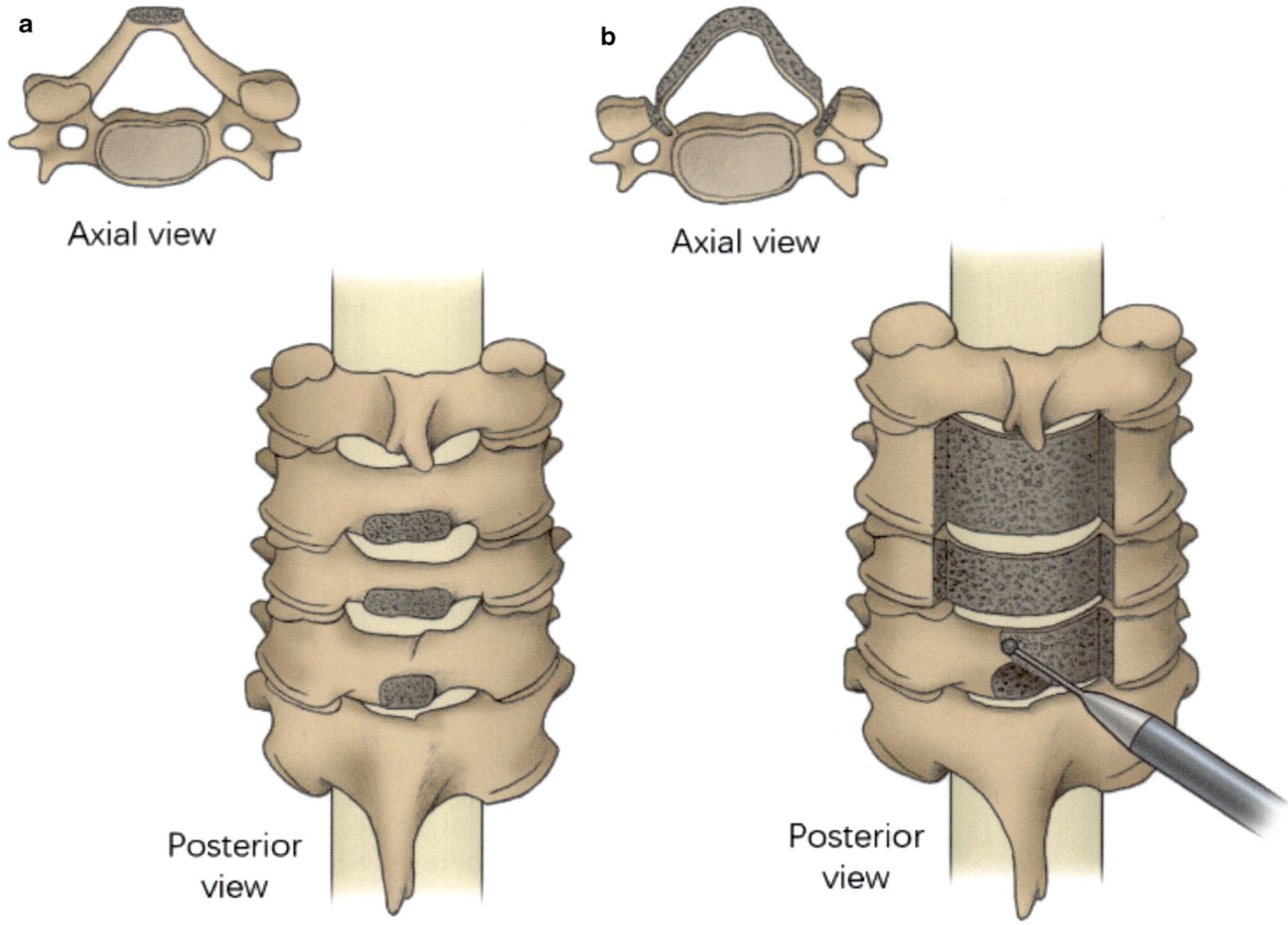

Fig. 7.1 (**a**) The spinous processes of the operative vertebral segments are resected. (**b**) The lamina is then thinned using a high-speed burr, and (**c**) a trough is made at the junction of the lamina and the lateral mass on both sides. (**d**) Finally, the lamina is cut in a Z-shaped fashion and then lifted, and the cut site is then sutured and secured

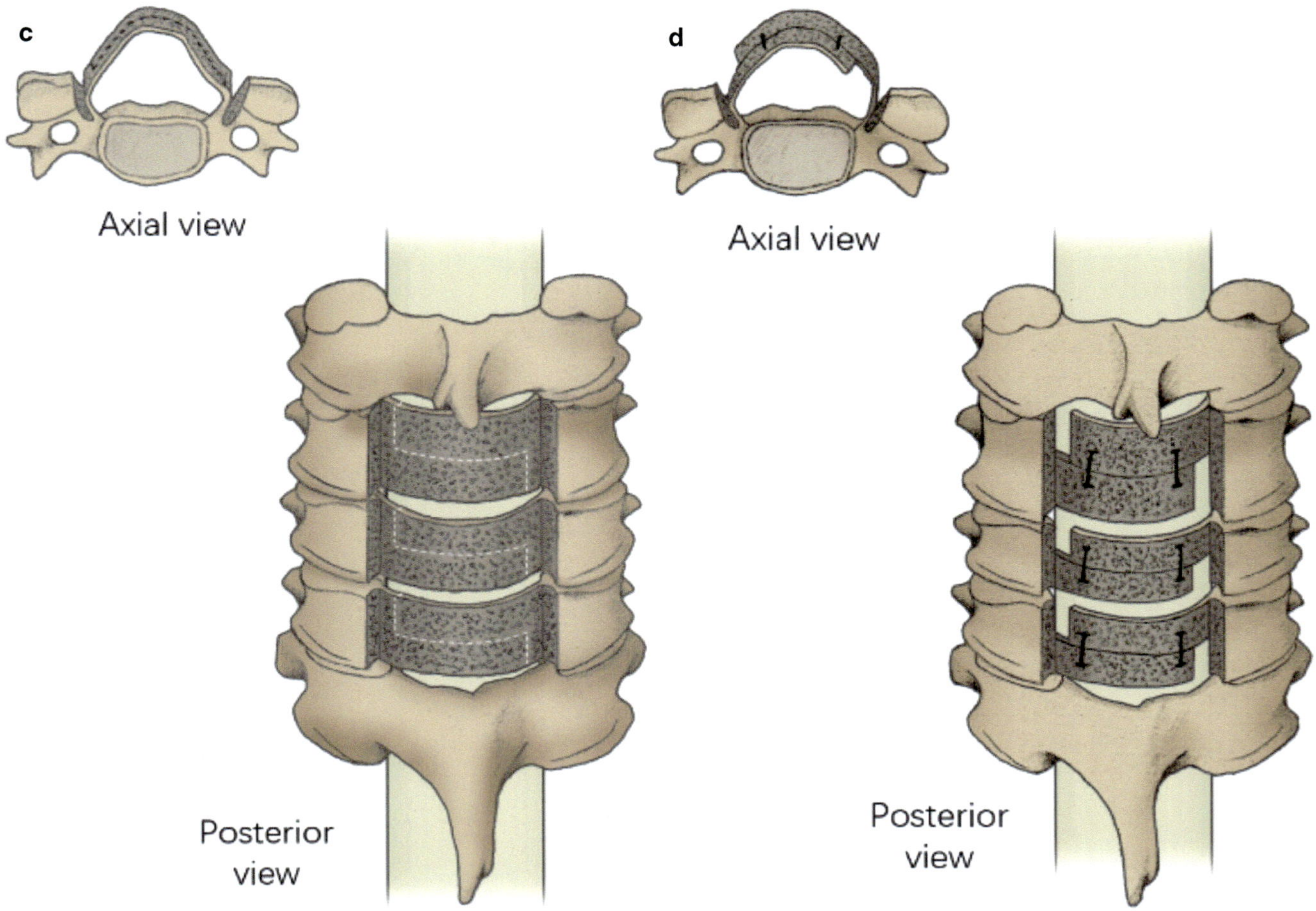

Fig. 7.1 (continued)

The oval-shaped center screw hole in the graft plate allows for fine adjustments of the plate on the allograft plate (Fig. 7.6).

3. Lateral hole plate (open-door or graft plate)

The medial/lateral orientation of the lateral mass screw holes allows for flexible screw placement in the event that the surface area of the lateral mass has been reduced in its cranial-caudal dimension, especially following supplemental foraminotomies (Fig. 7.7).

4. Hinge plate

A hinge plate is suitable for a floppy or displaced hinge (Fig. 7.8).

5. Wide mouth plate

A wide laminar shelf is designed to accommodate thick laminae (Fig. 7.9).

6. Screws

Screws include self-tapping screws that come in 2.6 and 3 mm in diameter and 5, 7, 9, and 11 mm in length (Fig. 7.10).

7.3 System Features

1. The pre-cut, pre-contoured plate design allows ease of use.
2. Multiple screw hole options facilitate screw placement.
3. Color coding allows easy recognition and distinction.
4. Plate dimensions are uniform. The length ranges from 8 to 18 mm and each 2-mm increment represents a new dimension.

7.4 Indications and Contraindications

A. Indications

It is indicated for laminoplasty fixation via the posterior approach for cervical vertebra diseases:

1. Developmental cervical vertebra spinal stenosis

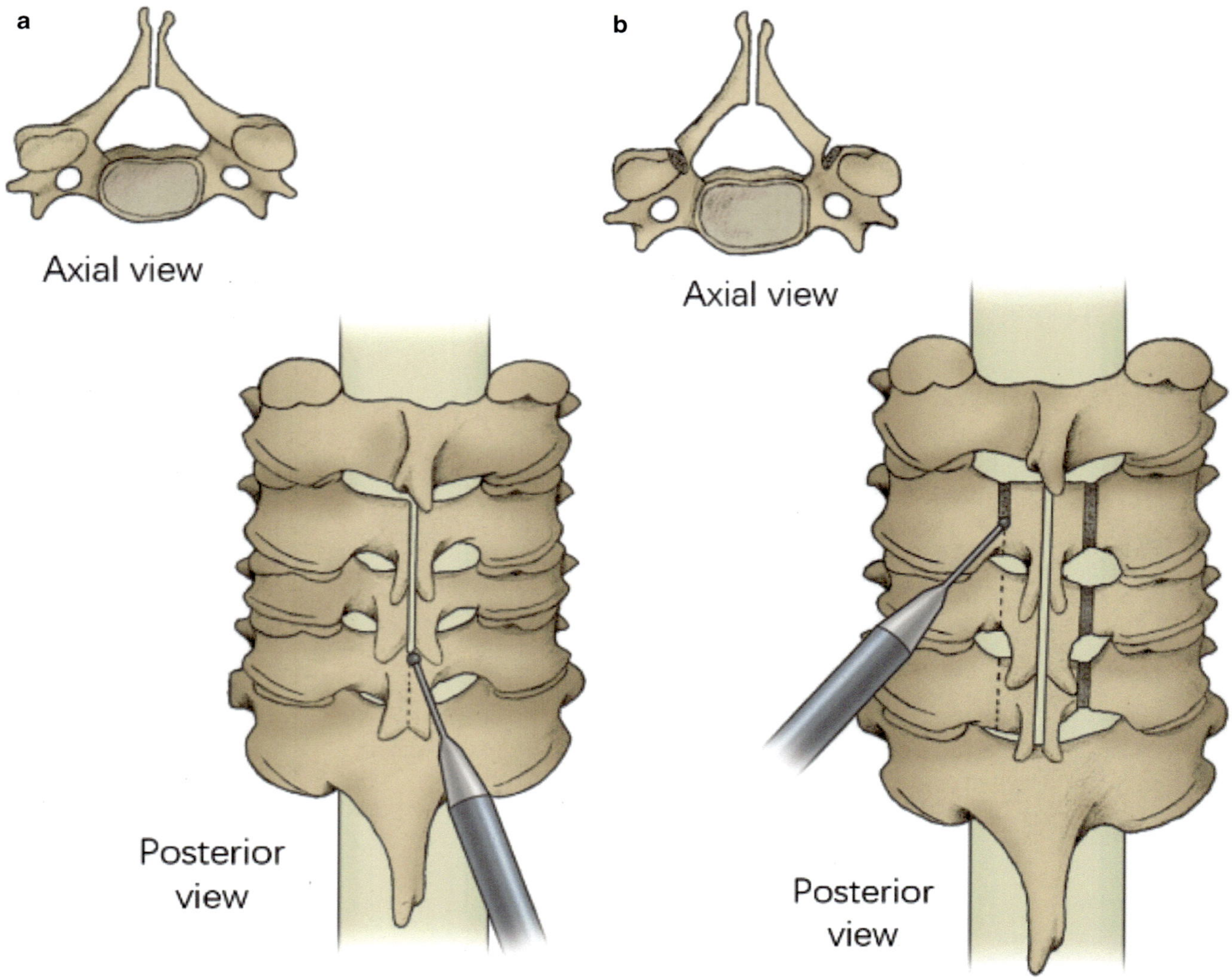

Fig. 7.2 (**a**) The spinous processes of the operative vertebral segments are vertically split using a high-speed burr or T-shaped saw. (**b**) Then, a trough is made at the junction of the lateral lamina and the facet joints on both sides, and (**c**) the bilateral spinous processes are lifted together with the lamina. (**d**) Finally, the appropriately sized allograft is inserted between the cut edge of the lamina and the split spinous process to act as support

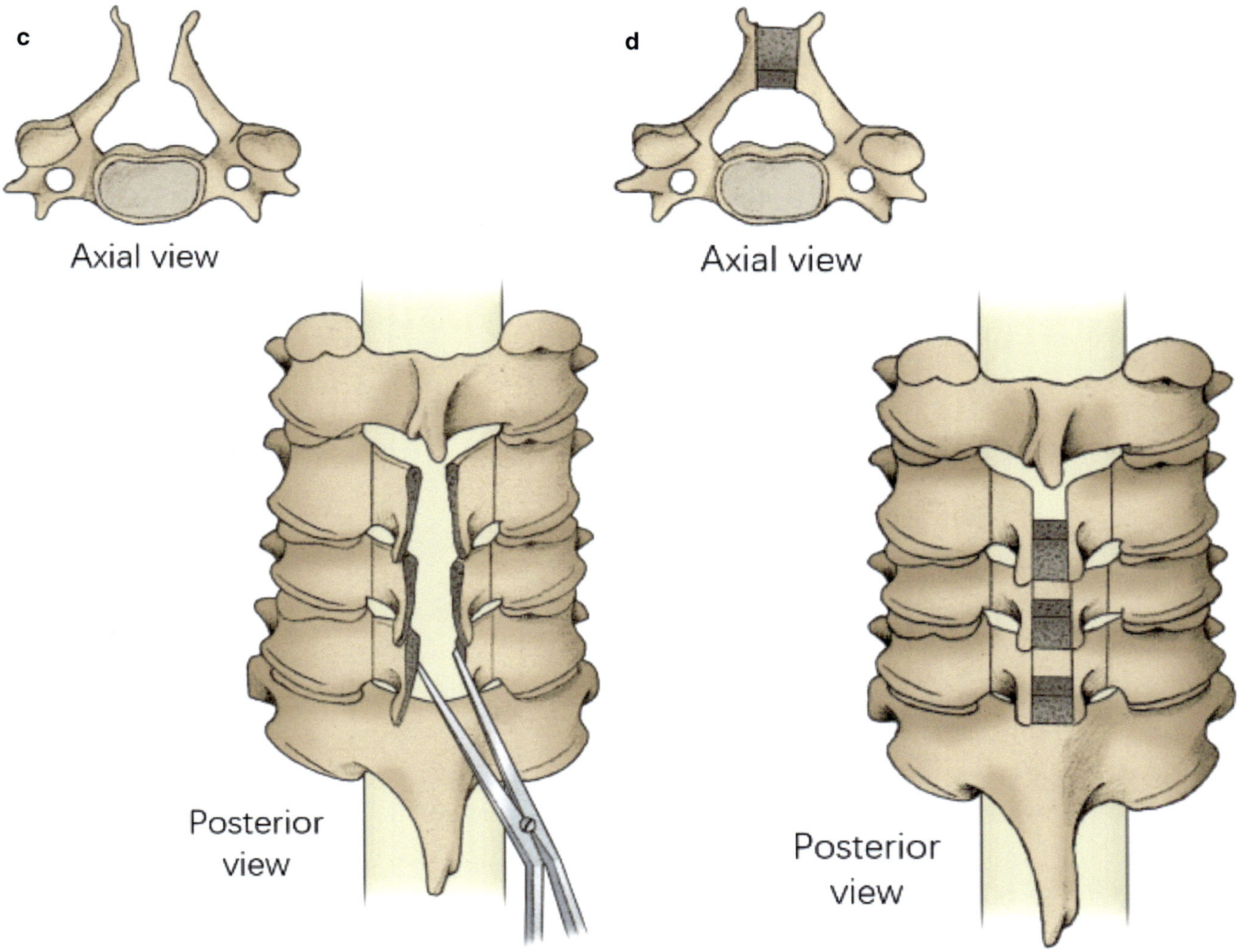

Fig. 7.2 (continued)

2. Multi-segmental cervical spine disorders with or without cervical vertebra spinal stenosis
3. Multi-segmental posterior longitudinal ligament ossification (Fig. 7.11)
4. Unsatisfactory outcome with cervical vertebra surgery via the anterior approach and requiring supplemental decompression via the posterior approach

B. Contraindications

Cervical spine kyphosis

7.5 Standard Imaging Features of Cervical Spinal Stenosis

1. A sagittal diameter of the spinal canal of 13–14 mm indicates mild stenosis, 10–12 mm moderate stenosis, and <10 mm absolute stenosis (Fig. 7.12).
2. The ratio of the sagittal diameter of the spinal canal to the midsagittal diameter of the vertebral body is normally 1:1, and a ratio less than 0.82 suggests spinal stenosis and less than 0.75 confirms spinal stenosis.
3. The cross-sectional area of the vertebral canal is normally above 200 mm^2. The maximal cross-sectional area of the vertebral canal is 185 mm^2 in spinal stenosis patients with a mean reduction of 72 mm^2 (Fig. 7.12).

7.6 Surgical Procedures

The key surgical techniques lie in two aspects: how to properly carry out open-door laminoplasty and how to prevent door closing.

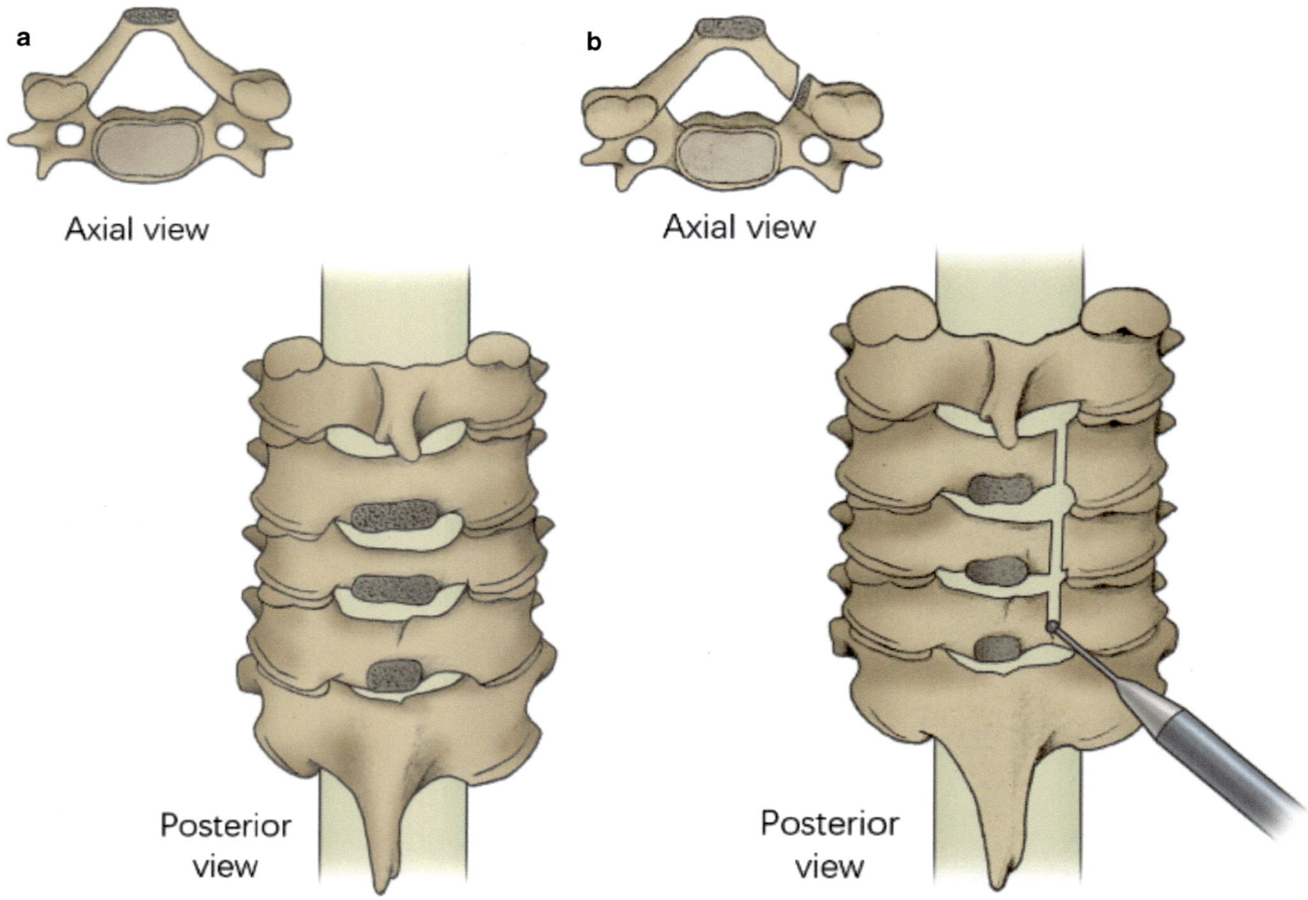

Fig. 7.3 (**a**) The spinous processes of the operative vertebral segments are resected. (**b**) Then, a trough is made at the junction of the lamina and small facet joint on both sides. (**c**) A thin layer of bone is preserved on the side of the door shaft, and (**d**) then the lamina is lifted, and the lamina and the small facet joint are secured with sutures. The procedure is also called Hirabayashi expansive laminoplasty

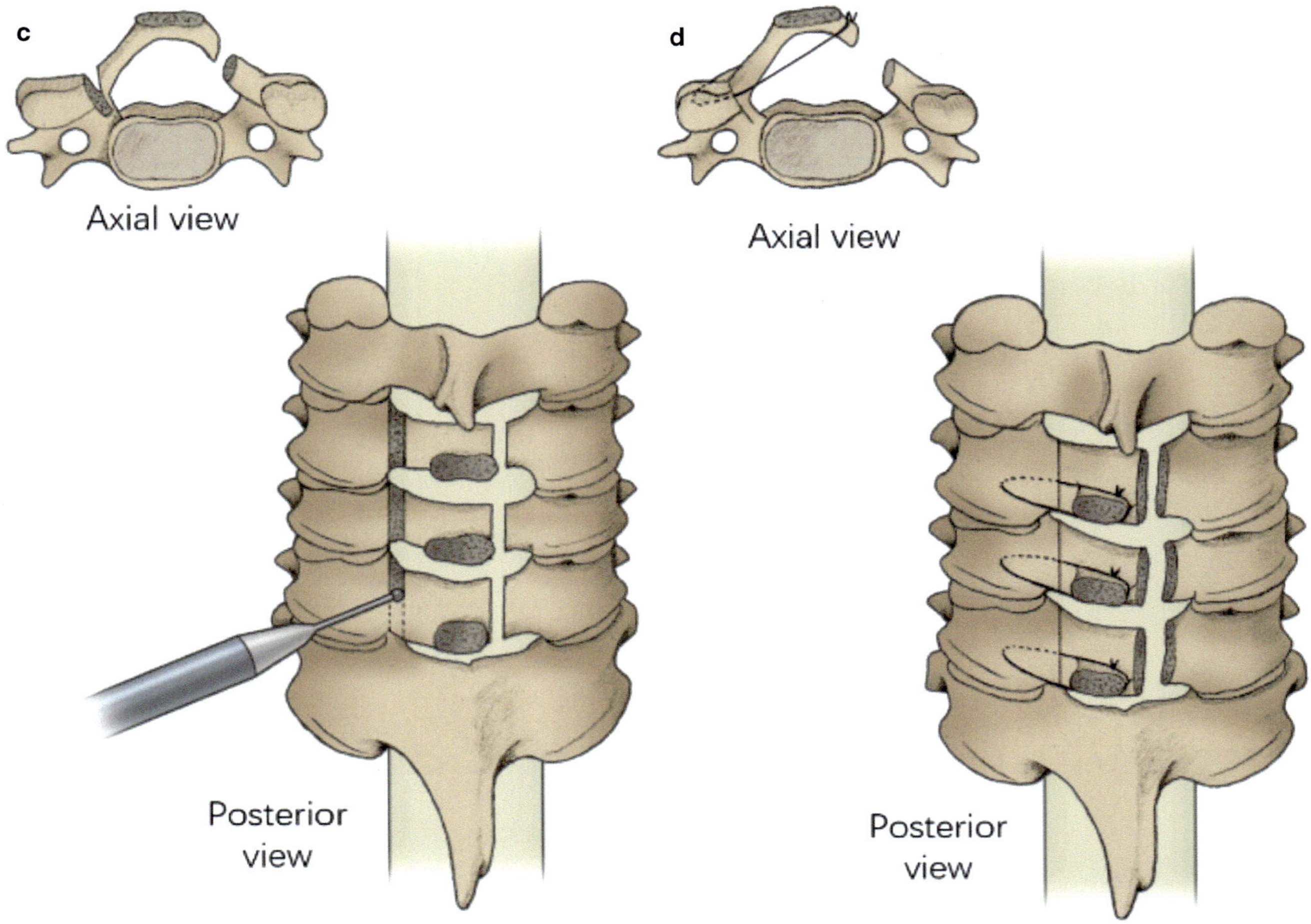

Fig. 7.3 (continued)

7.6.1 Surgical Exposure

Using C3–C7 single-door laminoplasty as an example, the surgeon performs a midline posterior exposure from the inferior aspect of C2 to the superior aspect of T1 (Figs. 7.13 and 7.14). The lateral dissection follows the subperiosteal plane out to the midportion of the lateral masses. The insertion of the extensor muscles is only detached from the lower laminar margin of C2 to allow access to the C2–C3 interlaminar space.

Caution: The muscle origins and insertions over the medial and lateral half of the lateral masses are in general not dissected and are preserved. This will minimize intraoperative bleeding.

If the condition of the patient requires that decompression be extended to C2 segment, this can be accomplished by preserving the integrity of C2 posterior arch and the majority of muscle origins and insertions: a Kerrison rongeur and a burr can be used to remove the lower margin of C2, and then the middle cancellous bone and ventral cortex, rendering the lamina dome-shaped (Fig. 7.15).

Caution: Preservation of muscle origins and insertions is very critical to reduction of postoperative axial pain.

7.6.2 Proper Techniques for Open Door

7.6.2.1 The Open Side and Direction

1. If myelopathy is symmetric, the side of the spinal canal to be opened can be at the discretion of the surgeon. A right-hand dominant surgeon may prefer standing on the left side of the patient and open the left side for decompression. Therefore, open door is carried out on the left side (Fig. 7.16).
2. If myelopathy is asymmetric, the side of the spinal canal with a greater maneuvering space can be chosen for open door. The contents in the spinal canal are less likely to be disturbed, and the spinal cord is less prone to injuries (Fig. 7.17).

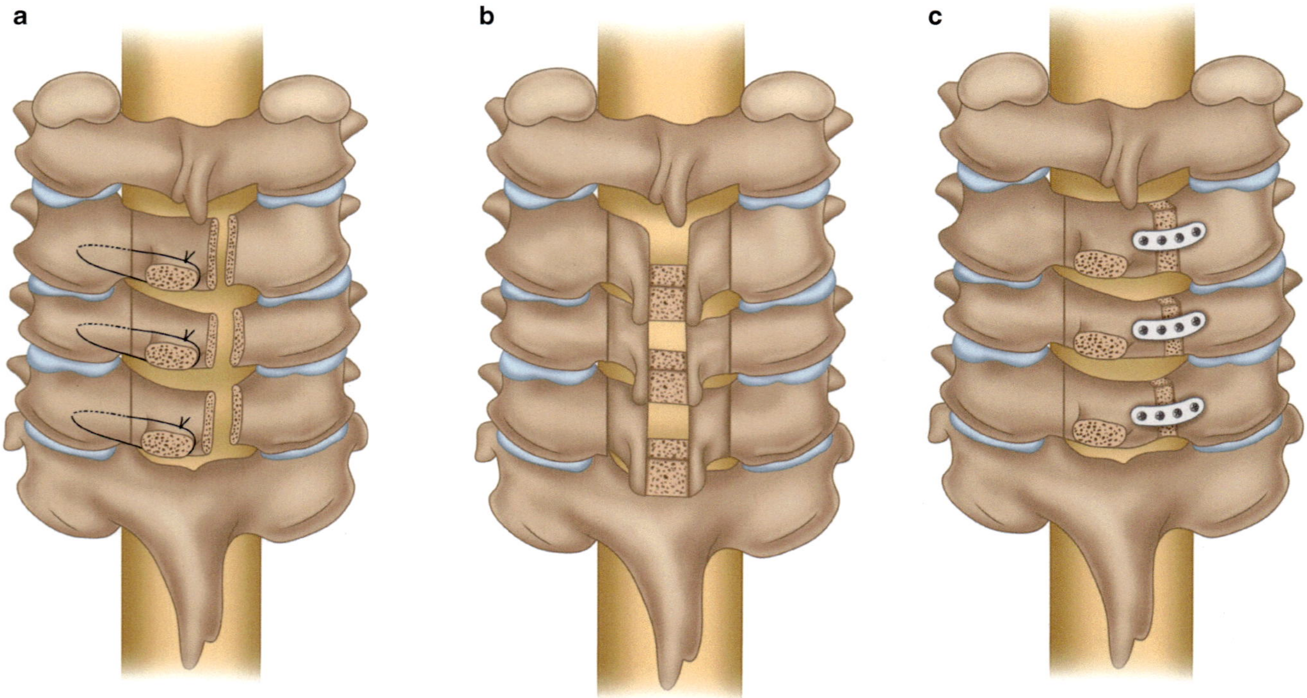

Fig. 7.4 Illustrations of the laminoplasty. (**a**) Hirabayashi technique. (**b**) Kurokawa-type technique. (**c**) Plate-augmented Hirabayashi technique

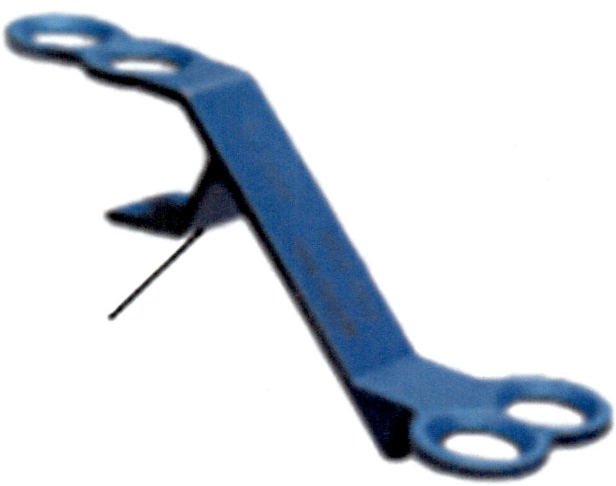

Fig. 7.5 Open door plate

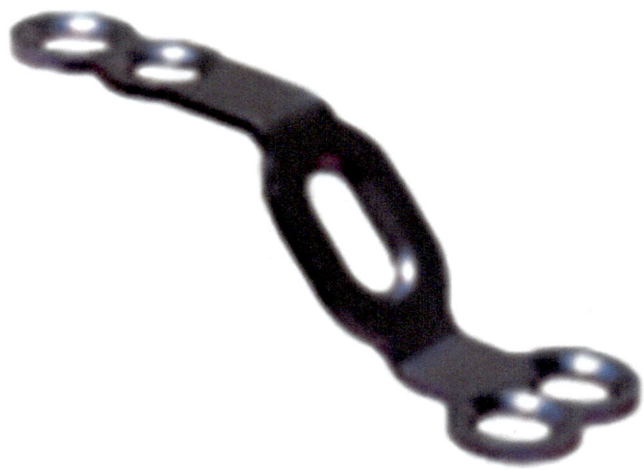

Fig. 7.6 Graft plate

3. If the condition of the patient requires that supplemental foraminotomies be done for decompression, the open side should be ipsilateral to the foraminotomies.

7.6.2.2 Trough Preparation and Hinge Position

The trough should be made at the junction of the lamina and the lateral mass, and the outer edge of the trough should be oriented toward the interior margin of the pedicle (Fig. 7.18).

The location of the hinge should be symmetrical to the trough (Fig. 7.19).

7.6.2.3 Trough and Hinge Shape

The trough is longitudinal.

The hinge can be opened into a wedge-shaped trough, with an optimal angle of 45–50°. The cancellous bone, 1 mm in thickness, and the inner cortex are preserved (Fig. 7.20).

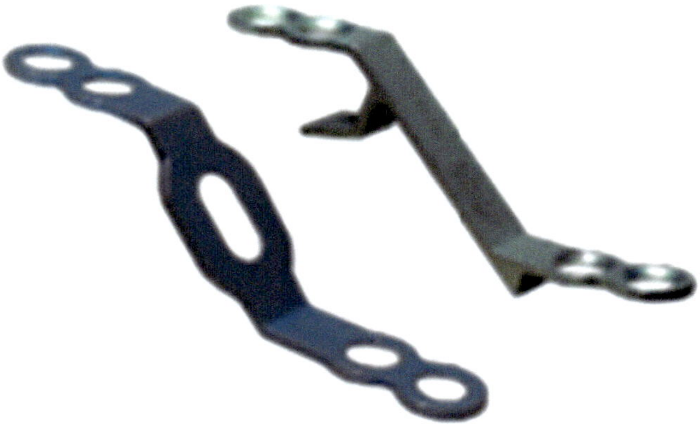

Fig. 7.7 Lateral hole plate

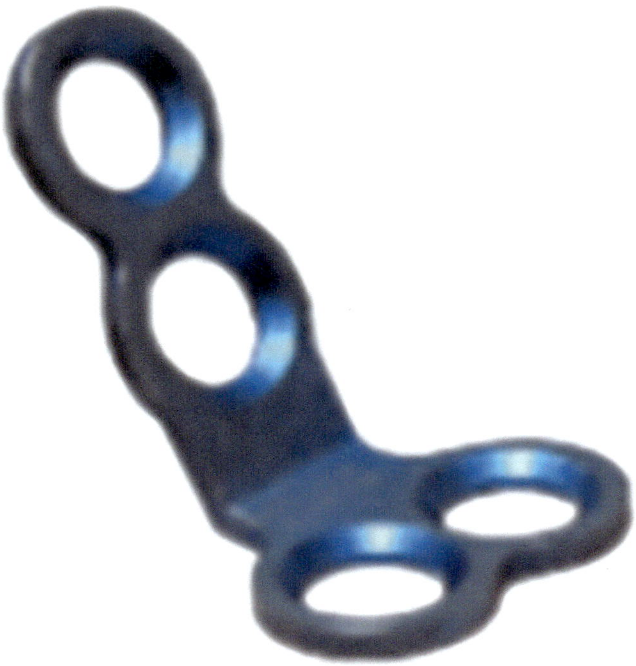

Fig. 7.8 Hinge plate

7.6.2.4 Tools for Open-Door Laminoplasty

The outer cancellous bone and then the cortex on the open side are first partially removed using a 3-mm burr. The remaining interior bone is removed using a 1-mm Kerrison rongeur (Fig. 7.21).

The outer cortex bone and then parts of the cancellous bone on the hinge side are removed using the 3-mm burr.

7.6.2.5 Size of the Open Door

The wider the open door (the distance of the cut end of the lamina to the lateral mass) is, the larger the increase in the sagittal diameter of the spinal canal of the operative segment is. For each 1-mm increase in open-door width, there is a 0.5-mm increase in the sagittal diameter. In general, the minimal size of the open door is 8–10 mm, and the distance from the lamina to the dural sac increases by 4–5 mm. The size of the open door can be appropriately increased depending on the severity of spinal stenosis (Fig. 7.22).

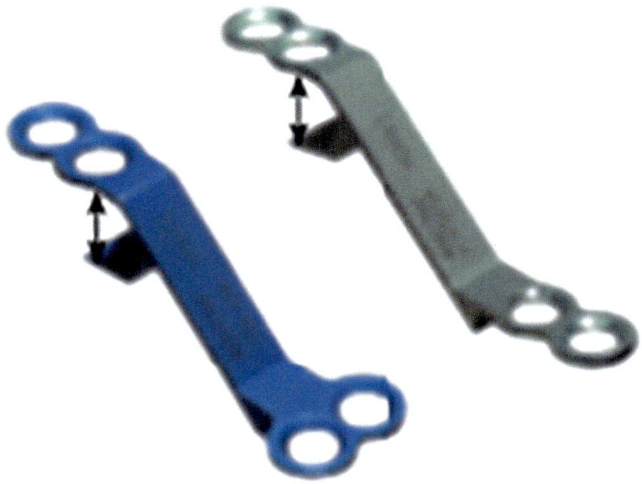

Fig. 7.9 Wide mouth plate

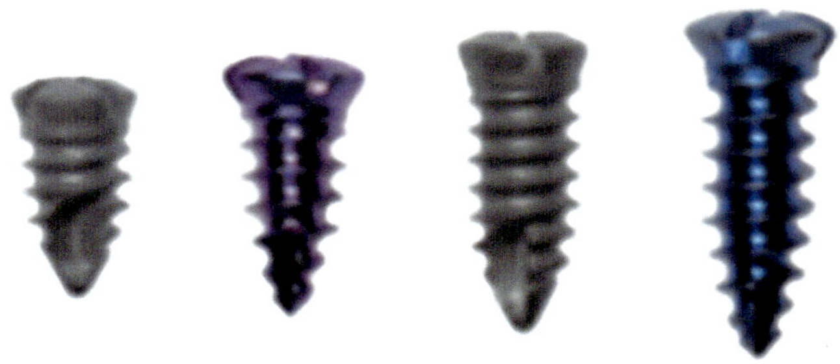

Fig. 7.10 Screws

7.6.2.6 Extent of the Open Door

The area of the open door should include full or partial laminae of the stenosed segment and the segment immediately above and immediately below the stenosed segment (Fig. 7.23a, b). In the illustrations below, MRI reveals stenosis at C3–C6 and that the area of the open-door covers C3–C7. C2 is typically not chosen.

7.6.2.7 Methods for Open-Door Laminoplasty

After a trough is prepared on the hinge side, the ligamentum flavum is cut superior and inferior to the open door. After the dural sac tissues and the epidural veins are divided, a 2- or 3-mm Kerrison punch is used to excise the ligamentum flavum at C2–C3 and C7–T1. While the laminae are gently opened, a nerve hook is used to separate the veins from the dura (Fig. 7.24), and then the laminae are sequentially opened from one end to the other. Before fully opening the

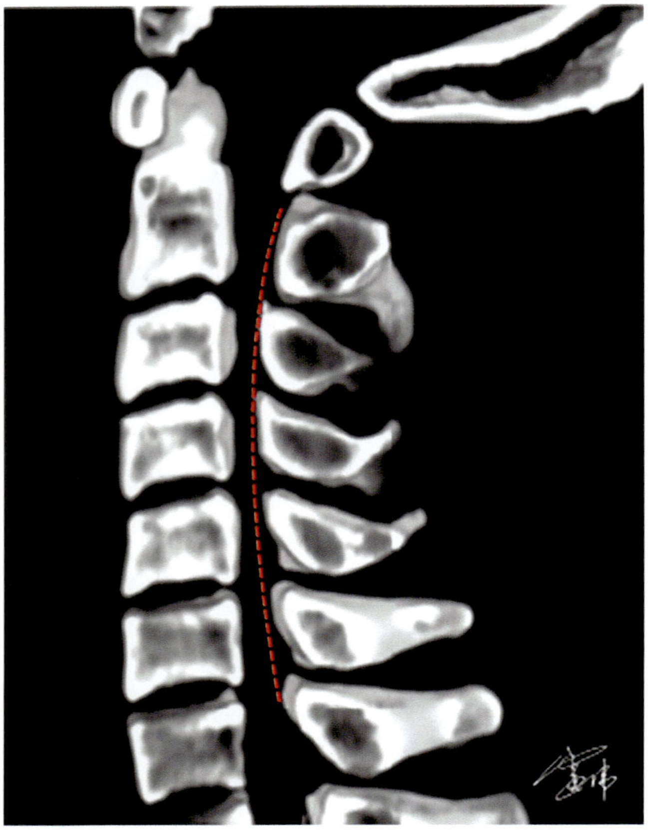

Fig. 7.11 Posterior longitudinal ligament ossification

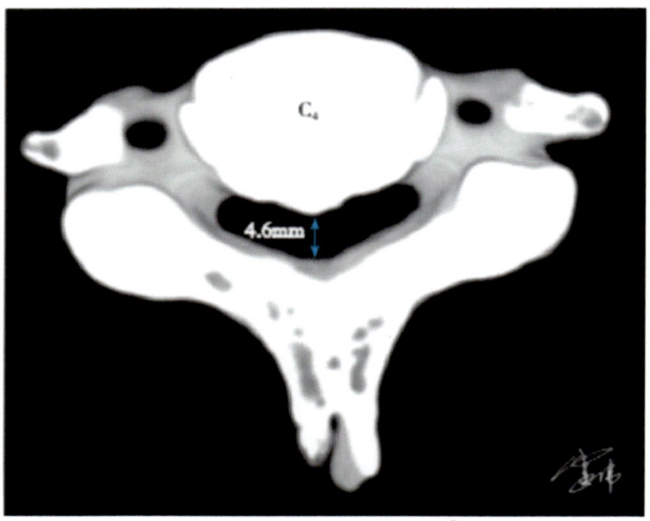

Fig. 7.12 Spinal stenosis. Spinal canal area = 90 mm^2

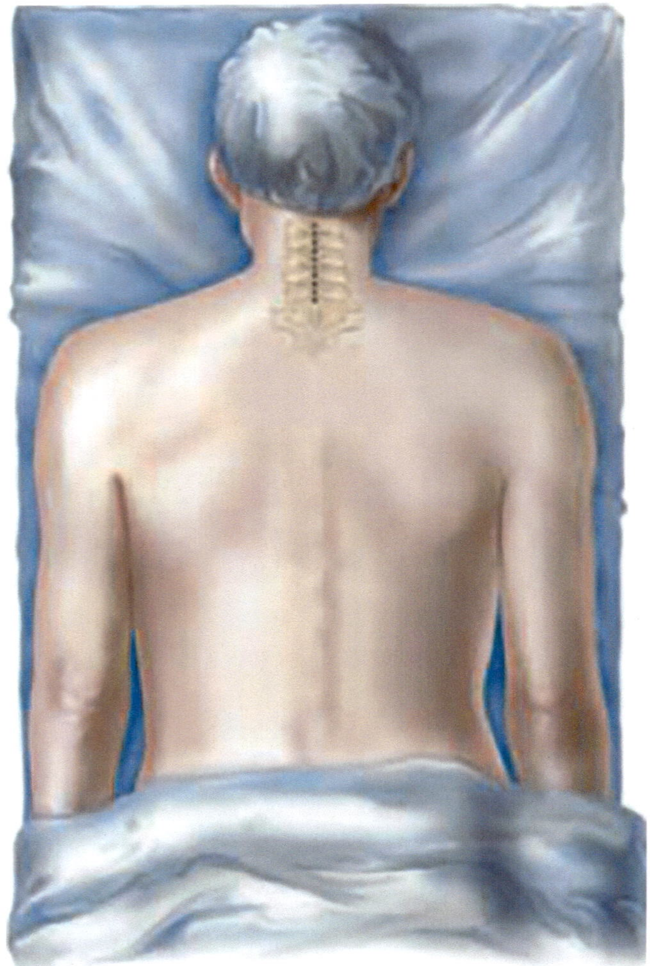

Fig. 7.13 Midline incision

lamina, an angled probe is used to ensure that any epidural adhesions have been lysed beneath the laminae.

7.6.3 Keeping the Door Open

Keeping the door open: using the open-door plate (Fig. 7.25)

1. Plate positioning: The appropriate size of the open-door plate is determined for each segment using bone trials (Fig. 7.26). The plate is then secured using the plate holder into the laminar shelf of the plate, and then the lateral portion of the plate is seated down onto the edge of the lateral mass (Fig. 7.27).

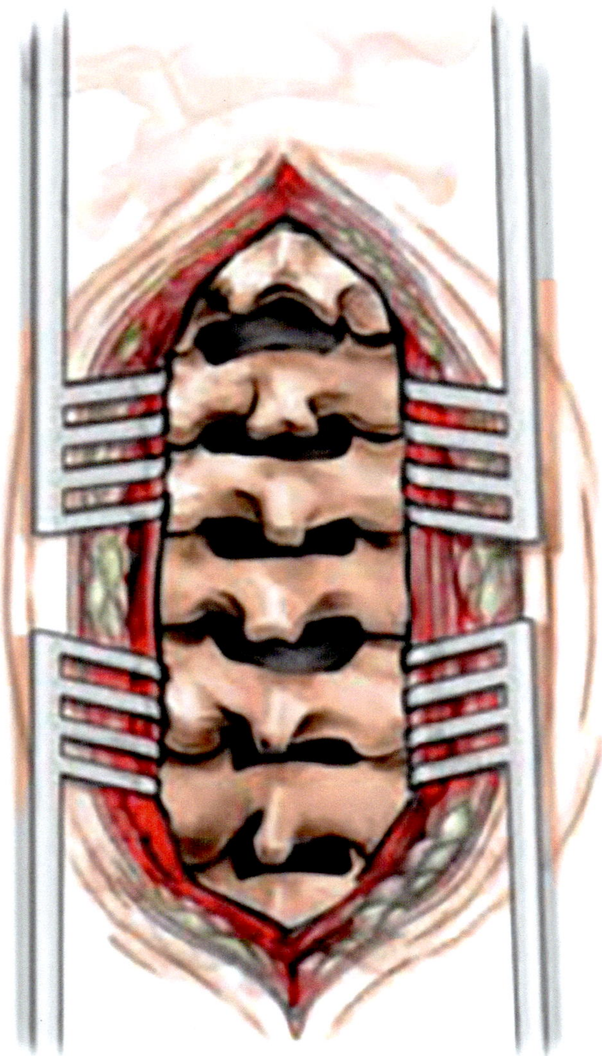

Fig. 7.14 Extent of exposure

Caution: The etched line on the plate holder should be aligned with the axis of the laminoplasty plate.

2. Drill and screw insertion: Each of the lateral mass screw holes is made using the 1.9 × 5.5-mm depth-stopped drill bit. Drilling is done manually or using a power drill (Fig. 7.28a). The plate is secured to the lateral mass with self-tapping screws using the self-holding screwdriver (Fig. 7.28b). The screwdriver sleeve can be used, and during insertion of the screws, screws are secured on the screwdriver and function as one piece, which facilitates maneuvering. The screwdriver and the sleeve are separate parts (Fig. 7.28c).

The laminar hole is then drilled using the same 1.9 × 5.5-mm depth-stopped drill bit and secured with a self-tapping screw (Fig. 7.29). While the screws are inserted, an assistant may hold the lamina with a clamp to prevent damage to the hinge; if necessary, a second screw may be placed in the lamina.

Two types of plate can be chosen in the process: the lateral hole plate and the wide mouth plate.

1. Lateral hole plate: The lateral hole plate can be used when the cranial-caudal diameter of the lateral mass is relatively small or the surface area of the lateral mass becomes diminished as a result of foraminotomies (Fig. 7.30). Except that the two fixation screws on the lateral mass are parallel to the long axis of the plate, the size measurement and insertion methods for the lateral hole plate are identical to those for the open-door plate and the graft plate. The exposure of the segment to be secured with the lateral hole plate should be relatively wider.
2. Wide mouth plate: The wide mouth plate can be used if the lamina is relatively thick (Fig. 7.31). Size selection and placement methods are identical to those of the standard open-door plate.

7. Inserting the wedge: using the graft plate

The graft plate allows for the placement of allograft on the open side of laminoplasty. After the laminoplasty is opened, the appropriately sized allograft is selected using the bone trials (Fig. 7.32a). As an example, a 10-mm trial corresponds to a 10-mm allograft. By inserting a 2.6 × 5-mm screw through the pre-drilled center hole in the allograft, the allograft is attached to the graft plate and secured (Fig. 7.32b, c). The oval-shaped center screw hole in the graft plate allows for fine adjustments of the plate on the allograft. The allograft/graft plate construct is inserted between the cut edge of the lamina and the lateral mass. The insertion methods are the same as for the open-door plate.

The graft plate can be used at each open-door segment (Fig. 7.33a), or the graft plate and the open-door plate can be used in combination (Fig. 7.33b, c).

8. Locking the hinge: the hinge plate

The hinge plate may be needed on occasion to secure a floppy or displaced hinge which threatens to impinge upon a nerve root or the dura (Fig. 7.34).

If the hinge plate is necessary, it should be stabilized before opening the laminoplasty. The loose lamina should be grasped and stabilized with a suitable clamp (e.g., a ligamentum flavum clamp). It is held firmly while the screw holes are drilled on the lamina with the 1.9 × 5.5-mm depth-stopped

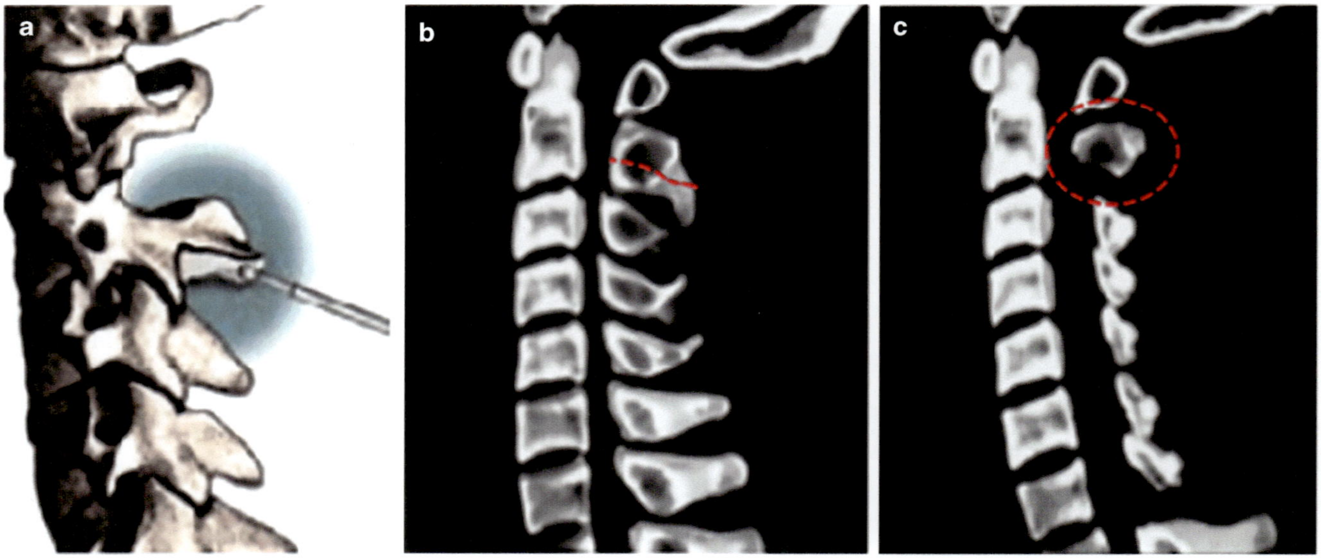

Fig. 7.15 C2 decompression. (**a**) Milling; (**b**) Extent of removal of the ventral cortex; (**c**) Removal of the ventral cortex

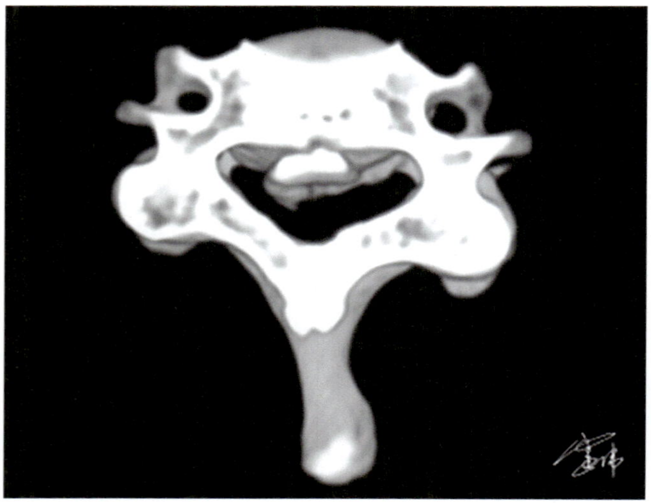

Fig. 7.16 The occupying lesion is symmetric

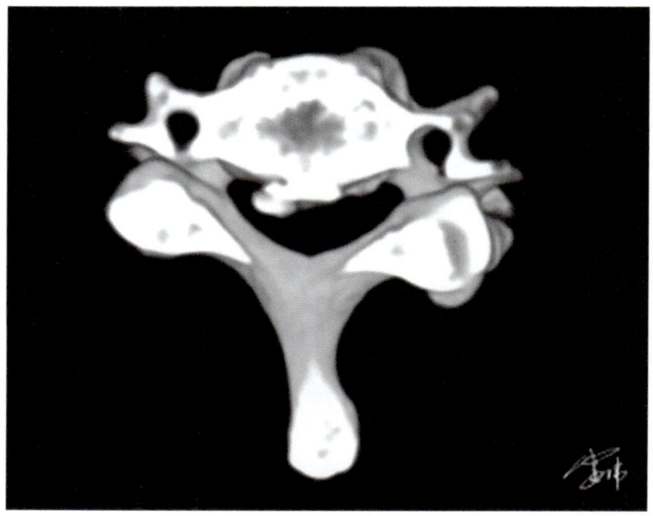

Fig. 7.17 The occupying lesion is asymmetric

drill bit, and the hinge plate is held firmly to the lamina with two screws. The laminoplasty is opened, and the lateral mass screw holes for the hinge plate are then drilled for two additional screws, firmly fixing the hinge in place.

9. Welding the hinge: the hinge graft

In general, the allograft is not placed in the hinge. If the cervical spine is unstable, the allograft can be placed in the hinge to maintain cervical spine stability (Fig. 7.35).

7.7 Clinical Cases

Case 1

Patient: A 44-year-old male complained of neck pain with numbness and weakness of the extremities for 3 years that had been aggravated for 3 months.

Diagnosis: Cervical myelopathy, cervical spine posterior longitudinal ligament ossification, and cervical vertebral spinal stenosis.

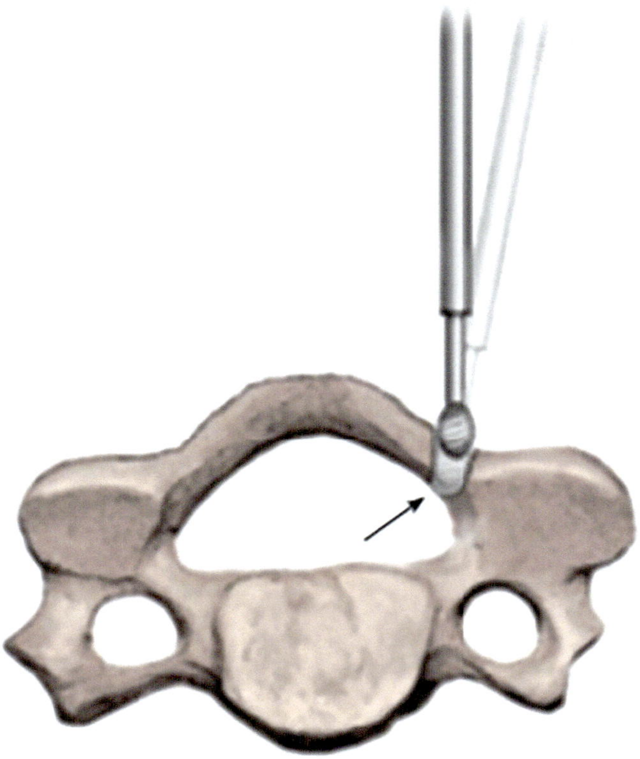

Fig. 7.18 Trough location

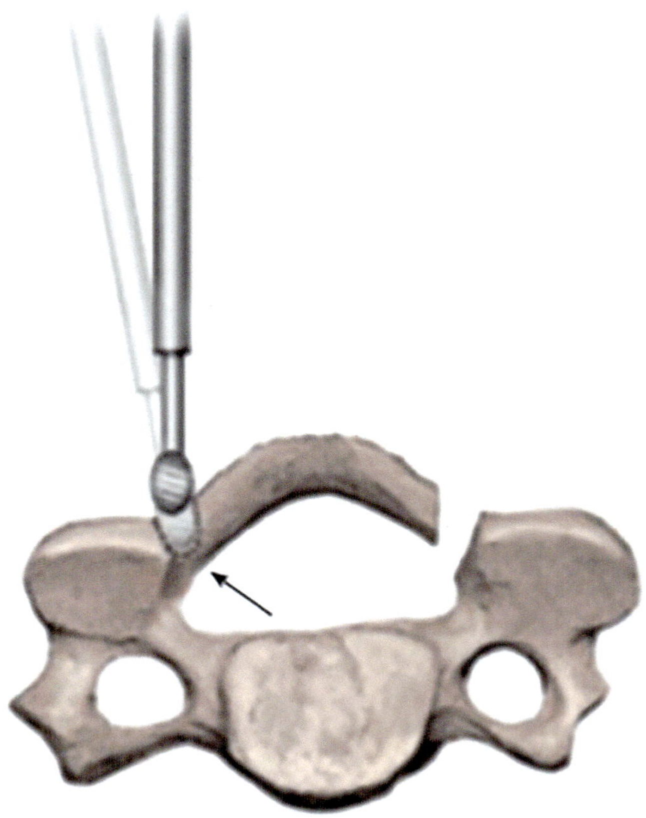

Fig. 7.19 Hinge location

Surgery: Cervical vertebral laminoplasty via the posterior approach, C3–C7 CENTERPIECE internal fixation.

Imaging data: See Figs. 7.36, 7.37, 7.38, 7.39, 7.40, 7.41, and 7.42.

Caution: The excised cervical spinous processes are longitudinally split and trimmed and cut into allograft blocks.

Case 2

Patient: A 67-year-old male complained of limited range of motion of the extremities for 28 hours following trauma.

Diagnosis: Cervical myelopathy and cervical vertebral spinal stenosis.

Surgery: Cervical vertebral laminoplasty via the posterior approach and C3–C6 CENTERPIECE internal fixation.

Imaging data: See Fig. 7.43.

Case 3

Patient: A 2-year-old male complained of numbness of the extremities and difficulty walking for 6 months.

Diagnosis: Developmental cervical spinal stenosis.

Surgery: Cervical vertebral laminoplasty via the posterior approach and C3–C7 CENTERPIECE internal fixation (Figs. 7.44, 7.45, 7.46, 7.47, 7.48, 7.49, and 7.50).

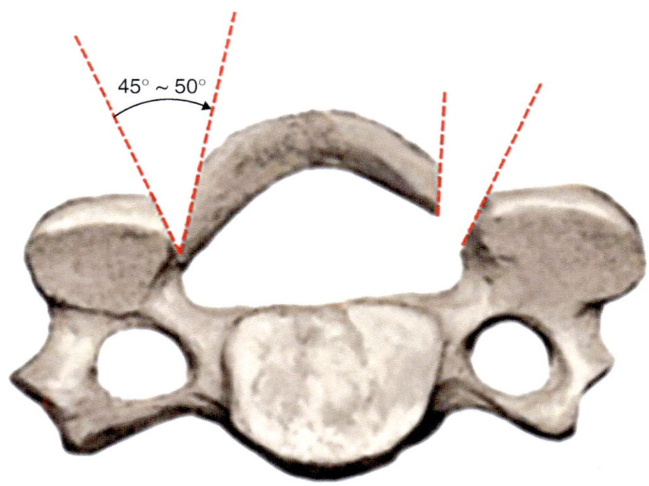

Fig. 7.20 Trough and hinge shape

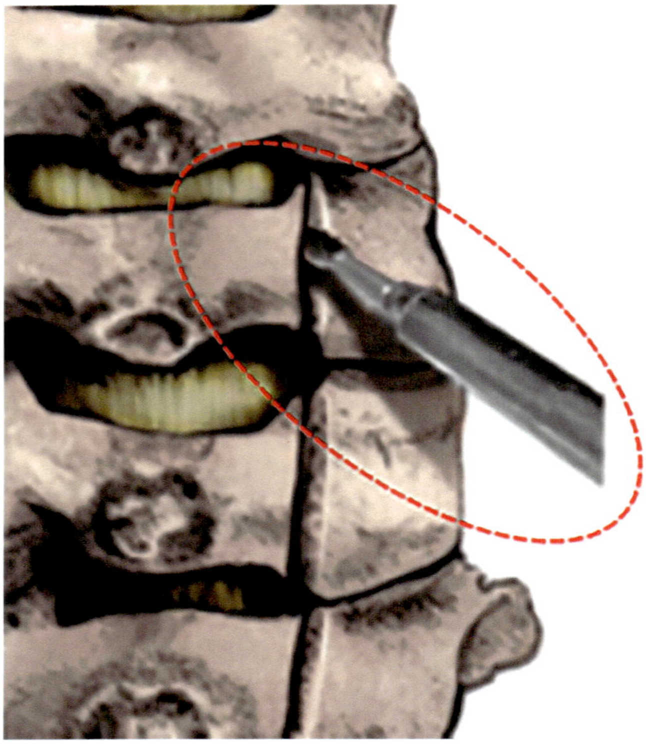

Fig. 7.21 Milling with a burr

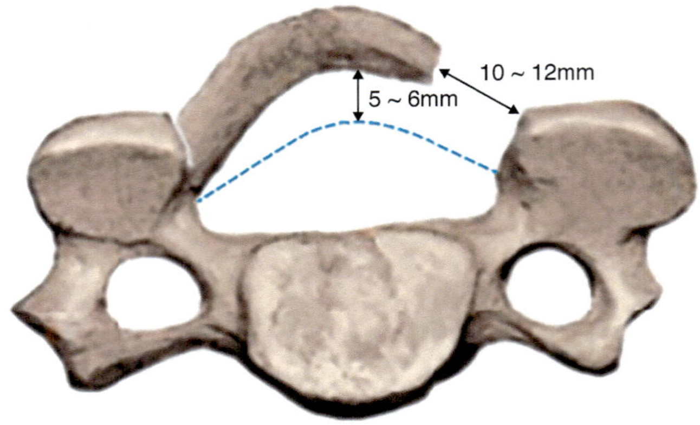

Fig. 7.22 The relationship between the open-door size and the spinal canal diameter. The ratio is approximately 2:1

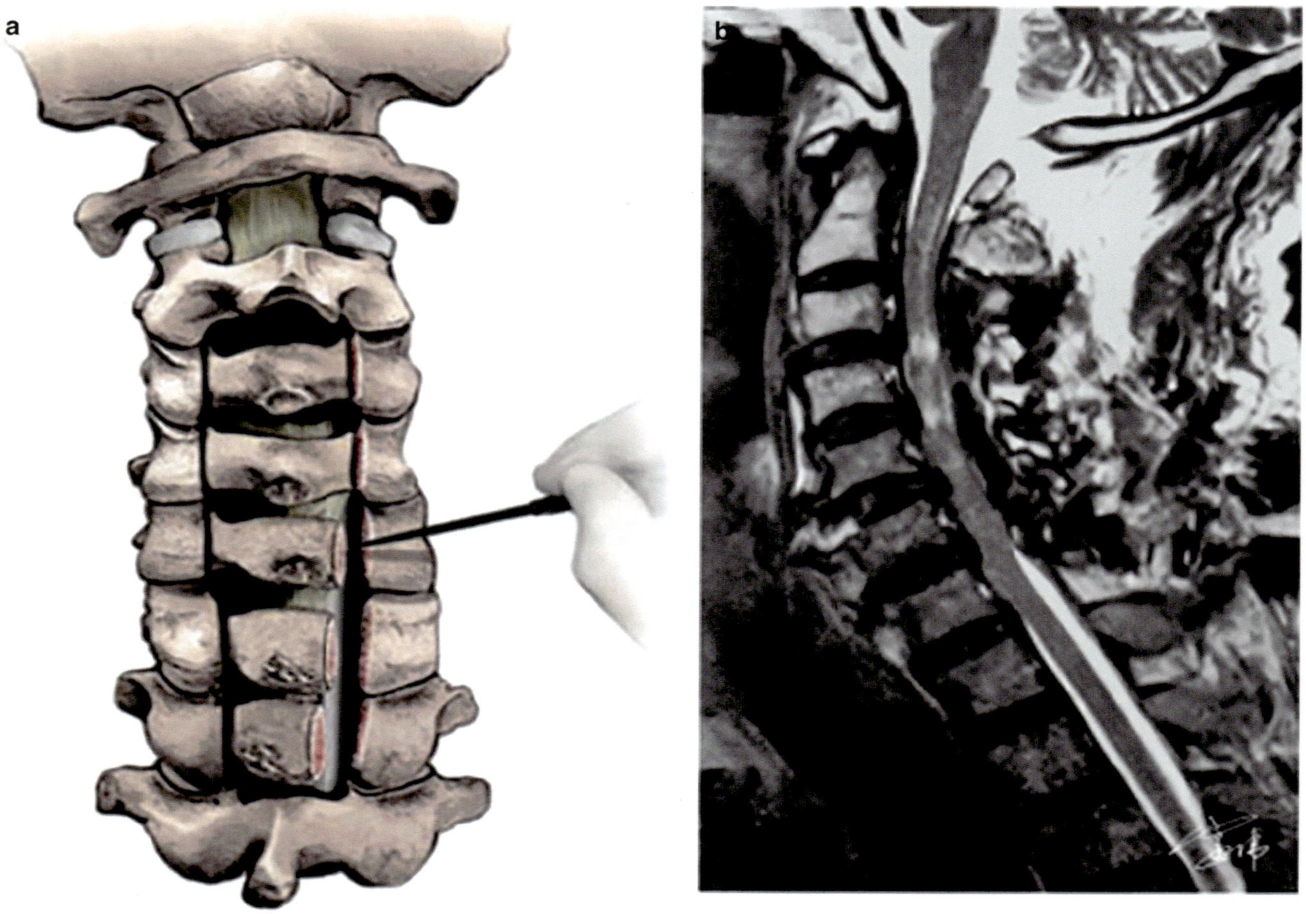

Fig. 7.23 Extent of the open door. (**a**) Open-door segments; (**b**) Diseased segments

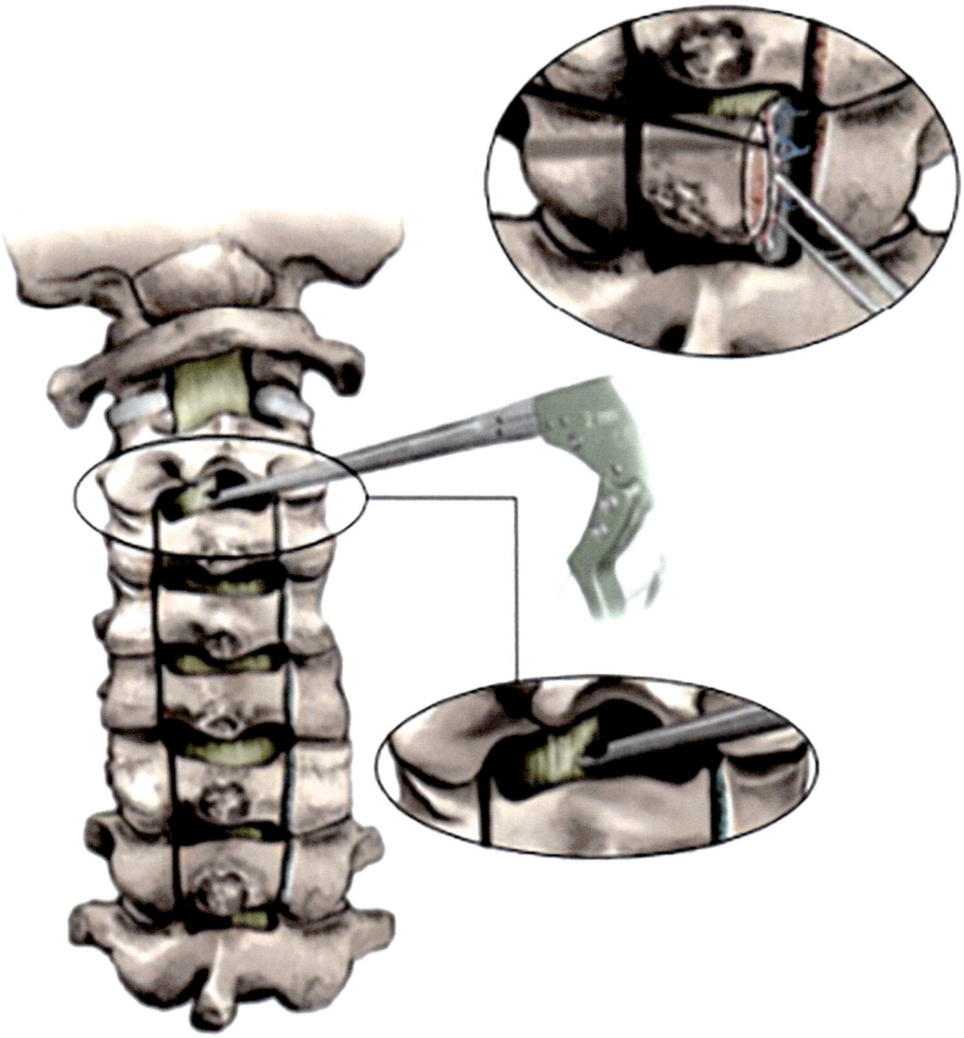

Fig. 7.24 Dissection of soft tissues

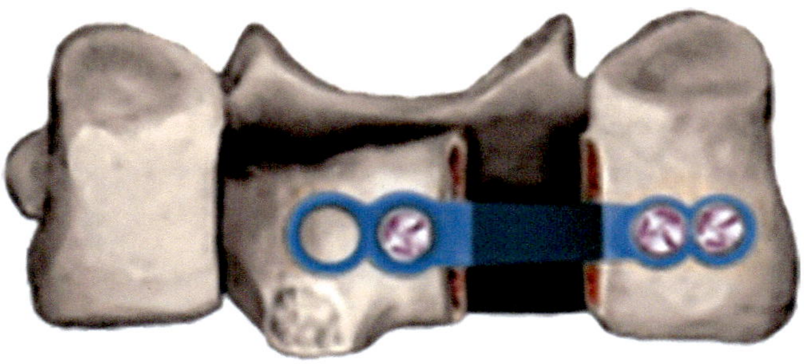

Fig. 7.25 Using the open-door plate

7.8 Intraoperative Cautions and Clinical Pearls

1. If the lamina has central break during removal of the spinous process with a Kerrison rongeur, the lamina can be excised for decompression or double-door laminoplasty can be done.

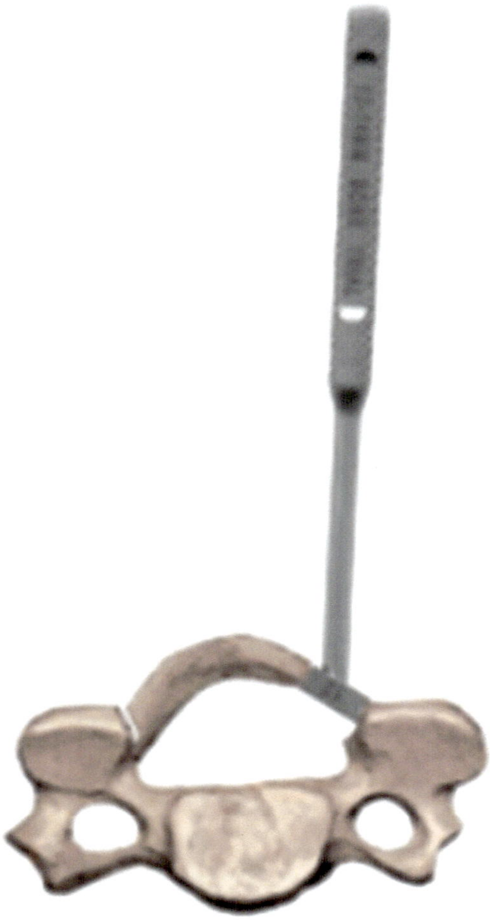

Fig. 7.26 Bone trials

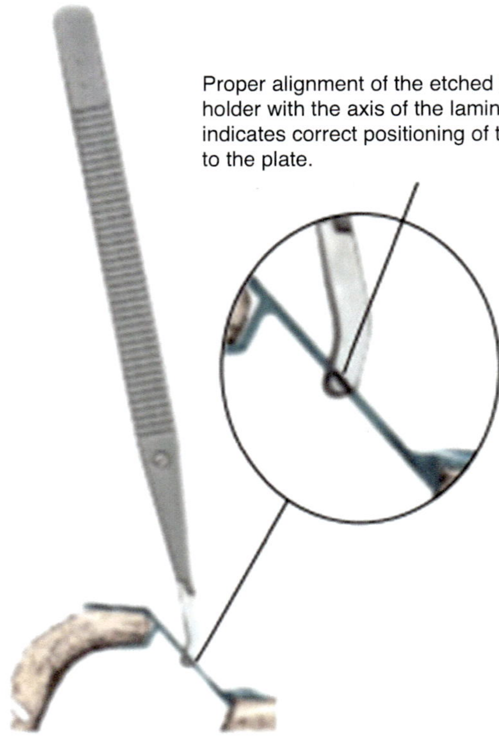

Fig. 7.27 Plate placement

2. If hinge breakage occurs or if breakage is impending, the hinge plate can be used for stabilization. Otherwise, the open door is prone to collapse and leads to surgical failure.
3. Complete open-door laminoplasty or alternative open-door and complete laminectomy for decompression can be performed during the surgery depending on the condition of the spinal canal.
4. The open-door plate or the graft plate or the two in combination can be used during the surgery depending on the condition of the spinal canal.
5. The position of the open door and the hinge should be properly selected in order to avoid abnormalities in spinal canal shape due to wrong open-door position and excessive elevation of the lamina (Fig. 7.51).

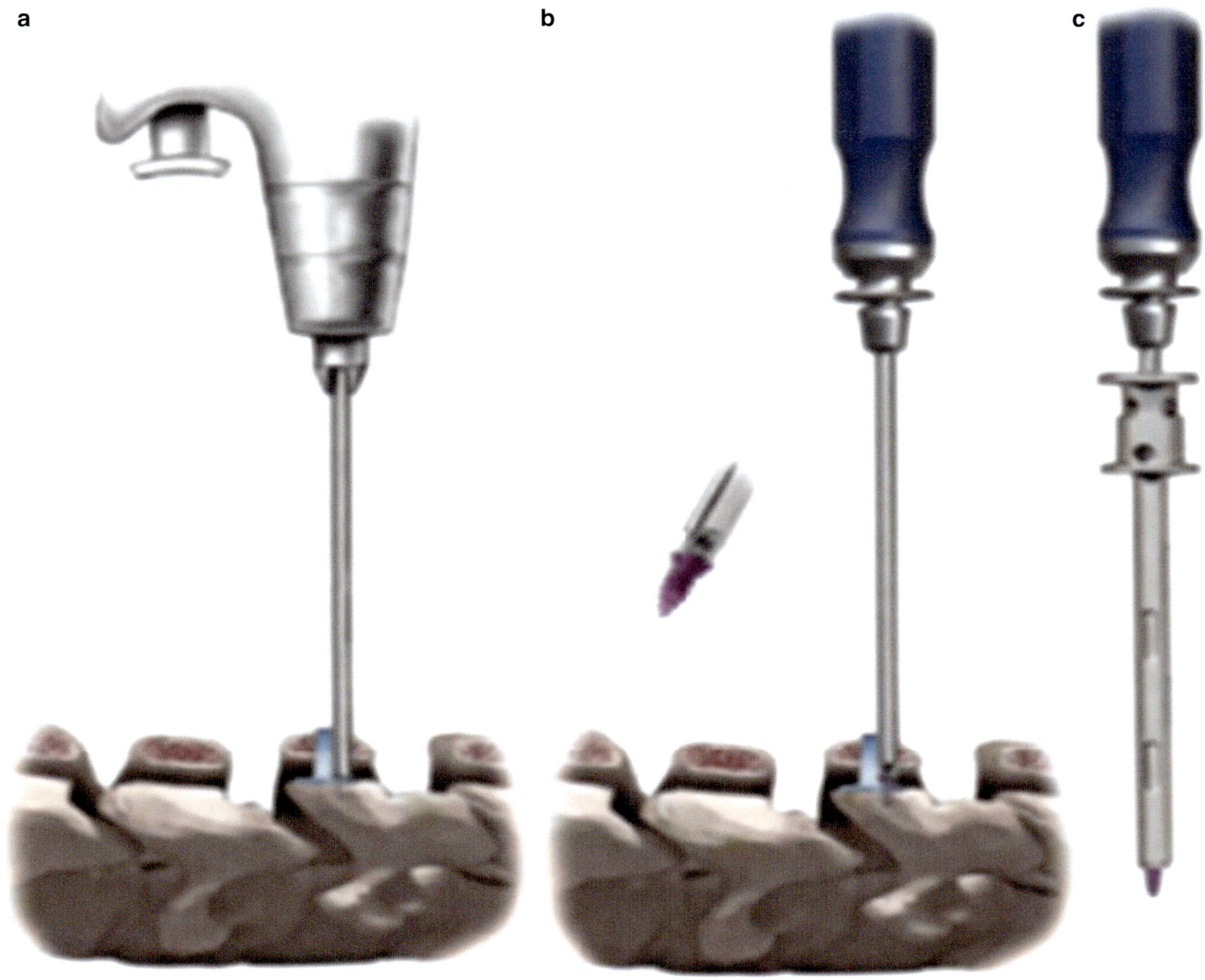

Fig. 7.28 Drill and screw insertion. (**a**) Drilling a hole; (**b**) Fixing the plate; (**c**) The screwdriver and sleeve

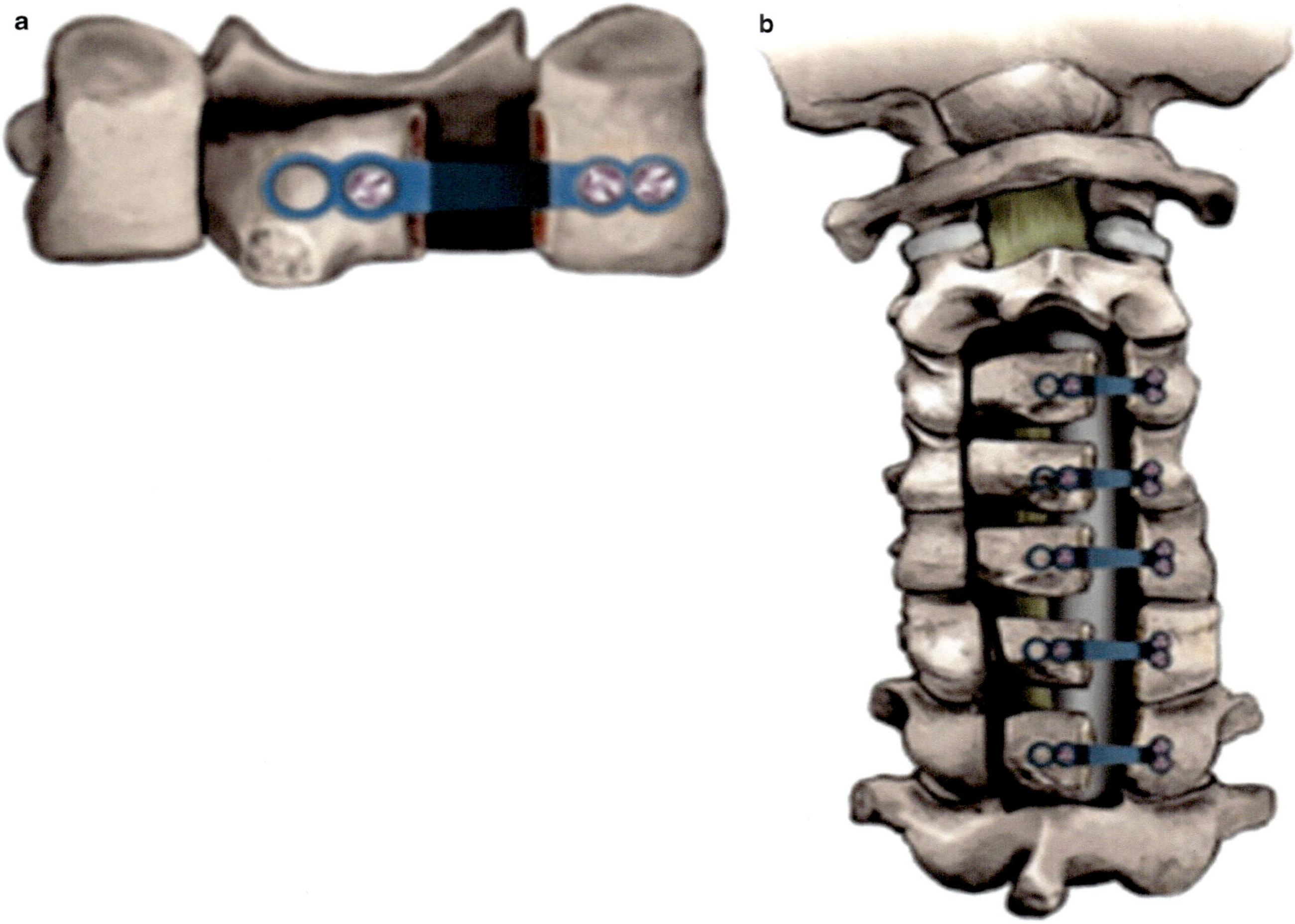

Fig. 7.29 Plate fixation. (**a**) The open-door plate; (**b**) The range of the open door

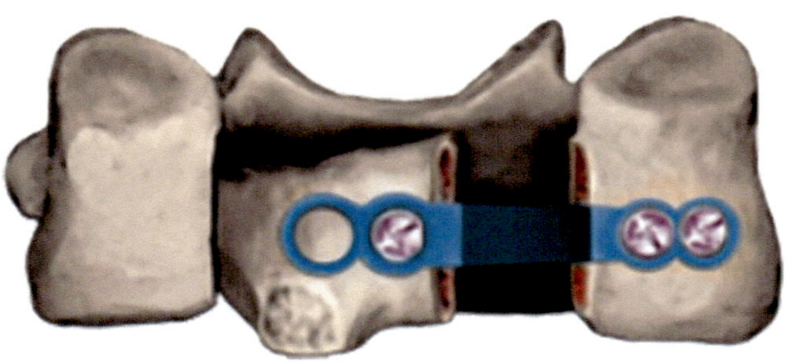

Fig. 7.30 The lateral hole plate

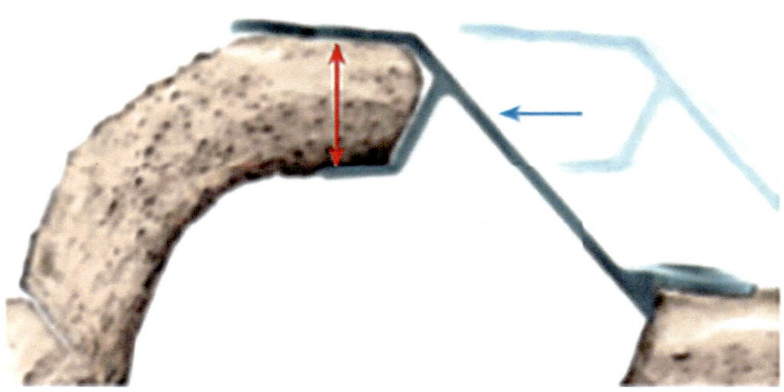

Fig. 7.31 The wide mouth plate

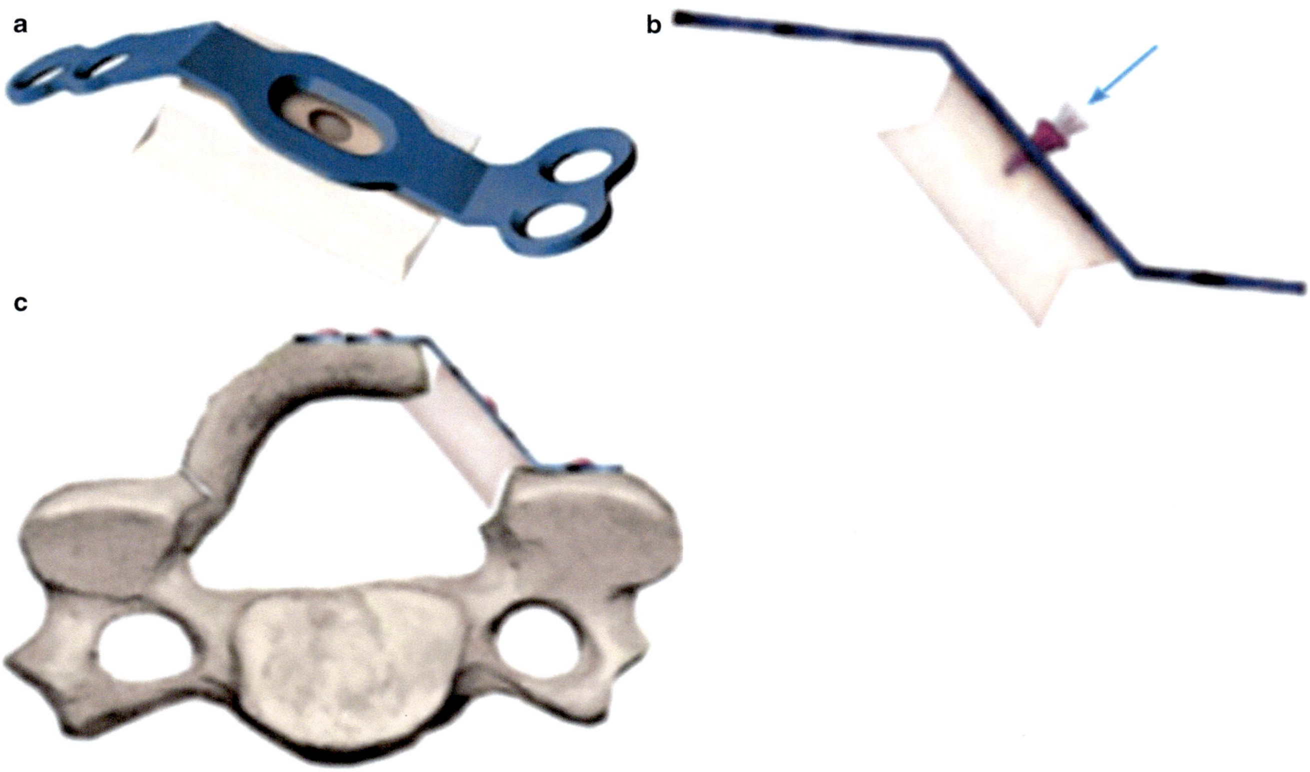

Fig. 7.32 Using the graft plate. (**a**) Choosing the allograft; (**b**) Securing the allograft; (**c**) Inserting the plate and allograft

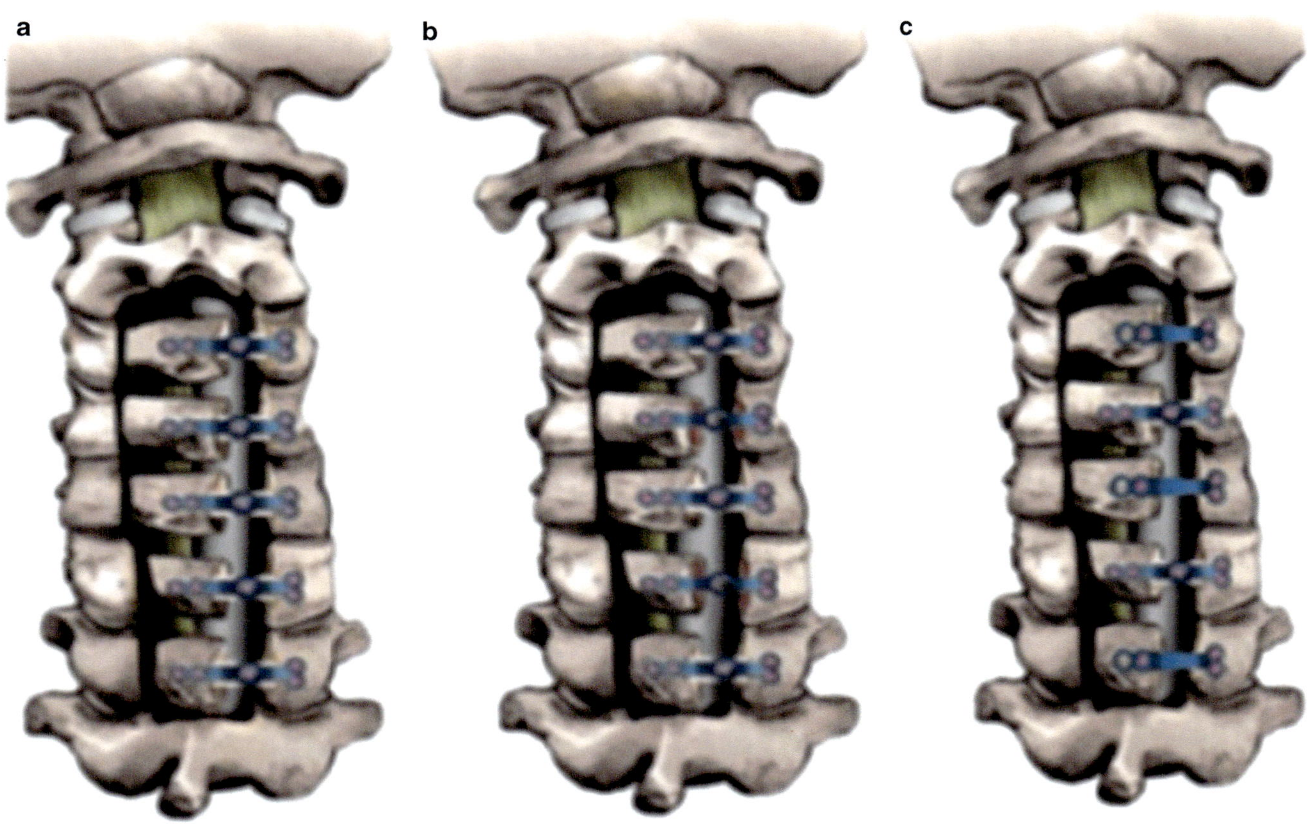

Fig. 7.33 Using the open-door plate. (**a**) The graft plate; (**b**) The graft plate in combination with the open-door plate; (**c**) The graft plate in combination with the open-door plate

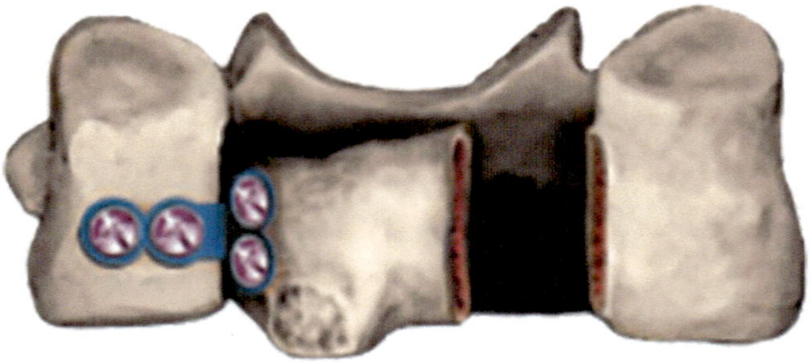

Fig. 7.34 Using the hinge plate

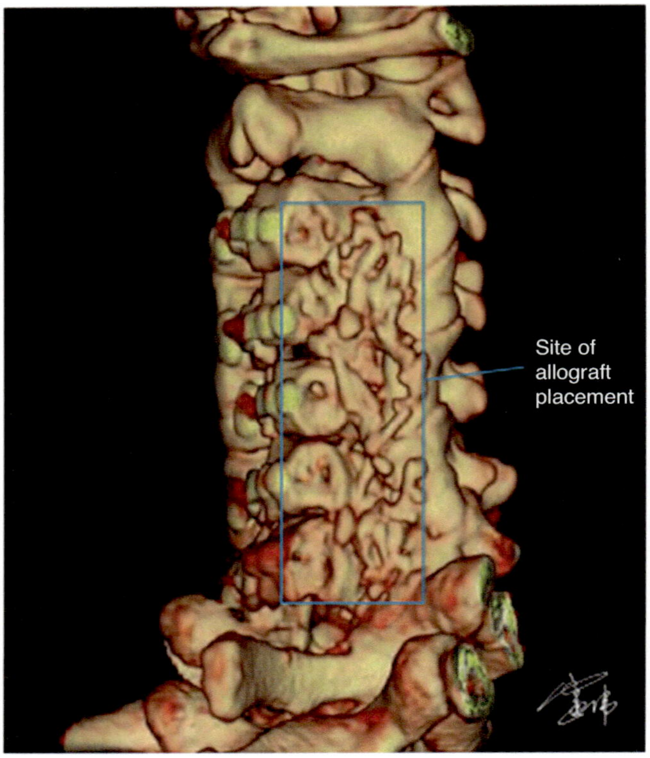

Fig. 7.35 The hinge graft

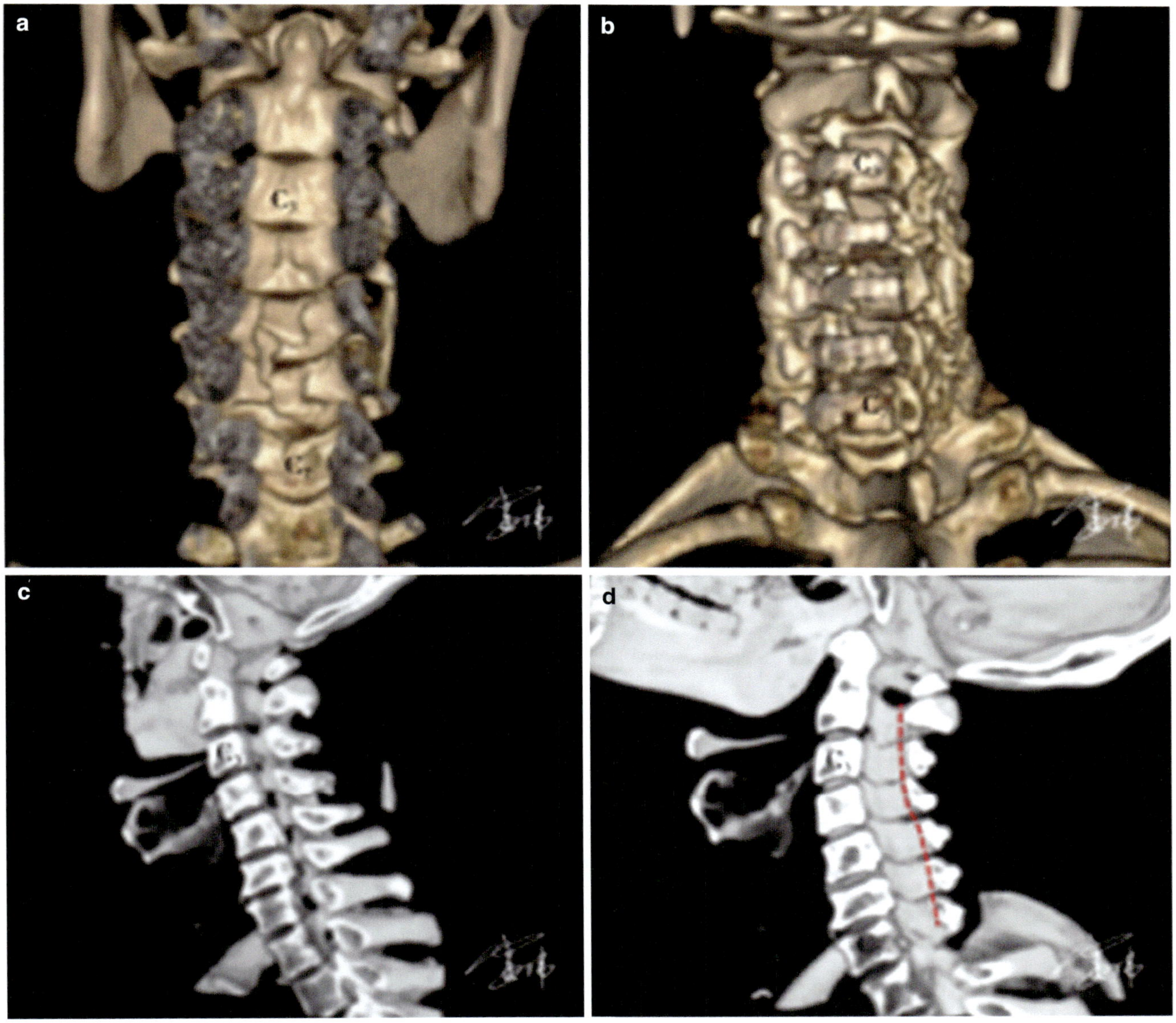

Fig. 7.36 Preoperative and postoperative CT 3D reconstruction images. (**a**) Preoperative split coronal view of the spine canal showing ossified longitudinal ligaments at C3–C7; (**b**) The posterior structures of the cervical spine postoperatively; (**c**) The preoperative split sagittal view of the spine canal; (**d**) The postoperative coronal view shows an enlarged spinal canal

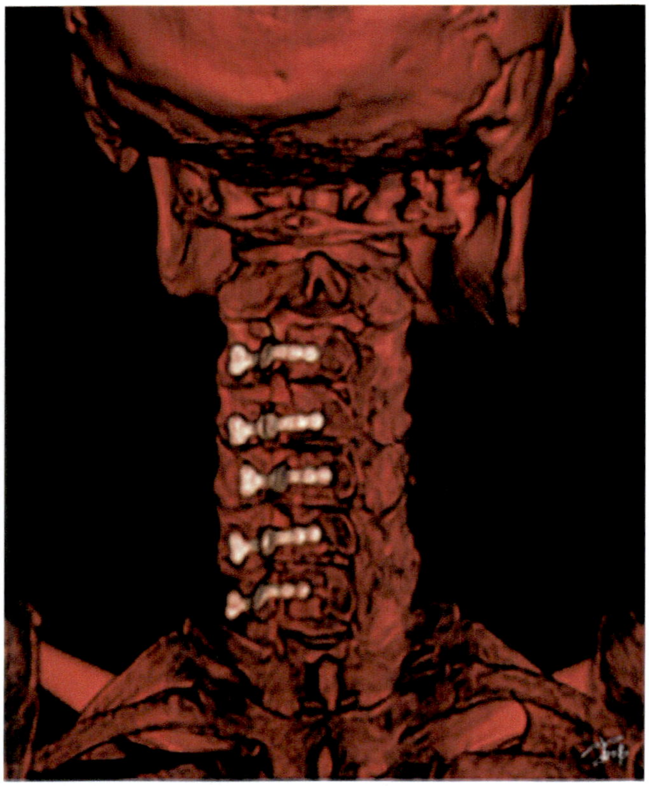

Fig. 7.37 Postoperative 3D reconstruction

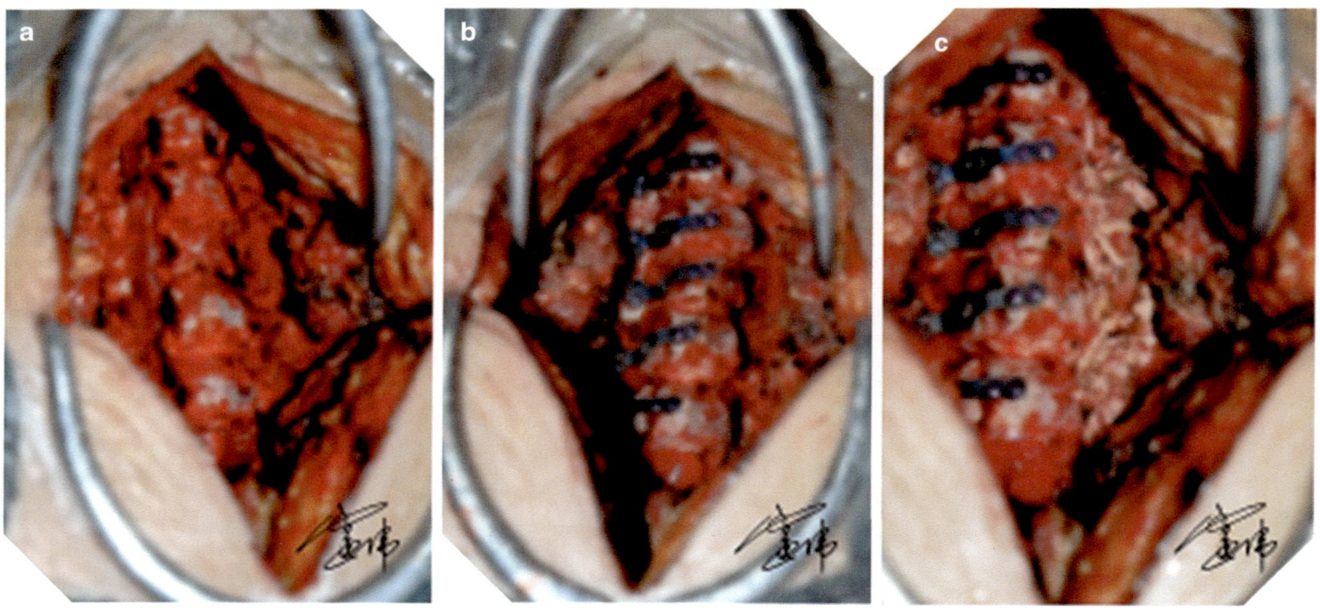

Fig. 7.38 Intraoperative images. (**a**) C3–C7 open door on the left side; (**b**) Graft and steel plate fixation; (**c**) Graft on the hinge side

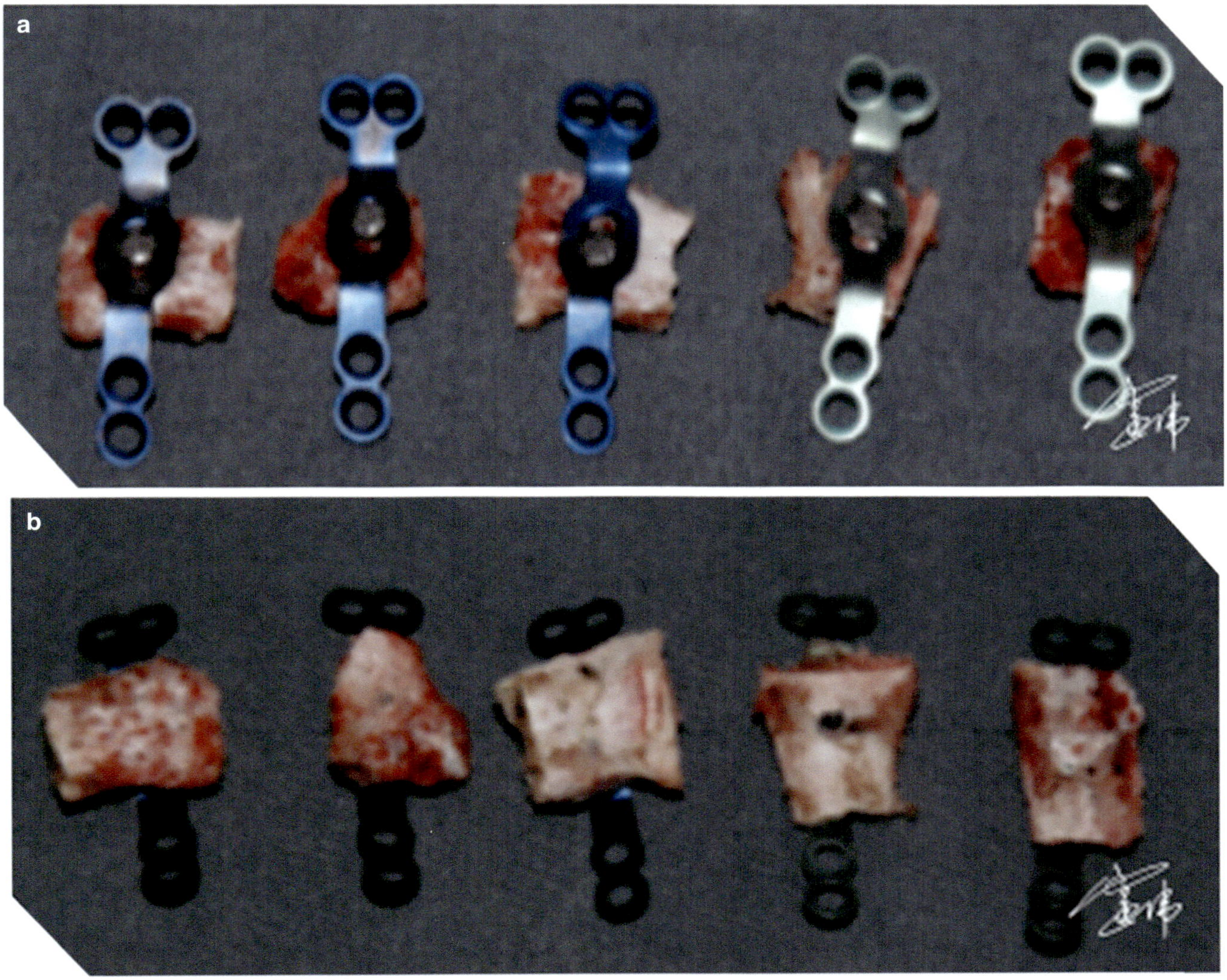

Fig. 7.39 The graft plate and allografts. (**a**) The dorsal view; (**b**) The ventral view

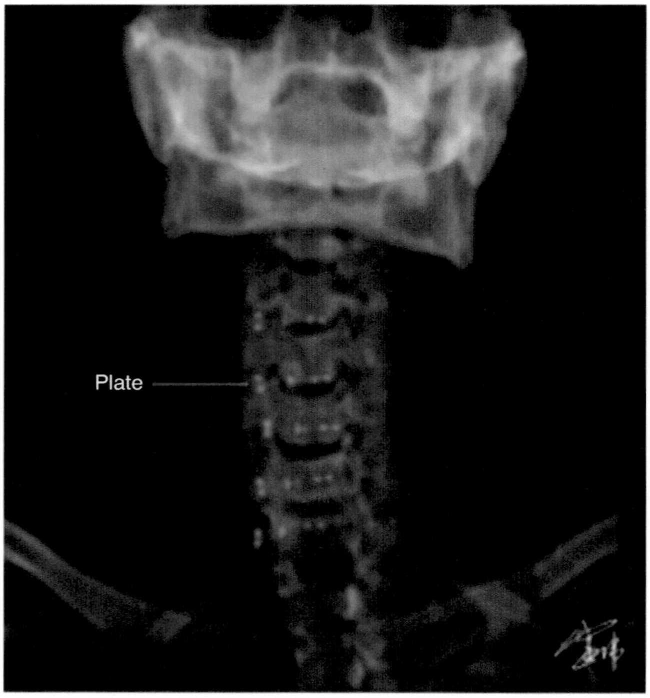

Fig. 7.40 CT 3D reconstruction (*front view*)

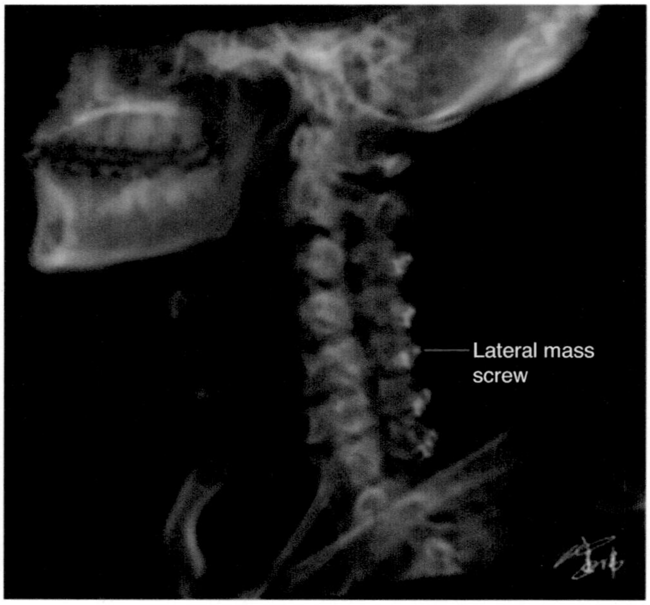

Fig. 7.41 CT 3D reconstruction (*lateral view*)

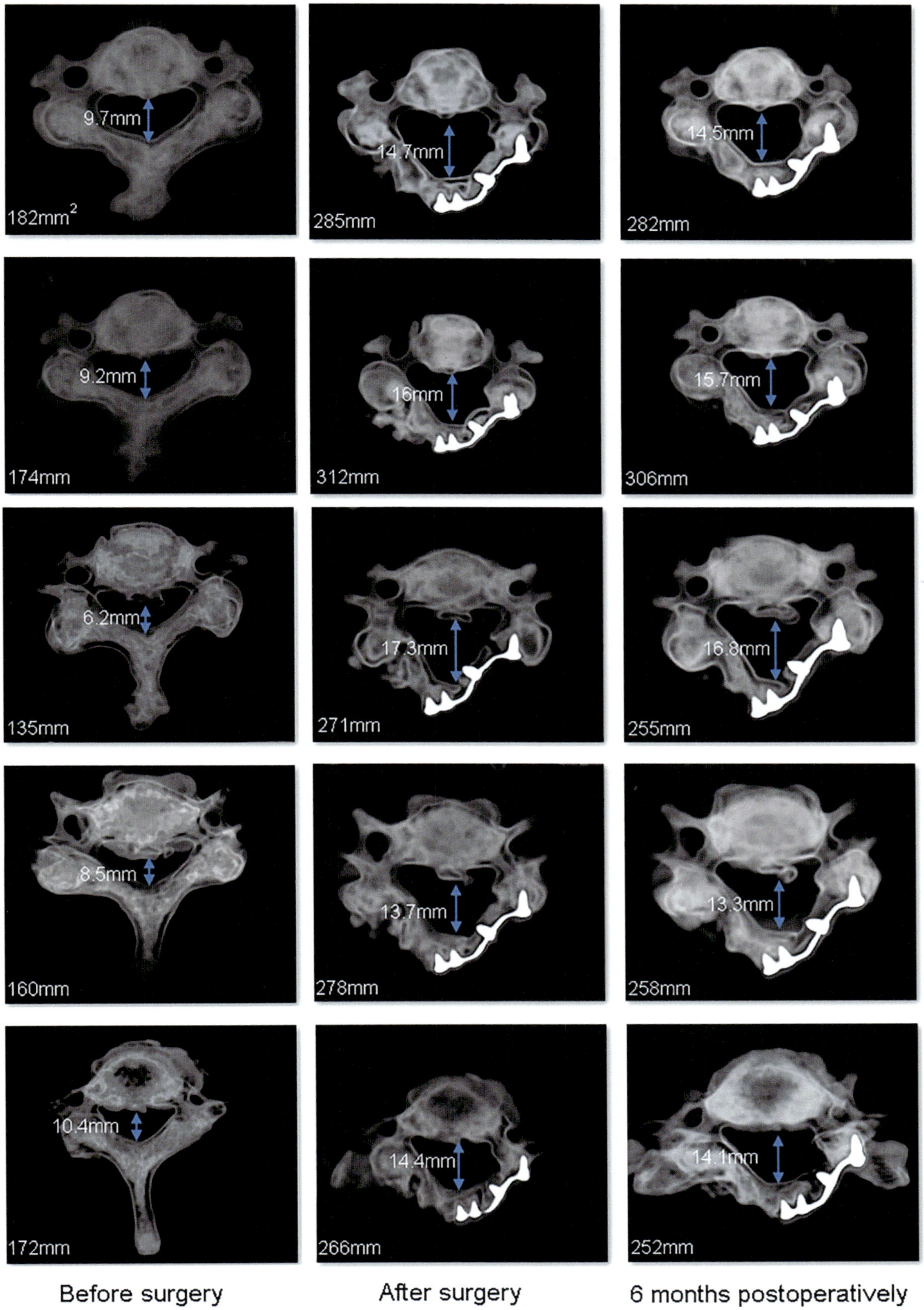

Fig. 7.42 Preoperative and postoperative spinal canal diameter and area

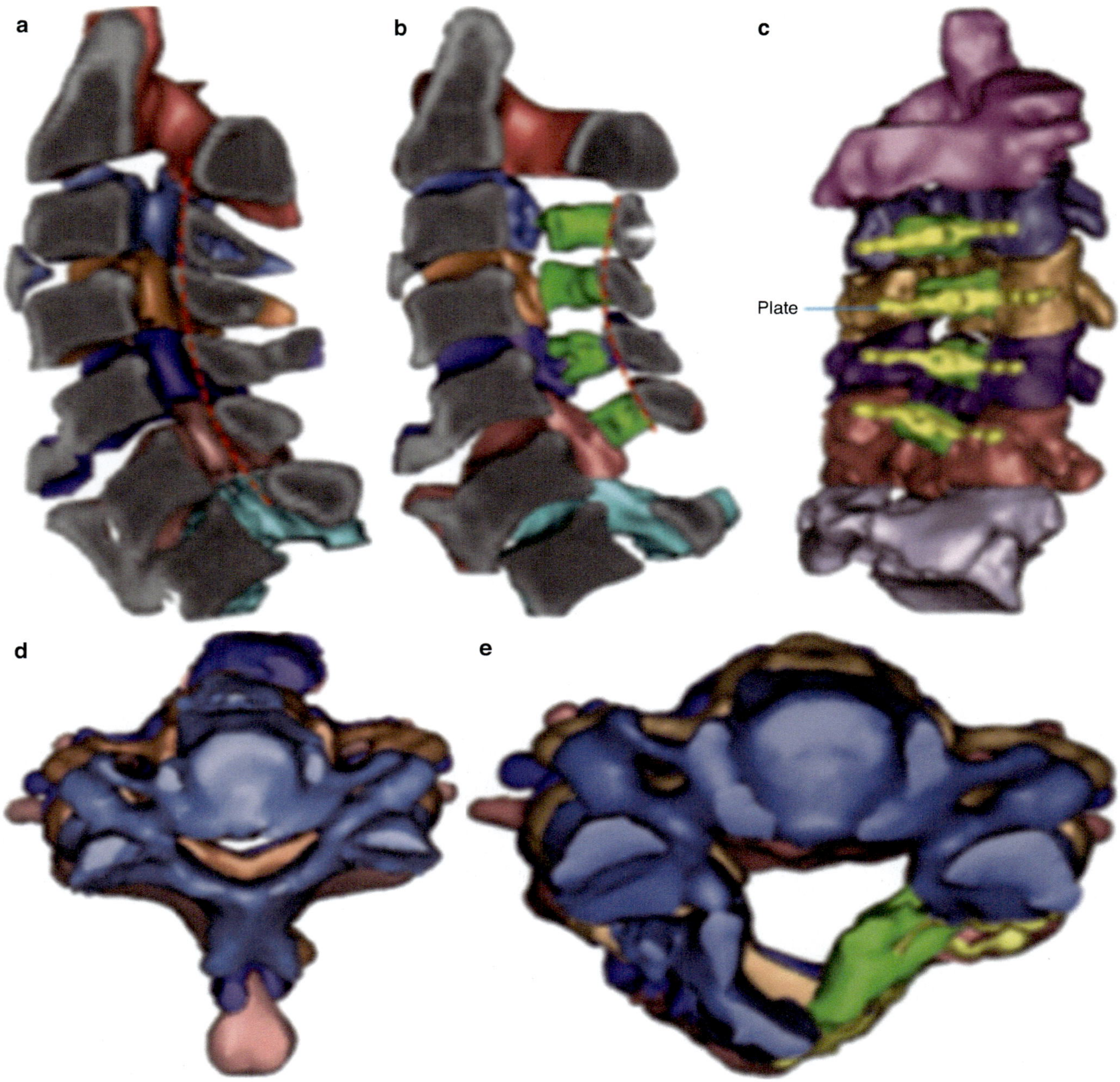

Fig. 7.43 Preoperative and postoperative CT 3D reconstruction images. (**a**) The sagittal split view of the spinal canal preoperatively. (**b**) The sagittal split view of the spinal canal postoperatively. (**c**) The complete view of the open-door vertebra postoperatively (*oblique view*). (**d**) The overlooking view of C3–C6 spinal canal preoperatively and (**e**) postoperatively

2. Ito M, Nagahama K. Laminoplasty for cervical myelopathy. Global Spine J. 2012;2(3):187–94.
3. Heller JG, Raich AL, Dettori JR, Riew KD. Comparative effectiveness of different types of cervical laminoplasty. Evid Based Spine Care J. 2013;4(2):105–15.
4. Benglis DM, Guest JD, Wang MY. Clinical feasibility of minimally invasive cervical laminoplasty. Neurosurg Focus. 2008;25(2):E3.
5. Duetzmann S, Cole T, Ratliff JK. Cervical laminoplasty developments and trends, 2003–2013: a systematic review. J Neurosurg Spine. 2015;23(1):24–34.
6. Kurokawa R, Kim P. Cervical Laminoplasty: the history and the future. Neurol Med Chir (Tokyo). 2015;55(7):529–39.

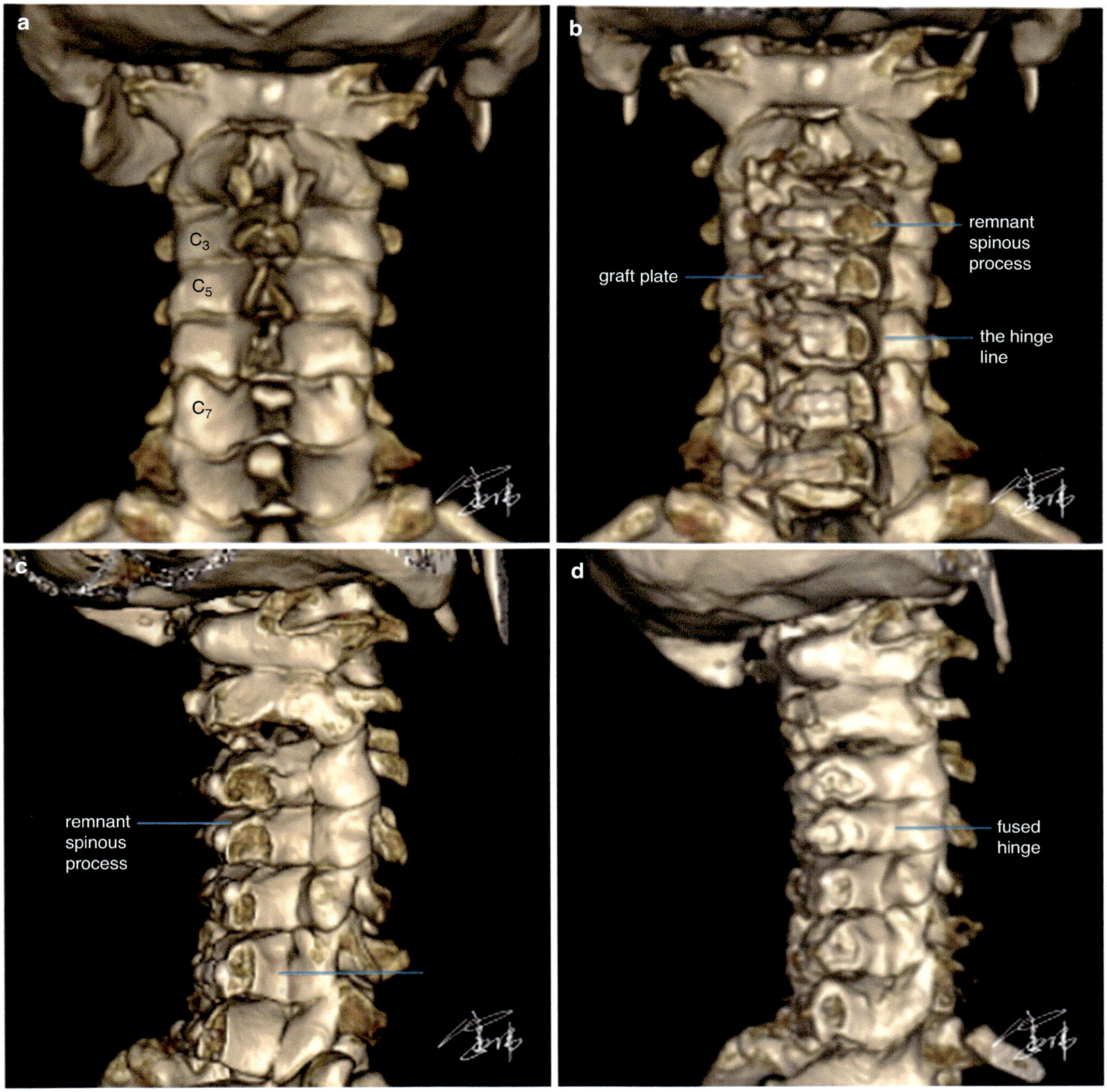

Fig. 7.44 Preoperative CT 3D reconstruction images (**a**) and CT 3D reconstruction images of posterior structures of the cervical spine postoperatively (**b**, **c**, **d**)

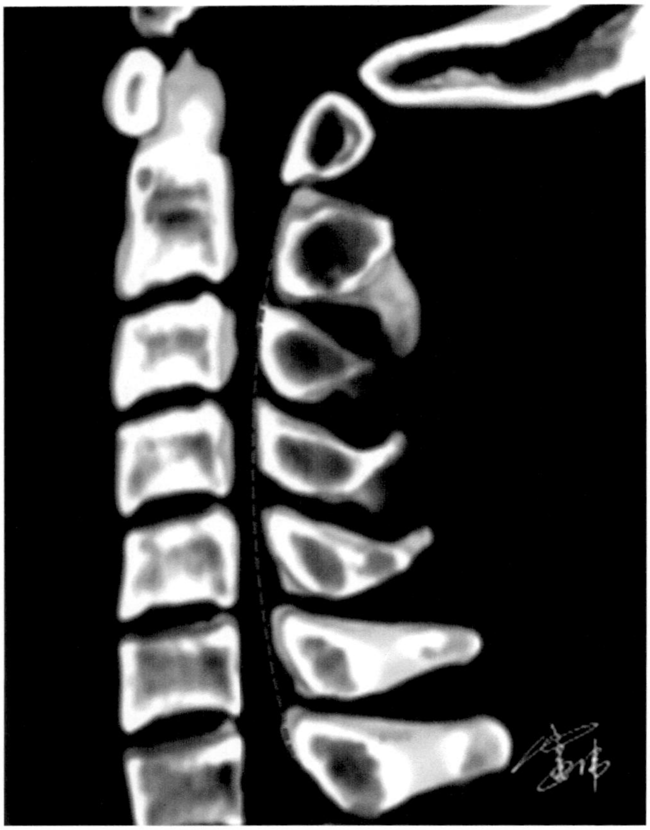

Fig. 7.45 Spinal stenosis before surgery

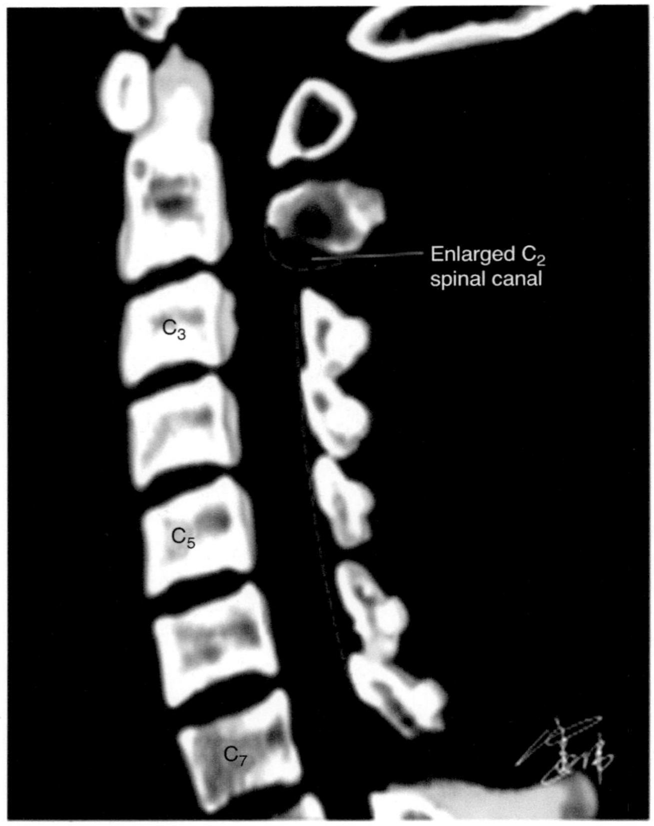

Fig. 7.46 The enlarged spinal canal following surgery (C3–C7 open-door plasty and C2–C7 partial laminoplasty open-door decompression)

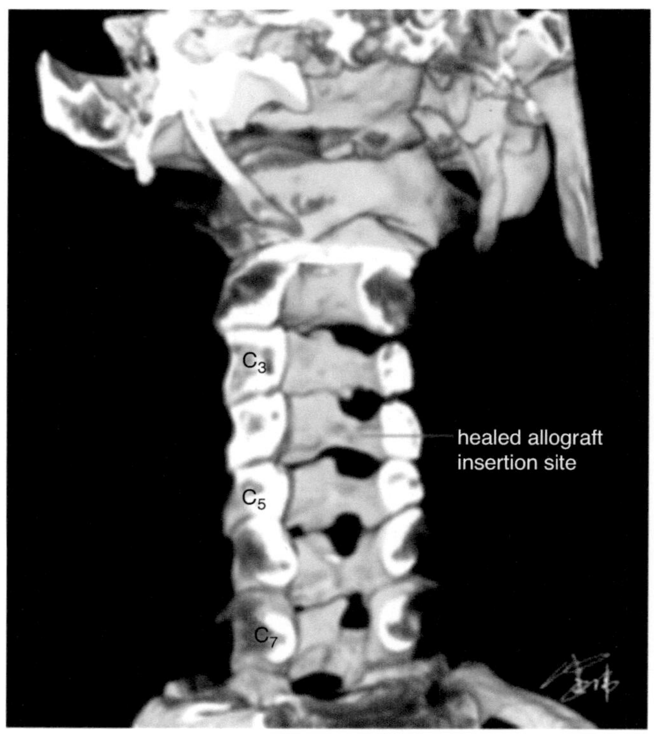

Fig. 7.47 The C3–C7 allograft has healed 6 months following surgery (the split coronal view of the spinal canal rotated 30°)

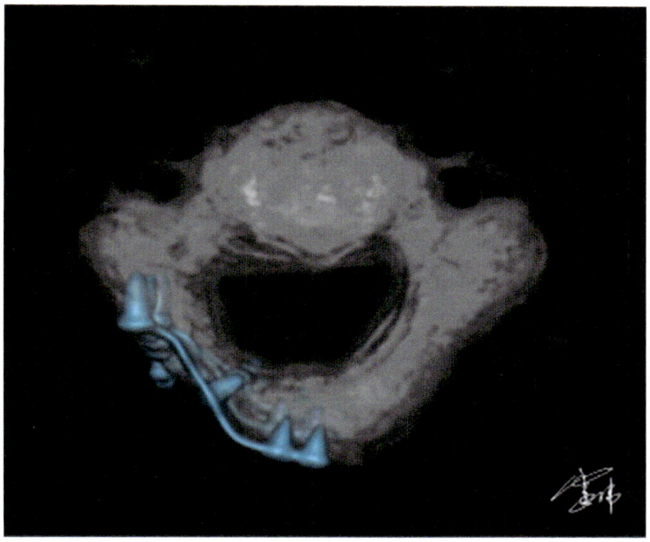

Fig. 7.48 The overlooking view of C3–C7 spinal canal

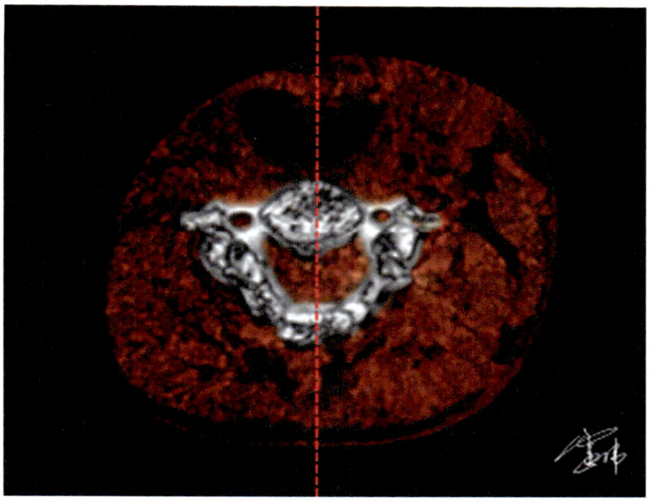

Fig. 7.49 Complete symmetrical spinal canal reconstruction helps reduce the occurrence of postoperative axial pain of the cervical spine

Fig. 7.50 Preoperative and postoperative anteroposterior diameter and area of the spinal canal

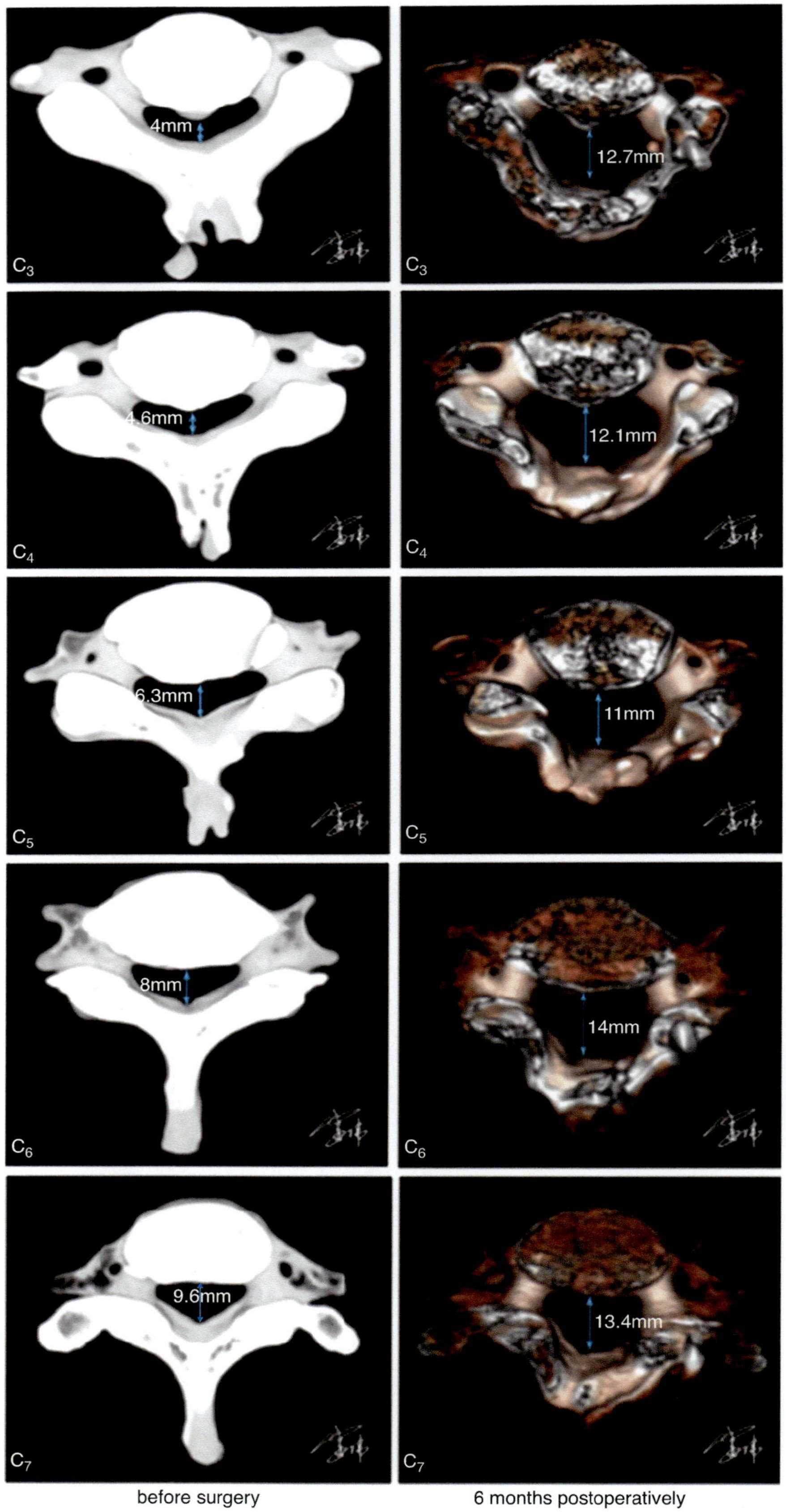

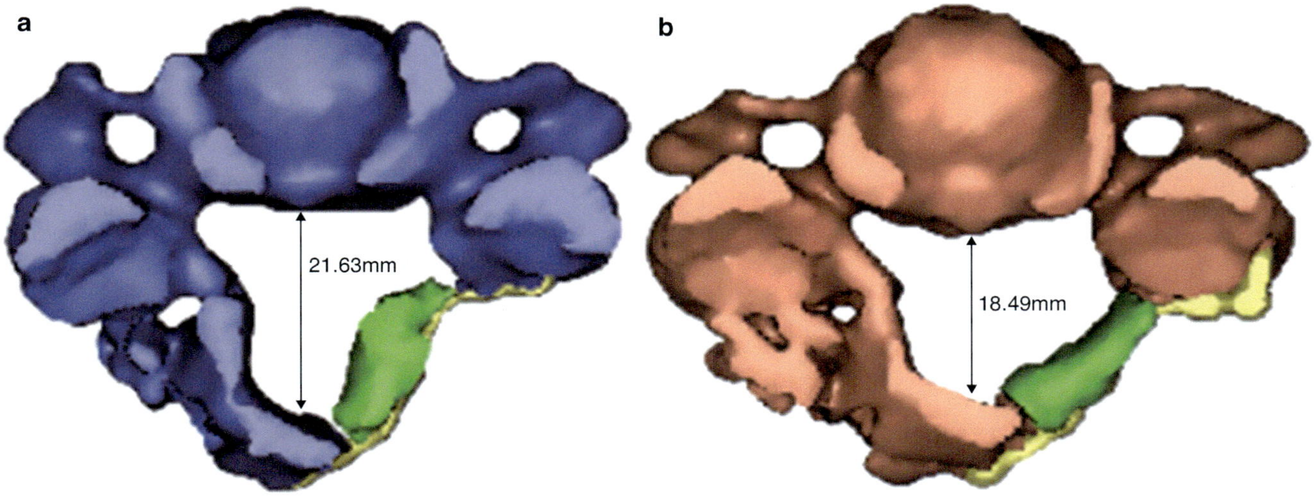

Fig. 7.51 Inappropriately shaped spinal canal and excessive elevation of the lamina. (**a**) C3 postoperatively; (**b**) C4 postoperatively

7.9 Postoperative Management

The postoperative patient can be placed in the supine position and wear neck collar to prevent undue pressure on the posterior cervical region. The patient can ambulate 2–3 days postoperatively under the protection of the neck collar and after removal of the drainage tube and start rehabilitation training. The neck collar is removed approximately 6 weeks postoperatively.

Reference

1. Ratliff JK, Cooper PR. Cervical laminoplasty: a critical review. J Neurosurg. 2003 Apr;98(3 Suppl):230–8.

8 Surgical Techniques for Pedicle Screw Fixation of the Thoracic Spine

Xiong Zhao, Yi Huan, and Wei Lei

Abstract

The technique of posterior thoracic spine screw fixation was developed to reconstruct the stability of the thoracic spine after decompression, tumor resection, trauma, or congenital scoliosis. This technique is an essential method for spine surgeon. There are several different screw entry methods for thoracic spine. In this chapter, we review the screw entry method and propose our own method for thoracic spine. At the same time through the combination of specific cases explained in the operation of the detailed steps and precautions.

Keywords

Thoracic spine · Pedicle screw · Entry site

8.1 Pedicle Screw Fixation Technique for the Thoracic Spine: A Historical Perspective

1. In 1976, Roy-Camille [1] developed the thoracic screw placement technique, which is now called the Roy-Camille technique (Fig. 8.1a, b).
2. In 2004, Kim et al. [2] reviewed the data of 394 patients who received totally 3204 thoracic pedicle screws and listed the recommended placement sites for all thoracic pedicle screws. The screw entry site in the lower thoracic spine (T10–T12) lies at the junction of the bisected transverse process and lamina at or just medial to the lateral aspect of the pars pedicle. The screw entry site in the mid-thoracic spine (T7–T9) lies at the junction of the vertical line to the lateral edge of the midportion of the base of the superior articular process and the horizontal line of the proximal edge of the transverse process. The entry site moves toward a more lateral position as one proceeds toward the more proximal thoracic region. The screw entry site in the lower thoracic spine (T10–T12) lies at the junction of the horizontal line of the bisected transverse process and the vertical line to the lateral edge of the lateral pars (Fig. 8.2).
3. In 2014, Fennell [3] proposed a novel method for thoracic pedicle screw placement. The key technical points are as follows: The uniform entry point for pedicle screw of any segment of the thoracic spine pedicle is 3 mm caudal to the junction of the lateral margin of the superior articular facet and the transverse process. The screw trajectory/direction is vertical in the sagittal plane to the physiological curve in the plane of the vertebral body. The medial inclination angle of the pedicle screw is approximately 30° at T1 and T2 and 20° at T3–T12 (Figs. 8.3 and 8.4).

8.2 Surgical Anatomy of the Pedicles of the Thoracic Spine (Figs. 8.5, 8.6, 8.7, and 8.8)

8.3 Data in Relation to the Pedicles of the Thoracic Spine

The thoracic pedicle is projected superoposterior to the vertebral body and its height is larger than its width (Tables 8.1 and 8.2). The medial wall of the thoracic pedicle is the thickest. The axis of the pedicle is projected medial to the lateral margin of the superior articular facet and superior to the bisected line of the transverse process. In general, the pedicle medial inclination progressively declines from T1 to T12. The articulate thoracic articular facet is obviously different from that of the cervical spine and the lumbar spine and is more coronal. Because the diameter of the thoracic pedicle is

X. Zhao · W. Lei (✉)
Department of Orthopedics, Xijing Hospital, Air Force Medical University, Xi'an, Shaanxi, China
e-mail: zhangyang@fmmu.edu.cn; leiwei@fmmu.edu.cn

Y. Huan
Department of Radiology, Xijing Hospital, Air Force Military Medical University, Xi'an, China

W. Lei, Y. Yan (eds.), *Internal Fixation of the Spine*, https://doi.org/10.1007/978-981-16-1562-7_8

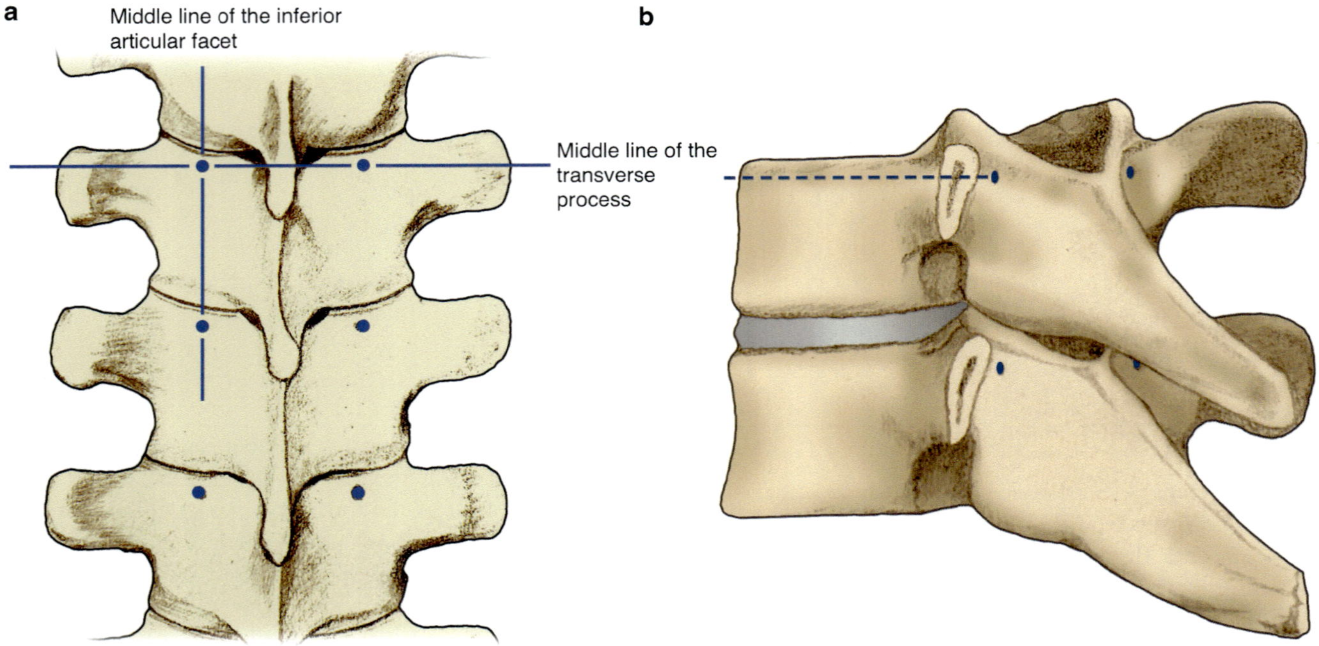

Fig. 8.1 Pedicle entrance point in the thoracic spine is situated at the crossing of two lines, at the middle of the inferior articular facet, and the middle of the insertion of the transverse process. This point is 1 mm below the facet joint

noticeably smaller than that of the lumbar pedicle, the transverse process has wide variations. After thoracic pedicle screw placement, there is a high risk of penetration through or disruption of the cortex, especially above T10, and the risk of injury to the spinal cord also likely markedly increases. Apart from inappropriately sized screw diameter, these increased risks may be related to inappropriate selection of screw entry points and direction (Figs. 8.9, 8.10, 8.11, 8.12, and 8.13).

8.4 Determination of Thoracic Pedicle Screw Entry Points (Fig. 8.14)

There are many methods for thoracic pedicle screw placement, and currently there is not a consensus approach. The following two methods are commonly used:

In the Roy-Camille method, the entry point lies at the junction of the transverse line bisecting the transverse process and an imaginary line bisecting the superior articular facet joint or the inter-articular space. This technique is suitable for vertical screw insertion. The medial inclination angle is small and the method is surgically challenging.

Our methods: Because the thoracic transverse process is not level and has a certain angle with the midline of the spine, and because it also has wide variations, the transverse process can be viewed as an entity from the base to the lateral margin. The transverse process can be divided into equal parts. The junction of the mid- and upper one third and an imaginary line from the lateral margin of the inferior articular facet joint of the adjacent superior vertebral body can be used as the screw entry point.

Thoracic pedicle screw placement typically starts from the most distally and neutrally rotated spine and progresses cephalad. The starting screw entry point of T12 is at the junction of the bisected transverse process and lamina at the lateral border of the pars. As one proceeds upward toward the mid-thoracic region (T7_T9), the screw entry points become more medial and cephalad and are at the junction of the line traversing the superior margin of the transverse process and the lateral edge of the midportion of the base of the superior articular process. Finally, the screw entry point of T1 is at the junction of the bisected transverse process and lamina at the lateral border of the pars A screw is placed at each level in succession from distal to proximal in the thoracic spine, and fine adjustments are made to the trajectory of the next screw base on the previous level screw or the contralateral screw.

Though the transverse process is a reliable marker for pedicle placement in the lumbar spine, this is only moderately reliable in the thoracic spine as the transverse processes are varied widely. Therefore, partial laminectomy and pedicle screw placement under direct vision can be a safe choice.

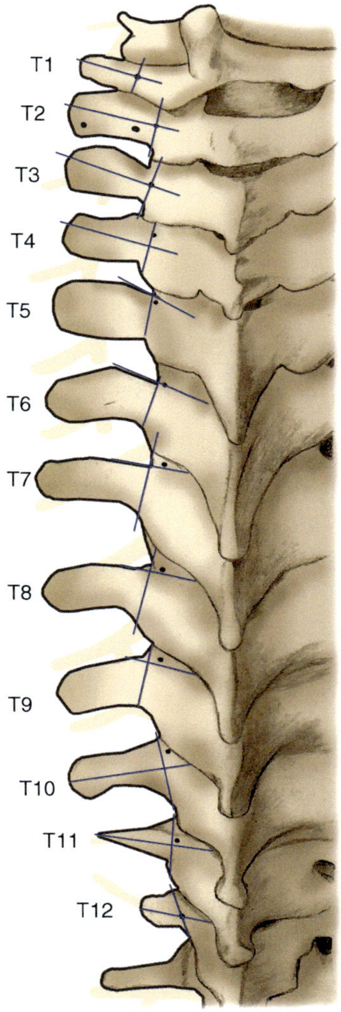

Fig. 8.2 Pedicle screw starting points distribution in the thoracic vertebral body. Proximal thoracic, junction of the bisected transverse process and lamina at the lateral pars; mid-thoracic, junction of the proximal edge of the transverse process and lamina, where it meets the lamina and superior facet, just lateral to the midportion of the base of the superior articular process; lower thoracic, junction of the bisected transverse process and lamina at or just medial to the lateral aspect of the pars

8.5 Thoracic Pedicle Screw Entry Angles

The pedicle medial inclination angle progressively declines from T1 to T12. The upper thoracic pedicle screw should form a medial inclination angle of 10–20° in the sagittal plane, and the mid- and lower thoracic pedicle screw should form a medial inclination angle of 0° in the sagittal plane.

Ebraheim proposed that T1_T2, T3_T11, and T12 pedicle screws should form a medial inclination angle of 30–40, 20–25, and 10° in the sagittal plane, respectively. The horizontal plane is parallel to the superior and inferior endplate (Figs. 8.15, 8.16, and 8.17).

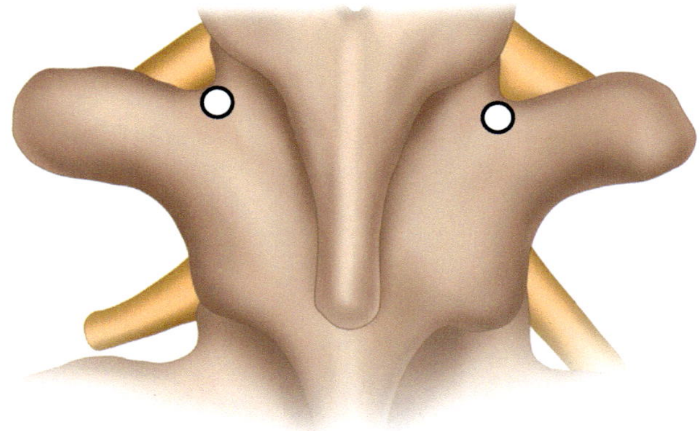

Fig. 8.3 The entry point is 3 mm caudal to the junction of the lateral margin of the superior articulating process and the transverse process

8.6 Thoracic Pedicle Screw Entry Depths

The thoracic pedicle screw entry depth gradually increases as one proceeds down the spine. In general, an entry depth of 35–40 mm should be chosen. Intraoperative probing and lateral X-ray examination allows precise determination of screw entry depth, which should not exceed 80% of the anteroposterior diameter of the vertebral body (Fig. 8.18).

8.7 Determination of the Diameters of Thoracic Pedicle Screws

The following screw diameters are chosen: 3.5–4.0 mm for T1_T5, 4.0–5.0 mm for T6_T10, and 5.5–6.5 mm for T11_T12.

8.8 Surgical Procedures

1. Selection of entry sites (Figs. 8.19, 8.20, 8.21, 8.22, and 8.23).
2. Other procedures and cautions: Please refer to the section on lumbar pedicle screw techniques.

8.9 Imaging Features of Standard Pedicle Screws (Figs. 8.24, 8.25, 8.26, 8.27, 8.28, 8.29, 8.30, 8.31, 8.32, 8.33, 8.34, 8.35, 8.36, and 8.37)

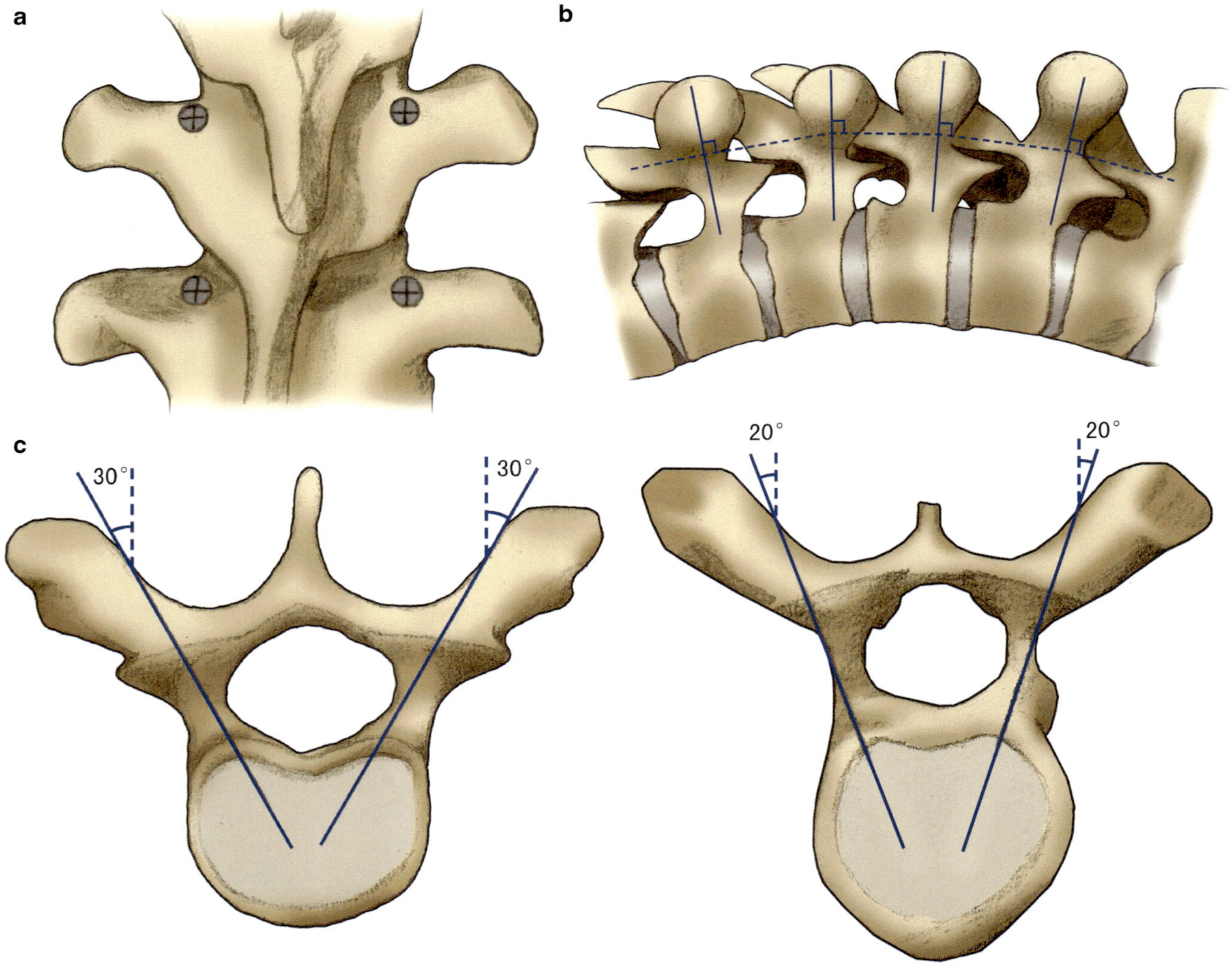

Fig. 8.4 Free-hand thoracic pedicle screw placement. (**a**) 3 mm caudal to the junction of the transverse process-superior articulating process; (**b**) Orthogonal to the sagittal curvature of the dorsal spine; (**c**) Axial trajectory of thoracic spine

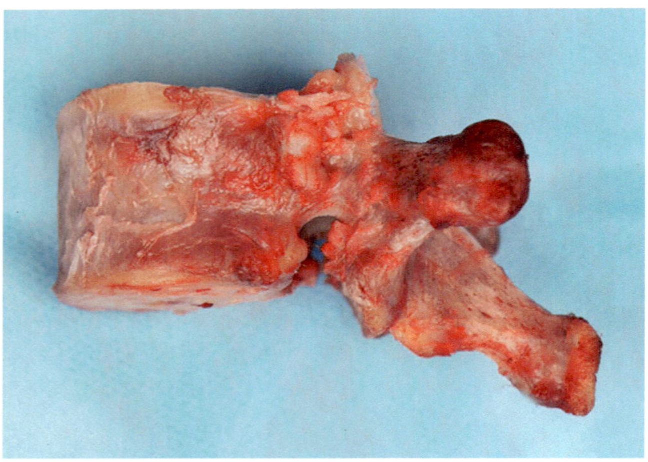

Fig. 8.5 The lateral view of the thoracic vertebral body

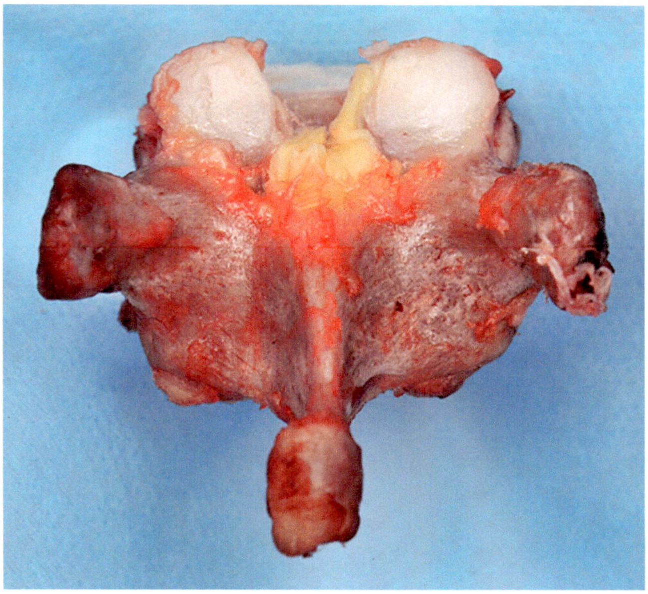

Fig. 8.6 The posterior view of the thoracic vertebral body

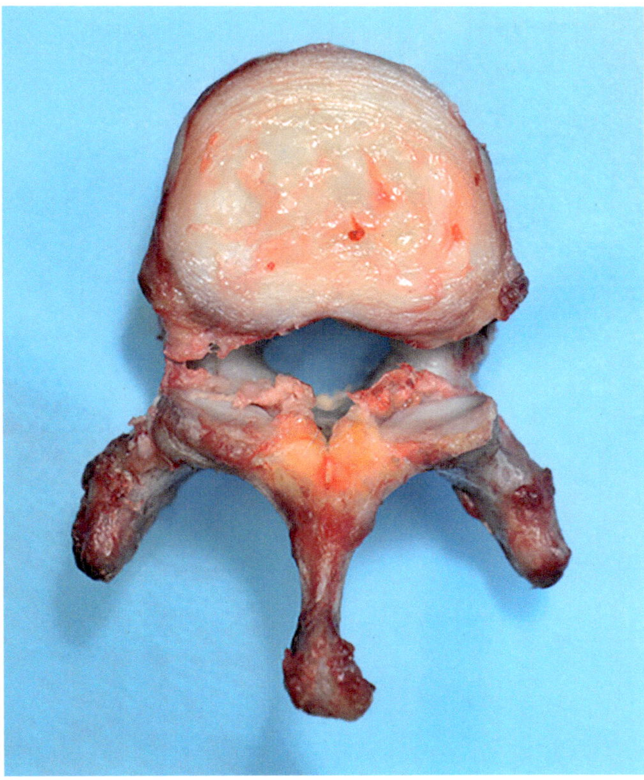

Fig. 8.7 The inferior view of the thoracic vertebral body

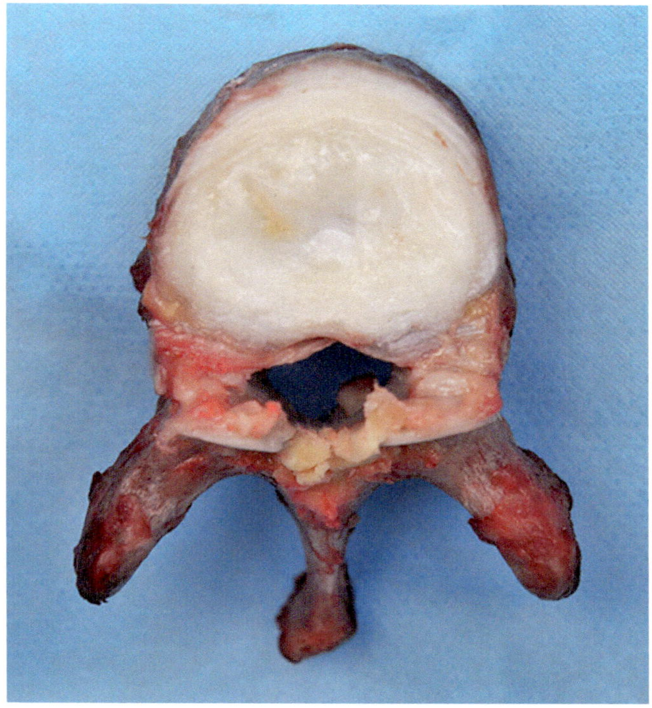

Fig. 8.8 The superior view of the thoracic vertebral body

Table 8.1 Height and width (mm) of thoracic pedicles (mean ± SD)

	Zindrick		Panjabi		Ebraheim	
	Height	Width	Height	Width	Height	Width
T1	9.9 ± 2.0	7.9 ± 1.4	9.6 ± 0.5	8.5 ± 0.5	8.2 ± 0.8	9.6 ± 1.2
T2	12.0 ± 1.2	7.0 ± 1.8	11.4 ± 0.4	8.2 ± 1.1	9.7 ± 0.9	6.4 ± 0.7
T3	12.4 ± 1.3	5.6 ± 1.4	11.9 ± 0.3	6.8 ± 0.7	10.0 ± 1.1	4.7 ± 0.9
T4	12.1 ± 1.0	4.7 ± 1.3	12.1 ± 0.5	6.3 ± 0.6	10.4 ± 0.7	3.7 ± 0.8
T5	11.9 ± 1.4	4.5 ± 0.9	11.3 ± 0.5	6.0 ± 0.5	10.4 ± 0.8	4.3 ± 0.8
T6	12.2 ± 1.0	5.2 ± 1.0	11.8 ± 0.5	6.0 ± 0.9	9.4 ± 1.1	3.8 ± 0.8
T7	12.1 ± 1.0	5.3 ± 1.0	12.0 ± 0.3	5.9 ± 0.7	10.4 ± 0.8	4.6 ± 0.7
T8	12.8 ± 1.2	5.9 ± 1.6	12.5 ± 0.5	6.7 ± 0.5	11.2 ± 0.7	4.8 ± 0.5
T9	13.8 ± 1.3	6.1 ± 1.5	13.9 ± 0.7	7.7 ± 0.6	12.8 ± 1.0	5.4 ± 0.9
T10	15.2±2.0	6.3±1.7	14.9 ± 0.4	9.0 ± 0.8	14.0 ± 1.0	5.8 ± 0.7
T11	17.4 ± 2.5	7.8 ± 2.0	17.4 ± 0.4	9.8 ± 0.6	16.1 ± 0.8	8.6 ± 0.6
T12	15.8 ± 2.4	7.1 ± 2.3	16.7 ± 0.8	8.7 ± 0.8	15.2 ± 0.9	8.7 ± 0.7

Table 8.2 The medial inclination angle of thoracic pedicles (degrees) (mean ± SD)

	Zindrick		Panjabi		Ebraheim	
	Left	Right	Left	Right	Left	Right
L1	15.4 ± 2.8	8.7 ± 2.3	15.9 ± 0.8	8.6 ± 0.9	14.1 ± 1.3	7.5 ± 1.5
L2	15.0 ± 1.5	8.9 ± 2.2	15.0 ± 0.5	8.3 ± 0.7	14.0 ± 1.2	8.2 ± 1.3
L3	14.9 ± 2.4	10.3 ± 26	14.4 ± 0.6	10.2 ± 0.6	13.9 ± 1.4	9.8 ± 1.1
L4	14.8 ± 2.1	12.9 ± 2.1	15.5 ± 0.6	14.1 ± 0.4	12.8 ± 1.7	12.7 ± 1.9
L5	14.0 ± 2.3	18.0 ± 4.1	19.6 ± 0.8	18.6 ± 1.0	11.4 ± 1.4	18.0 ± 2.4

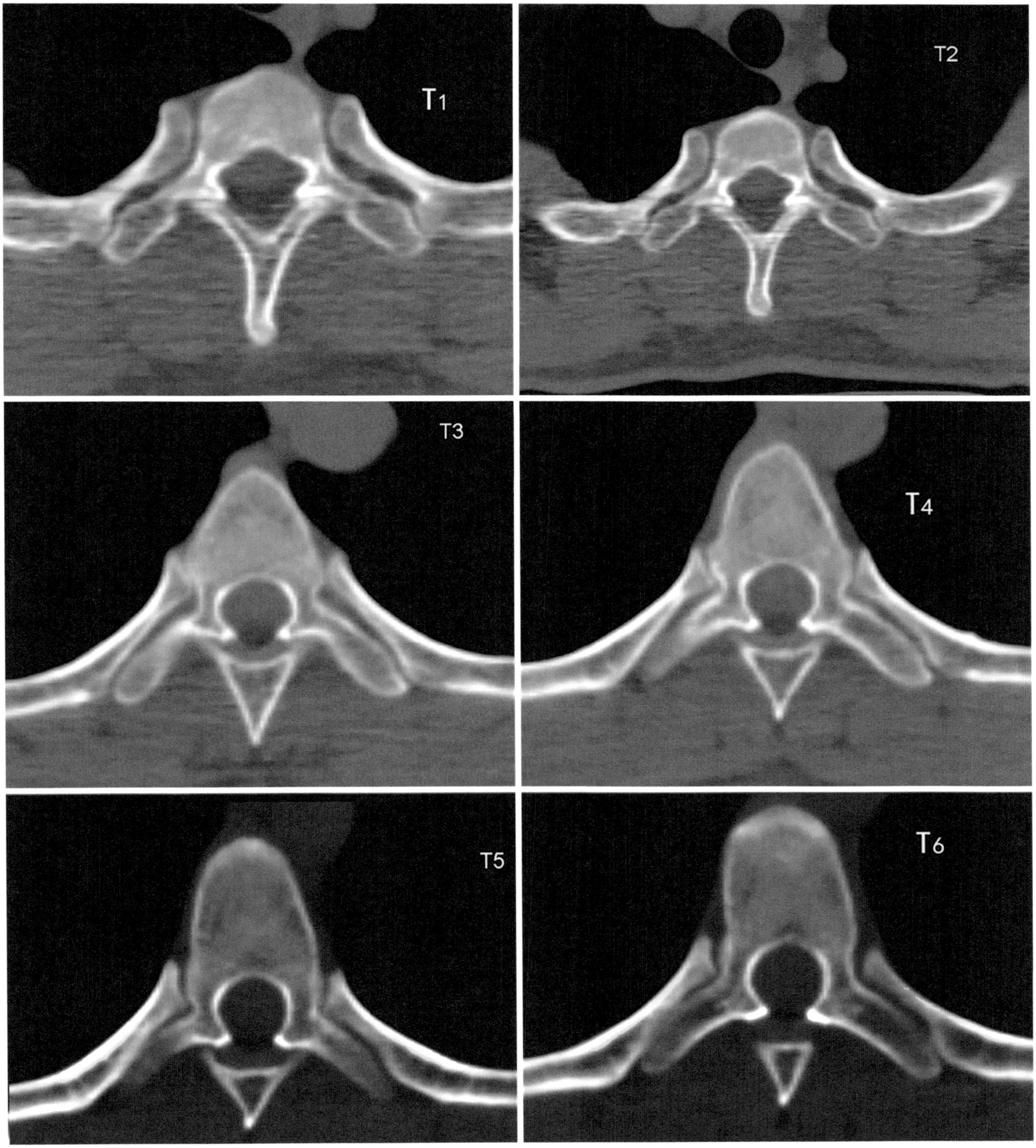

Fig. 8.9 Pedicle width (T1–T6)

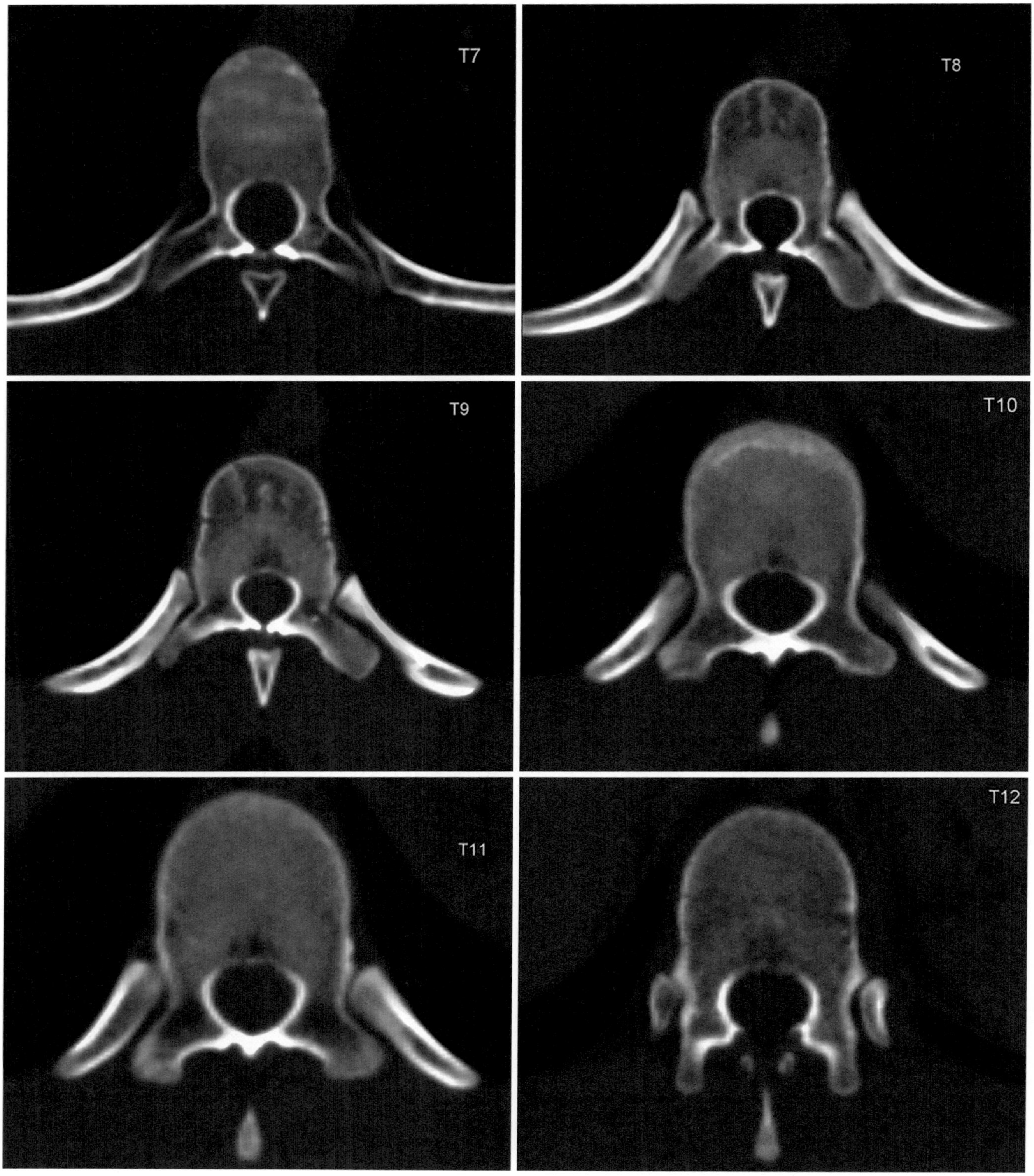

Fig. 8.10 Pedicle width (T7–T12)

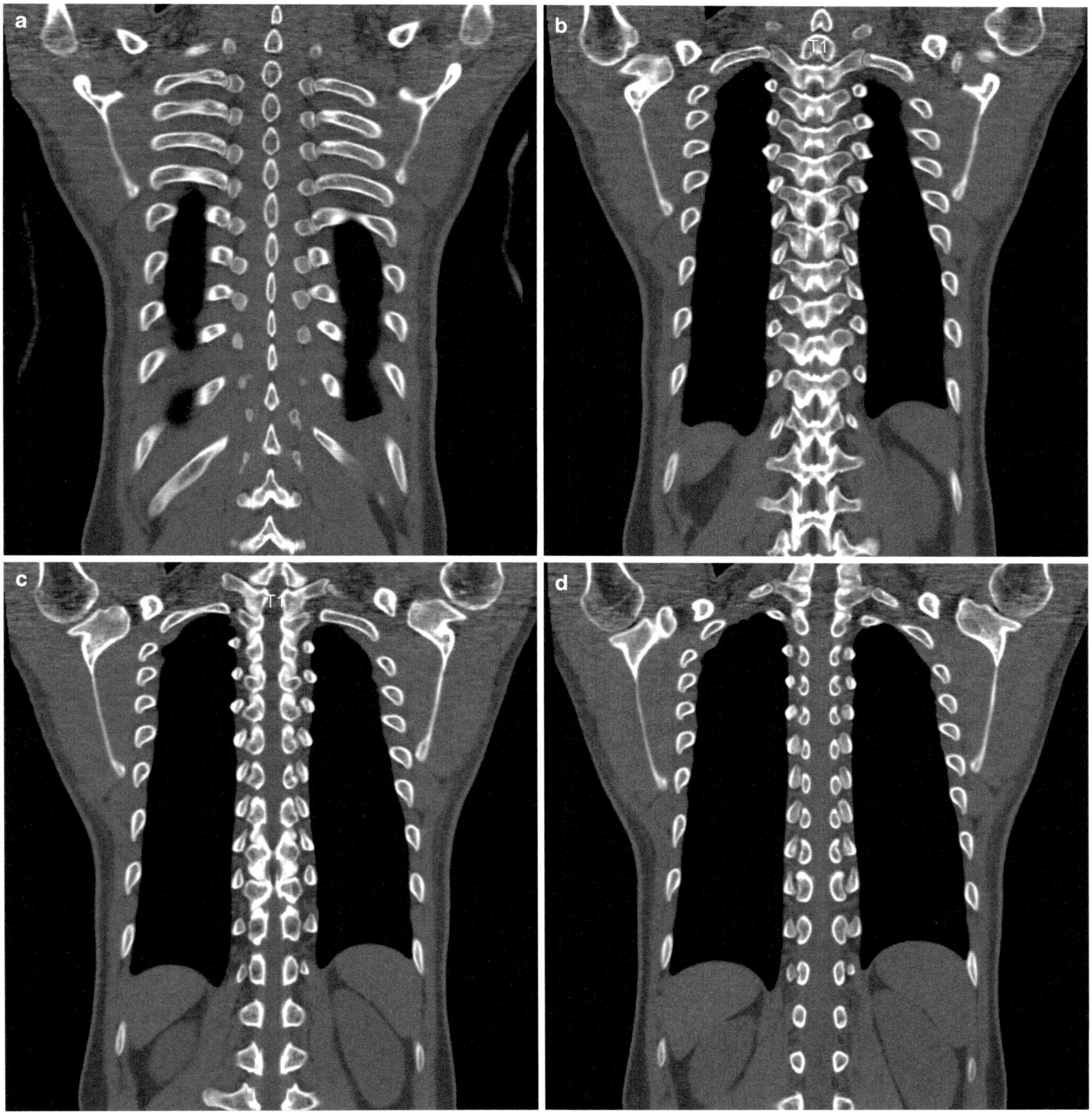

Fig. 8.11 Pedicle height

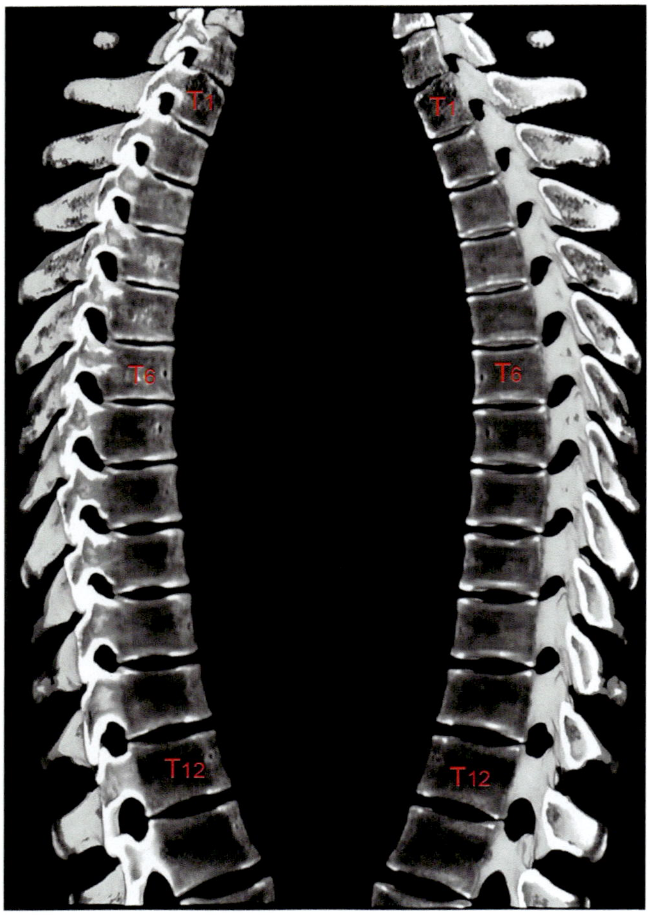

Fig. 8.12 The sectional view of the pedicles

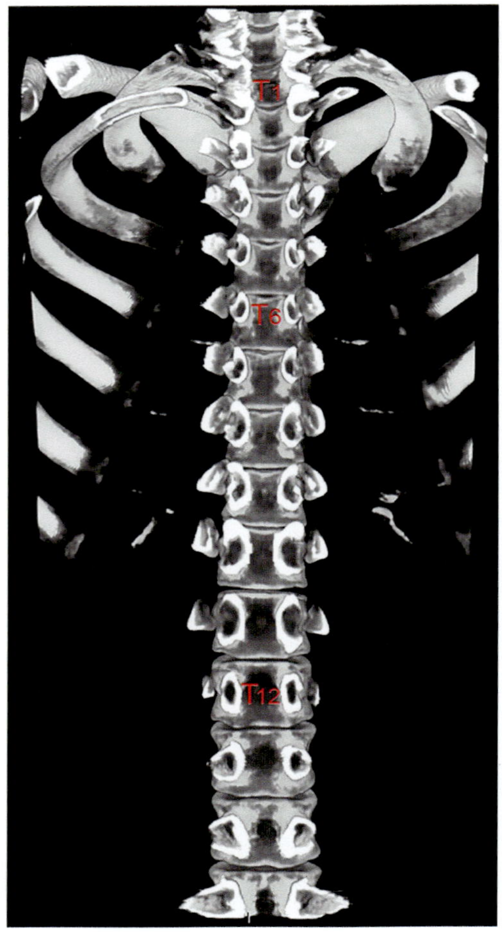

Fig. 8.13 The sectional view of the pedicles (the coronal section)

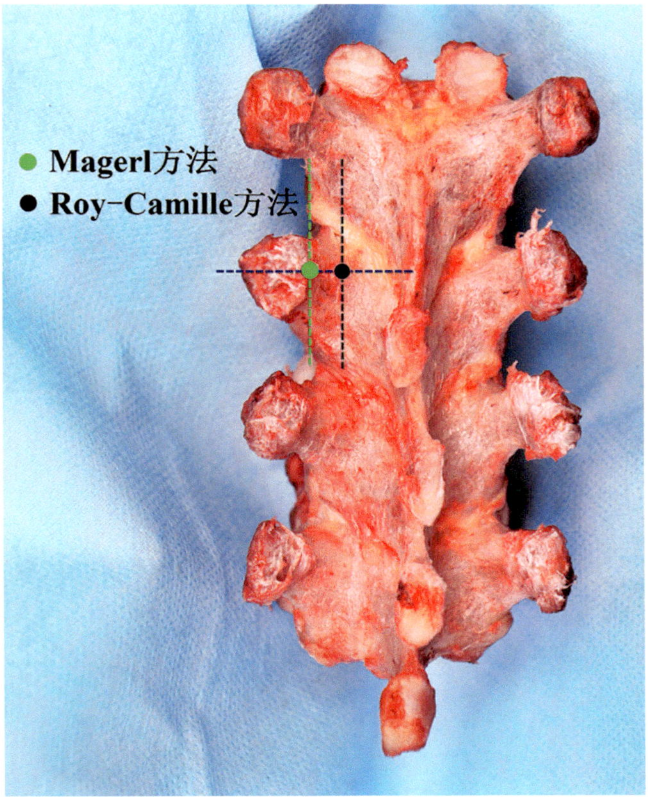

Fig. 8.14 Method for determining screw entry points

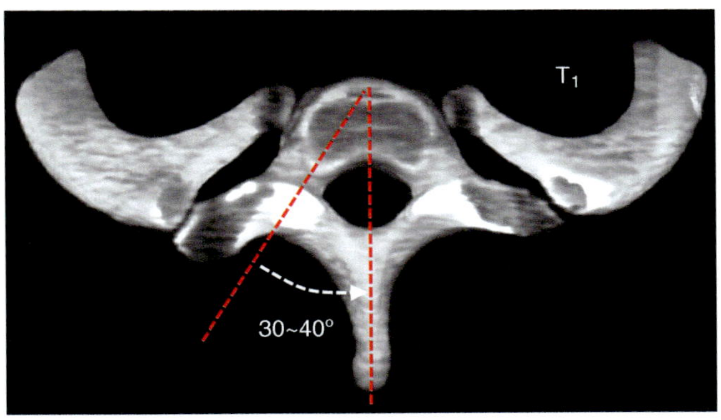

Fig. 8.15 The screw entry angle in the upper thoracic spine

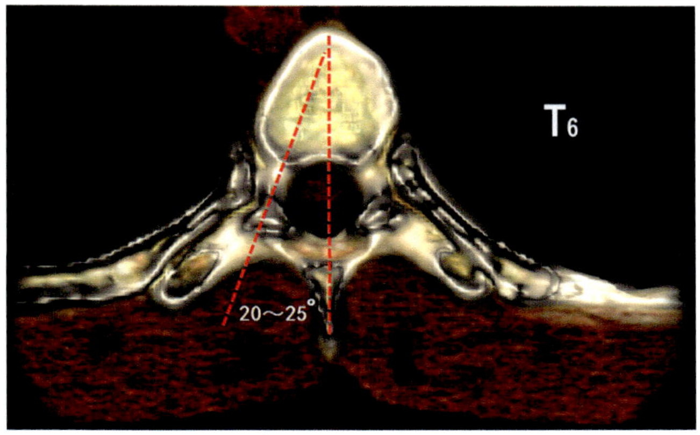

Fig. 8.16 The screw entry angle in the mid-thoracic spine

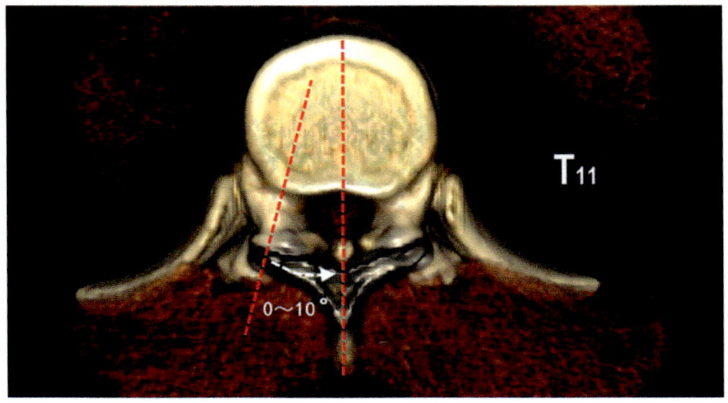

Fig. 8.17 The screw entry angle in the lower thoracic spine

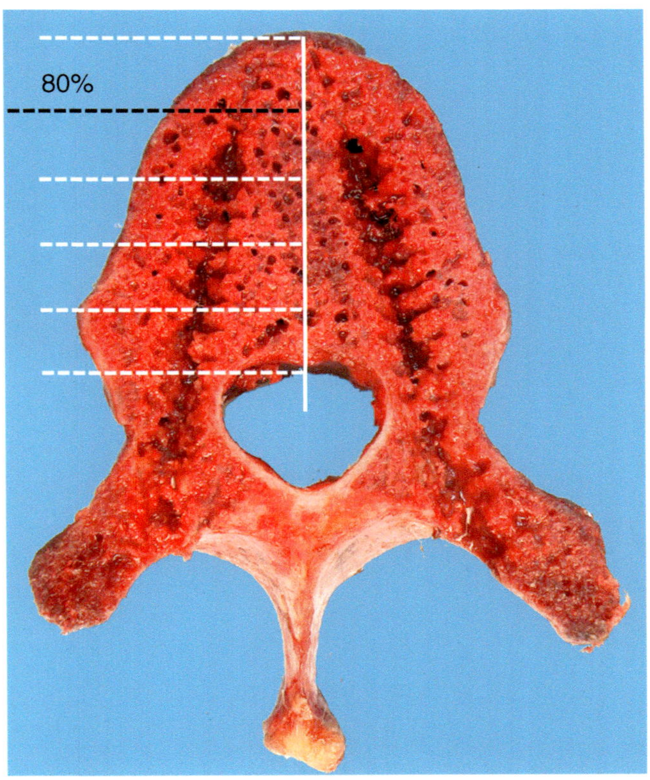

Fig. 8.18 Entry depths of the thoracic screw

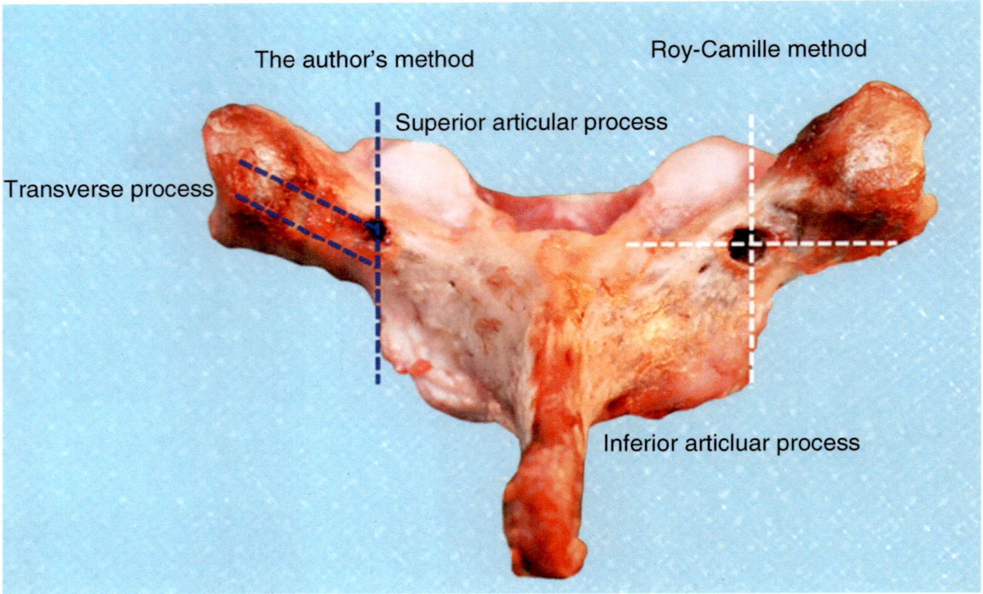

Fig. 8.19 Determination of screw entry sites in the upper thoracic spine (T1–T4)

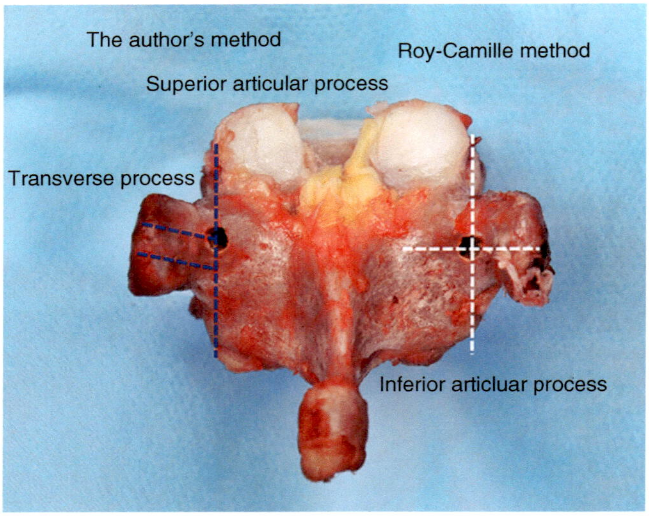

Fig. 8.20 Determination of screw entry sites in the mid-thoracic spine (T5–T8)

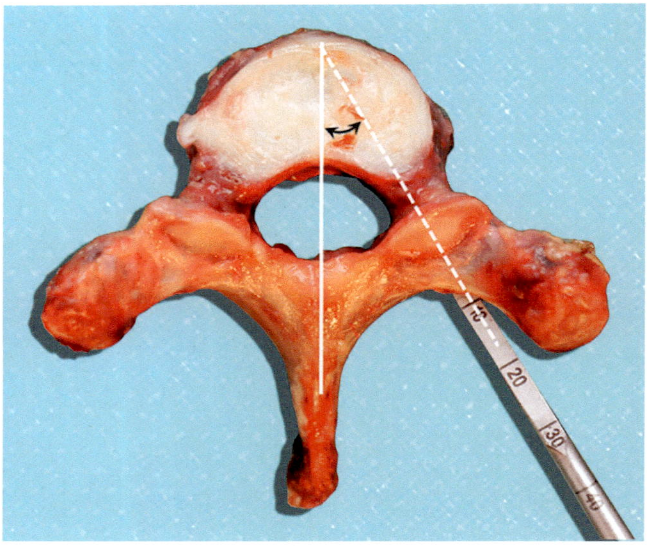

Fig. 8.22 The screw entry path should have a certain medial inclination angle in the horizontal plane

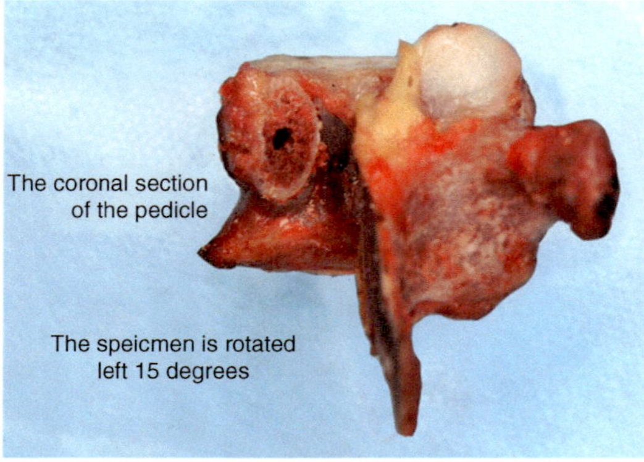

Fig. 8.21 The sectional view of the pedicle screw trajectory

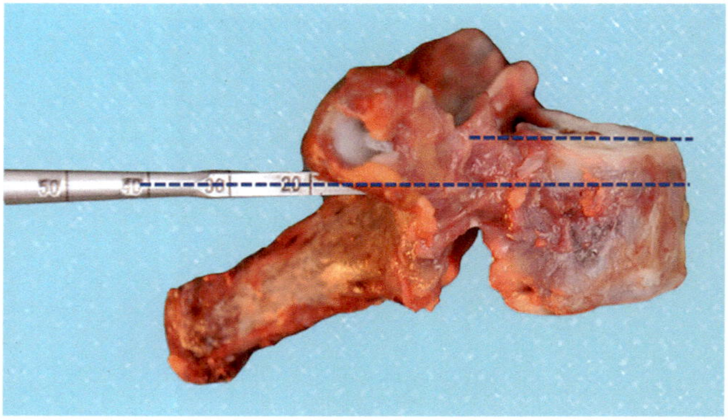

Fig. 8.23 The screw entry angle should best be parallel to the endplate in the sagittal plane

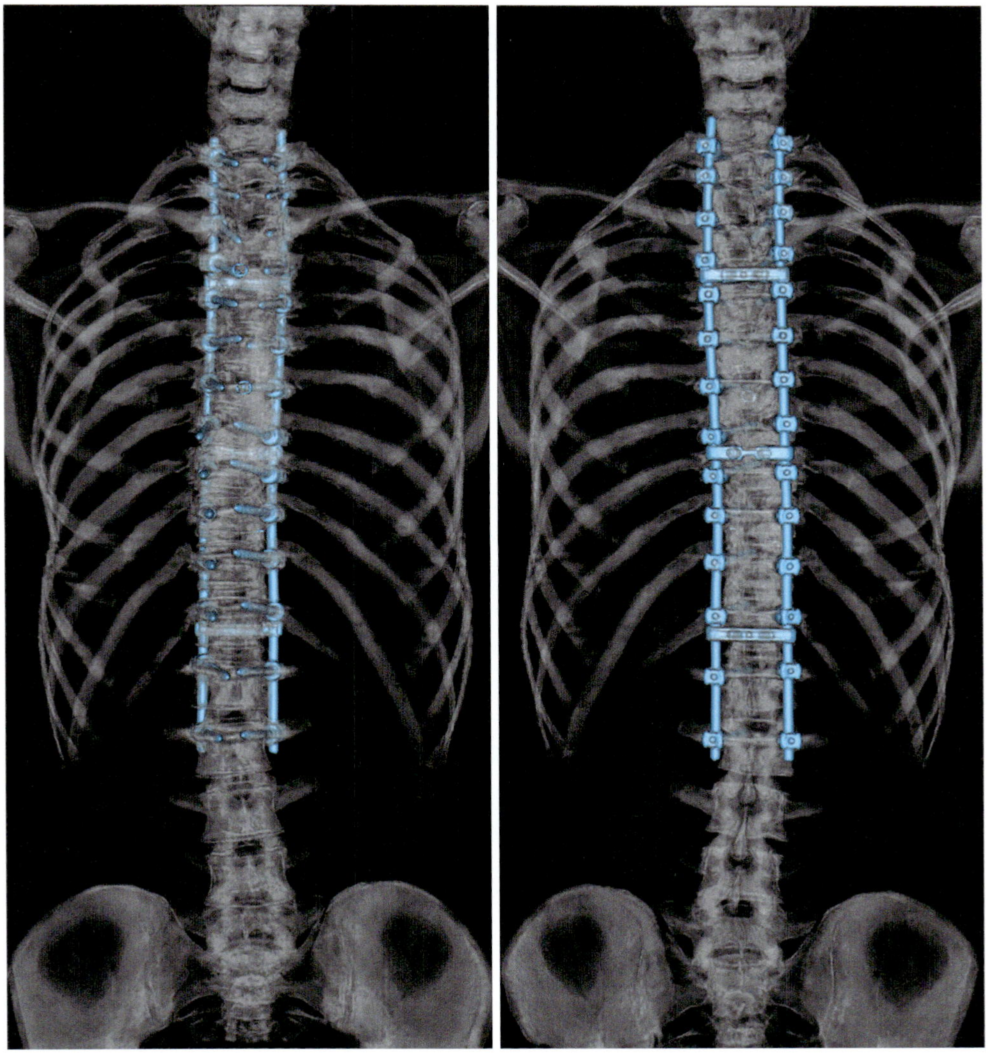

Fig. 8.24 Thoracic pedicle screw. *Left*: the front view; *Right*: the posterior view

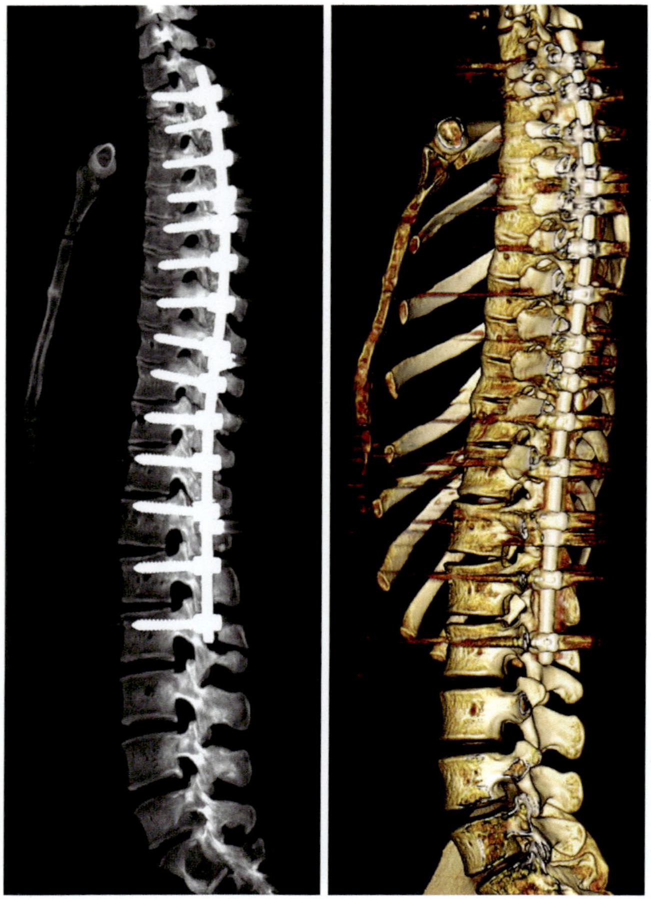

Fig. 8.25 The thoracic pedicle screw (*lateral view*)

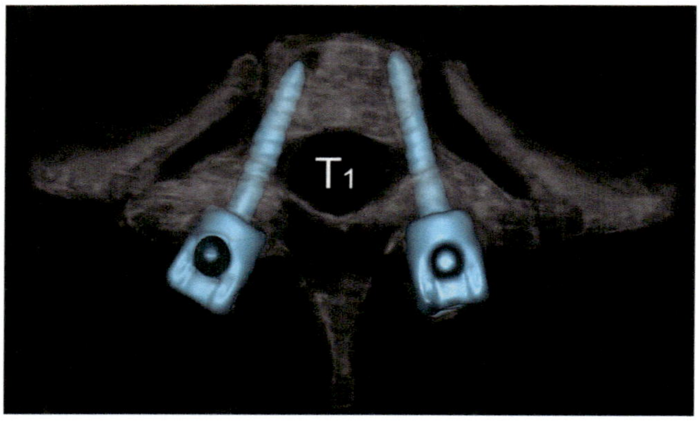

Fig. 8.26 T1 pedicle screw

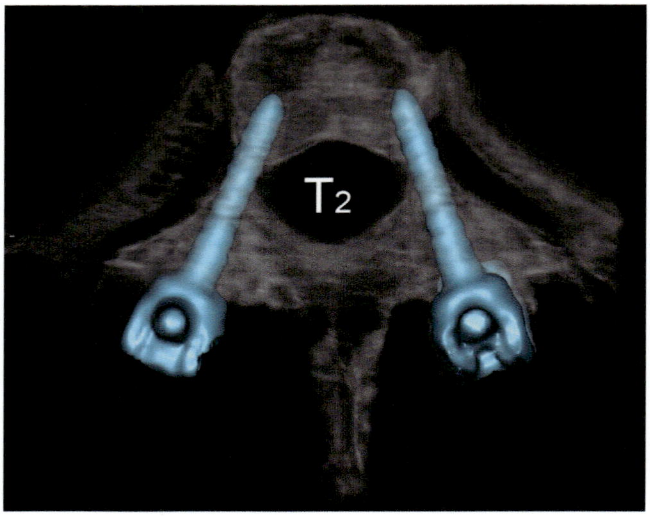

Fig. 8.27 T2 pedicle screw

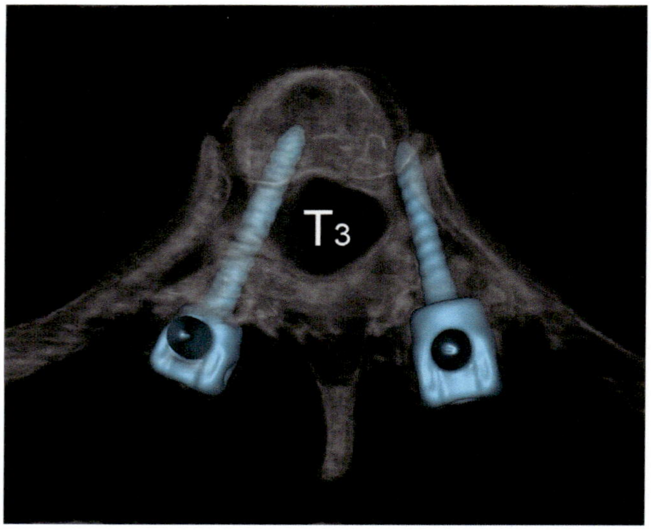

Fig. 8.28 T3 pedicle screw

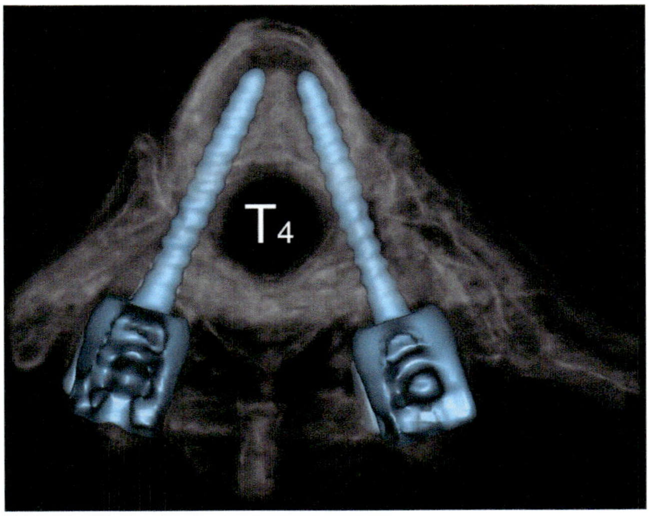

Fig. 8.29 T4 pedicle screw

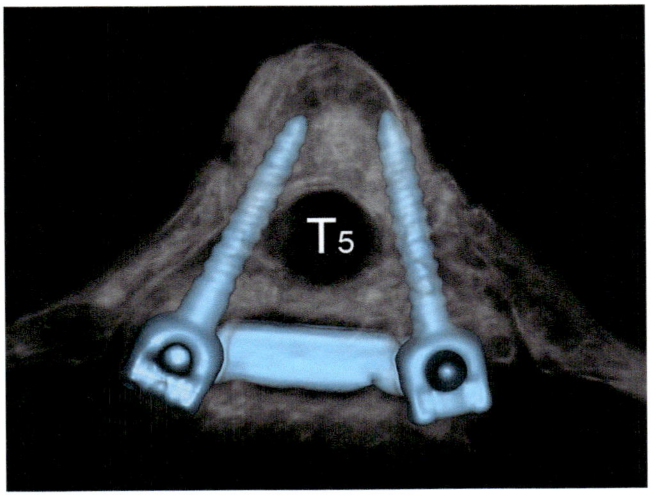

Fig. 8.30 T5 pedicle screw

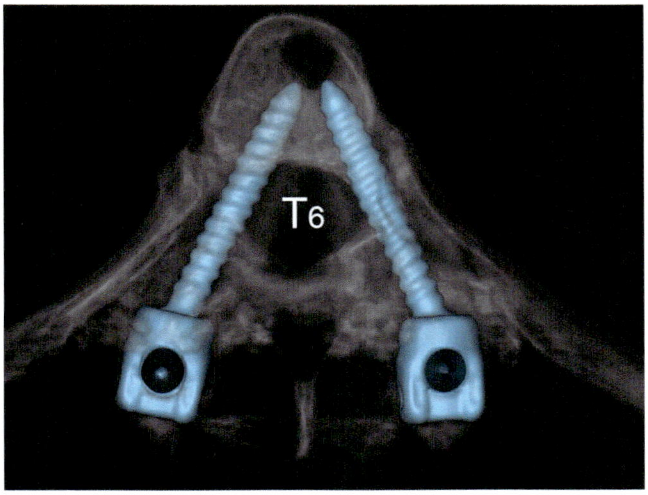

Fig. 8.31 T6 pedicle screw

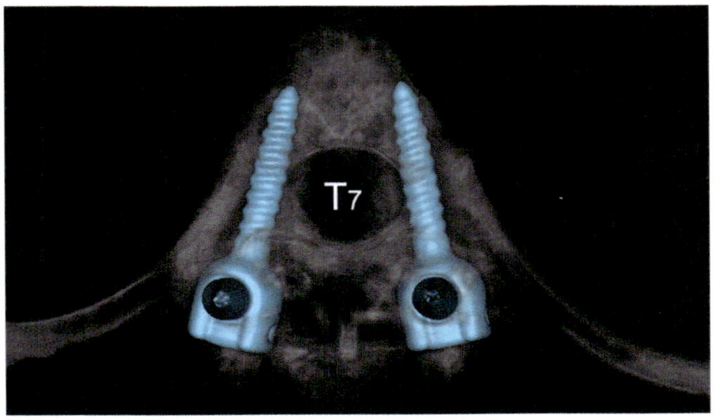

Fig. 8.32 T7 pedicle screw

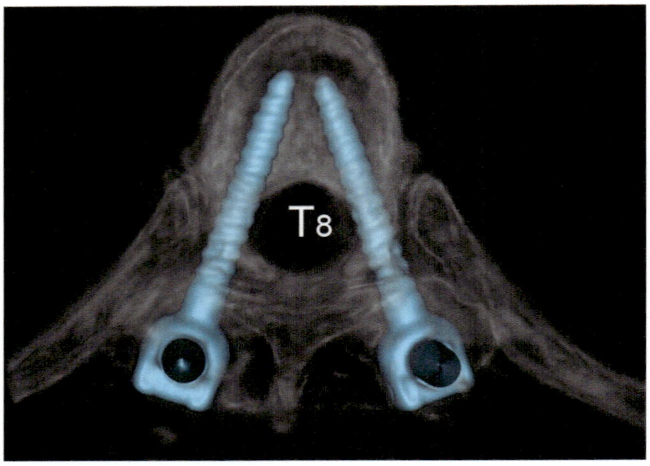

Fig. 8.33 T8 pedicle screw

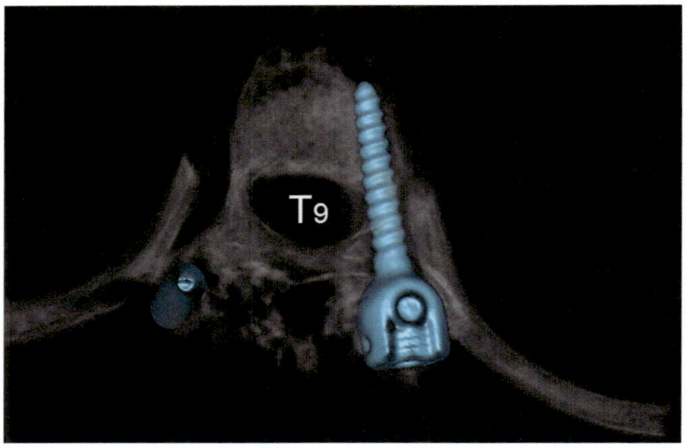

Fig. 8.34 T9 pedicle screw

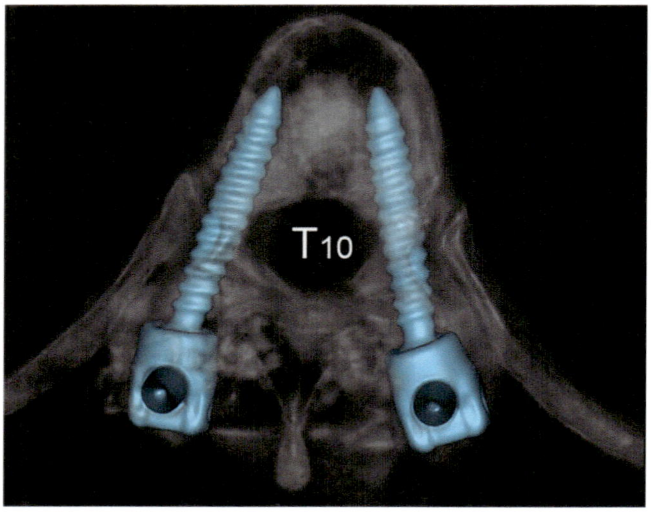

Fig. 8.35 T10 pedicle screw

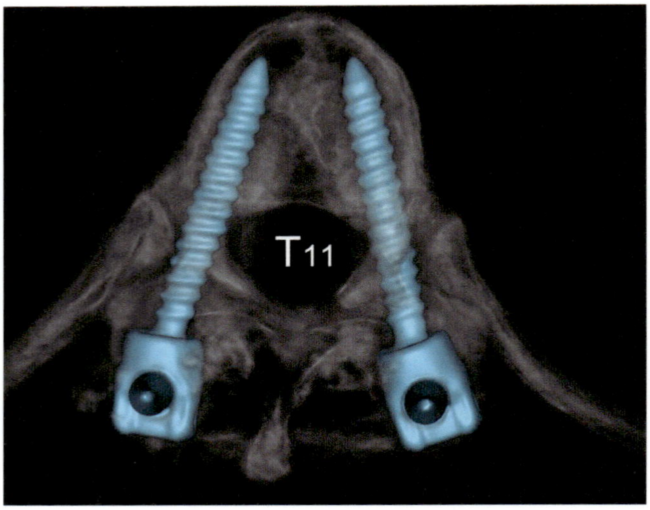

Fig. 8.36 T11 pedicle screw

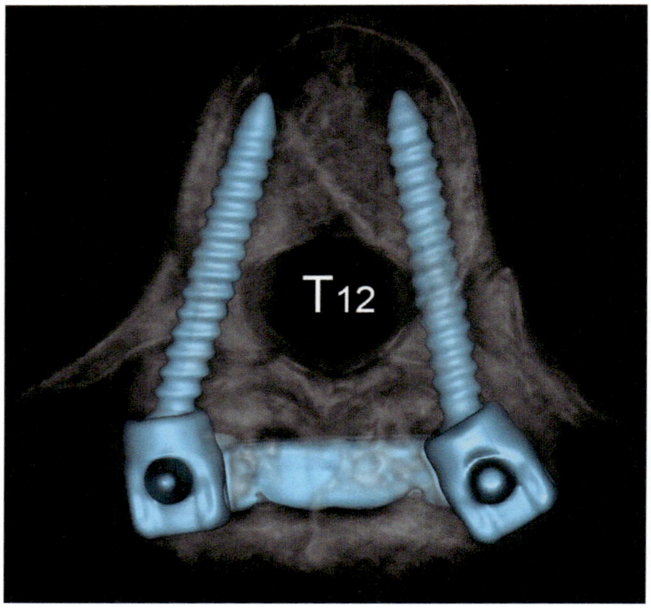

Fig. 8.37 T12 pedicle screw

References

1. Roy-Camille R, et al. Osteosynthesis of thoraco-lumbar spine fractures with metal plates screwed through the vertebral pedicles. Reconstr Surg Traumatol. 1976;15:2–16.
2. Kim YJ, Lenke LG, Bridwell KH, Cho YS, Riew KD. Free-hand pedicle screw placement in the thoracic spine: is it safe? Spine (Phila Pa 1976). 2004;29(3):333–42.
3. Fennell VS, Palejwala S, Skoch J, Stidd DA, Baaj AA. Freehand thoracic pedicle screw technique using a uniform entry point and sagittal trajectory for all levels: preliminary clinical experience. J Neurosurg Spine. 2014;21(5):778–84.

Lumbar Pedicle Screw Fixation Techniques and Their Applications

9

Xinxin Wen, Yabo Yan, and Wei Lei

Abstract

All three columns of the lumbar spine are stabilized in the posterior lumbar transpedicular internal fixation technique. This technique has been widely used in the treatment of lumbar degenerative disease and lumbar fracture. Anatomic characteristics of the lumbar vertebral body, the entry point, entry angle, entry depth of the lumbar pedicle screw, and operative details are demonstrated to guarantee proper positioning of the screw. The characteristics, clinical indications and contraindications, and the surgical technique of CD HORIZON LEGACY internal fixation system are introduced in detail. The applications of these techniques are presented in typical clinical cases. Pearls and pitfalls of lumbar pedicle screw fixation are summarized at the end of this chapter.

Keywords

Lumbar spine · Pedicle screw fixation · Surgical technique

9.1 Unit 1: Lumbar Pedicle Screw Fixation Techniques and Their Applications

9.1.1 A Historical Review and Anatomic Parameters

9.1.1.1 A Historical Review of Lumbar Pedicle Screw Techniques

Reconstruction of lumbar stability evolved from wire technique and hook and rod technique to pedicle screw technique, with the following milestones:

In 1891, Hadra first used silver wire to internally fix the spine in a patient with vertebral fracture and Pott's disease [1].

In 1945, Harrington used Harrington rod for correction of idiopathic scoliosis, which has ever since offered an effective treatment for vertebral scoliosis [2].

In 1949, Michele and Krueger reported the anatomic features of pedicles and described transpedicular screw entry into the vertebral body via a posterior approach [3] (Figs. 9.1 and 9.2).

In 1961, the French surgeon Raymond Roy-Camille initiated the treatment of unstable thoracolumbar fracture by internal fixation with pedicle screws and also developed a complete pedicle screw and plate system for treating unstable thoracolumbar fractures [4] (Fig. 9.3).

In 1983, Denis proposed the "three-column theory" in which the vertebra is divided into the "anterior, middle, and posterior columns." The pedicle is a channel that runs through and connects the three columns. This theory has exerted far-reaching effects on the development of pedicle screw techniques [5].

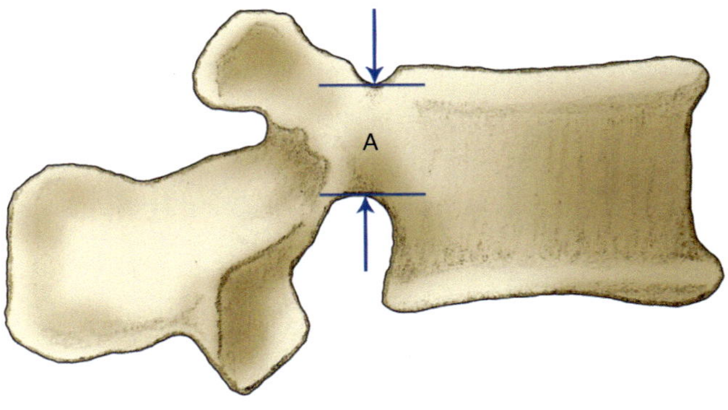

Fig. 9.1 Anatomic features of the lumbar pedicle: (*a*) vertical diameter, 0.7–1.5 cm

X. Wen · Y. Yan · W. Lei (✉)
Department of Orthopedics, Xijing Hospital, Air Force Medical University, Xi'an, Shaanxi, China
e-mail: leiwei@fmmu.edu.cn

W. Lei, Y. Yan (eds.), *Internal Fixation of the Spine*, https://doi.org/10.1007/978-981-16-1562-7_9

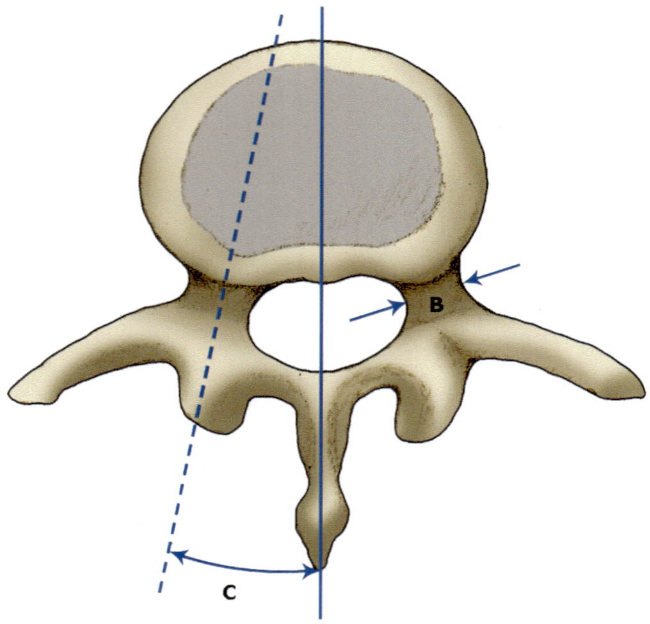

Fig. 9.2 Anatomic features of the lumbar pedicle: (*b*) horizontal diameter, 0.7–1.6 cm; (*c*): the angle between the two lines is less than 10°

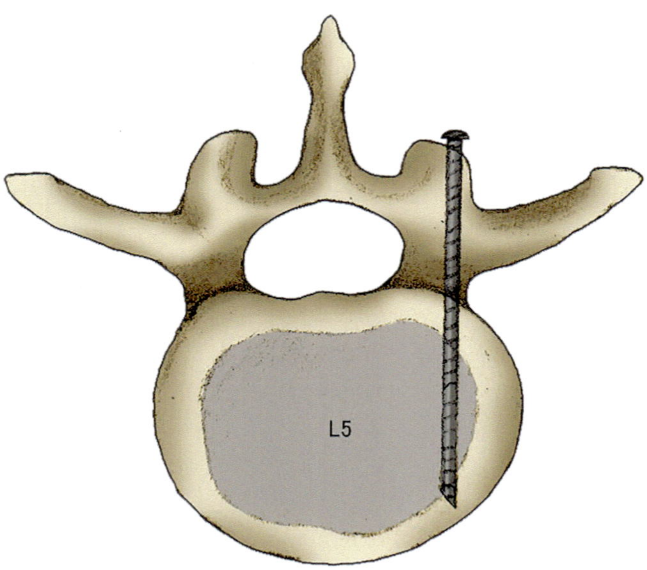

Fig. 9.3 The pedicle screw and plate system developed by Raymond Roy-Camille

In 1983, Steffee introduced the variable screw placement system as a means of transpedicular fixation of the unstable spine [6].

In 1983, French surgeons Cotrel and Dubousset invented Cotrel-Dubousset instrumentation, which replaces laminar hook with pedicle screws for lumbar fixation. The double-rod system was recommended for scoliosis patients, from which the concept of vertebral three-dimensional correction evolved [7].

The appearance of pedicle screws is an important milestone in the history of vertebral internal fixation surgery. Biomechanically, compared to hook and wire fixation, internal fixation with pedicle screws could provide three-column stabilization. Therefore, the technique provides powerful mechanical action in fracture reduction and correction; meanwhile, it does not need to enter the vertebral canal such as infralaminar wire and laminar hook, lessening the risk of nerve injury. In 1999, the US FDA approved this technique as one of the classical vertebral internal fixation techniques via the posterior approach.

9.1.1.2 Anatomy of the Lumbar Pedicle

Gross Anatomy

The gross anatomy of the lumbar vertebra is shown in Fig. 9.4.

Anatomic Data of the Lumbar Pedicle

The width of the lumbar pedicle gradually increases from L1 to L5, but variations exist among individuals (Fig. 9.5) [8–10]. In Zindrick's study [8], the height of the lumbar pedicle is 15.4 ± 2.8, 15.0 ± 1.5, 14.9 ± 2.4, 14.8 ± 2.1, and 14.0 ± 2.3 mm from L1 to L5. The width of the lumbar pedicle is 8.7 ± 2.3, 8.9 ± 2.2, 10.3 ± 2.6, 12.9 ± 2.1, and 18.0 ± 4.1 mm from L1 to L5. In Panjabi's study [9], the height of the lumbar pedicle is 15.9 ± 0.8, 15.0 ± 0.5, 14.4 ± 0.6, 15.5 ± 0.6, and 19.6 ± 0.8 mm from L1 to L5. The width of the lumbar pedicle is 8.6 ± 0.9, 8.3 ± 0.7, 10.2 ± 0.6, 14.1 ± 0.4, and 18.6 ± 1.0 mm from L1 to L5. In Ebraheim's study [10], the height of the lumbar pedicle is 14.1 ± 1.3, 14.0 ± 1.2, 13.9 ± 1.4, 12.8 ± 1.7, and 11.4 ± 1.4 mm from L1 to L5. The width of the lumbar pedicle is 7.5 ± 1.5, 8.2 ± 1.3, 9.8 ± 1.1, 12.7 ± 1.9, and 18.0 ± 2.4 mm from L1 to L5.

There is a medial inclination angle in the axial plane of the pedicle, which gradually increases from L1 to L5 [9, 11]. The medial inclination angle steadily rises in the cephalad-caudal direction. The range of the angle is from 0° to 10°, and the maximum medial inclination angle is approximately 27°, and is found at the L5 vertebral body in the horizontal

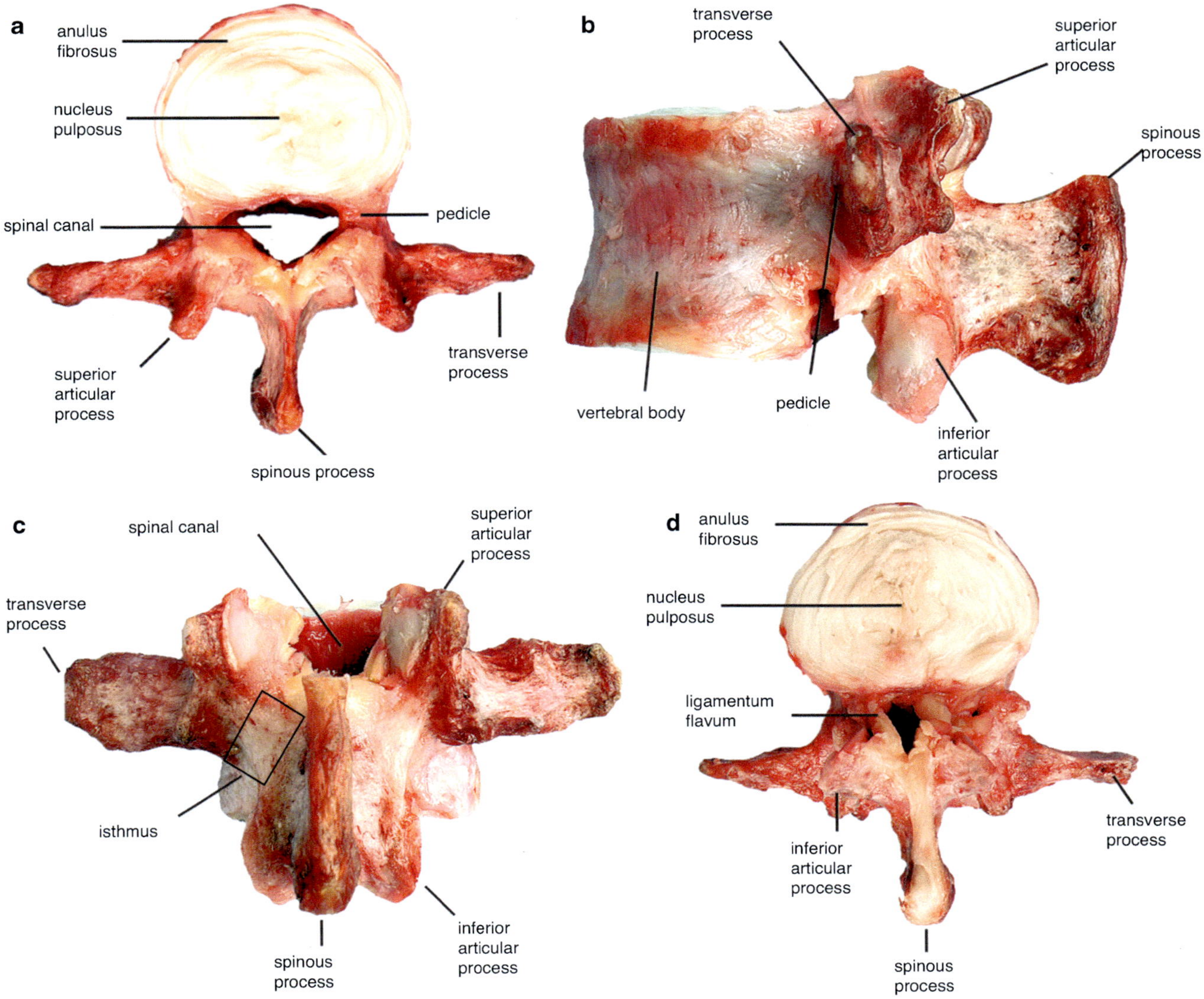

Fig. 9.4 The anatomic structures of the lumbar vertebra. (**a**) Superior view; (**b**) Inferior view; (**c**) Lateral view; (**d**) Posterior view

plane. In Panjabi's study [9], the medial inclination angle of the right lumbar pedicle is 16.5 ± 5.02°, 17.1 ± 3.75°, 19.8 ± 2.33°, 18.4 ± 1.66°, and 25.9 ± 1.73° from L1 to L5. The medial inclination angle of the left lumbar pedicle is 12.4 ± 1.87°, 11.2 ± 2.02°, 17.1 ± 1.56°, 14.7 ± 2.16°, and 23.2 ± 1.48° from L1 to L5.

9.1.1.3 Lumbar Pedicle Screw Techniques

Determining the Entry Point of Lumbar Pedicle Screws

1. Intersection method

The screw entry point is located at the intersection of a horizontal line passing through the midpoint of the transverse process and a vertical line tangential to the lateral border of the superior articular process. The approach requires partial exposure of the transverse process. Because of greater stripping and abundance of adjacent vessels, bleeding is more profuse [12] (Fig. 9.6).

2. The ^ vertex point method

There is a specific anatomic feature in the posterior lumbar spine-^ vertex point. ^ vertex point is the entry point of pedicle screw (Fig. 9.7). This method does not require exposure of the transverse process.

Entry Angle of Lumbar Pedicle Screws

The pedicle screw should have a medial inclination of 5°–10° relative to the sagittal plane at L1–L3 and a medial inclination of 10°–15°at L4–L5 [12] (Fig. 9.8).

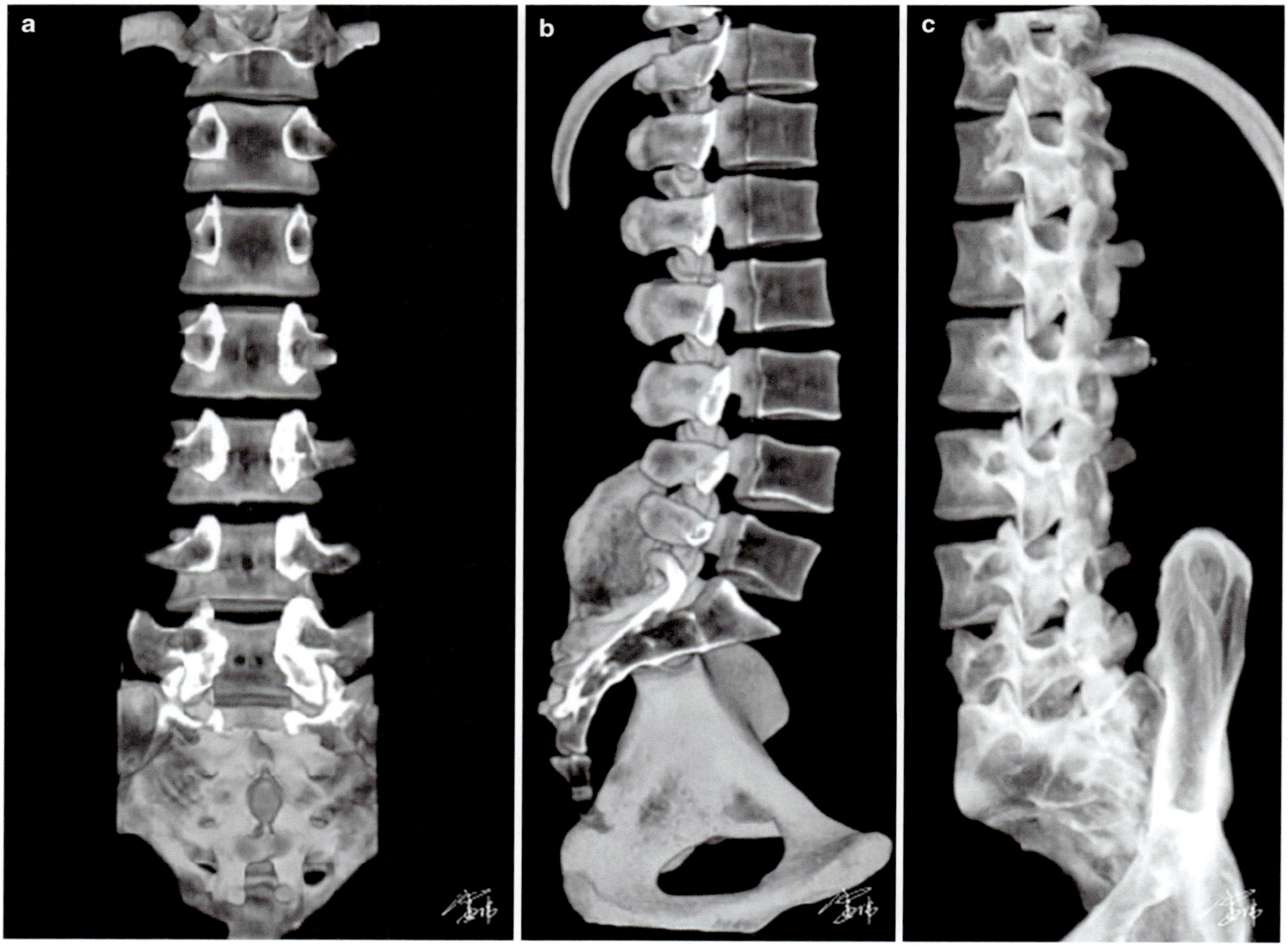

Fig. 9.5 Three-dimensional (3D) CT reconstruction of the lumbar pedicle. (**a**) The coronal section; (**b**) The sagittal section; (**c**) The oblique position

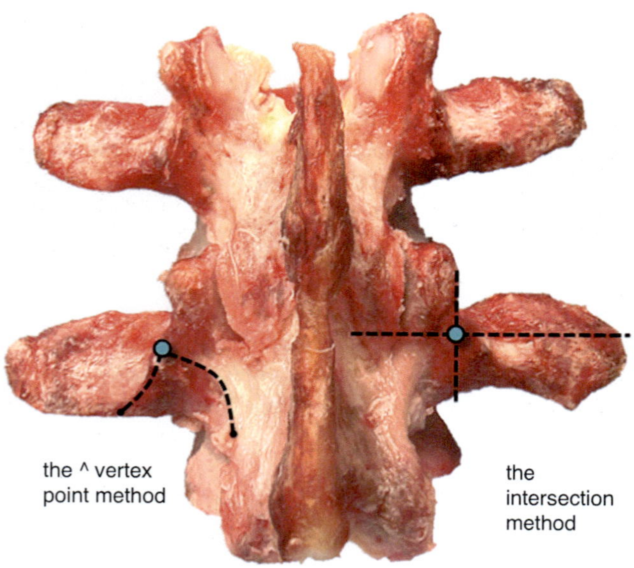

Fig. 9.6 Methods for determining screw entry points

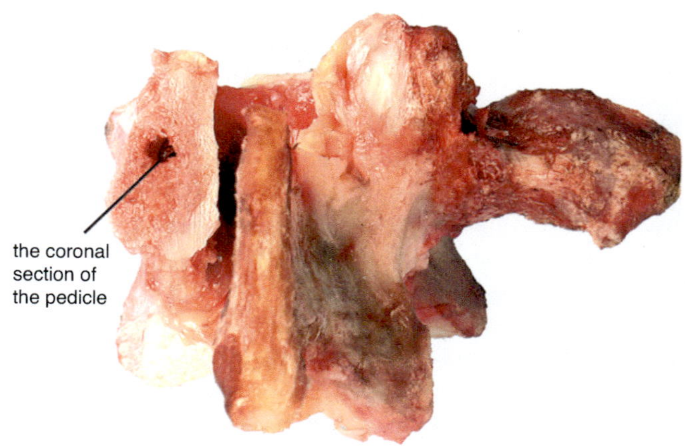

Fig. 9.7 The coronal section of the pedicle

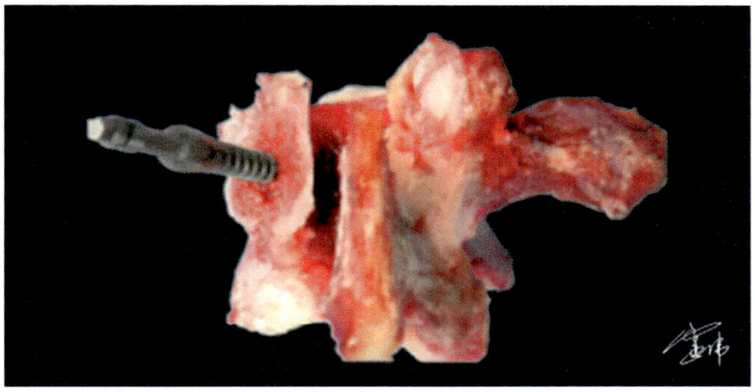

Fig. 9.8 Screw entry angle

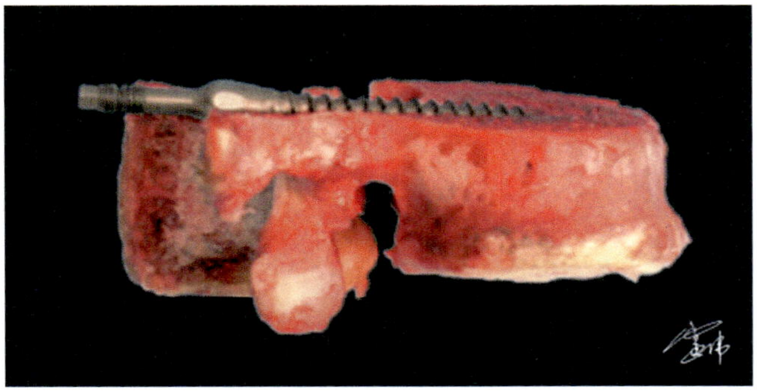

Fig. 9.9 The pedicle screw is parallel to the endplate

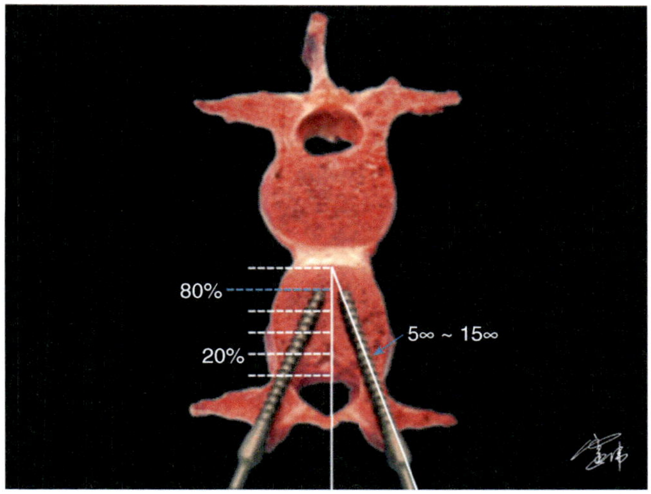

Fig. 9.10 Entry depth of lumbar pedicle screws

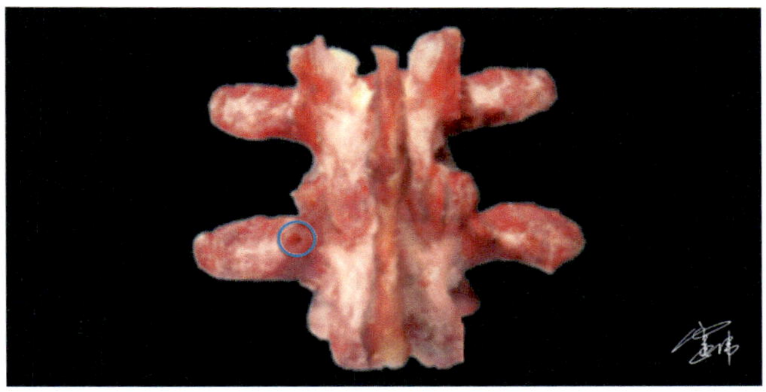

Fig. 9.11 Determining the screw entry point

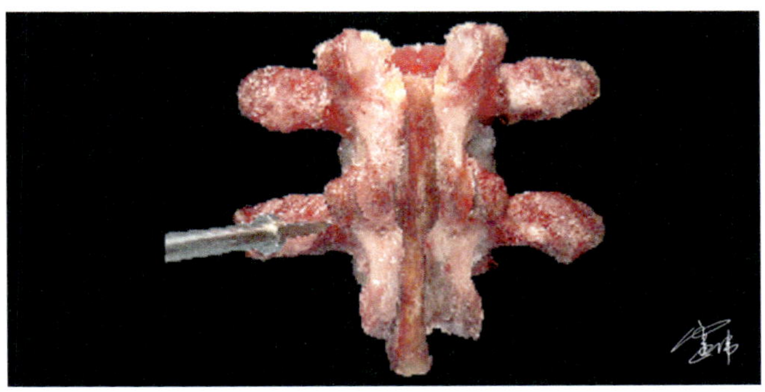

Fig. 9.12 Disrupting the bone cortex

At L1–L4, the pedicle screw should be parallel with the lumbar endplate, that is, vertical to the center of gravity line of the vertebral body. Because the L5 vertebral body is oblique, the entry direction should be inclined toward the caudal direction and has an angle of 10° relative to the horizontal plane [12] (Fig. 9.9).

Entry Depth of Lumbar Pedicle Screws

The entry depth is generally around 45 mm. On lateral X-ray, the depth of the positioning pin should not exceed 80% of the anteroposterior diameter of the vertebral body. The most commonly used screws are 6.5 mm in diameter (Fig. 9.10).

9.1.1.4 Surgical Steps

Determine Screw Entry Point (Fig. 9.11)

Prepare Screw Trajectory

1. Disrupt the bone cortex: A mill, a rongeur, or a burr is used to disrupt the cortical bone at the screw entry point (Fig. 9.12).
2. Drill the screw hole: A screw hole is gradually drilled in the cancellous bone of the pedicle and vertebral body using a drill bit with a drill guide at the above-mentioned angle and depth. During drilling, the surgeon should have an obvious manual feedback of having entered into the cancellous bone. If resistance is encountered, the surgeon should consider whether the entry point or entry angle is correct. If the surgeon con-

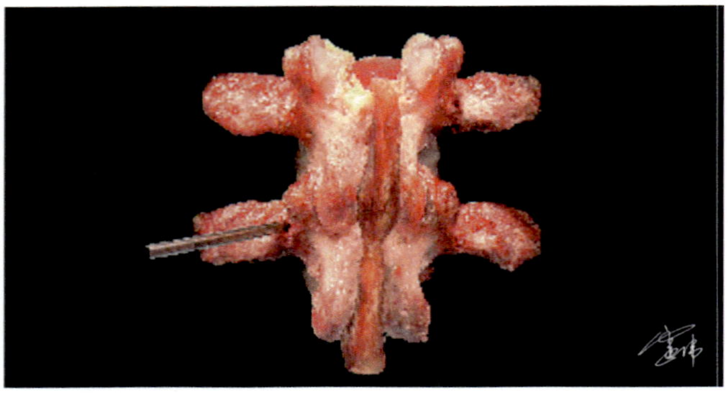

Fig. 9.13 Drilling the screw hole

tinuously feels resistance or changes in bone density during insertion, the surgeon should determine by X-ray whether the burr has disrupted the lateral wall of the pedicle (Fig. 9.13).

3. Probe insertion depth: A blunt pedicle probe is advanced into the vertebral body via the pedicle screw path. When the walls of the screw path are probed, the surgeon should have the manual feedback of probing the cancellous bone and make sure that the integrity of the walls is not violated. If resistance or discontinuity is encountered during probing, the surgeon should consider whether the entry angle is correct and verify by X-ray that the probe is within the pedicle under fluoroscopic guidance (Fig. 9.14).
4. Determining the location: After the hole is drilled, a metal probe is put in the screw hole and located under fluoroscopic guidance. Adjustment is made until satisfaction is achieved under fluoroscopic guidance (Fig. 9.15).

Screw Insertion

Appropriate screws are selected based on the screw trajectory and intraoperative need for correction. Suitable screws are inserted into the prepared screw path using a screwdriver. Screws should be fully inserted and enter 80% of the vertebral body; the screw path should be parallel to the endplates (Fig. 9.16).

9.2 Unit 2: The CD HORIZON LEGACY Plate Internal Fixation System via a Lumbar Posterior Approach

9.2.1 Implants

1. Screws (Fig. 9.17)
   a. Fixed angle screws
   b. Variable angle screws

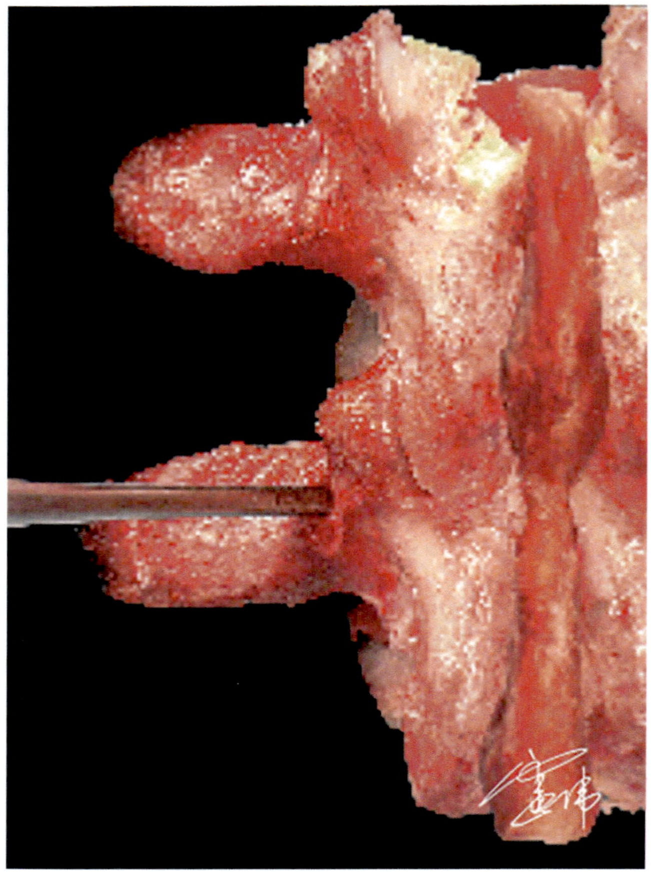

Fig. 9.14 Probing insertion depth

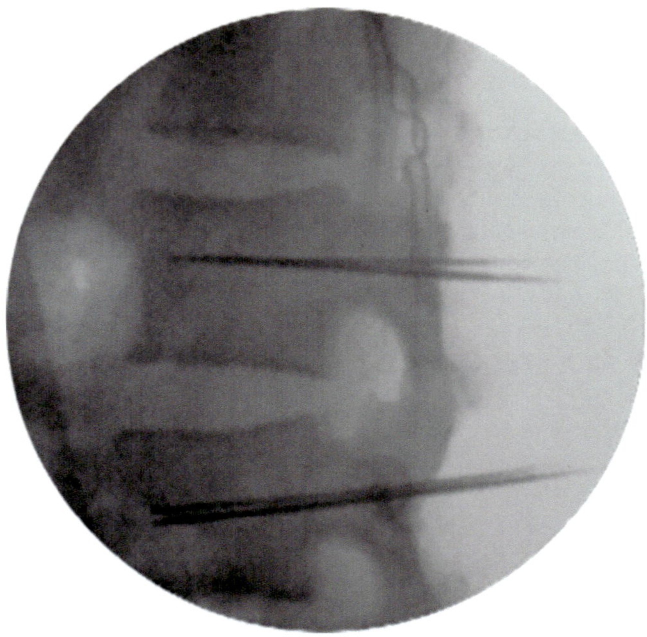

Fig. 9.15 Determining the location

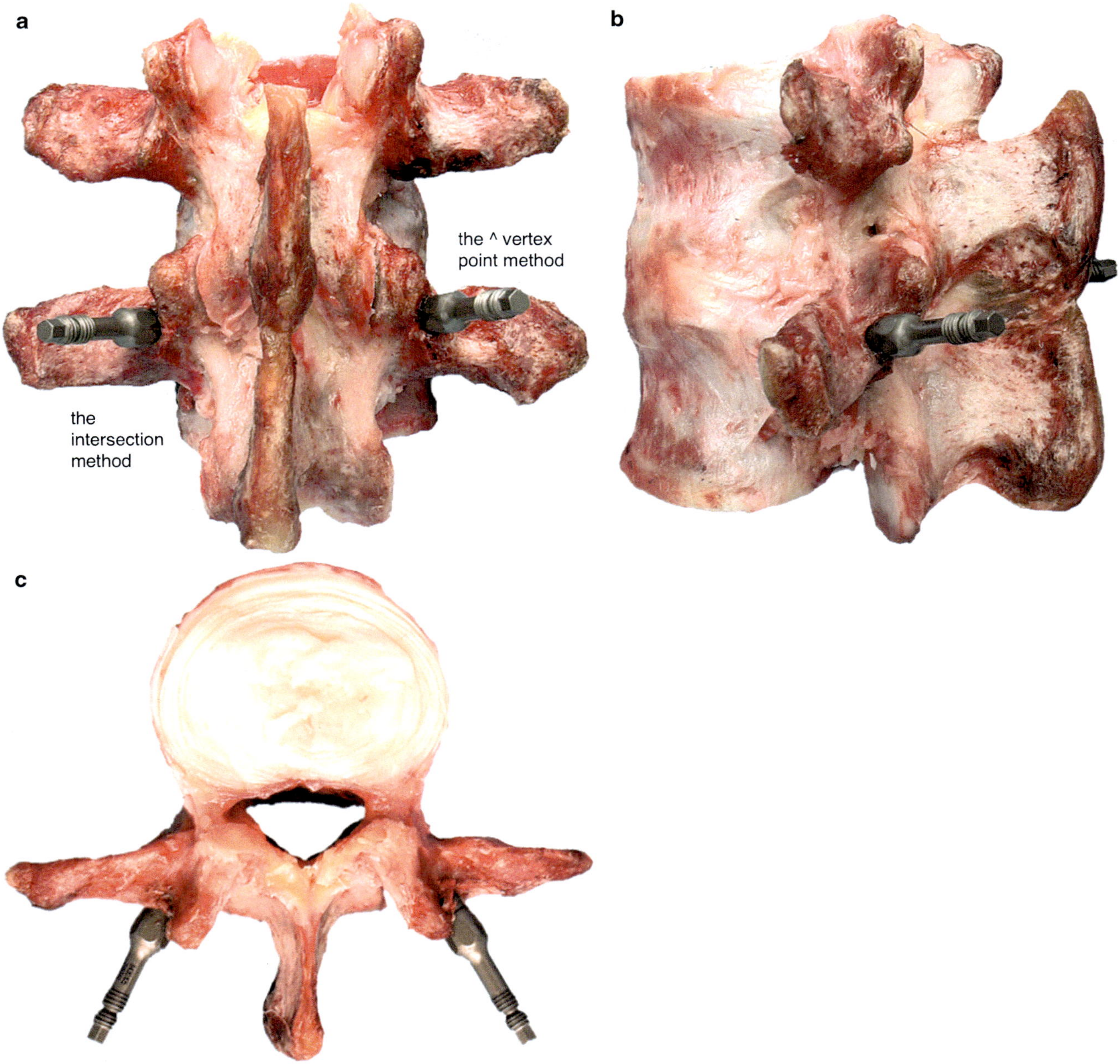

Fig. 9.16 Screw insertion. (**a**) Posterior view; (**b**) Oblique view; (**c**) Axial view

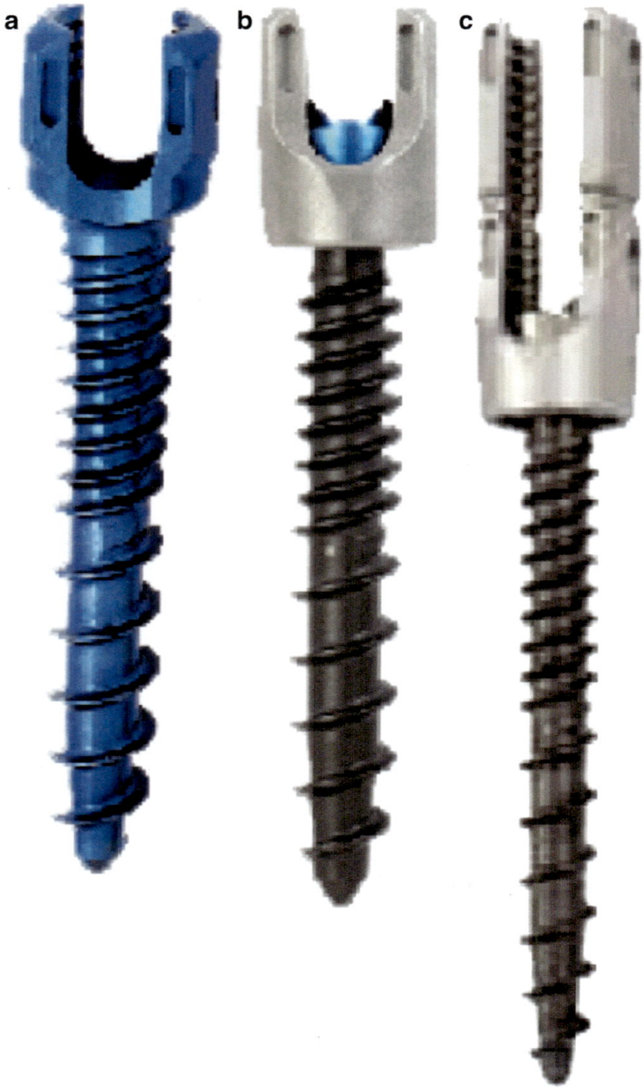

Fig. 9.17 Screws. (**a**) Fixed angle screw; (**b**) Multi-axial screw; (**c**) Multi-axial Reduction Screw

2. Laminar hooks (Fig. 9.18)
   a. Pedicle hook: For use for segments above T_{10}.
   b. Wide blade hook: It is the most frequently used hook type and is for use in the vertebral lamina or the transverse process.
   c. Thin blade hook: For use in the vertebral lamina or patients with a smaller spinal canal.
   d. Angled blade hook: It is mainly for use in the upper thoracic segments or patients with a smaller spinal canal.
   e. Angled laminar hook: For use in the infralaminar position, mainly in L_3, L_4, and L_5.
   f. Extended body hook: It is for use as a reverse hook, mainly in the infralaminar position.
   g. Thoracic laminar hook: It is for use in combination with pedicle hook at T_1, T_2, or T_3.
   h. Offset hook: It is for use in combination with pedicle screws.

9.2.2 Features of the System

1. The system uses patented G4 locking technology-reverse angle locking screws, which is easy to assemble and has a strong holding power, and a smaller implant notch (Figs. 9.19 and 9.20). Its clinical adoption has been increasing, with the following distinct features of the system:
   a. The entire system has a smaller profile.
   b. The adjacent superior articular process is preserved.
   c. It allows greater space for bone graft.
2. The design features of this system are its effectiveness, ease of use, and excellent handgrip of the silicone handle.
3. The system offers many options for the surgeon who can choose different combinations according to individual patient characteristics. The variety of implants include straight or curved rods of different diameters, fixed angle and universal angle screws of different diameters, bone hook, fixed angle, and universal screws. This system can be used for the thoracolumbar spine.

9.2.3 Clinical Indications and Contraindications

9.2.3.1 Indications

It is suitable for posterior thoracic, lumbar, and lumbosacral fixation.

1. Trauma
   a. Fracture and traumatic spondylolisthesis
   b. Correction of fracture malunion
2. Degenerative diseases
   a. Severe or recurrent lumbar disc hernia
   b. Vertebral instability or spondylolisthesis
   c. Stability reconstruction following laminectomy for spinal stenosis

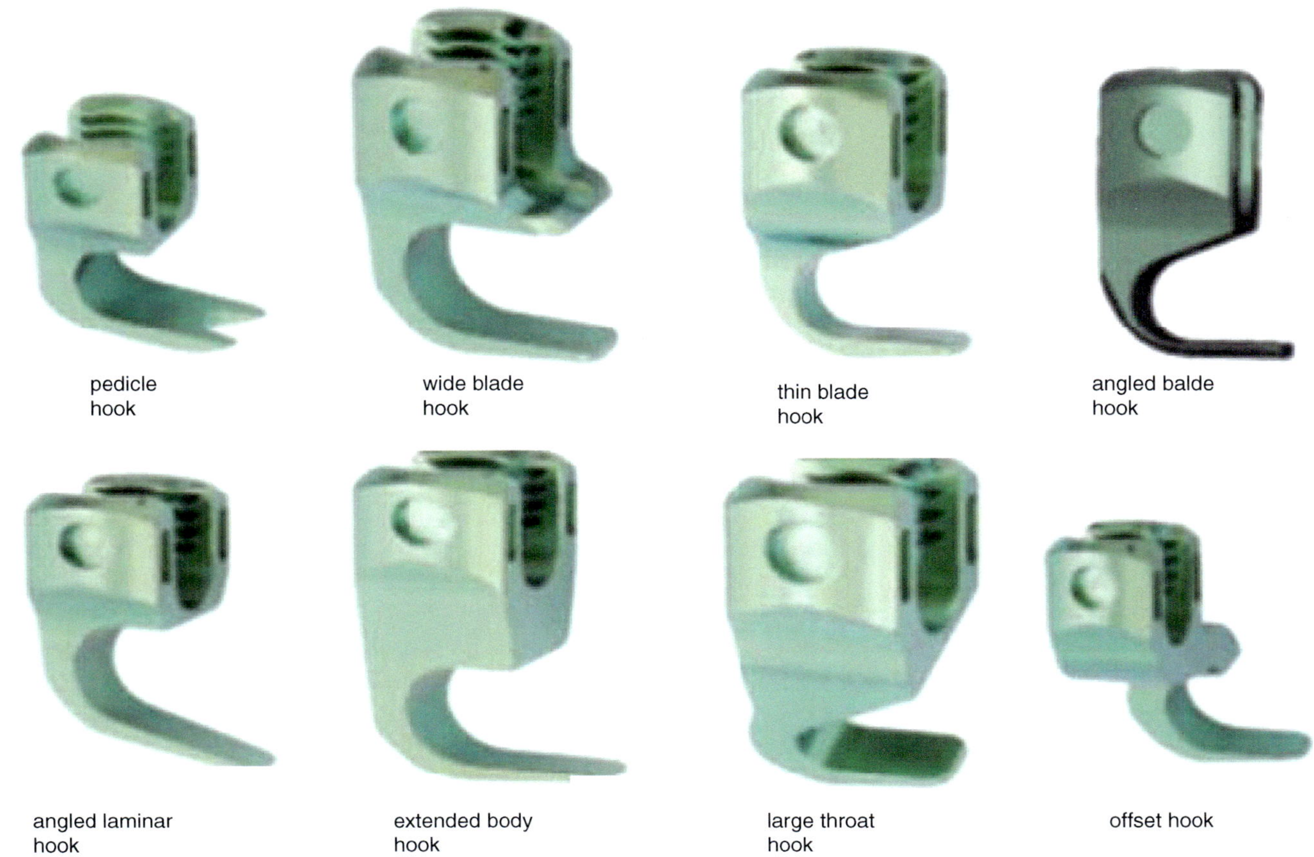

Fig. 9.18 Types of laminar hooks

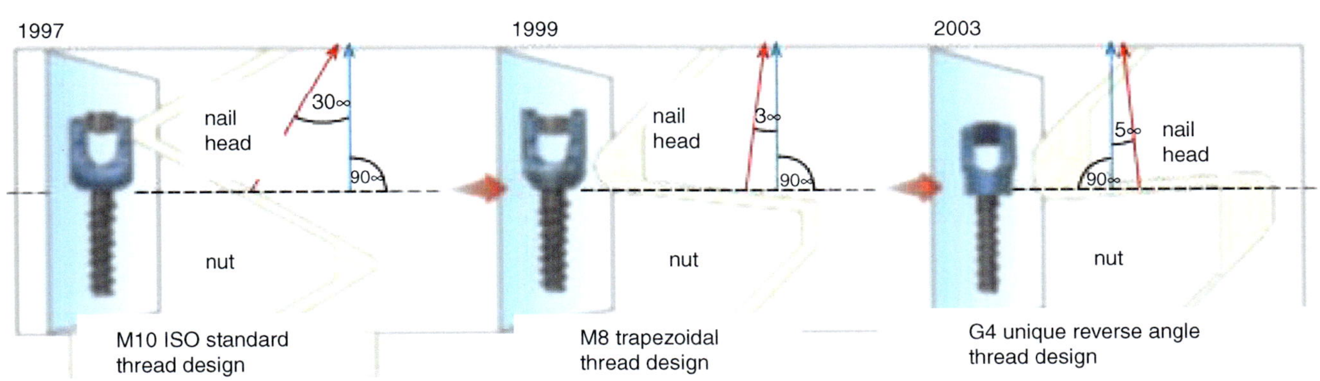

Fig. 9.19 G4 patented locking technology

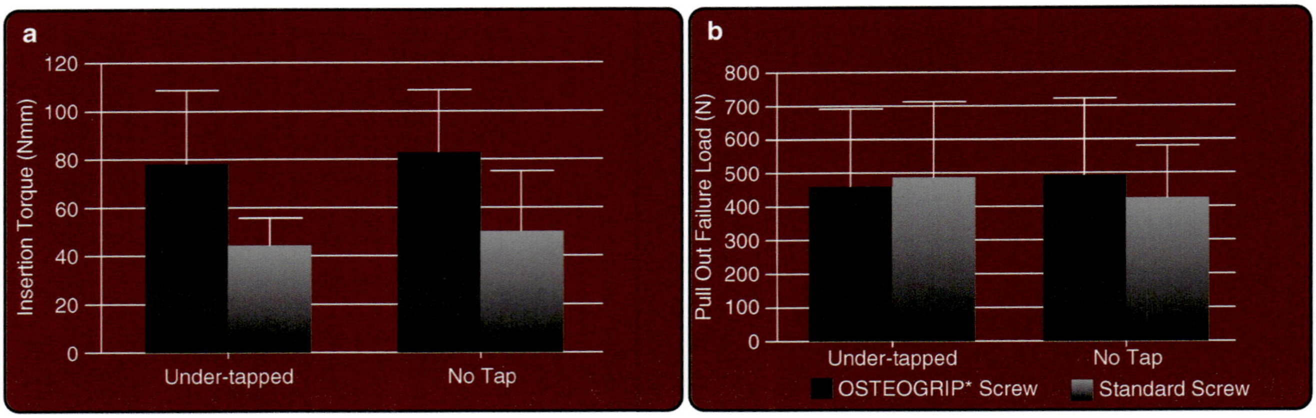

Fig. 9.20 Insertional torque (**a**) and pullout (**b**) study

3. Tumors
    a. Benign or malignant vertebral tumors or resection of metastatic tumor followed by reconstruction and posterior stabilization
    b. Laminectomy for intraspinal tumor followed by reconstruction and posterior stabilization
4. Infectious diseases
    a. Discitis or mild intervertebral disc space infection
    b. Vertebral tuberculosis debridement followed by reconstruction and posterior stabilization
5. Congenital diseases and malformations
    a. Correction of congenital vertebral scoliosis
    b. Correction of idiopathic vertebral scoliosis
    c. Correction of vertebral kyphosis

9.2.3.2 Contraindications

It cannot be used alone for anterior stabilization.

9.2.4 Surgical Techniques

9.2.4.1 CDH SOLERA Degenerative Surgical Technique

1. Universal screw placement

For pedicle preparation, screws of appropriate lengths are selected, and the hex head screwdriver is inserted into the screw head (Fig. 9.21a). Then, the screwdriver sleeve is rotated into the screw head (Fig. 9.21b). The hex head and thread sleeve provide durable support for universal screw placement. In addition, self-retaining screwdriver may also be used by inserting the inner hex head of the screwdriver into the screw head.

Screw position is assessed by fluoroscopy in the anteroposterior and lateral view. Intraoperative EMG monitoring may be undertaken if available. After a screw is fully placed, it should be parallel to the upper endplate and reaches 50–80% of the vertebral body height. For sacrum fixation, especially in patients with osteoporosis, screw fixation through two cortices can be employed. Some surgeons even recommend screw fixation through three cortices (to reach the anterior cortex via S1 endplate) in order to provide stronger fixation. The sleeve is withdrawn once a screw is properly placed.

9.2.4.2 Rod Contouring and Placement

Once correct screw placement has been verified radiographically, the selected rods were measured and contoured in the sagittal and coronal planes. To measure the rod length required for the construct, a rod template may be used (Fig. 9.22). A rod cutter (handheld or tabletop) may be used to cut the appropriate rod length.

The titanium alloy rods have an orientation line that serves as a reference point during contouring. To prevent the rod from rotating during contouring, it is helpful to clamp the rod with Dual Action Rod Grippers at both ends (Fig. 9.23). Note: Prior to implantation of the rod, break off the VERIFYI® Implant Tracking Tag and retain it in the Tag Sorter; thus, it can be scanned at the end of the surgery.

For non-hyperkyphotic deformities, the rod is first placed on the concave side. The contoured rod is then introduced into the previously placed screws. There are several methods and instruments for facilitating fully seating the rod into the saddle of the implant. Forceps Rocker Method: When only a slight height difference exists between the rod and the implant saddle, use of the Forceps Rocker is an effective method for reducing (or seating) the rod into the implant. To use the Forceps Rocker, the sides of the implant are grasped with the rocker cam above the rod and then lever backward over the rod (Fig. 9.24, left). Forceps

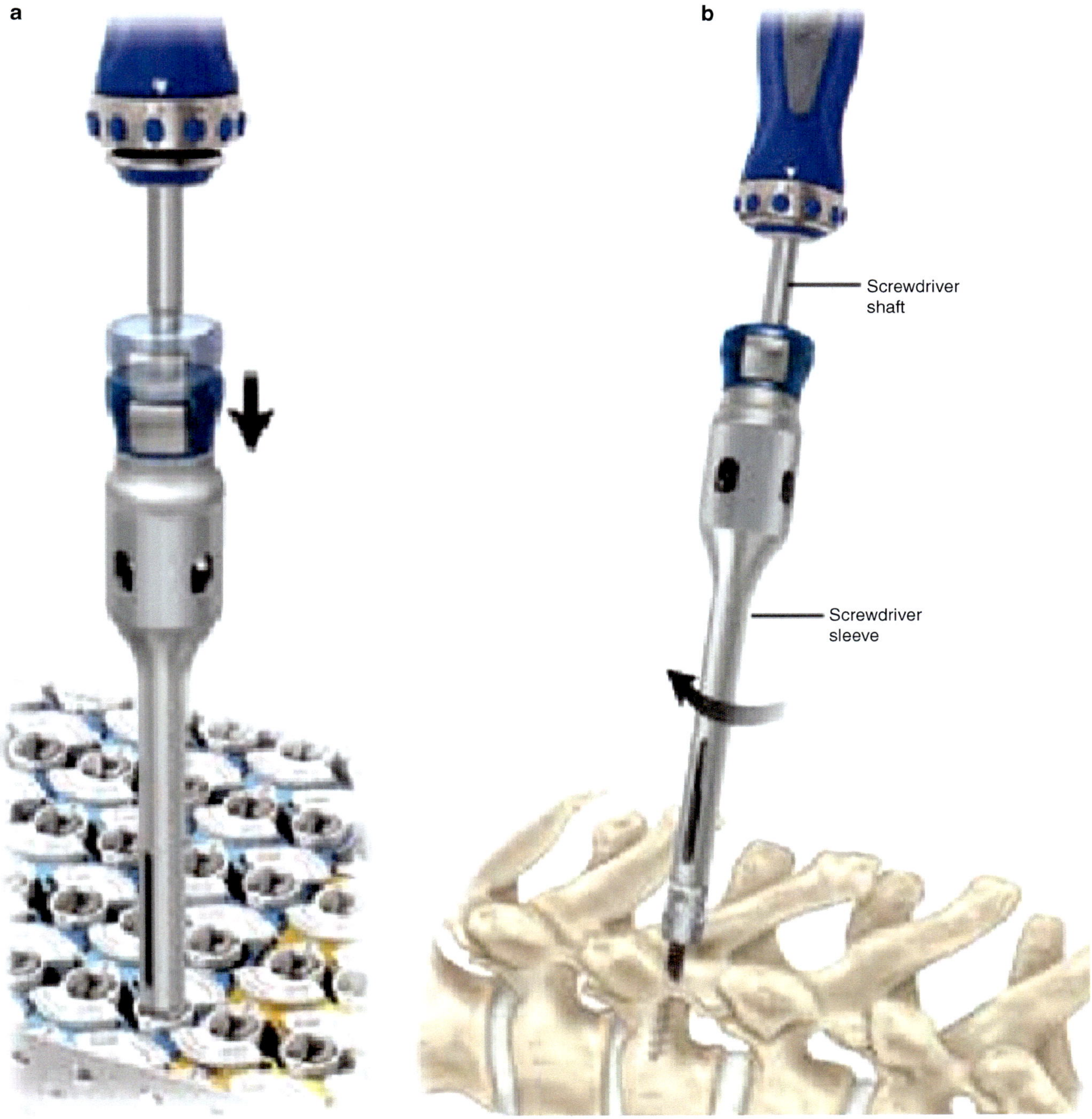

Fig. 9.21 Universal screw placement. (**a**) The screwdriver is inserted. (**b**) The sleeve is rotated into position

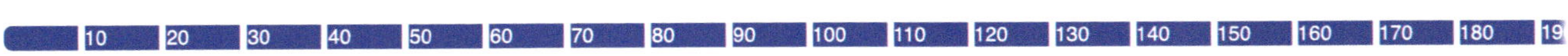

Fig. 9.22 Rod template

Rocker Method: The levering action allows the rod to be fully seated into the saddle of the implant. To introduce the set screw, the Dual Ended Set Screw Starter is then used (Fig. 9.24, right). Beale Rod Reducer: The Beale Rod Reducer may be used to seat the rod in situations where the rod rests at the top of the implant. The Beale Rod Reducer attaches to the four implant slots (Fig. 9.25, left). Once the Beale Rod Reducer is attached to the implant, the reducer handles are squeezed slowly, allowing the sleeve to slide down, and the rod is then seated into the implant saddle. Note: Prior to implantation of the set screw, break off the VERIFYI® Implant Tracking Tag and retain it in the Tag Sorter; thus, it can be scanned at the end of the surgery. The set screw is then placed through the reducer tube and into the implant head with the Provisional Driver or a Dual Ended Set Screw Starter. The set screw is provisionally tightened with the Provisional Driver in the extended position (Fig. 9.25, right).

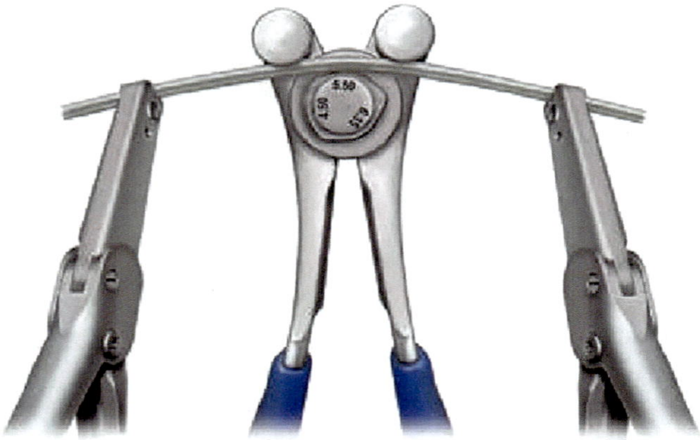

Fig. 9.23 Clamping the rod with Dual Action Rod Grippers

9.2.4.3 Compression/Distraction

Distraction and/or compression is performed to place the hooks in their final position once the rod is secured in the implants. The Hinged Translator, Multilevel Hook Compressor, Distractor, and Provisional Driver are used to perform these maneuvers (Fig. 9.26). Compression maneuvers are most often carried out directly on two hooks (Fig. 9.27). Another option is to use the Hinged Translator for compression. To ensure that the foot of either instrument is placed against the implant body and not against the set screw, care should be taken. It is preferable that compression

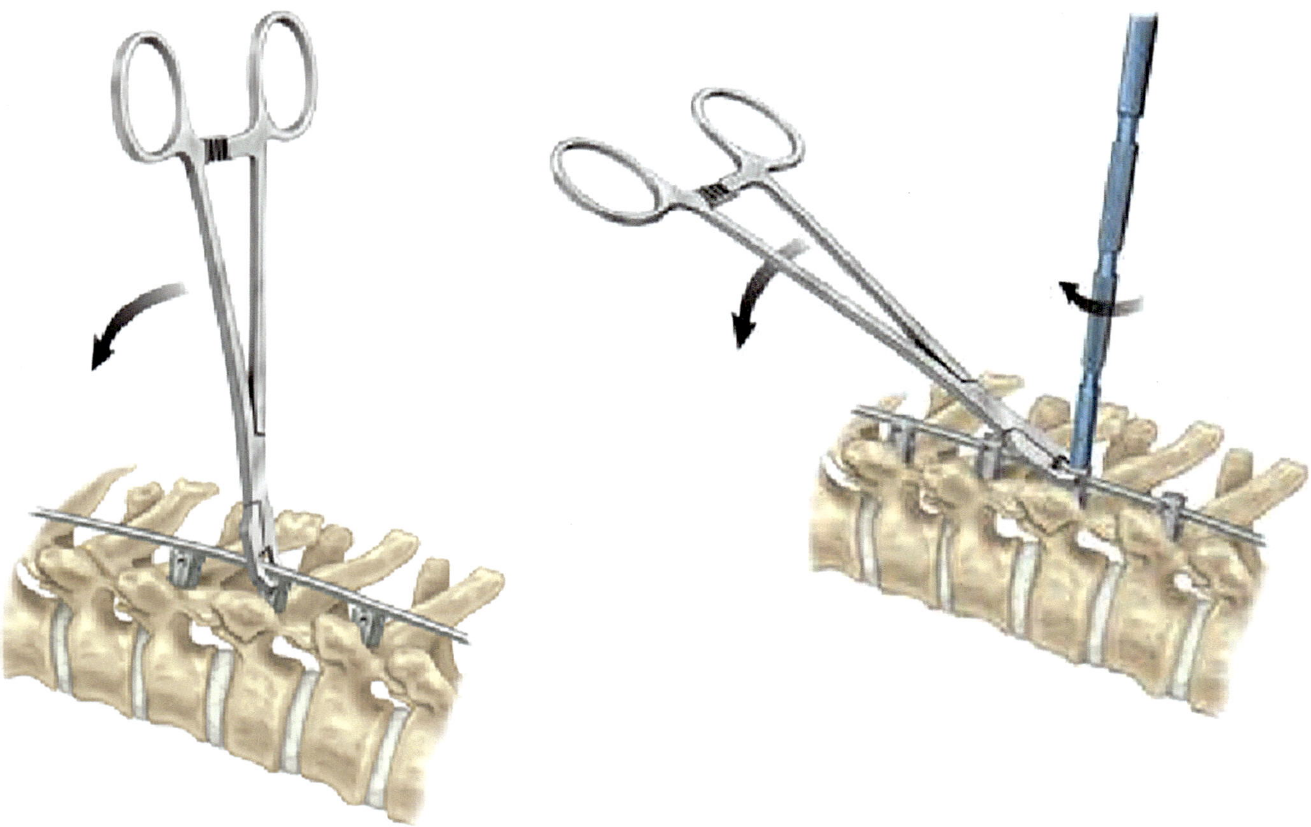

Fig. 9.24 Using the Forceps Rocker, *left*; Using the Dual Ended Set Screw Starter, *right*

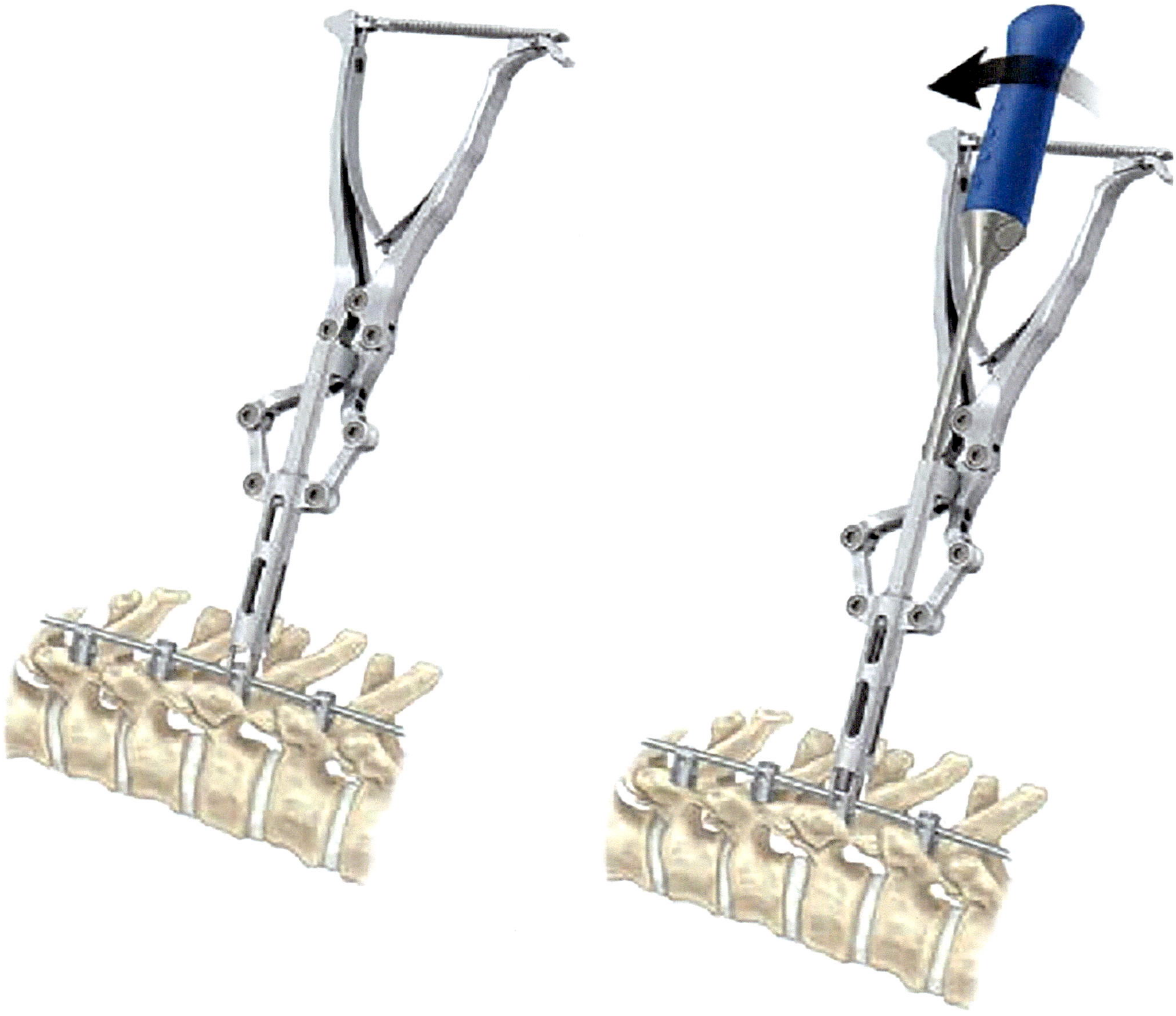

Fig. 9.25 *Left*, the Beale Rod Reducer attaches to the four implant slots. *Right*, the set screw with the Provisional Driver is provisionally tightened in the extended position

be released just prior to the set screw being broken off or finally tightened. This technique will help to ensure that the implant head and rod are normalized to one another and, therefore, allows for the rod to be fully seated in the implant head during final tightening. The set screw is tightened with the Provisional Driver after these maneuvers are completed. Note: Screw operation is similar to hook.

9.2.4.4 Final Tightening and Decortication

The set screws which lock the rods into place are sheared off using the Counter Torque and the Self-Retaining Break-Off Driver (Fig. 9.28). Having the appropriate locking torque built into it, the break-off set screw should not require additional tightening. The final tightening torque range is 9–10.5 Nm or 80–93 in-lbs for 4.75-mm implants and 10.50–12.50 Nm or 92–110 in-lbs for 5.5-/6.0-mm implants. To prevent overtightening of the set screw which could reduce the strength of the connection, the Torque Indicating Driver should be used if additional manipulation of the set screw is desired after the break-off is achieved. To use the 4.75-mm or the 5.5-/6.0-mm Torque Indicating Driver, the Quick Connect T-Handle is attached to the Torque Indicating Driver and passed through the Counter Torque and into the inner portion of the set screw (Fig. 9.29). The handle is turned until the slot reaches the line on the right side of the scale to ensure the correct torque limit has been achieved (Fig. 9.30). The

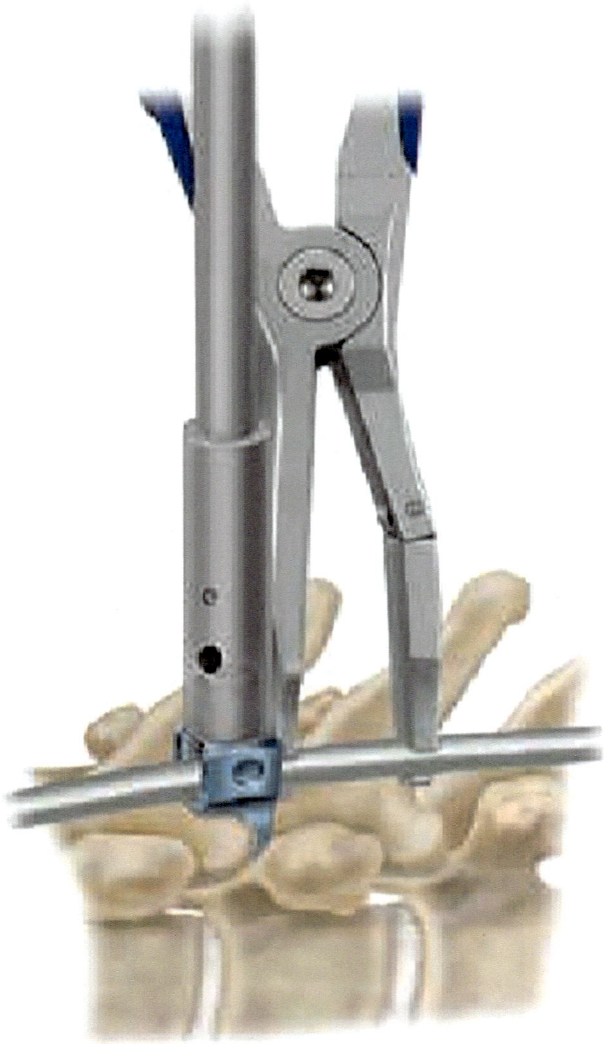

Fig. 9.26 The Hinged Translator, Multilevel Hook Compressor, Distractor, and Provisional Driver are used to carry out these maneuvers

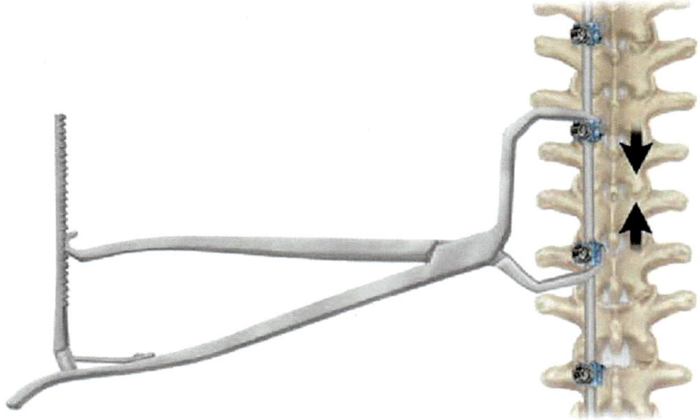

Fig. 9.27 Compression maneuvers are most often performed directly on two hooks

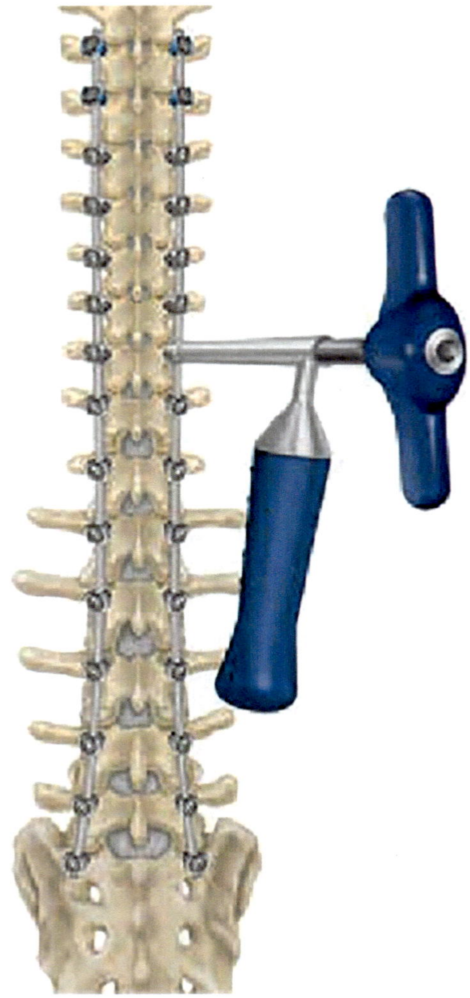

Fig. 9.28 Using the Counter Torque and the Self-Retaining Break-Off Driver

posterior elements are decorticated with a burr and the bone graft is placed.

9.2.4.5 Graft Placement

Despite internal fixation, bony fusion remains critical to the success of the surgical outcome. Careful decortication of the transverse processes, the facet joints, and the pars interarticularis should be accomplished using a high-speed burr. Some surgeons may choose to perform decortication prior to internal fixation in certain instances if poor visualization hampers decortications. Preservation of the facet capsules of the unfused adjacent levels is advantageous (Fig. 9.31).

Whether the autograft or allograft bone is utilized, precise placement of the graft onto the decorticated bone is essential. This can only be done with excellent visualization of the decorticated bone surfaces. Attention should be paid to the development of a pseudoarthrosis due to interposing muscle

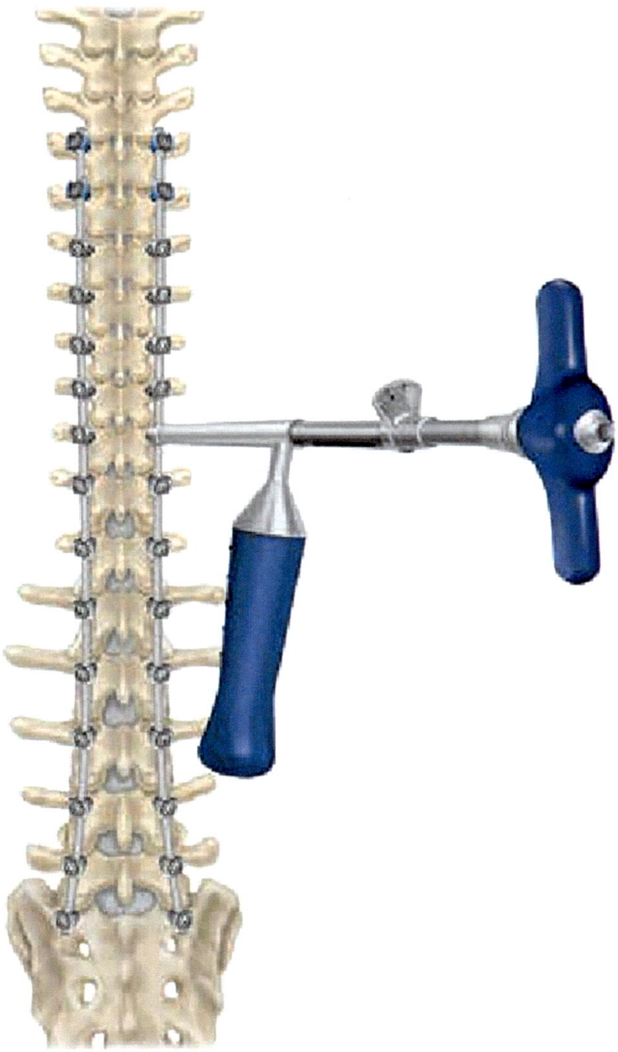

Fig. 9.29 The Quick Connect T-Handle is attached to the Torque Indicating Driver

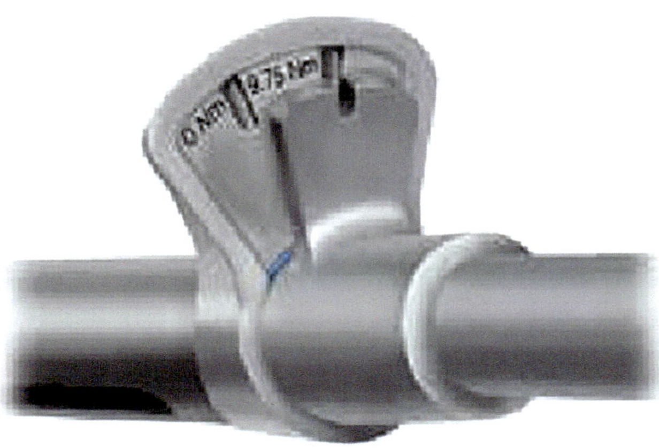

Fig. 9.30 The handle is turned until the slot reaches the line on the right side of the scale to ensure the Correct Torque limit has been achieved

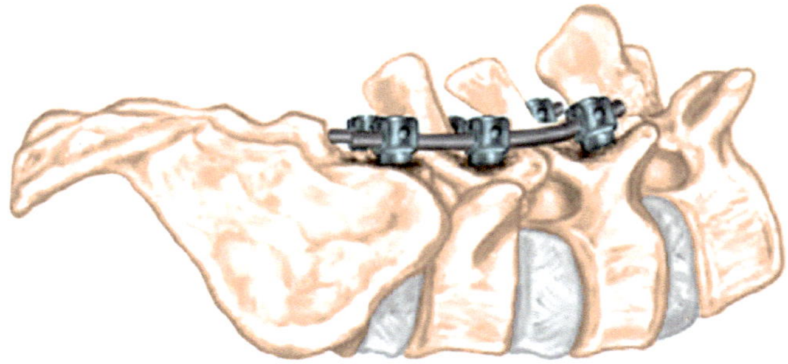

Fig. 9.31 Preservation of the facet capsules

tissues in fusion between transverse processes. If the facet architecture is not retained, the graft should be impacted into the facet to obtain a facet fusion. Once instrumentation is complete and the graft l is placed, the construct should be checked radiographically (Fig. 9.32).

9.2.4.6 X10 CROSSLINK Plate Placement

X10 CROSSLINK plates significantly increase the torsional stability of internal fixation. Internal fixation of longer segments necessitates placement of an X10 CROSSLINK plate at each end to increase construct rigidity. Two measuring devices are available to determine the proper length of X10 CROSSLINK plate for use: the measuring card (Fig. 9.33, left) and the measuring caliper (Fig. 9.33, right).

Prior to plate placement, the X10 CROSSLINK plate set screws are backed out to prevent binding onto the rods of the construct during placement. If the set screw is backed out too far, it will disengage from the plate, but it can easily be reinserted. A surgeon has several X10 CROSSLINK plate placement options.

9.2.4.7 In Line Plate Holder Method

The midline nut is provisionally tightened to facilitate X10 CROSSLINK plate placement. The In Line Plate Holder is used to select, grip, and position the plate to capture the far rod. In addition, the Torque-Limiting Set Screwdriver is used to tighten the ipsilateral set screws (Fig. 9.34). Thereafter, the midline nut is loosened, and a CROSSLINK plate is placed on the opposite end onto the other rod. Next, the midline nut is tightened on the screw head, and a 7-N·m torque is used to shear off the screw head. Finally, the midline nut is tightened using a 9-N·m torque (Fig. 9.35). Following placement of the plate onto one rod, the set screw is tightened using the 7/32″ Torque-Limiting Set Screwdriver until it is firmly attached to the rod.

Caution: The midline nut is *not* a break-off set screw.

9.2.4.8 Implant Positioner Method

With the use of Implant Positioners, appropriate X10 CROSSLINK plates are selected (Fig. 9.36). Ensure that both Implant Positioners fit securely onto both rod set screws.

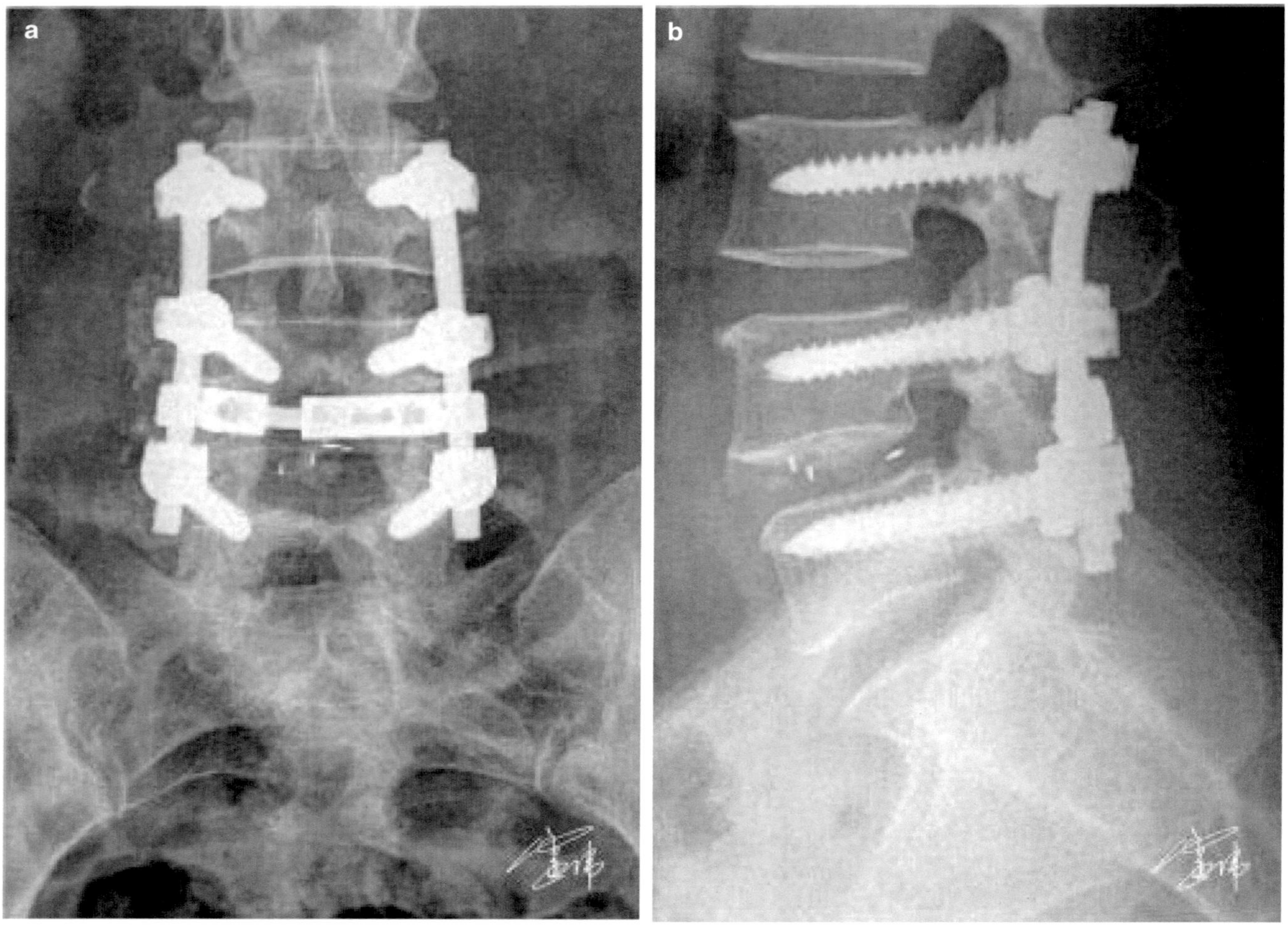

Fig. 9.32 The implant construct is checked radiographically. (**a**) Anteroposterior view. (**b**) Lateral view

The Implant Positioners can be used to sequentially articulate the CROSSLINK plate around the rod (Fig. 9.37).

9.2.4.9 Forceps Plate Holder Method

With the use of the Forceps Plate Holder, the appropriate X10 CROSSLINK Multi-Span Plate is selected and gripped (Fig. 9.38).

Ensure that both crossbars on the X10 CROSSLINK plate are gripped using the Forceps Plate Holder. The plate is then placed to capture the far rod (in relation to the surgeon) of the two rods to be stabilized. The far rod's set screw is provisionally tightened using the Torque-Limiting Set Screwdriver to anchor the device to this rod (Fig. 9.39).

The Forceps Plate Holder is removed from both crossbars and placed on the crossbar that is able to move. The second side of the plate to the rod is then anchored and the set screw is provisionally tightened. Next, after the Forceps Plate Holder is removed, the midline gut is provisionally tightened. To minimize torque transfer to the construct during final tightening, a Counter Torque may be placed on the X10 CROSSLINK Multi-Span Plate. The screwdriver shaft is introduced through the Counter Torque. Using the Torque-Limiting Set Screwdriver, the set screws are sheared off. The midline nut then undergoes final tightening with the same screwdriver.

If the CROSSLINK plate cannot be precisely seated against the rod, the set screw protrudes outward. Ensure that the CROSSLINK plate 1 abuts against the rod in the maneuvering space. The set screw can be manipulated and slightly backed out by rotating the Implant Positioners, allowing the rod to fully seat in the ventral opening. To provisionally

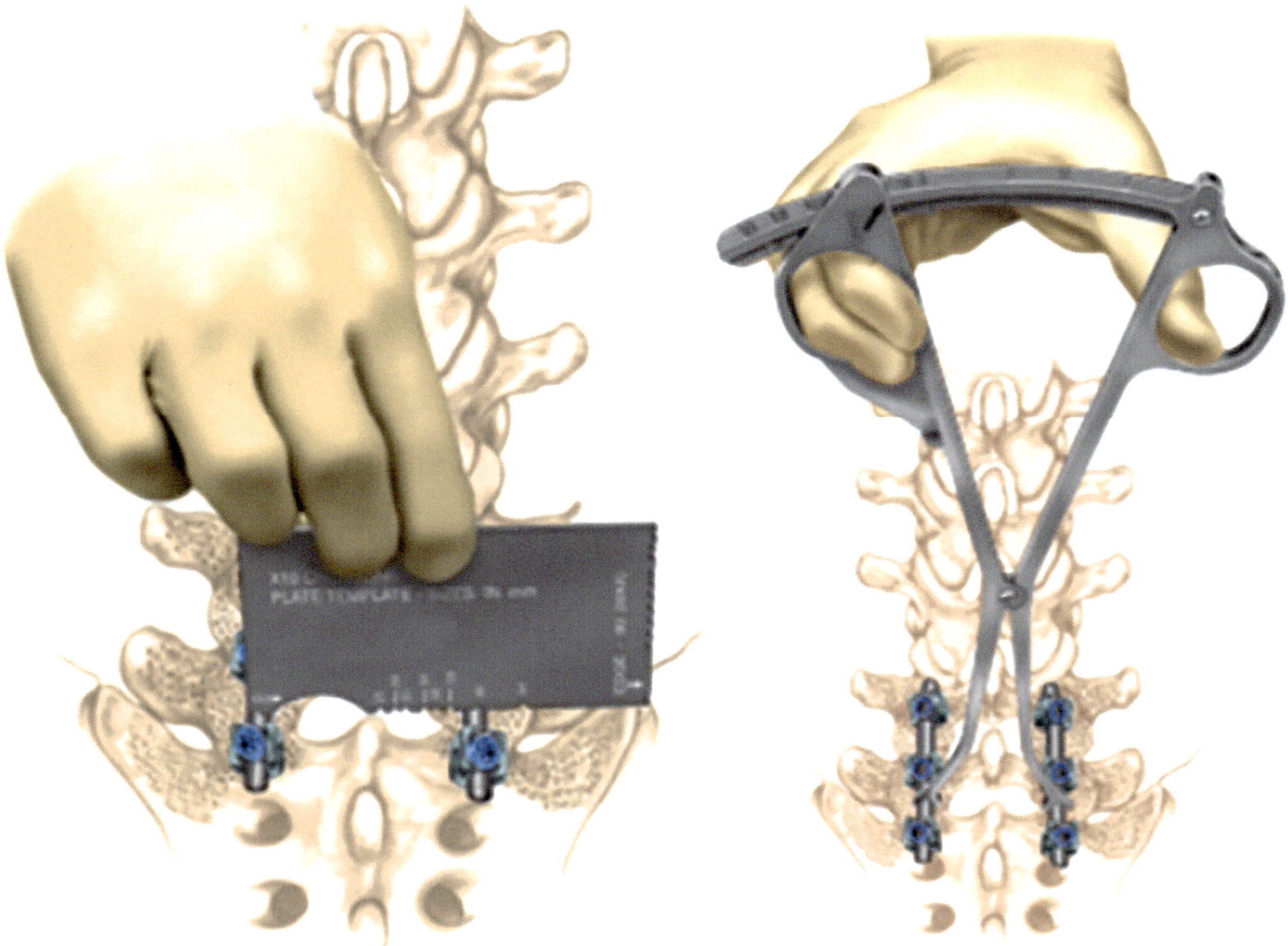

Fig. 9.33 The measuring card (*left*) and the measuring caliper (*right*)

tighten the X10 CROSSLINK plate to the rod, the Implant Positioners can be used once precise contact has been achieved between the plate and the rod. The same process is carried out for the other side of the plate. With the rod before final tightening and set screw break-off, both halves of the plate should precisely articulate (Fig. 9.40).

The Implant Positioner is removed, and the midline nut is provisionally tightened by the Torque-Limiting Set Screwdriver. To minimize torque transfer to the construct during final tightening, a Counter Torque may be placed on the X10 CROSSLINK Multi-Span Plate. The screwdriver shaft is introduced through the Counter Torque. The set screws are sheared off by using the screwdriver. The midline nut then undergoes final tightening with the same screwdriver. Before the wound is closed, ensure that the set screws are symmetrically seated in the screw heads, there is no bone graft displacement, and the number of screw heads that are sheared off is correct.

9.2.5 Pedicle Screw Surgery for Deformity Correction Using the SOLERA System

The set screws are kept loose (or only locked at one end); then with the left and right Coronal Benders, the concave rod is slowly straightened (Fig. 9.41). Each straightening of the concave rod is performed over a pedicle screw. In order for viscoelastic relaxation with subsequent curve correction to occur, several passes may be required. The apical set screws are tightened and appropriate compression or distraction is

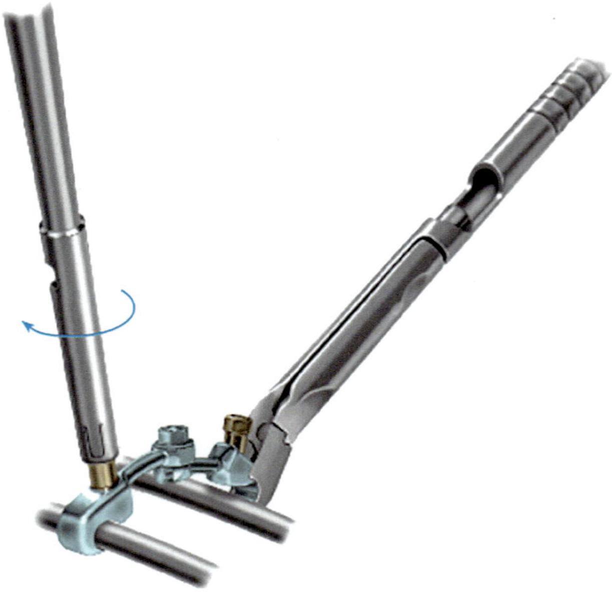

Fig. 9.34 The In Line Plate Holder Method

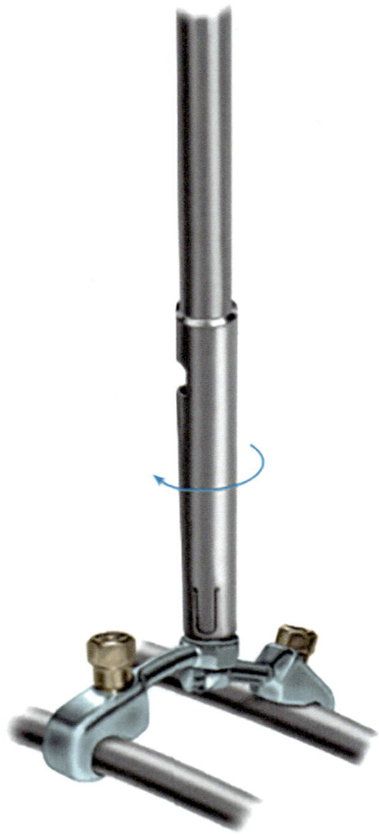

Fig. 9.35 The midline nut is tightened

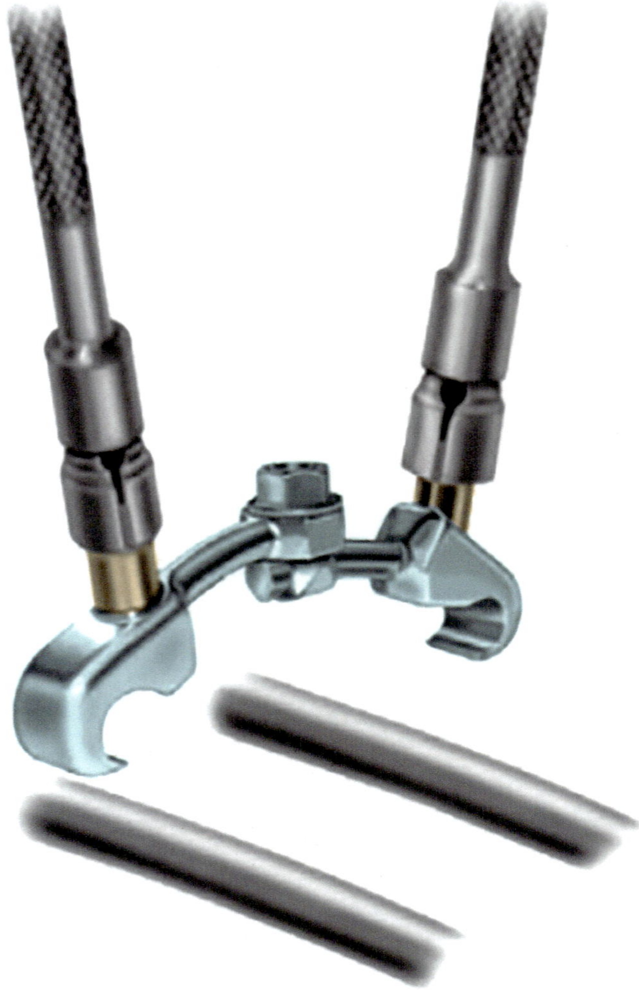

Fig. 9.36 CROSSLINK plate placement

performed. The bone-to-screw interface should be watched with all correction maneuvers.

9.2.5.1 Hinged Translator

During correction maneuvers, the Hinged Translator can be used in place of either a compressor or a distractor. The straight leg of the instrument will push the implant, while the hinged leg engages on the rod acting as rod gripper. Careful attention should be paid to the bone-to-screw interface during any correction maneuver.

To make hinged leg and straight leg touching each other, the rack is disengaged prior to placing the Hinged Translator on the rod (Fig. 9.42). A left and a right translator are included in the set for facilitating the compression and dis-

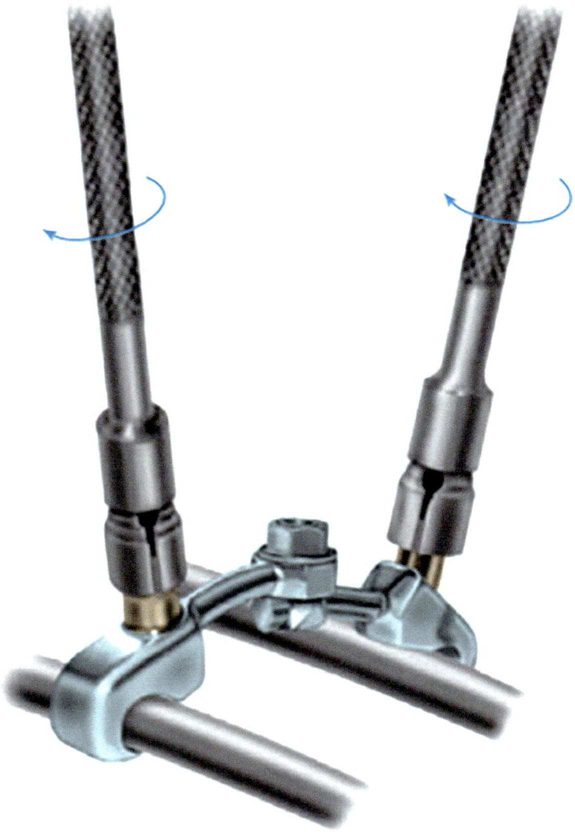

Fig. 9.37 Securing the CROSSLINK plate

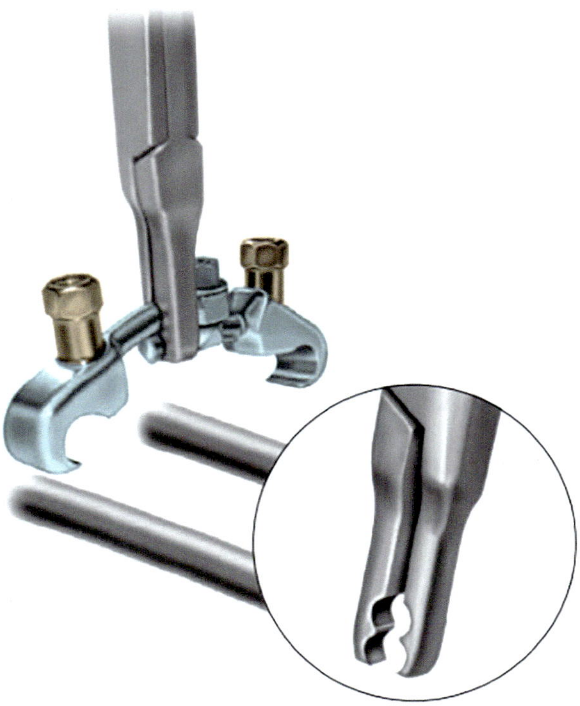

Fig. 9.38 Forceps Plate Holder method

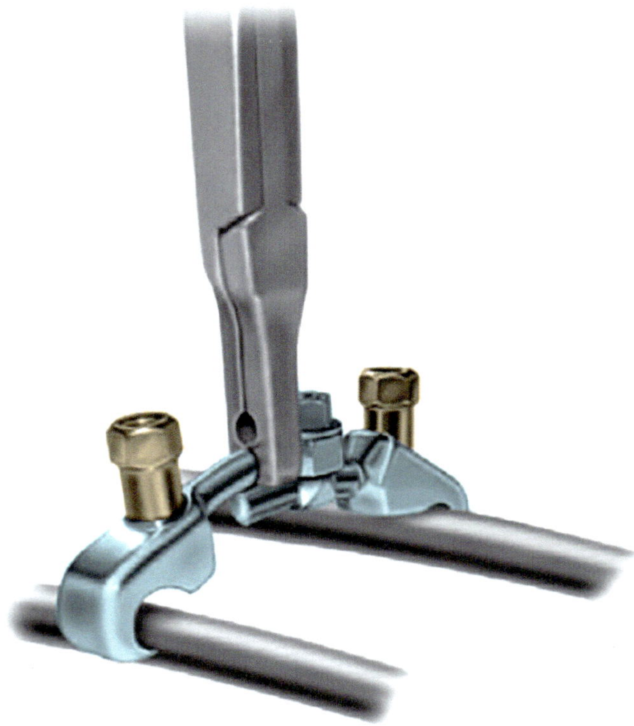

Fig. 9.39 CROSSLINK plate placement

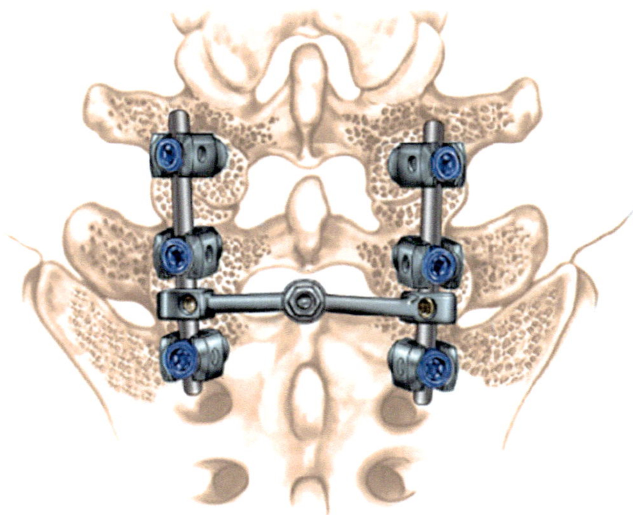

Fig. 9.40 Tightening the CROSSLINK plate

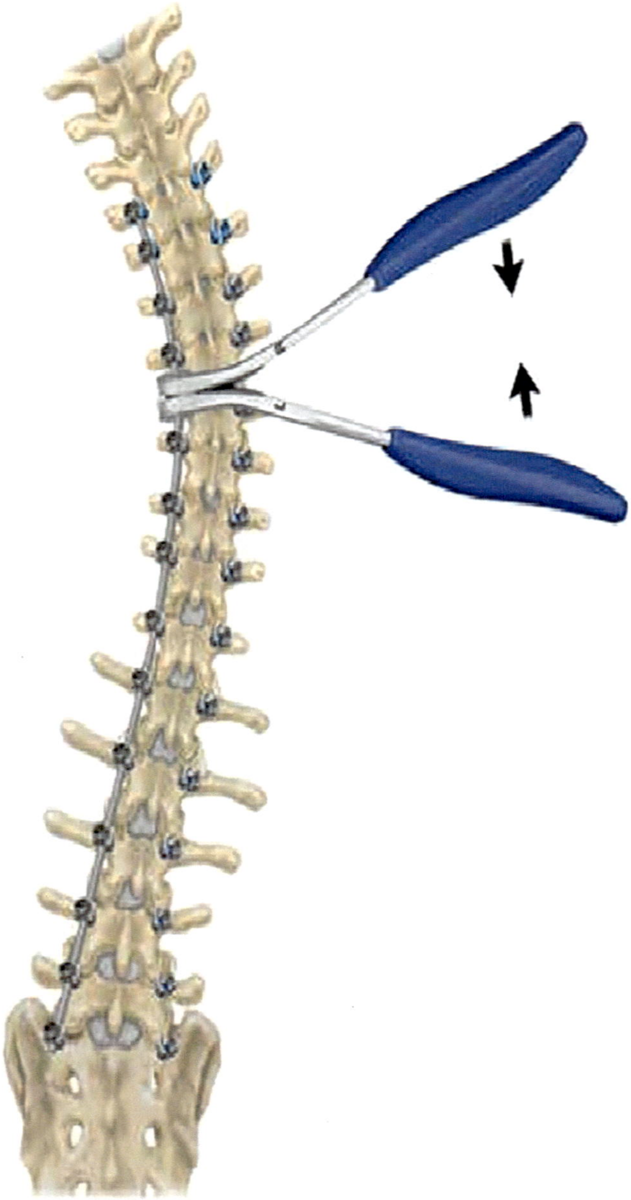

Fig. 9.41 Left and right Coronal Benders

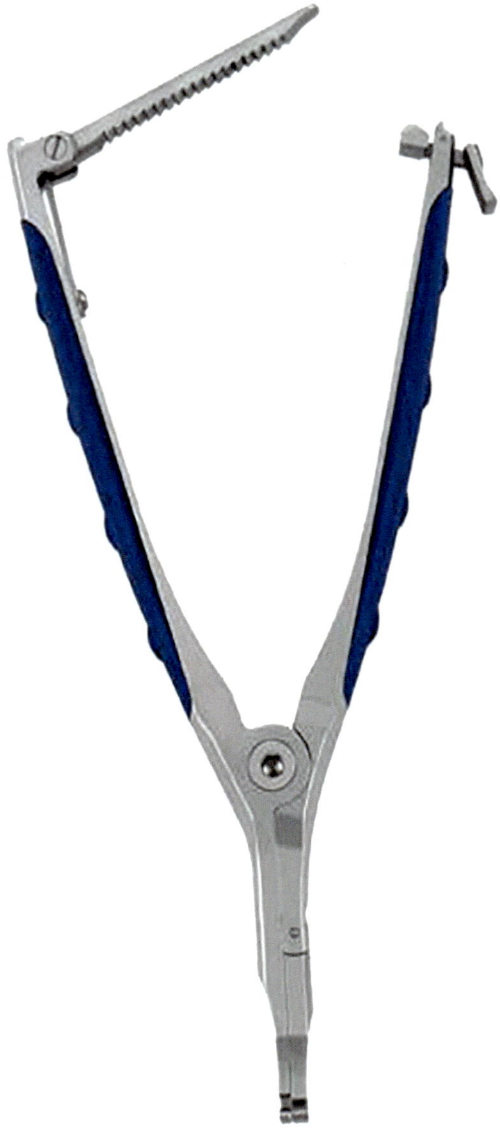

Fig. 9.42 Hinged Translator

traction maneuvers around the bony anatomy. The arrow on the rack of the Hinged Translator shows the direction in which the implant will be moved.

Example for Compressing the T8–T9 Segment: The T9 set screw is provisionally tightened. The instrument is placed along the rod with the straight leg below and immediately against the T9 screw prior to squeezing the handles (Fig. 9.43). The handles are squeezed to begin compression (Fig. 9.44). Example for Distracting the T8–T9 Segment: The T8 set screw is provisionally tightened. The instrument is placed along the rod with the straight leg below and immediately against the T8 screw prior to squeezing the handles (Fig. 9.45). The handles are squeezed to begin distraction (Fig. 9.46).

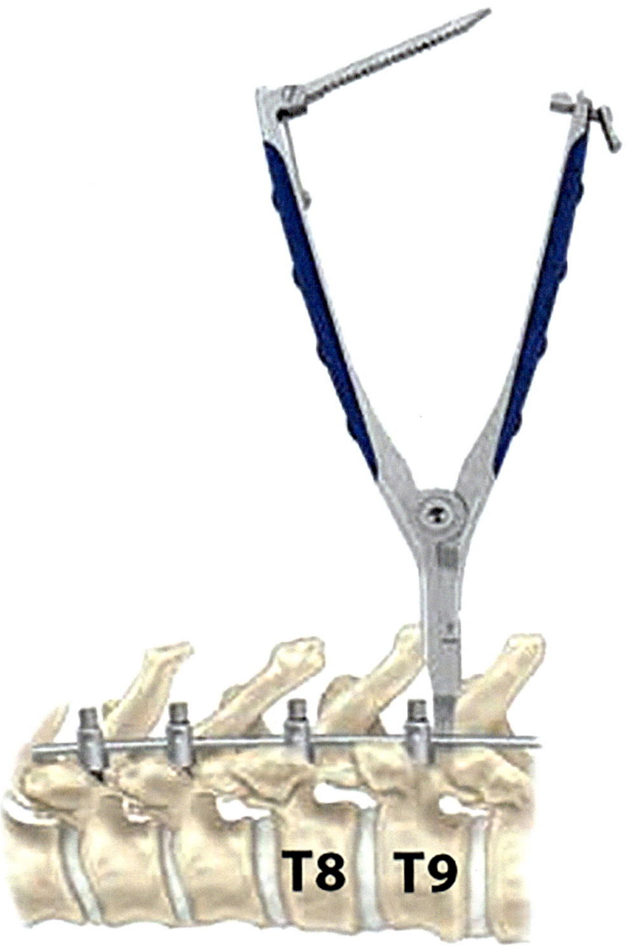

Fig. 9.43 Place the instrument

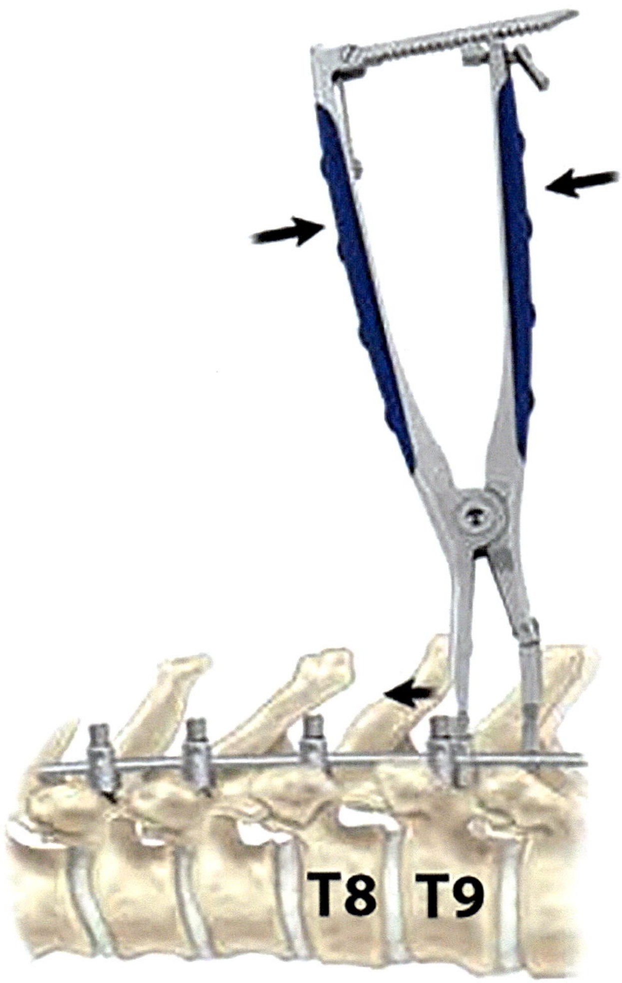

Fig. 9.44 Squeeze the handles

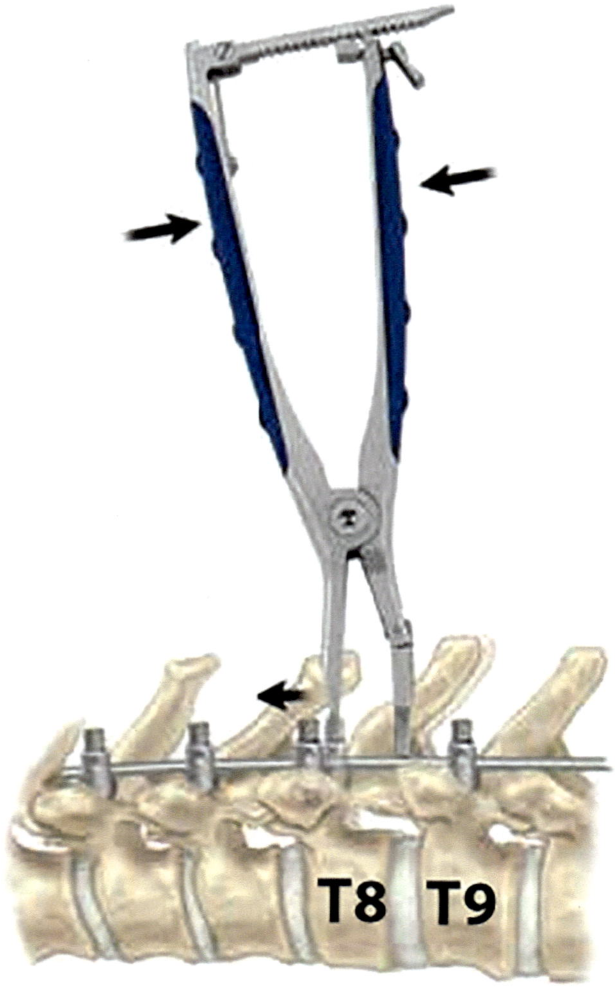

Fig. 9.45 The instrument is placed against the T8 screw

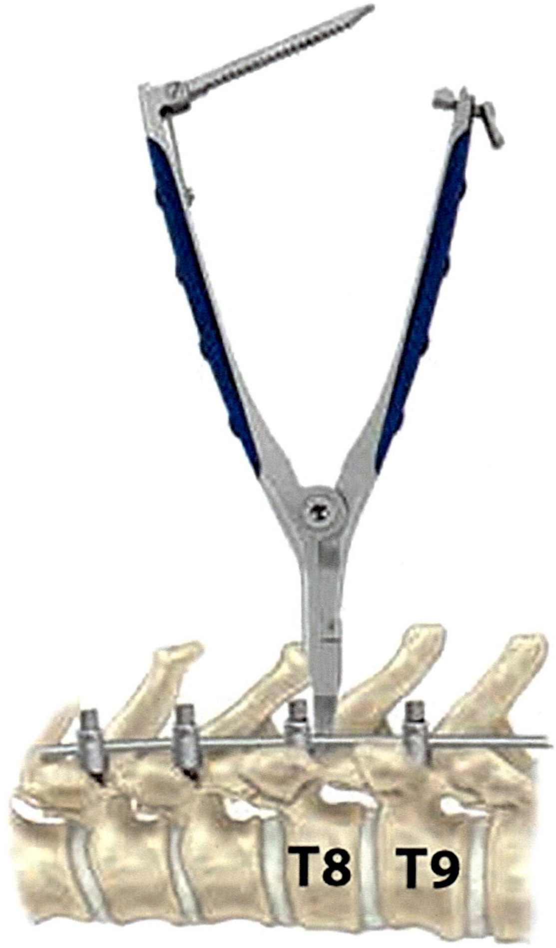

Fig. 9.46 Release the handles

9.2.5.2 Placing the Stabilizing Rod

Following placement of the second rod and set screws (Fig. 9.47), convex compressive forces are placed on the segments by using the compressor to horizontalize the lowest instrumented vertebra and mildly compress the convexity of the deformity (Fig. 9.48). It is preferable that compression be released just prior to the set screw being broken off or with final tightening. This technique will help to ensure that the implant head and rod are normalized to one another and therefore allow for the rod to be fully seated in the implant head during final tightening. To detect any potential neurologic deficits, NMEP and/or SSEP monitoring is performed. Fixation is verified with anteroposterior and lateral X-rays for confirmation of spinal correction and alignment.

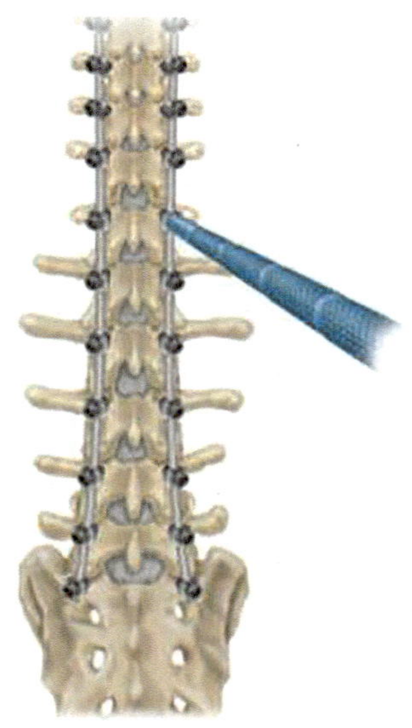

Fig. 9.47 Placement

9.2.5.3 Final Tightening and Decortication

Using the Counter Torque and the Self-Retaining Break-Off Driver, the set screws which lock the rods into place are sheared off (Fig. 9.49). Having the appropriate locking

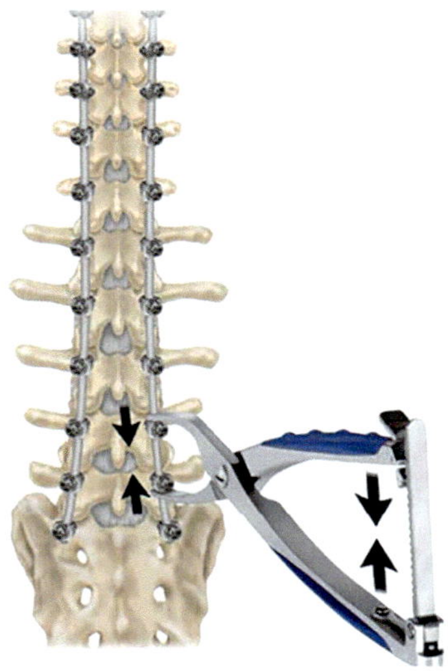

Fig. 9.48 Compression

torque built into it, the break-off set screw should not require additional tightening. The final tightening torque range is 9–10.5 Nm or 80–93 in-lbs for 4.75-mm implants and 10.50–12.50 Nm or 92–110 in-lbs for 5.5-/6.0-mm implants.

To prevent overtightening of the set screw which could reduce the strength of the connection, the Torque Indicating Driver should be used if additional manipulation of the set screw is desired after the break-off is achieved. To use the 4.75-mm or the 5.5-/6.0-mm Torque Indicating Driver, the Quick Connect T-Handle is attached to the Torque Indicating Driver and passed through the Counter Torque and into the inner portion of the set screw (Fig. 9.49). The handle is turned until the slot reaches the line on the right side of the scale to ensure the correct torque limit has been achieved (Fig. 9.50). The posterior elements are decorticated with a burr and the bone graft is placed.

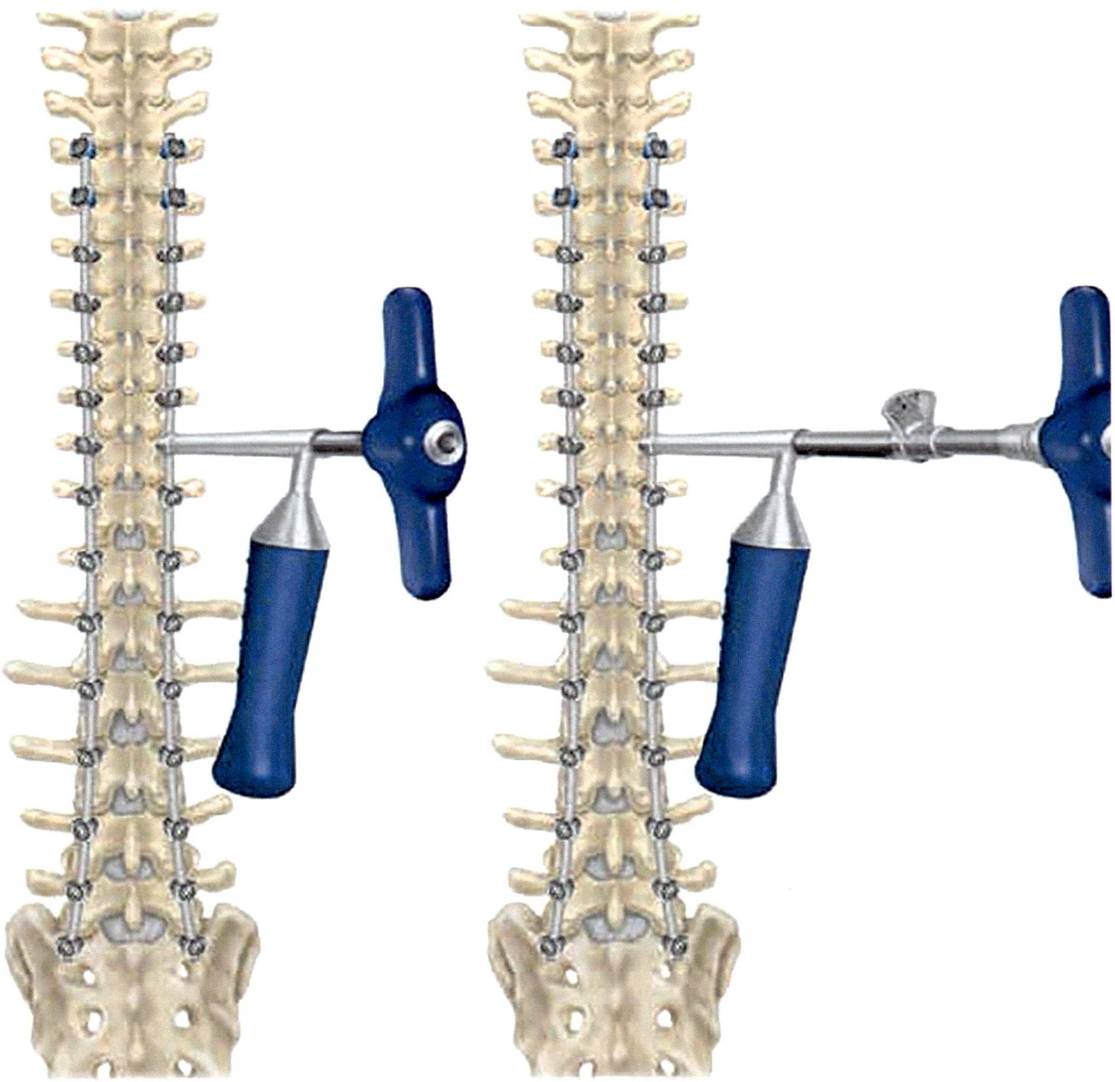

Fig. 9.49 Final tightening

9.2.6 Multi-axial Reduction Screw Techniques

9.2.6.1 Screw/Rod Placement

After the pedicles are prepared, multi-axial screws are placed horizontally at L4 and S1, and Multi-axial Reduction Screws are inserted at L5 (Fig. 9.51a). Multi-axial screws can be used at all segments to facilitate rod placement. The set screws are then inserted into the implants at L_4 and S_1 and provisionally tightened to facilitate seating the rod (Fig. 9.51b).

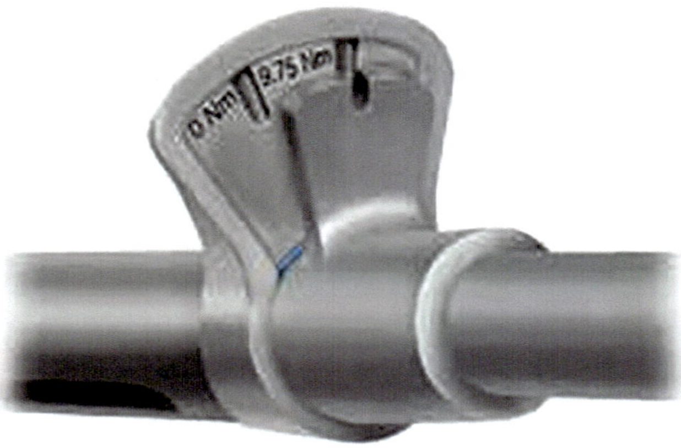

Fig. 9.50 Torque limit

9.2.6.2 Spondylolisthesis Reduction

1. Screw pulling reduction: The Ring Counter Torque is placed over the implant head throughout the reduction procedure. The reduction set screws are inserted into the reduction implant head using the self-retaining screw-driver. This will pull the implant to the rod, translating the vertebral body of L5 posteriorly and, therefore, reducing spondylolisthesis (Fig. 9.52).
2. Use of Forceps Rocker for reduction: The Forceps Rocker can be used to seat the rod and provide incremental reduction. The head of the implant is grasped with the Forceps Rocker and rocked down, applying pressure to the rod (Fig. 9.53).
3. Use of the Beale Rod Reducer for reduction: The Beale Rod Reducer can be used in conjunction with the Rod

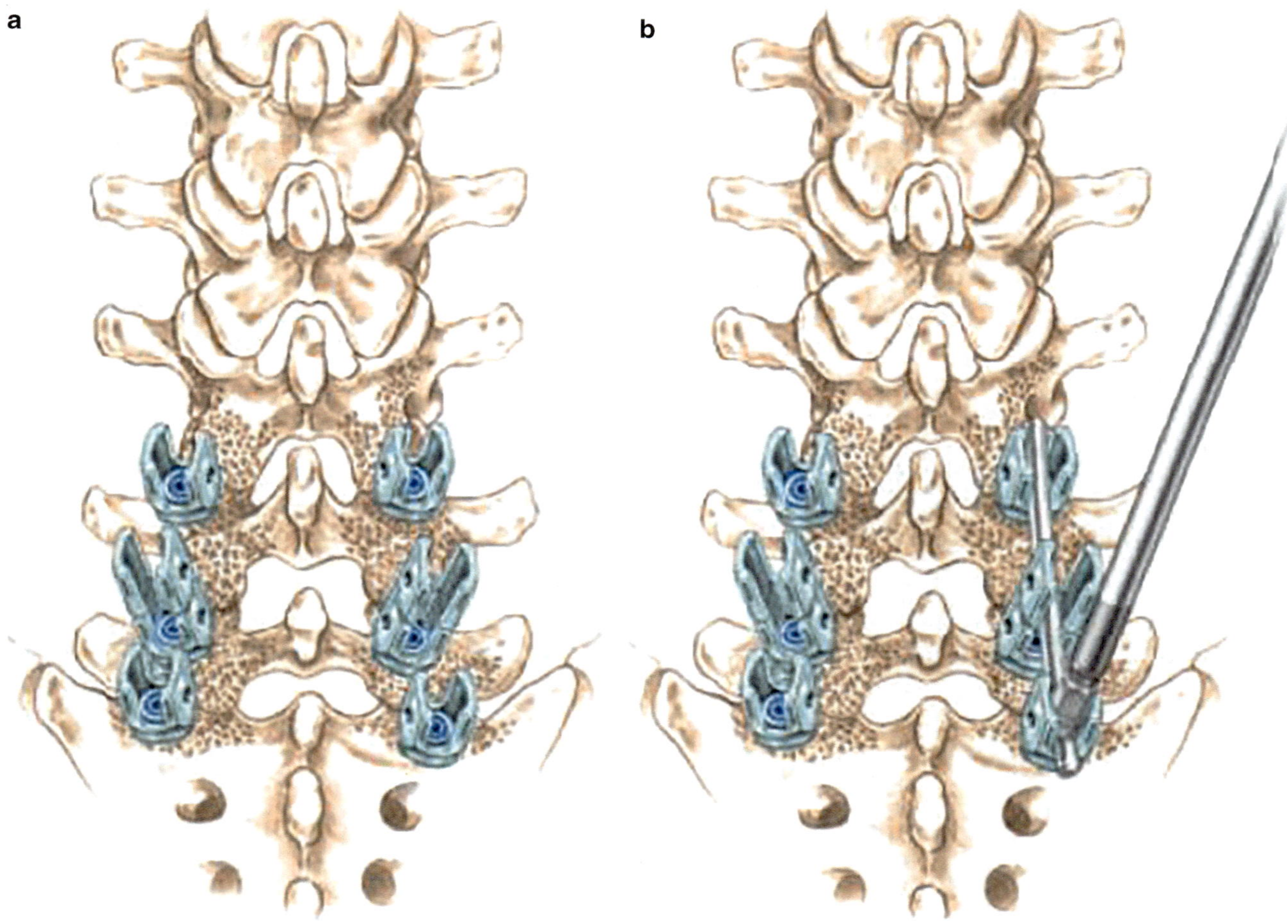

Fig. 9.51 The rod is placed and provisionally tightened. (**a**) Inserting the screw. (**b**) Rod is placed and provisionally tightened

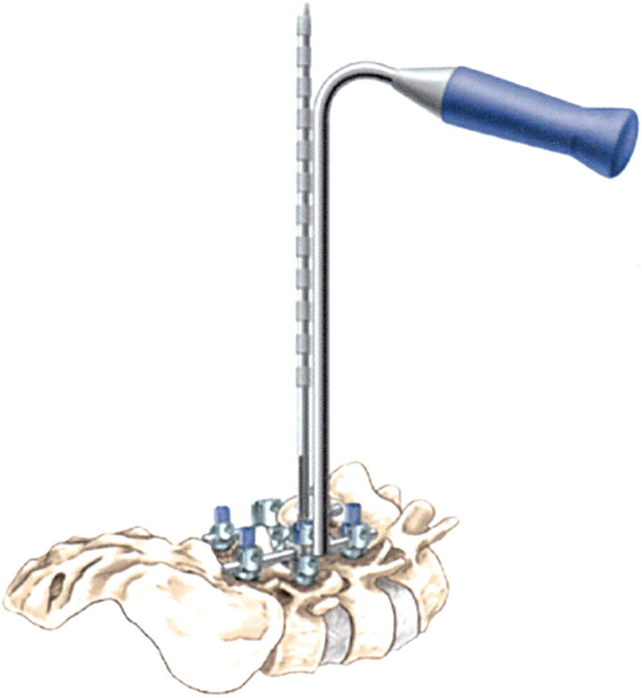

Fig. 9.52 Screw pulling reduction

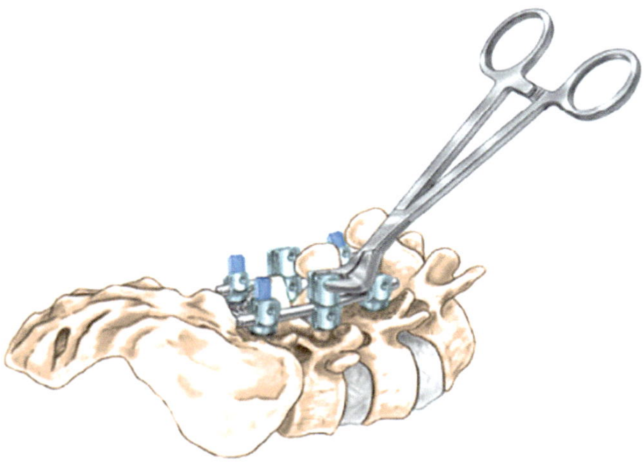

Fig. 9.53 Reduction by Forceps Rocker

Reducer Sleeves to reduce the rod into the extended implant head. To achieve full reduction with the Beale Rod Reducer, the surgeon incrementally reduces spondylolisthesis by graduating to the 7- and 14-mm sleeves (Fig. 9.54). When the rod is fully seated in the bottom of the implant head, reduction is complete. Bilateral reduction may be attained by simultaneously driving the set screws at L5 on both sides.

9.2.6.3 Final Tightening

Once the rod is secured in the implants, distraction and/or compression is performed to place the screws in their final position. Preferably, compression should be released immediately before the set screws are broken off or finally tightened. This technique helps to ensure that the implant head and rod are normalized to one another, thus allowing for the rod to be fully seated in the implant head during final tightening. Once these maneuvers are performed, the set screws at L4 and S1 should be broken off.

To break off the extended tabs of the Multi-axial Reduction Screw, the Ring Counter Torque is placed over the implant head with the handle of the Ring Counter Torque facing lateral. The Reduction Screw Tab Breaker is slid over the medial tab of the extended portion of the Multi-axial Reduction Screw. Air pressure is applied to break off the tabs medially (Fig. 9.55).

While the Ring Counter Torque remains in place, the tab is broken off (Fig. 9.56), which should be broken off medially (Fig. 9.57a). If the tabs do not bend and break off easily, the surgeon should examine if the set screw is fully advanced. If not, its threads will prevent the tabs from being broken off. The surgery is completed after final tightening (Fig. 9.57b).

9.3 Clinical Cases

Case 1

Patient: A 57-year-old female with back pain and radiating pain of the left lower leg for 1 year and worsening for 3 months.

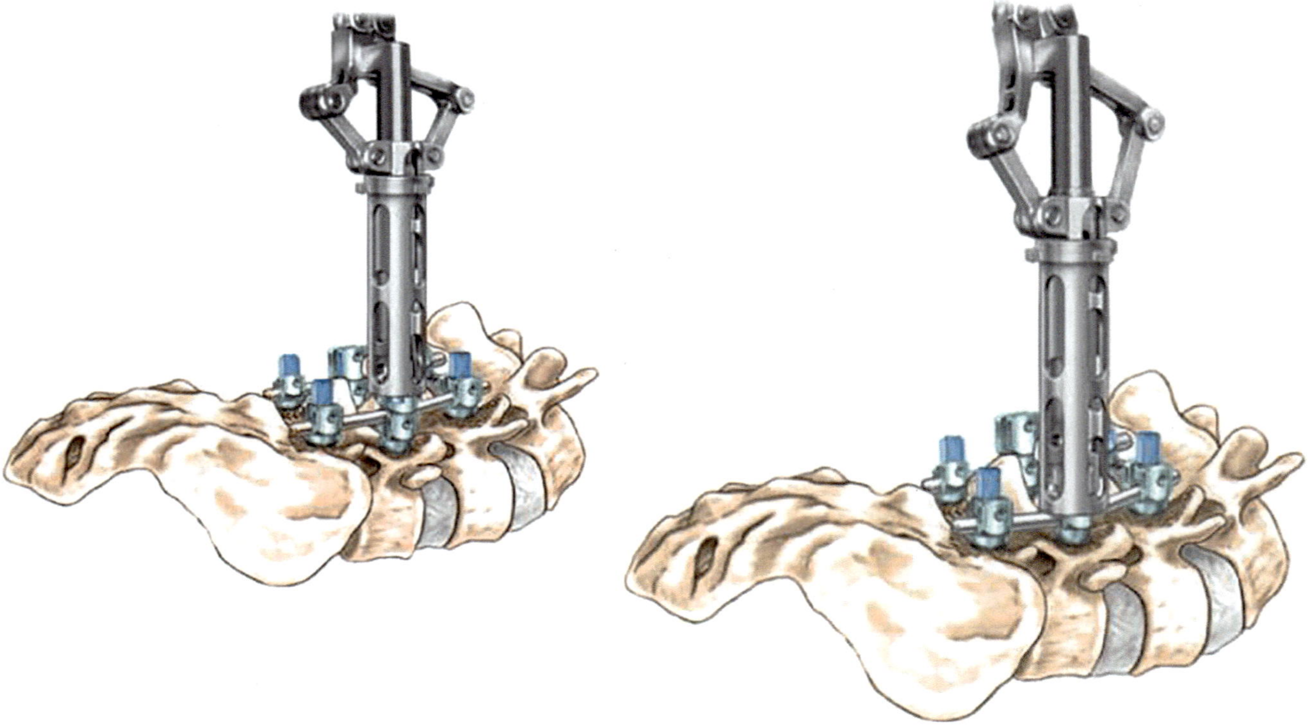

Fig. 9.54 Reduction with two types of sleeves. (**a**) 7-mm sleeve; (**b**) 14-mm sleeve

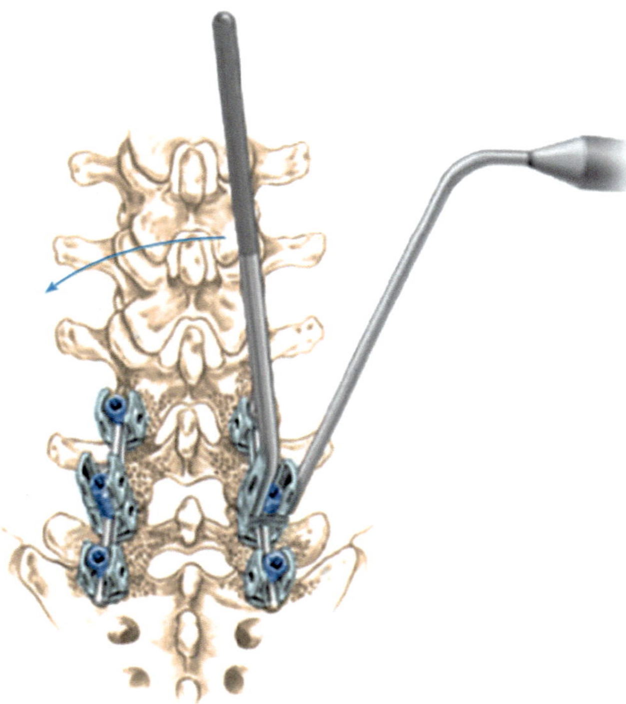

Fig. 9.55 Breaking off the tabs

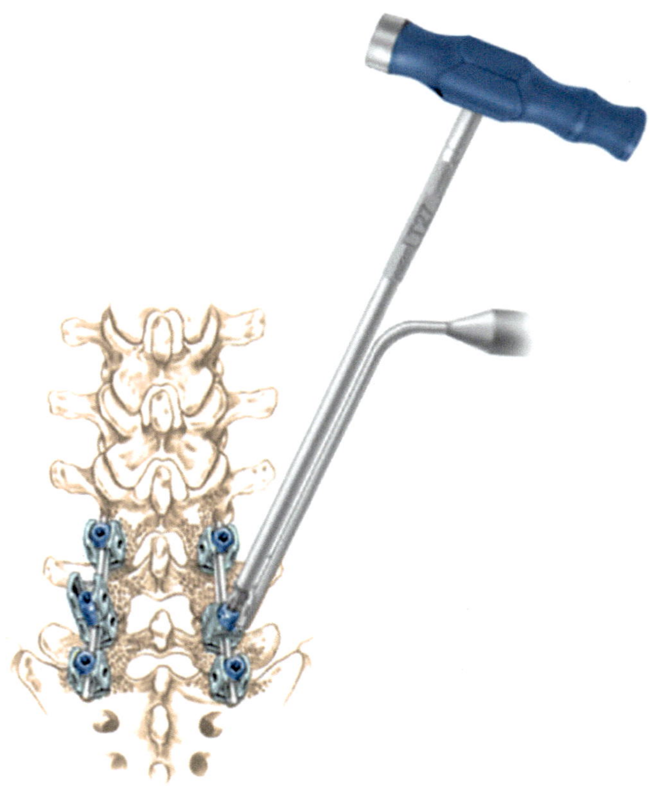

Fig. 9.56 Breaking off the tab with the Ring Counter Torque

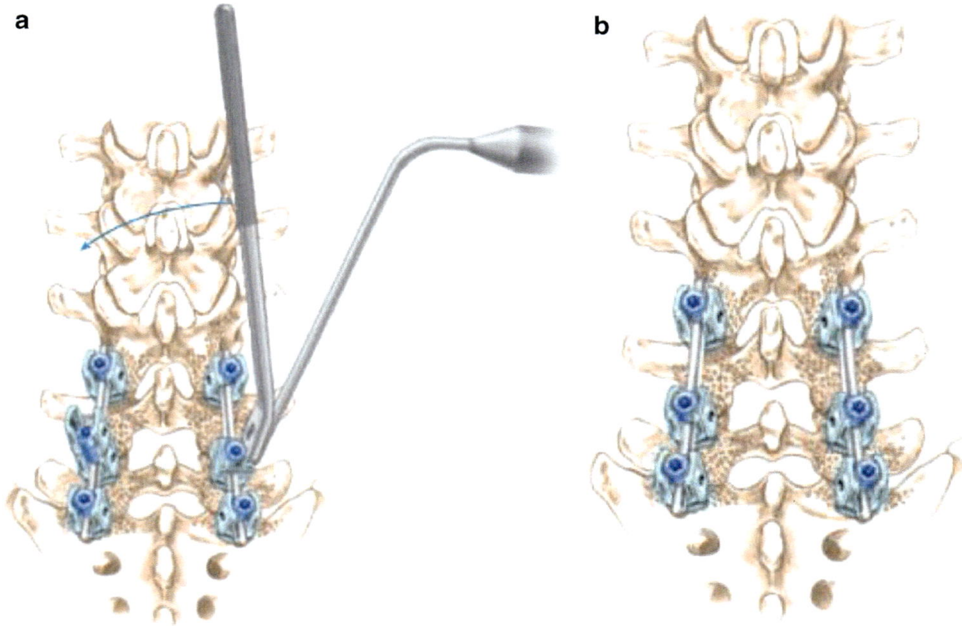

Fig. 9.57 (**a**) The tab is broken off medially. (**b**) Surgery is completed

Diagnosis: L5 isthmic spondylolisthesis.

Surgery: L5–S1 left intervertebral disc fenestration with removal of nucleus pulposus from the intervertebral disc, interbody fusion surgery, CAPSTONE placement, spondylolisthesis reduction, and L5 and S1 pedicle screw internal fixation.

Imaging studies: Preoperative (Fig. 9.58) and postoperative images (Fig. 9.59).

Case 2

Patient: A 16-year-old boy with back pain for 11 h due to trauma.

Diagnosis: L2–L3 fracture.

Surgery: Open reduction, posterior interbody fusion surgery, L1–L4 pedicle screw internal fixation.

Imaging studies: Preoperative (Fig. 9.60) and postoperative images (Fig. 9.61).

Case 3

Patient: A 35-year-old female complaining of lumbosacral pain due to trauma and defecation dysfunction for 7 days.

Diagnosis: L5 spondylolisthesis (grade V, posterior spondylolisthesis).

Surgery: L5, S1 open reduction, vertebral interbody fusion surgery, L4–L5, S1–S2 pedicle screw internal fixation.

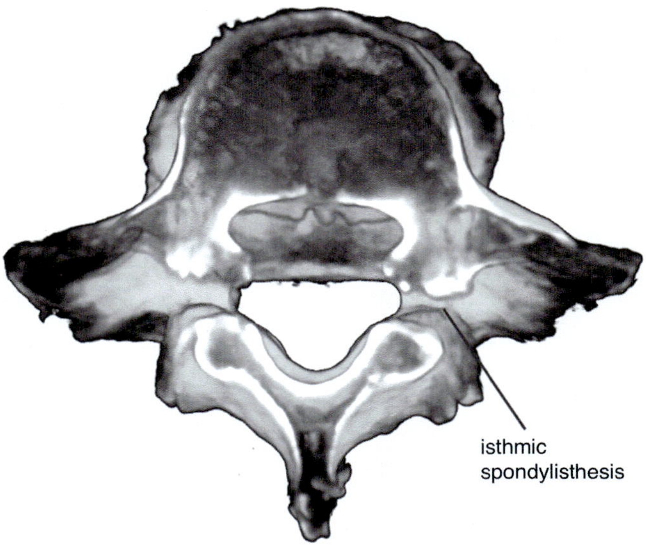

Fig. 9.58 Preoperative imaging studies. CT 3D reconstruction image (*horizontal*)

Imaging studies: Preoperative (Fig. 9.62) and postoperative images (Fig. 9.63).

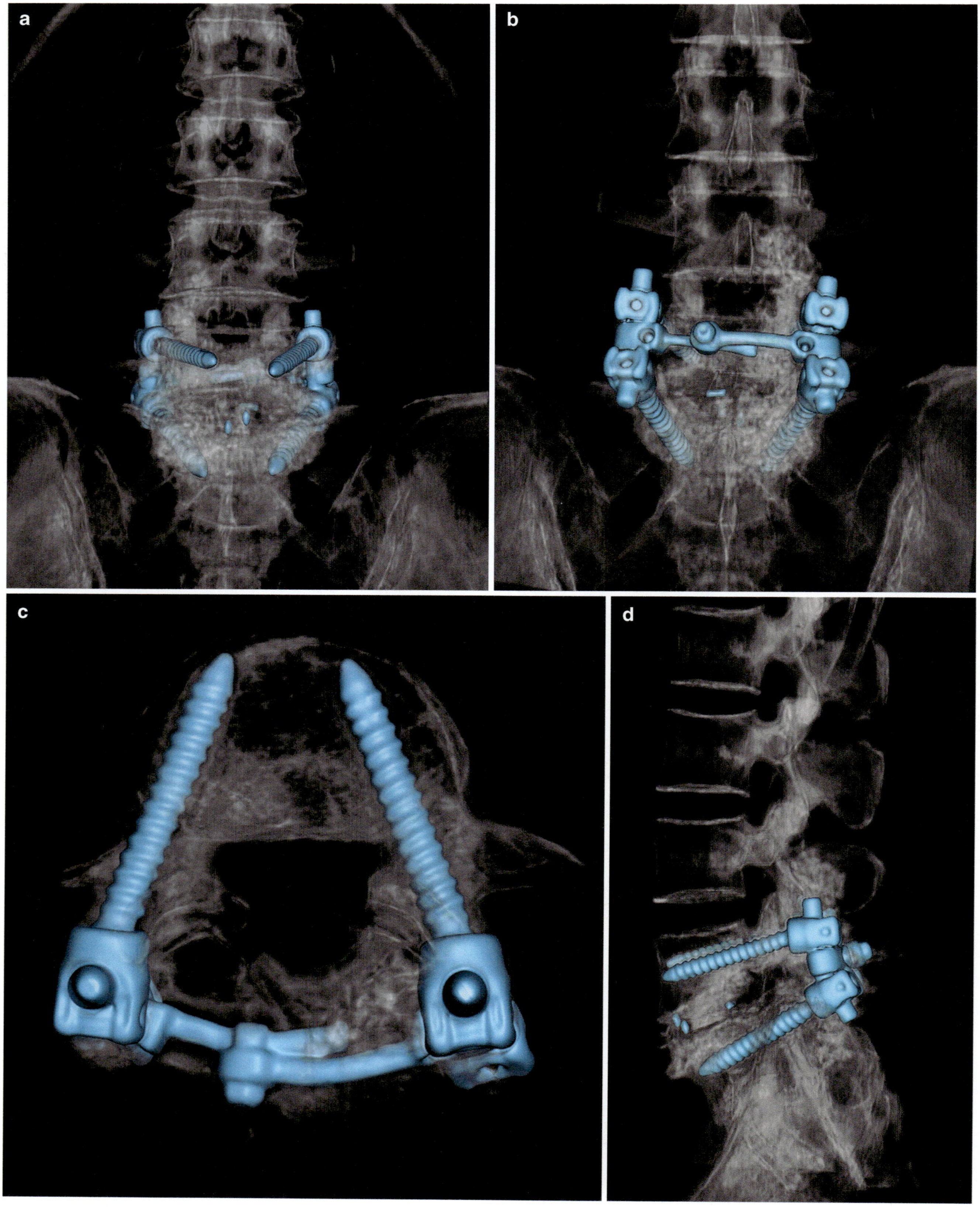

Fig. 9.59 Postoperative images. (**a**) CT 3D reconstruction (*anterior view*); (**b**) CT 3D reconstruction (*posterior view*); (**c**) CT 3D reconstruction (*axial view*); (**d**) CT 3D reconstruction (*lateral view*)

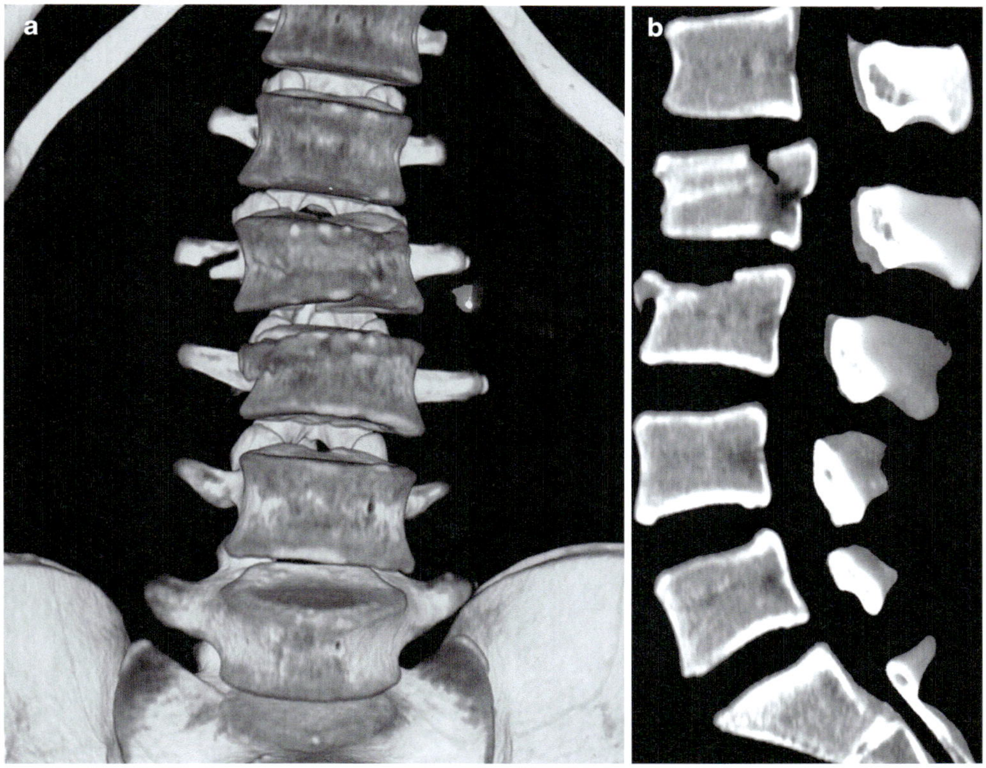

Fig. 9.60 Preoperative imaging studies. (**a**) CT 3D reconstruction (*anterior view*); (**b**) CT 3D reconstruction (*sagittal view*)

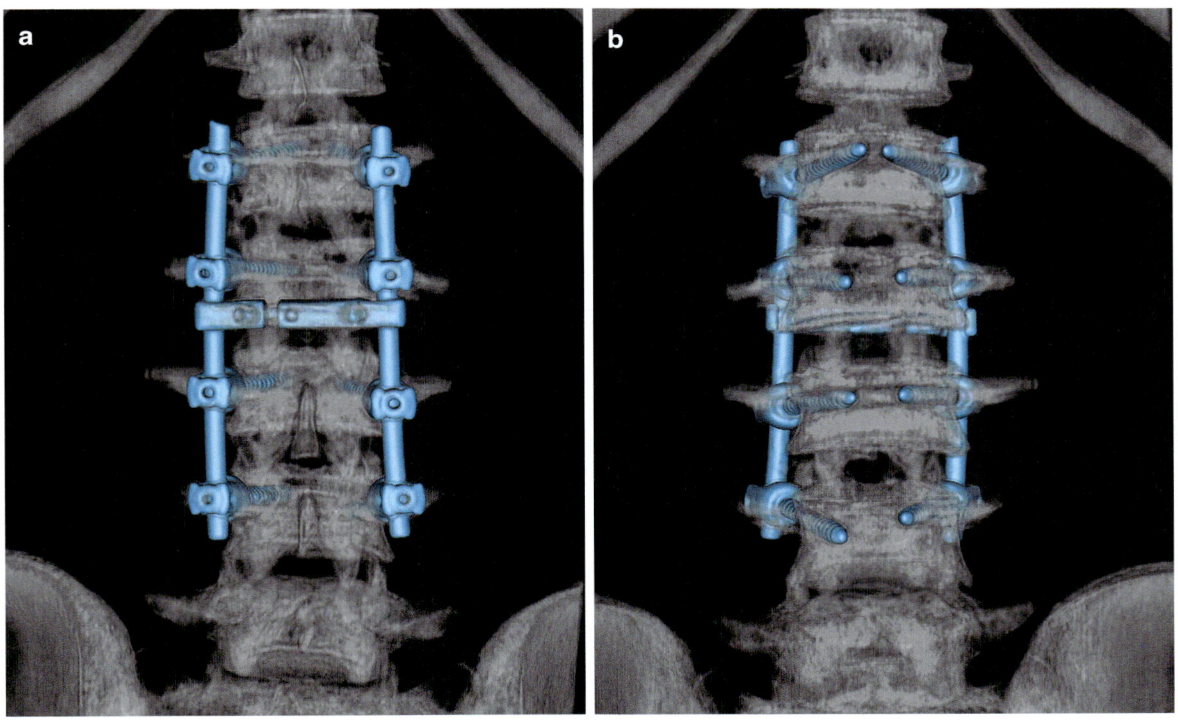

Fig. 9.61 Postoperative images. (**a**) CT 3D reconstruction (*posterior view*); (**b**) CT 3D reconstruction (*anterior view*); (**c**) CT 3D reconstruction (*sagittal view*); (**b**) CT 3D reconstruction (*lateral view*); (**e**) CT 3D reconstruction showing screw positions

Fig. 9.61 (continued)

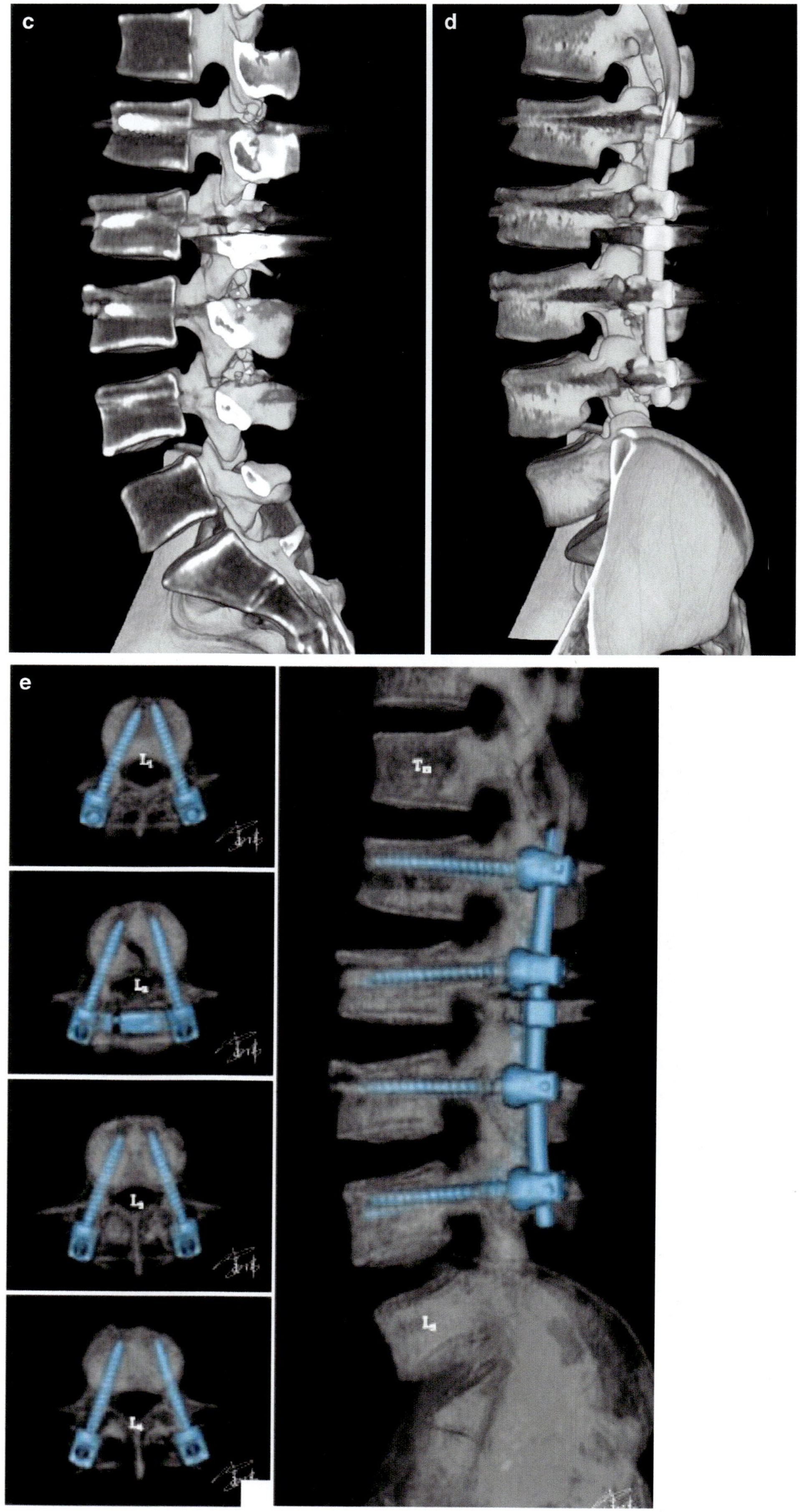

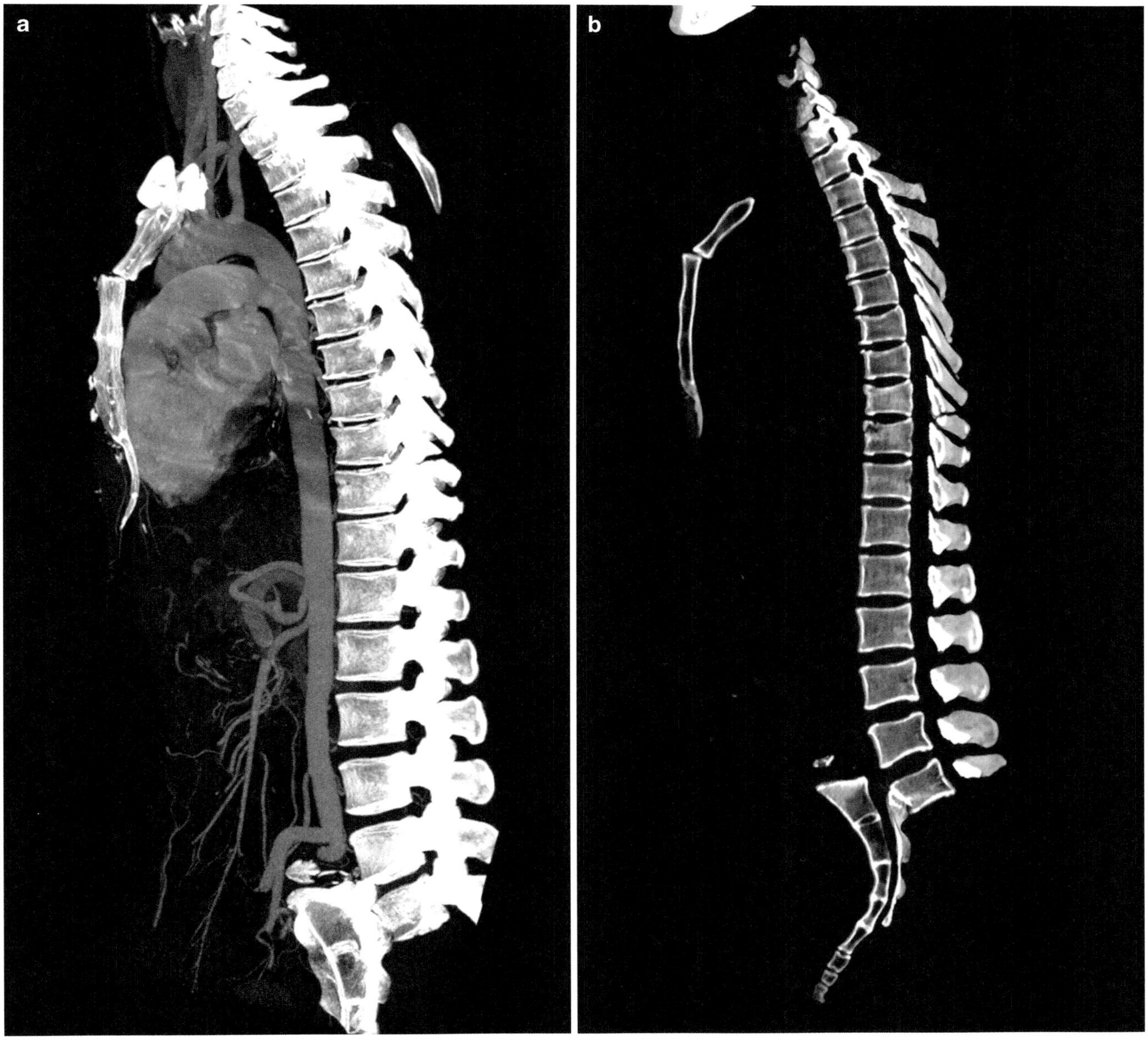

Fig. 9.62 Preoperative imaging studies. (**a**) CT 3D reconstruction (*lateral view*); (**b**) CT 3D reconstruction (*sagittal view*)

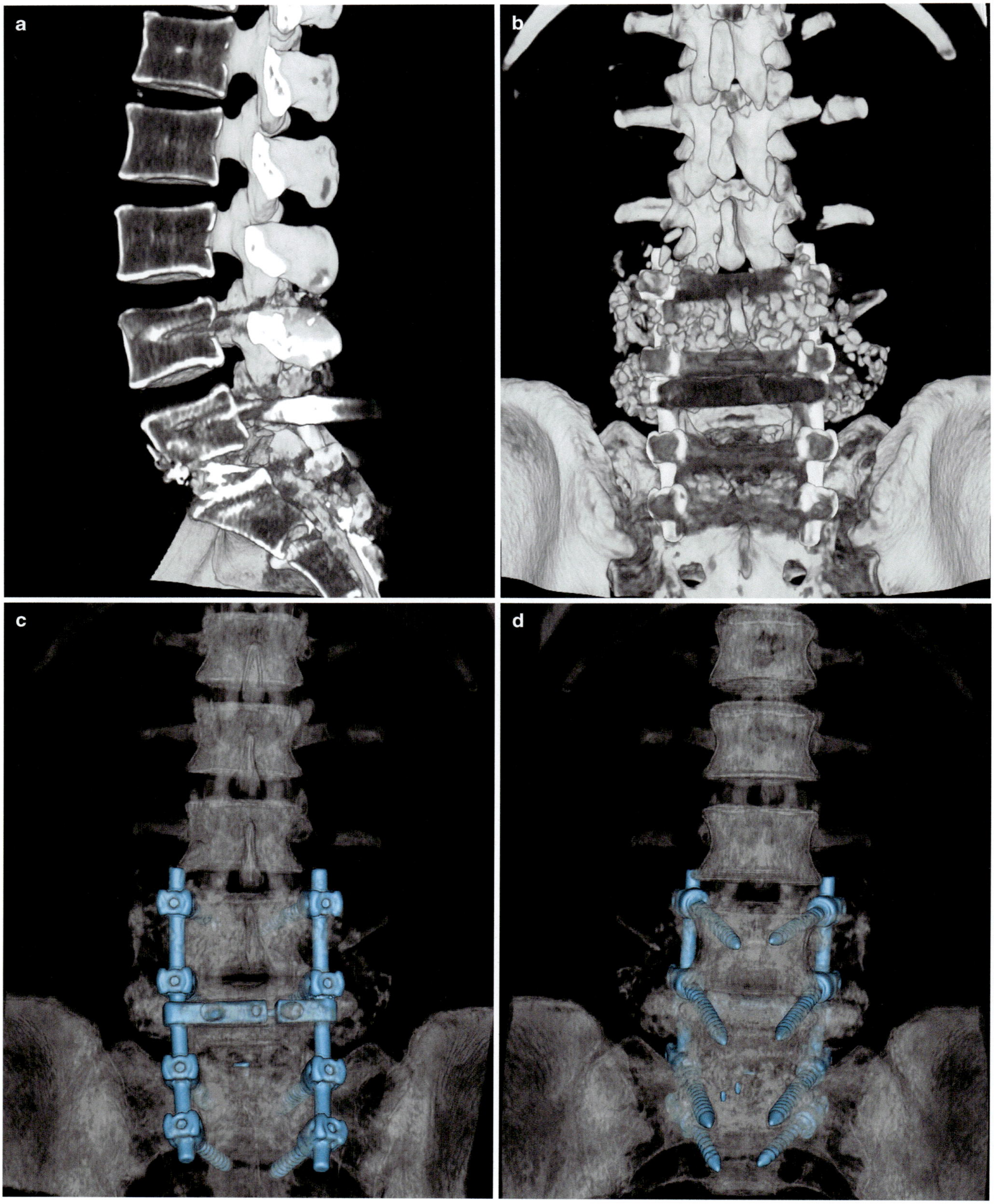

Fig. 9.63 Postoperative images. (**a**) CT 3D reconstruction (*sagittal view*); (**b**) CT 3D reconstruction (*posterior view*); (**c**) CT 3D reconstruction (*posterior view*); (**d**) CT 3D reconstruction (*anterior view*); (**e**) CT 3D reconstruction showing screw positions

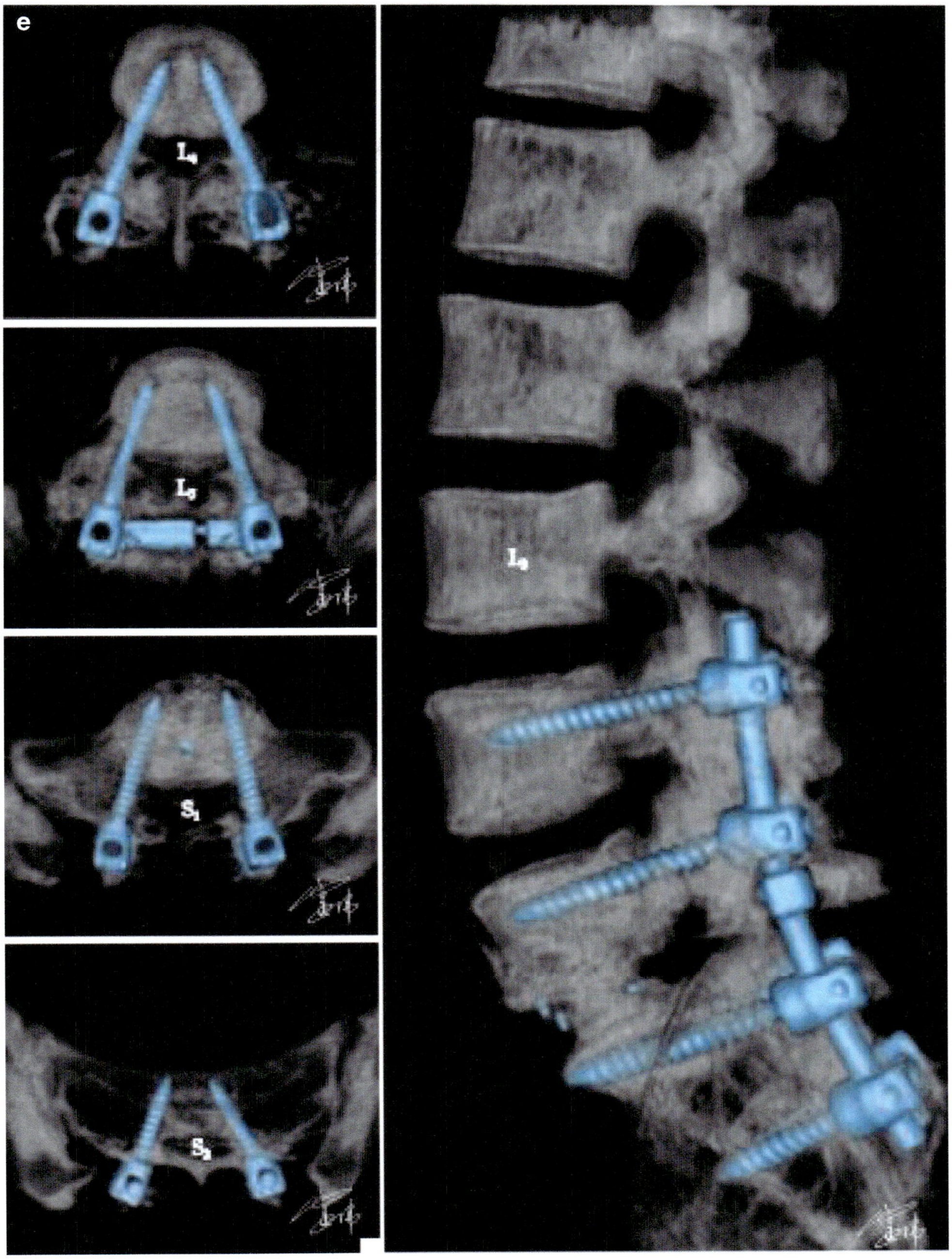

Fig. 9.63 (continued)

Case 4

Patient: A 20-year-old male with vertebral deformity for 3 years.

Diagnosis: Idiopathic vertebral scoliosis.

Surgery: T1–L2 posterior pedicle screw internal fixation and spine correction surgery, interbody fusion surgery.

Imaging studies: Preoperative (Fig. 9.64) and postoperative images (Fig. 9.65).

Case 5

Patient: A 10-year-old boy with vertebral deformity for 5 years.

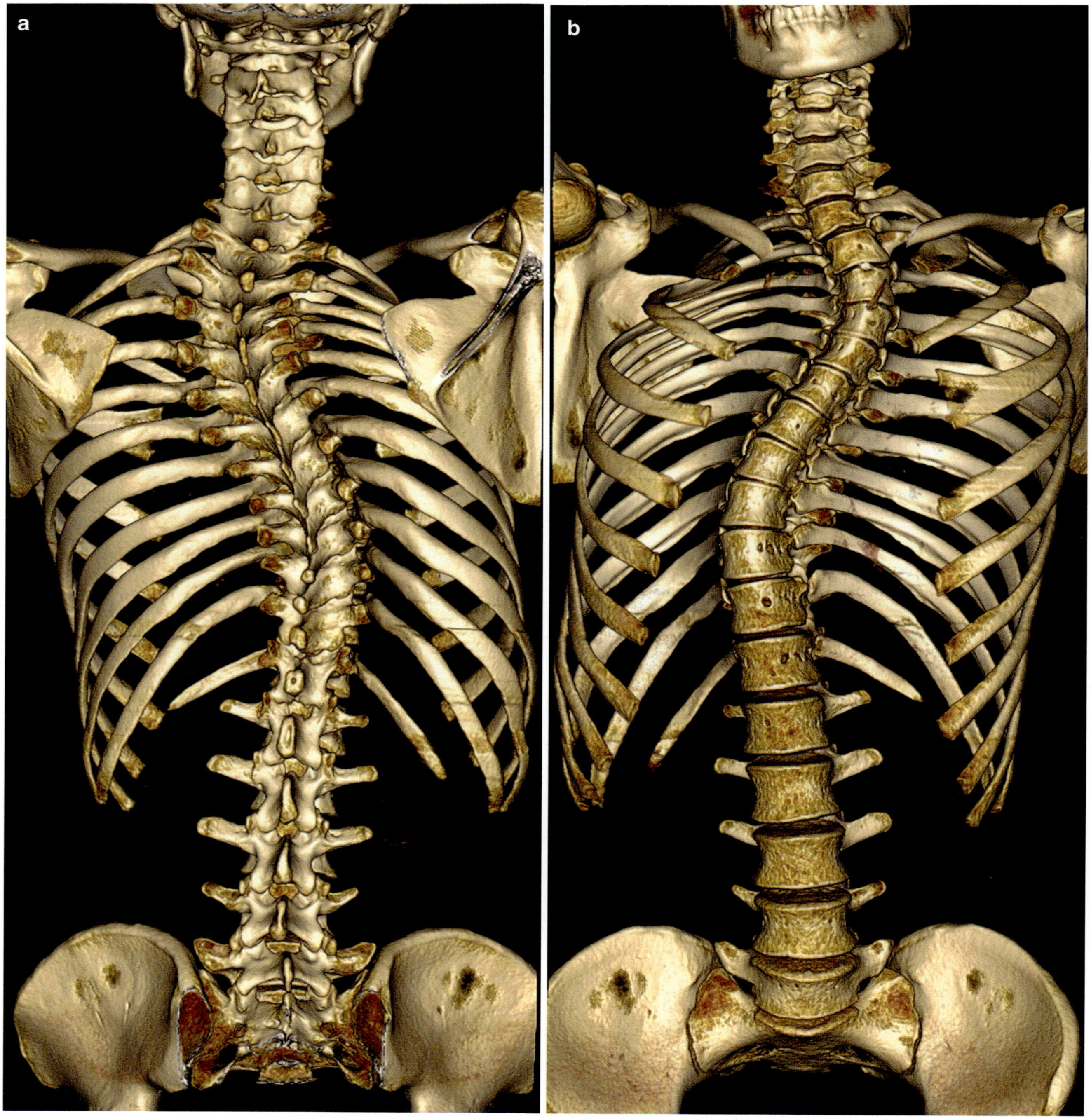

Fig. 9.64 Preoperative imaging studies. (**a**) CT 3D reconstruction (*posterior view*); (**b**) CT 3D reconstruction (*anterior view*)

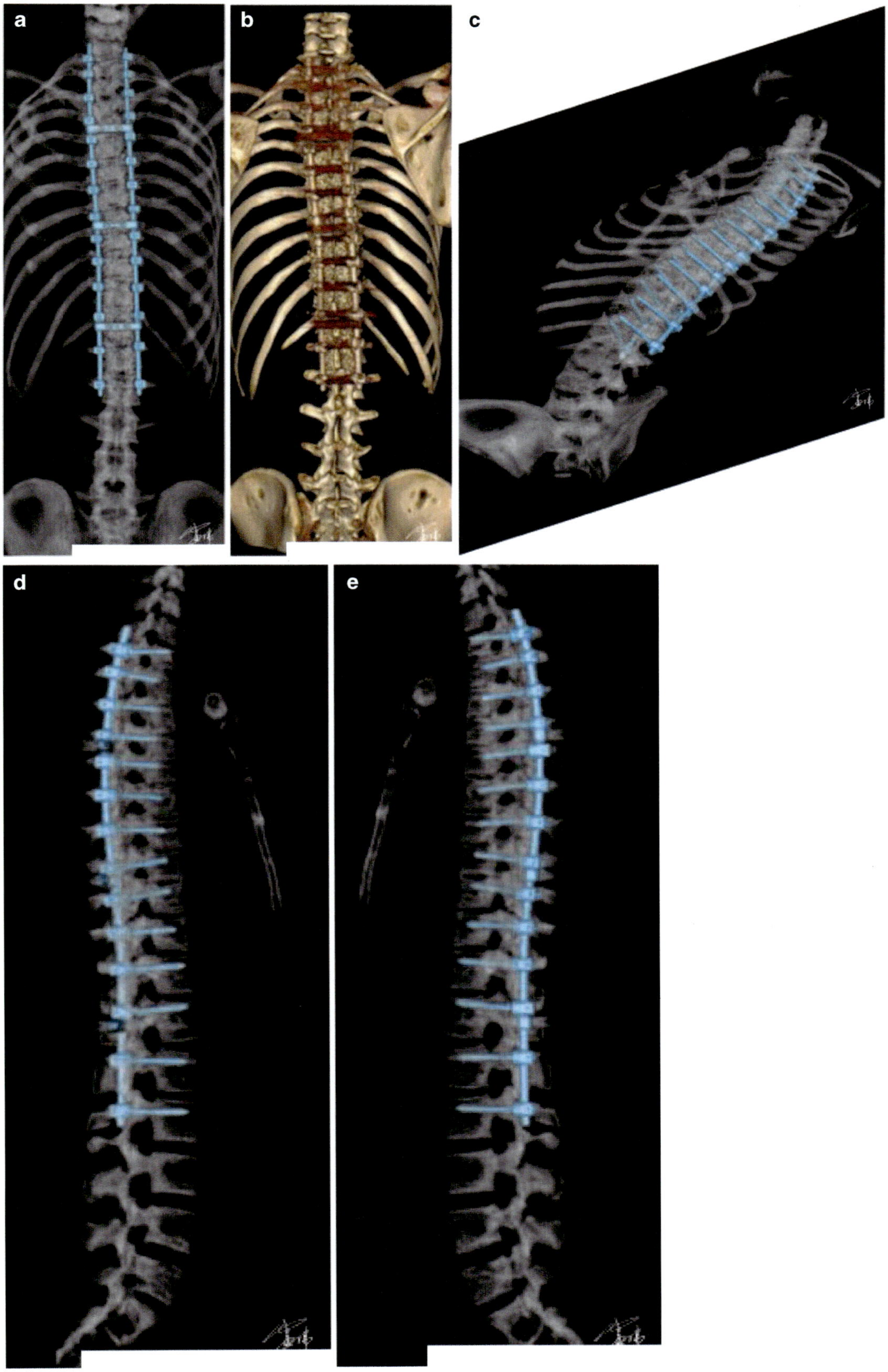

Fig. 9.65 Postoperative images. (**a**) CT 3D reconstruction (*posterior view*); (**b**) CT 3D reconstruction (*posterior view*); (**c**) CT 3D reconstruction showing screw positions; (**d**) CT 3D reconstruction (*right lateral view*); (**e**) CT 3D reconstruction (*left lateral view*)

Diagnosis: Vertebral scoliosis due to neurofibromatosis.

Surgery: Spine correction surgery with transverse process hook and pedicle screw internal fixation, interbody fusion surgery.

Imaging studies: Preoperative (Fig. 9.66) and postoperative images (Fig. 9.67).

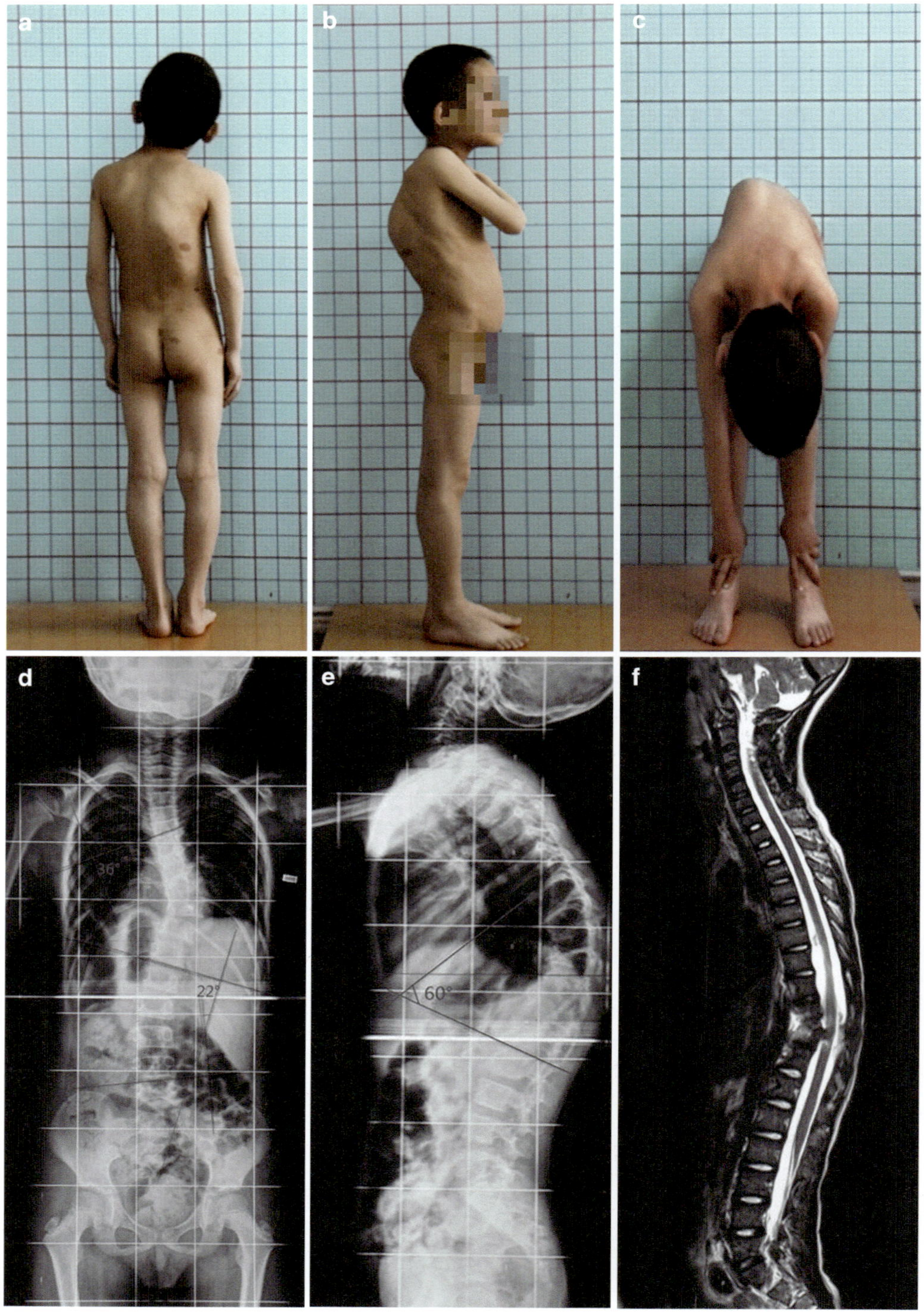

Fig. 9.66 Preoperative imaging studies. (**a**) The posterior view of the patient; (**b**) The lateral view of the patient; (**c**) The patient bending over; (**d**) X-ray image (*anteroposterior view*); (**e**) X-ray image (*lateral view*); (**f**) MRI (*sagittal view*)

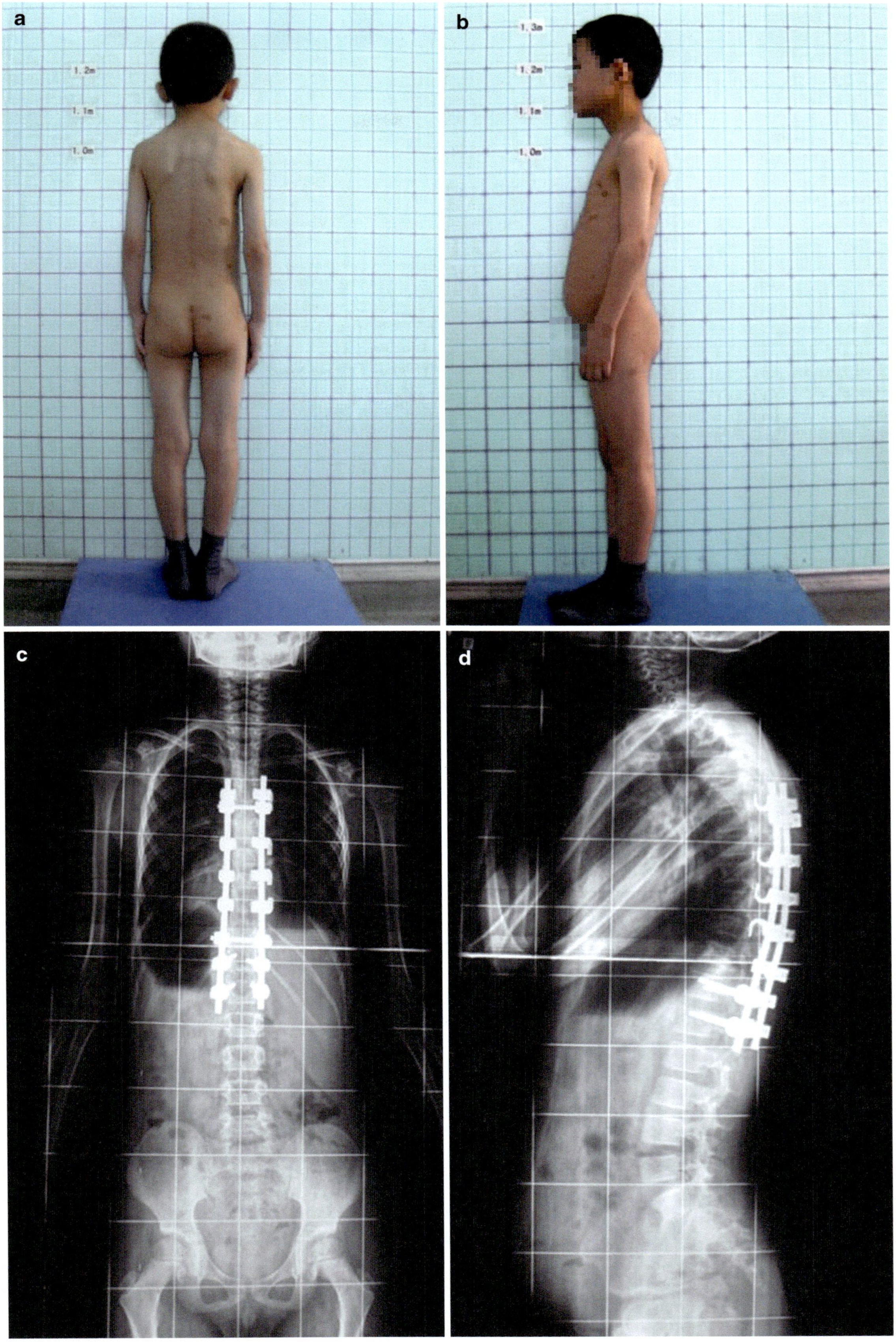

Fig. 9.67 Postoperative images. (**a**) The posterior view of the patient; (**b**) The lateral view of the patient; (**c**) X-ray image (*anteroposterior view*); (**d**) X-ray image (*lateral view*); (**e**) CT 3D reconstruction showing position of implants; (**f**) CT 3D reconstruction (*anterior view*); (**g**) CT 3D reconstruction (*lateral view*); (**h**) CT 3D reconstruction (*anterior view*); (**i**) CT 3D reconstruction (*posterior view*)

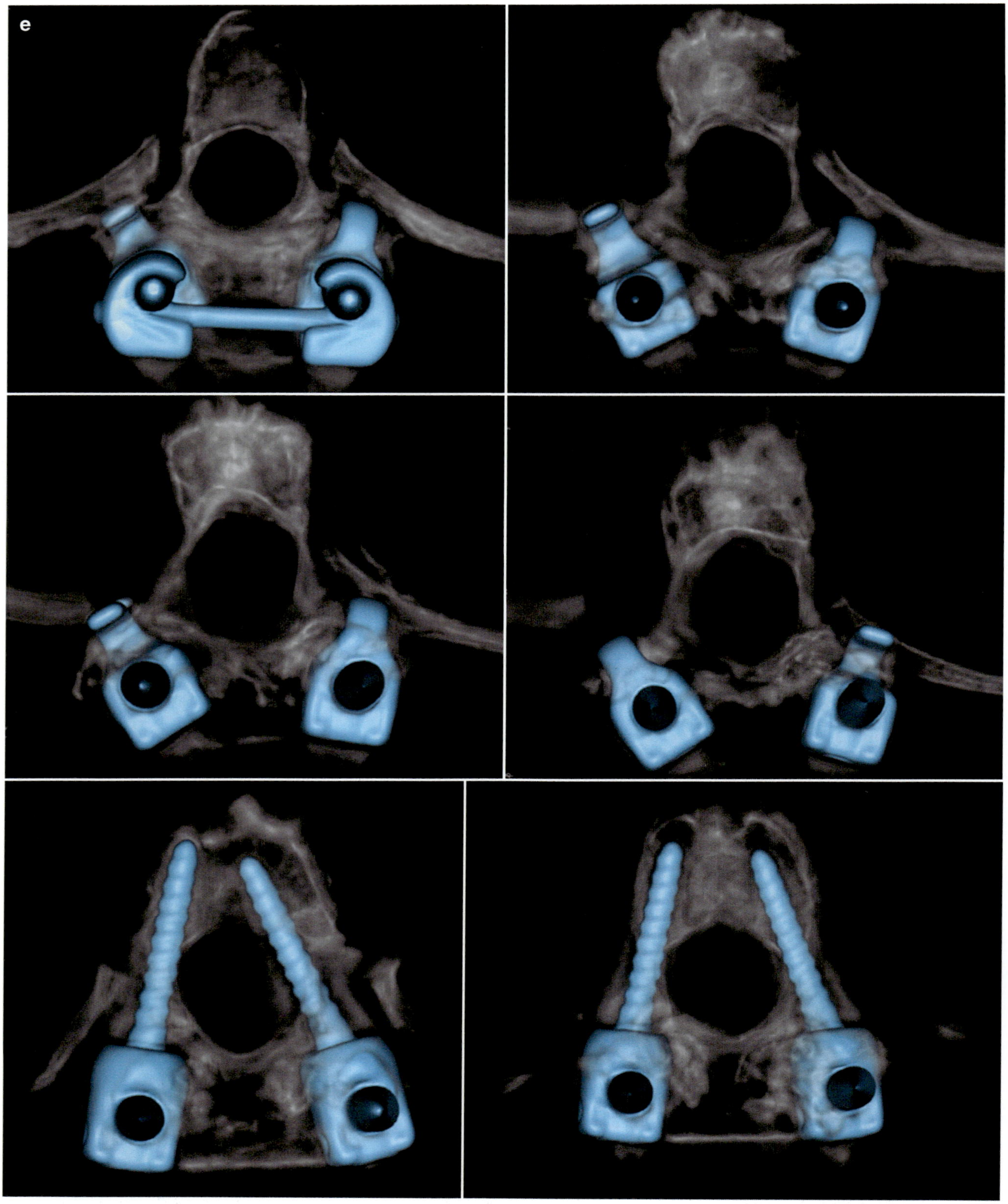

Fig. 9.67 (continued)

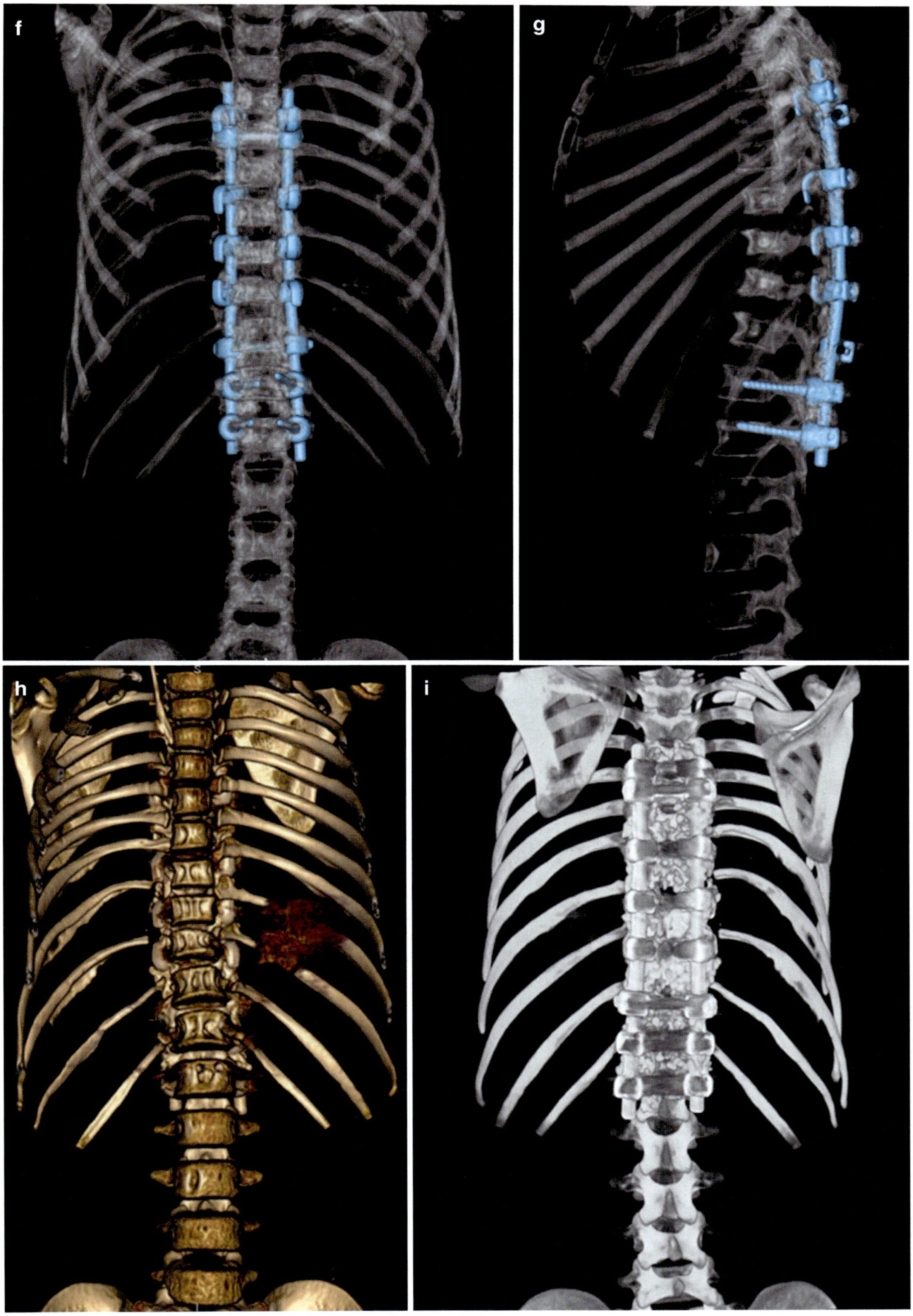

Fig. 9.67 (continued)

9.4 Common Pitfalls in Surgery of Vertebral Scoliosis due to Neurofibromatosis

9.4.1 Pitfall #1

In the presence of invasion by the capitulum costae into the vertebral canal, blind correction surgery may readily lead to paralysis of the patient (Fig. 9.68).

9.4.2 Pitfall #2

The use of screws for small pedicles may lead to multiple injuries (Fig. 9.69).

9.4.3 Pitfall #3

Mishandling of paravertebral soft tissue tumors may inadvertently cause massive bleeding (Fig. 9.70).

Cautions:

1. Preoperative reading of imaging results should focus on capitulum costae dislocation, pedicle diameter, size of the transverse process, and size of the spinal canal and the contents within and paravertebral tumor.
2. Surgery precautions: The capitulum costae invading the spinal canal should be first excised before correction surgery. The use of hook or screw is based on pedicle diameter and size of the transverse process. The likelihood of using hooks is greater. Besides, bone graft volume should be sufficient.

Case 6

Patient: A 13-year-old boy with vertebral deformity for 8 years with worsening for 2 years.

Diagnosis: Congenital vertebral scoliosis, L5 hemivertebra.

Surgery: Posterior L5 hemivertebrectomy, interbody fusion surgery, L1–L4, S1 pedicle screw internal fixation, posterior interbody fusion surgery.

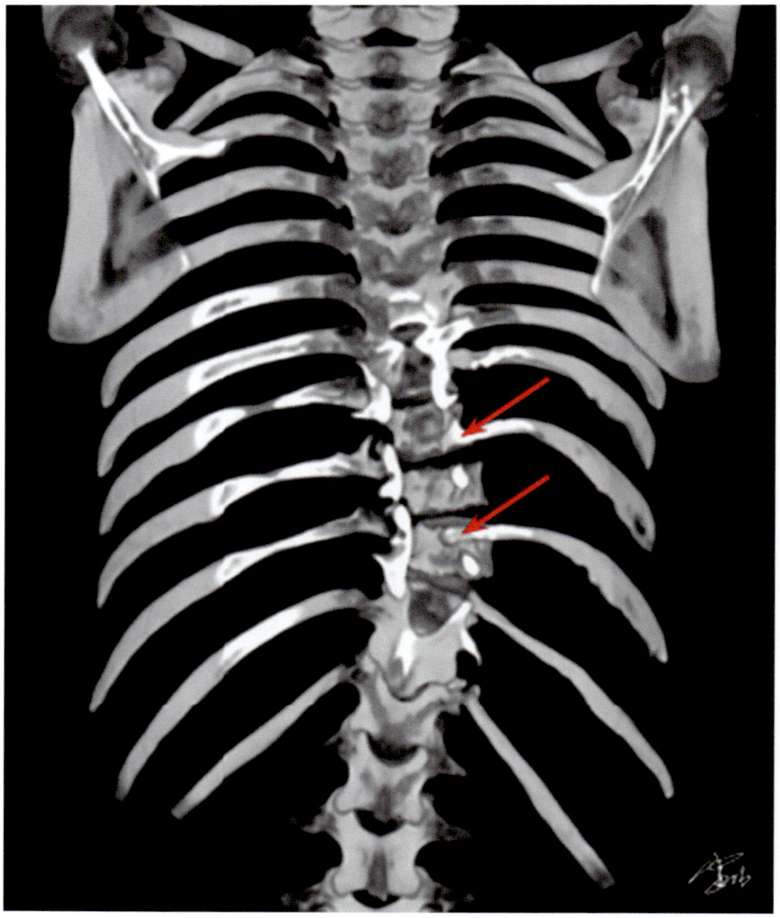

Fig. 9.68 Invasion by the capitulum costae into the vertebral canal

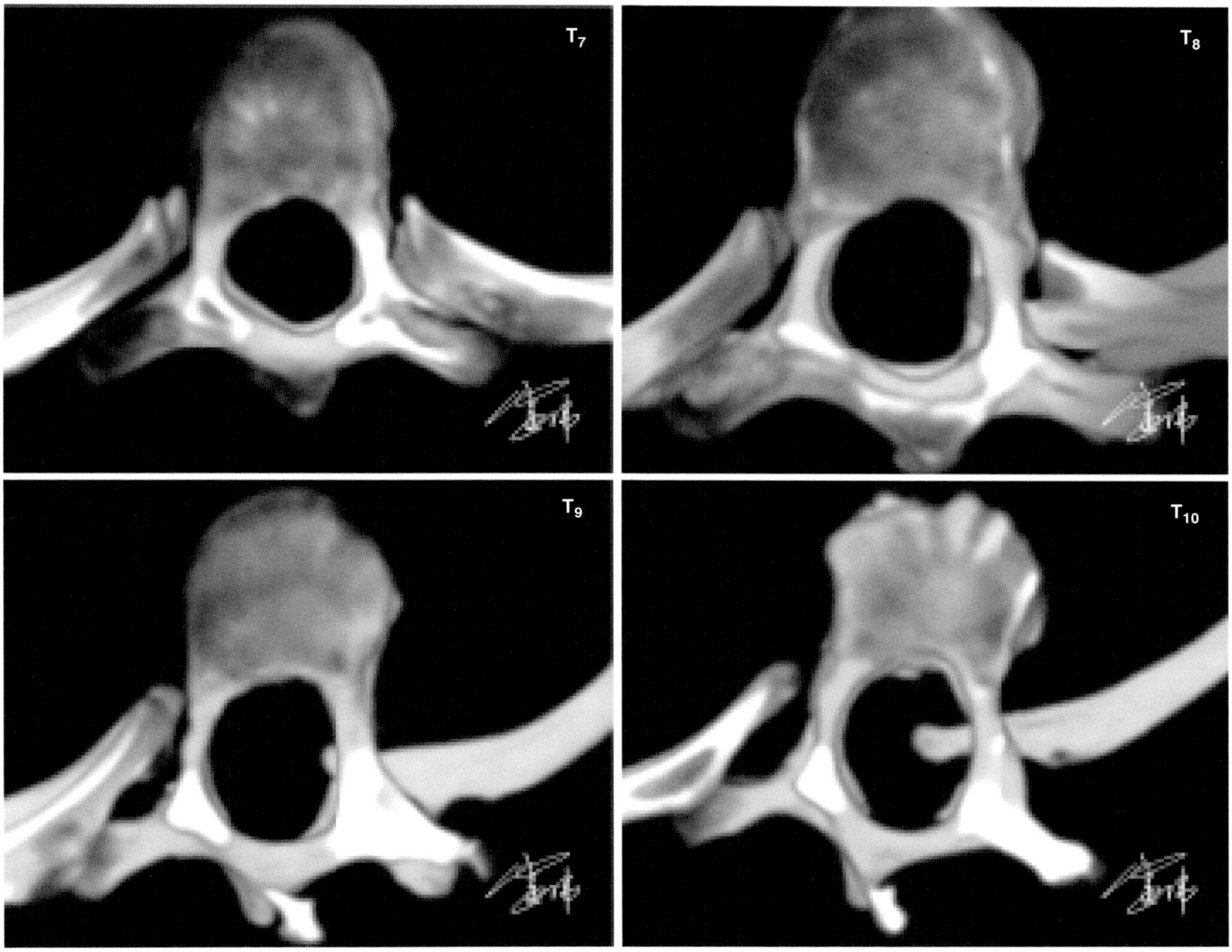

Fig. 9.69 Small pedicles

Imaging studies: Preoperative (Fig. 9.71) and postoperative images (Fig. 9.72).

Case 7

Patient: A 33-year-old female with lumbosacral deformity for 32 years and defecation and urinary dysfunction for 1 year.

Diagnosis: Congenital lumbosacral kyphosis.

Surgery: Correction surgery by posterior lumbosacral osteotomy; L1, L2, S2 pedicle screw internal fixation; sacroiliac screw internal fixation; and interbody fusion surgery.

Imaging studies: Preoperative (Fig. 9.73) and postoperative images (Fig. 9.74).

Case 8

Patient: A 43-year-old male complaining of back pain with right front thigh pain for 1 year.

Diagnosis: L3–L4 intervertebral disc herniation.

Surgery: L3–L4 posterior intervertebral disc fenestration with removal of the nucleus pulposus, CAPSTONE interbody fusion surgery, and L3–L4 pedicle screw internal fixation (PEEK rod).

Imaging studies: Preoperative (Fig. 9.75), intraoperative (Fig. 9.76), and postoperative images (Fig. 9.77).

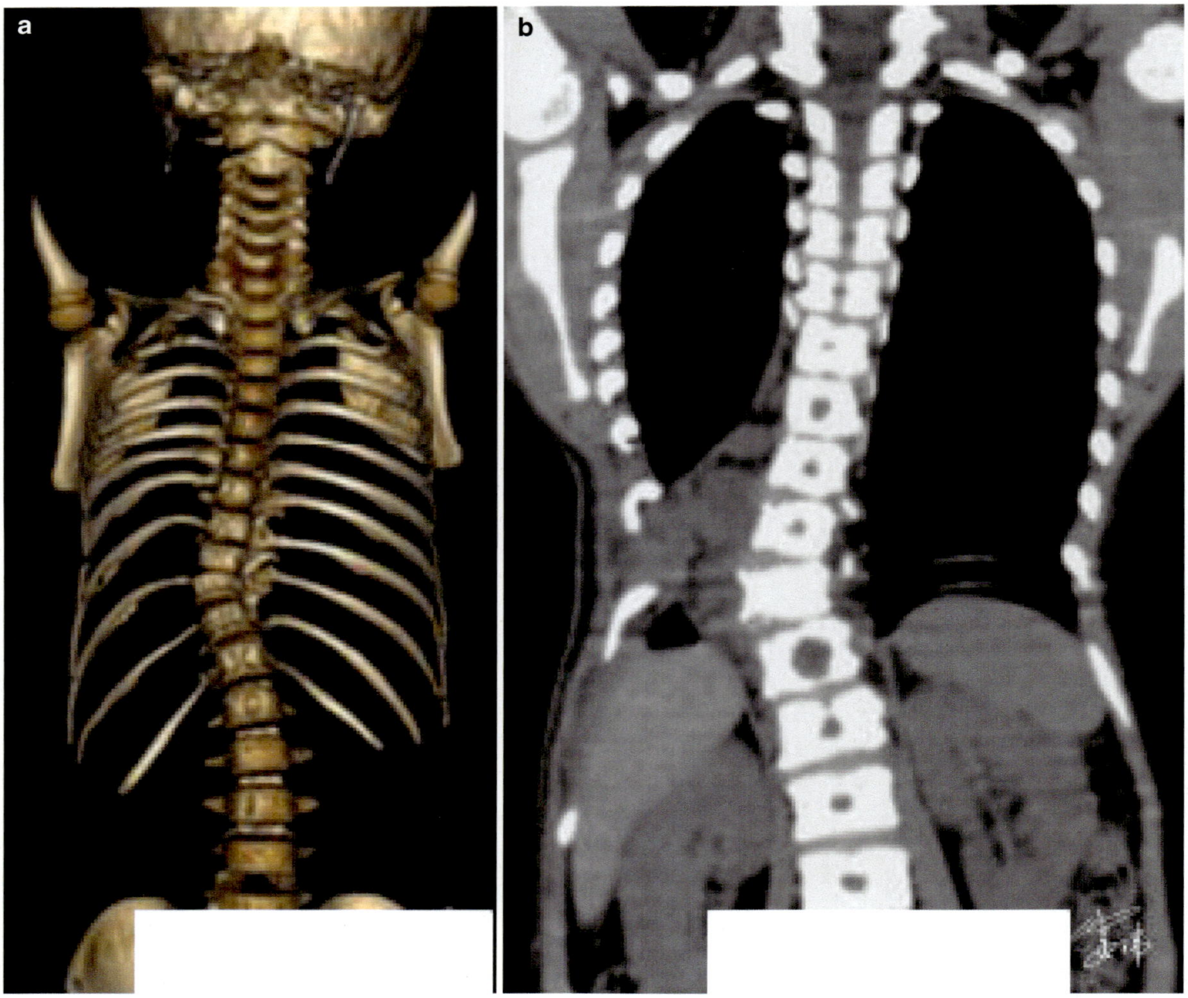

Fig. 9.70 Anatomical relationship of paravertebral tissues. (**a**) CT 3D reconstruction (*anterior view*); (**b**) CT 3D reconstruction (*sagittal view*)

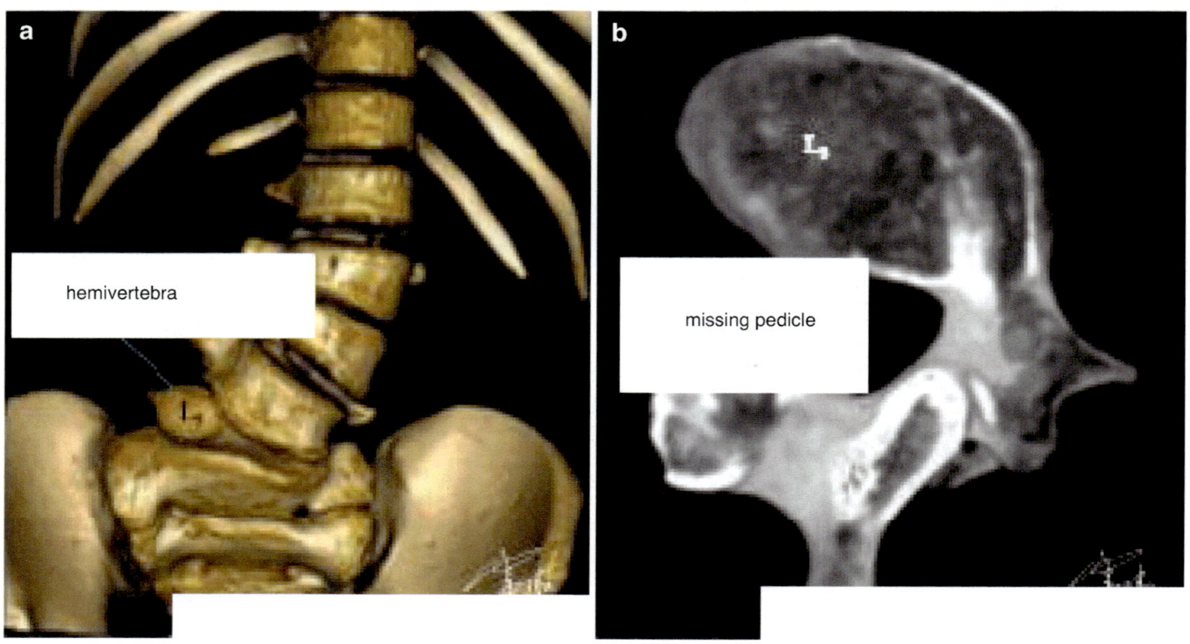

Fig. 9.71 Preoperative imaging studies. (**a**) CT 3D reconstruction (*anterior view*); (**b**) CT 3D reconstruction (*hemivertebra*)

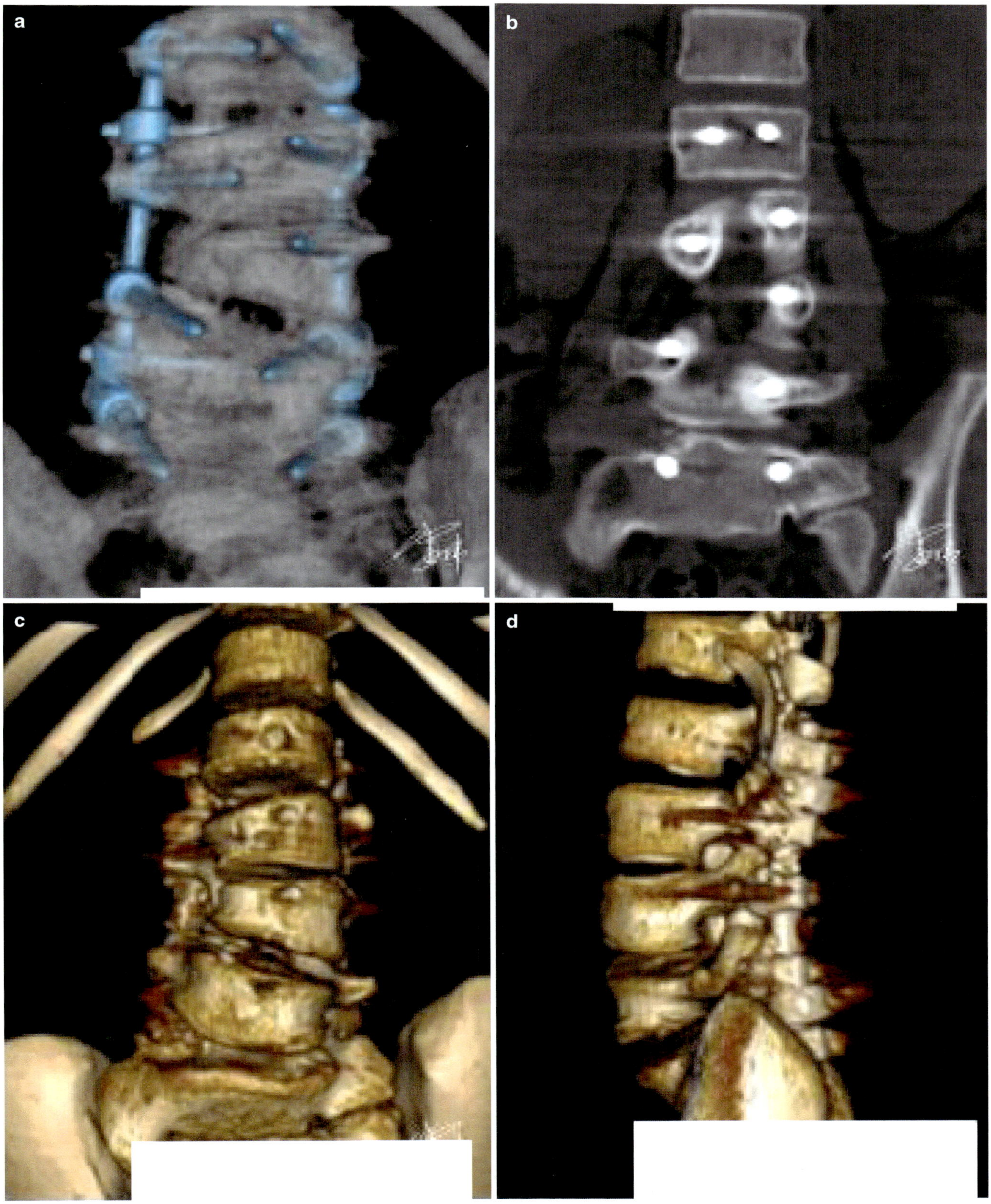

Fig. 9.72 Postoperative images. (**a**) CT 3D reconstruction (*anterior view*); (**b**) CT 3D reconstruction (*coronal view*); (**c**) CT 3D reconstruction (*anterior view*); (**d**) CT 3D reconstruction (*lateral view*); (**e**) CT 3D reconstruction showing screw position

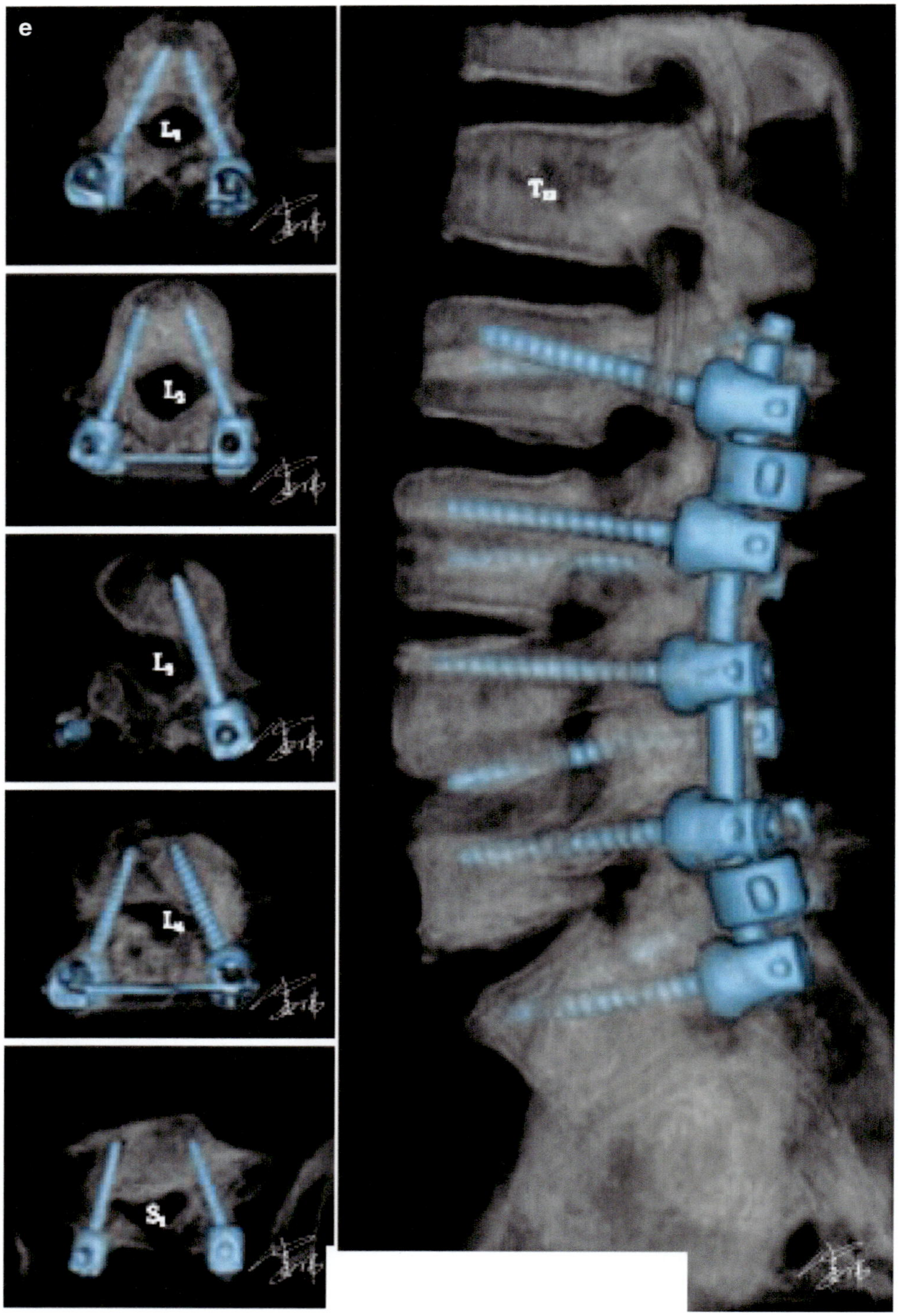

Fig. 9.72 (continued)

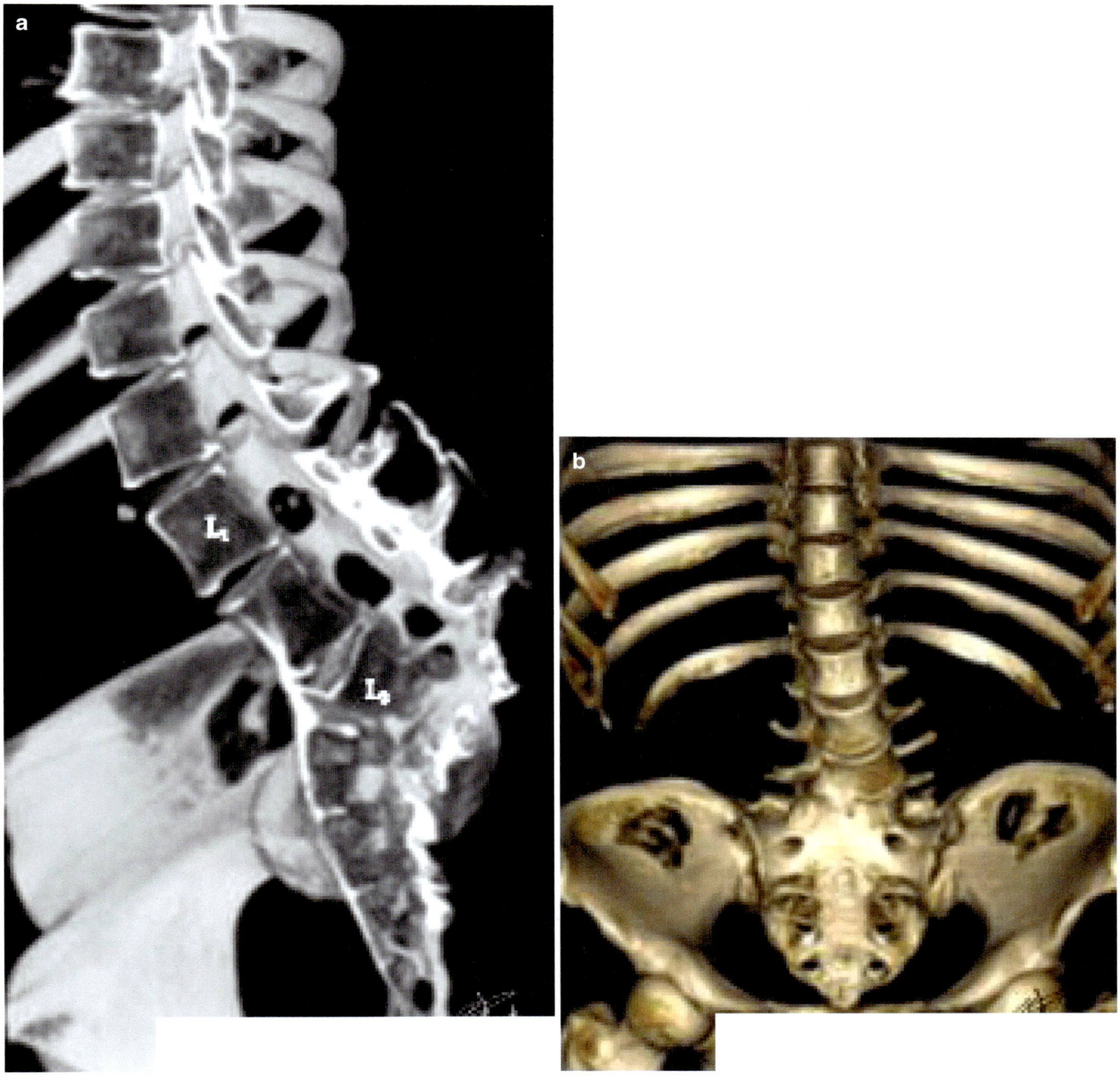

Fig. 9.73 Preoperative imaging studies. (**a**) CT 3D reconstruction (*sagittal view*); (**b**) CT 3D reconstruction (*anterior view*)

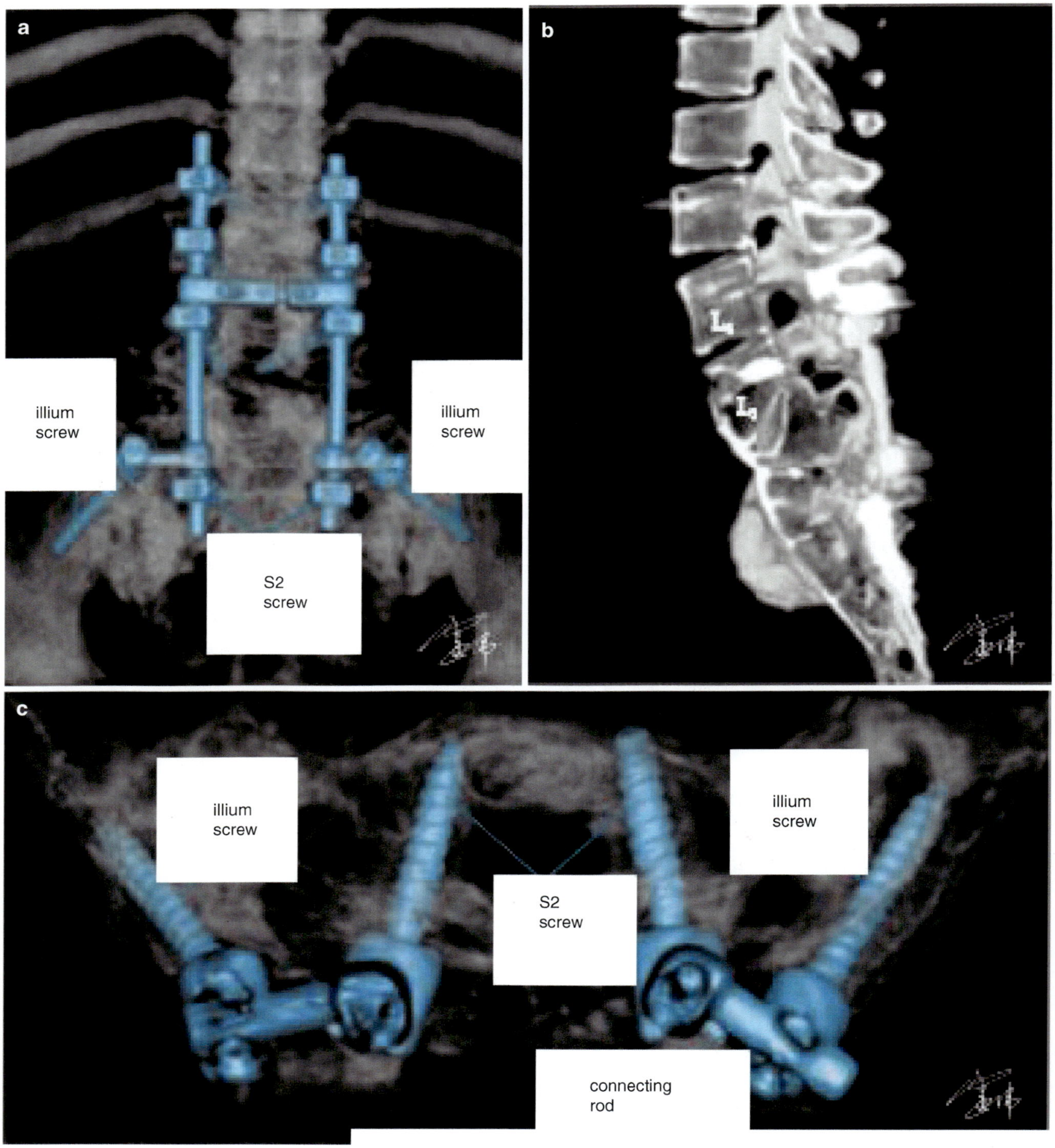

Fig. 9.74 Postoperative images. (**a**) CT 3D reconstruction (*posterior view*); (**b**) CT 3D reconstruction (*sagittal view*); (**c**) CT 3D reconstruction (*sagittal view*); (**d**) CT 3D reconstruction showing screw positions

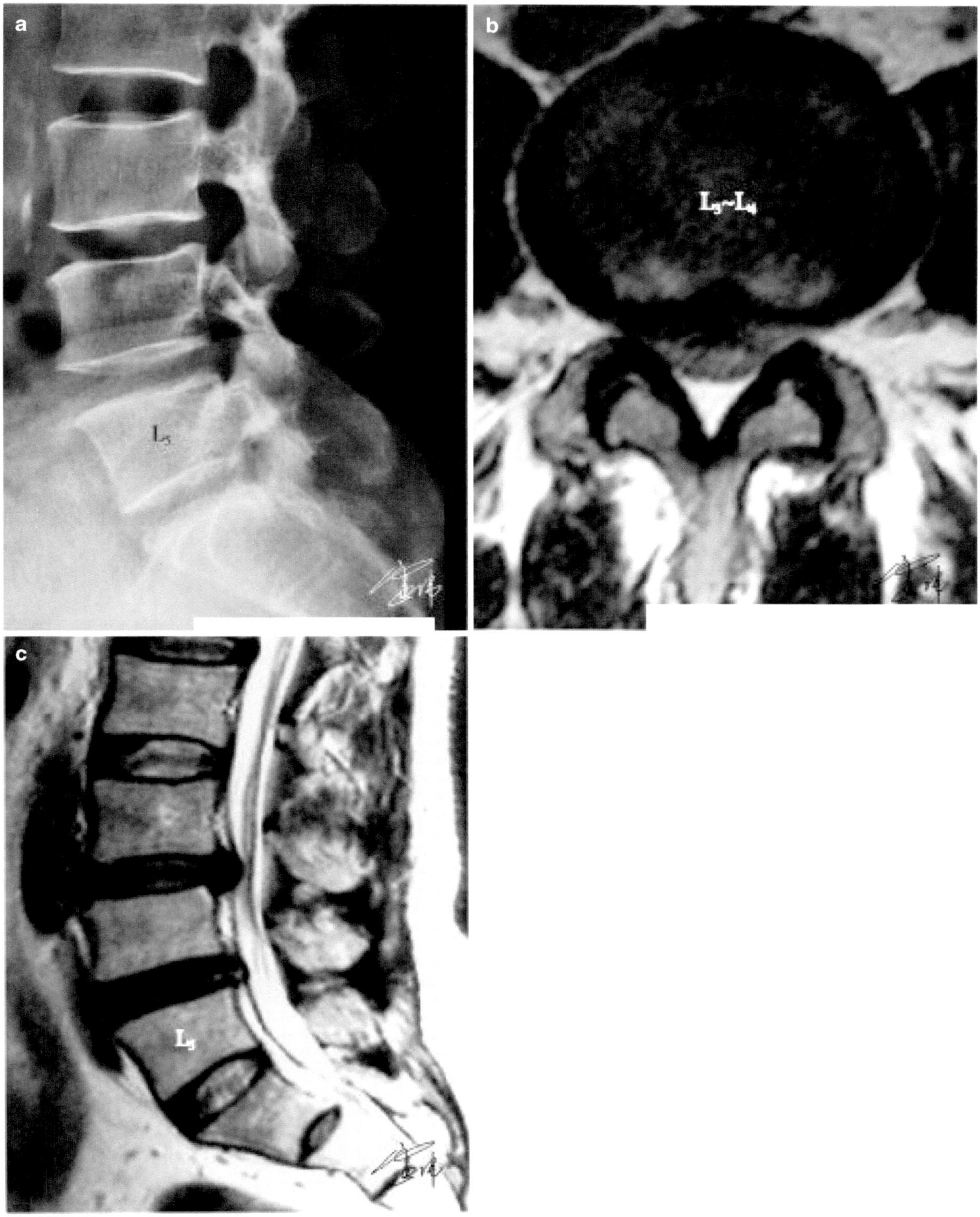

Fig. 9.75 Preoperative imaging studies. (**a**) X-ray (*lateral view*); (**b**) MRI (*horizontal view*); (**c**) MRI (*sagittal view*)

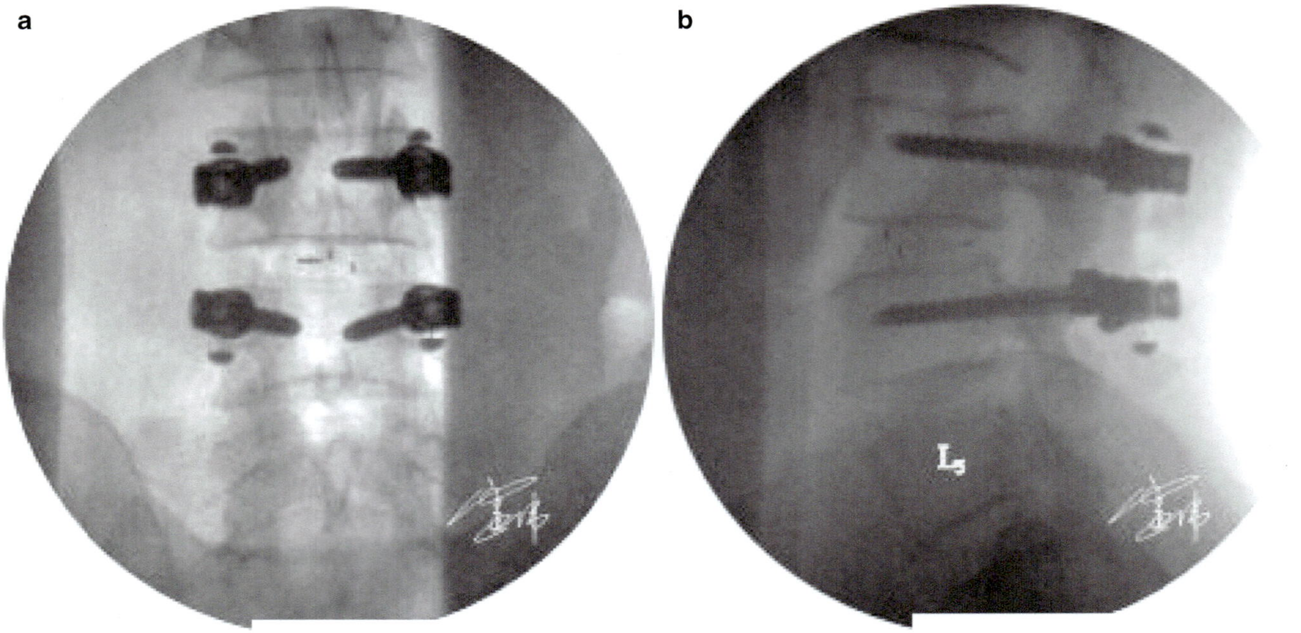

Fig. 9.76 Intraoperative images. (**a**) Fluoroscopy (*anteroposterior view*); (**b**) Fluoroscopy (*lateral view*)

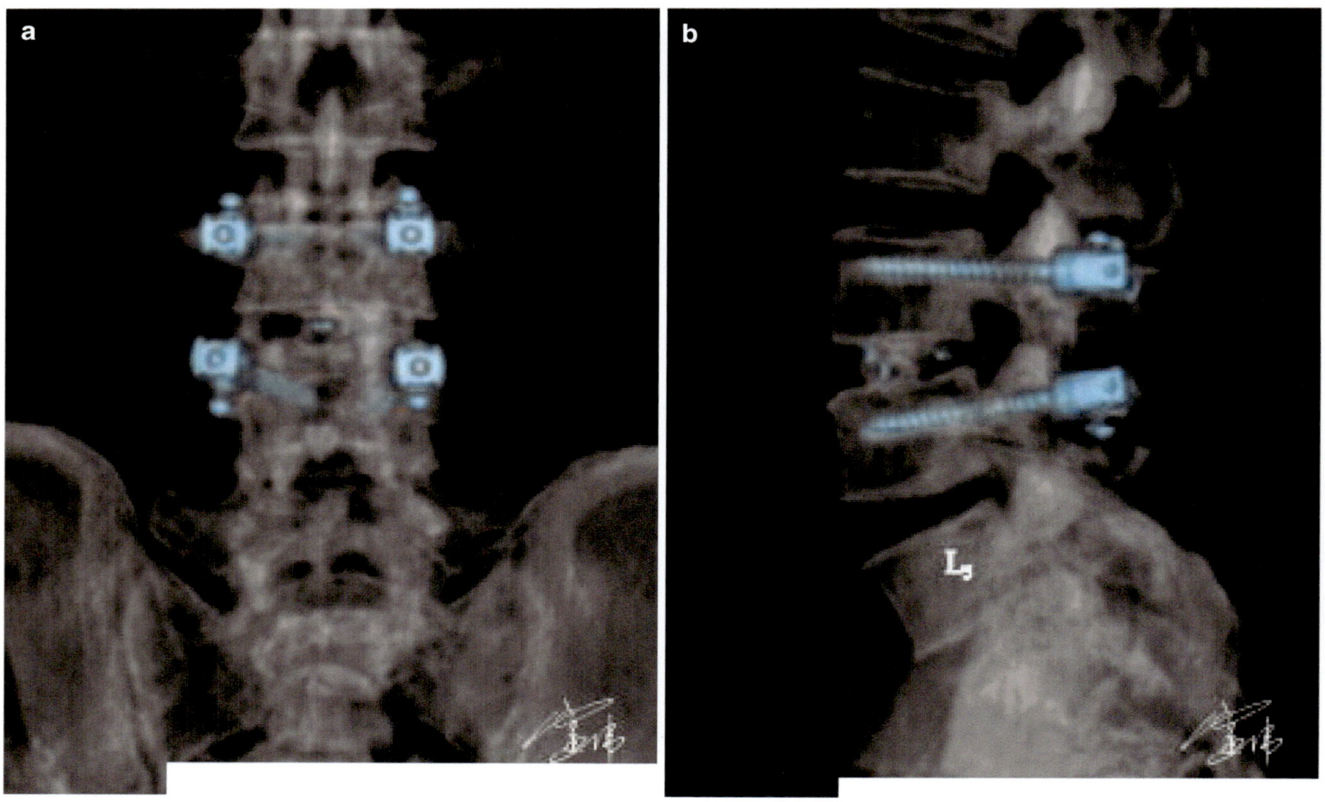

Fig. 9.77 Postoperative images. (**a**) CT 3D reconstruction (*posterior view*); (**b**) CT 3D reconstruction (*lateral view*)

9.5 Pearls and Pitfalls

1. Be cautious about the use of compressors and distractors

During compression and distraction, the feet of either the compressor or the distractor are placed securely against the implant body and not against the screw plug; otherwise, slippage of the implant or premature breaking of the plug may ensue.

2. Change of screw threads

The provisional screwdriver can be used to temporarily secure the rod. Temporary fixations can be done multiple times without damaging the screw plug or implant threads. If the screw plug has been cross-threaded, it should be replaced.

3. Caution in bending horizontally connected devices

The curvature on any plane cannot exceed 20 degrees; otherwise, breakage may occur.

4. The break-off of multi-axial reduction (lifting) screws

If soft tissues prevent the lateral break-off of the lengthened portion of the reduction screw, the medial lengthened proportion of the screw can be first broken off medially. Then, the Counter Torque can be used for break-off of the screw plug, and finally the lateral lengthened proportion of the screw can be broken off medially. If the lengthened portion cannot be easily bent and broken off, the screw plug should be examined to see it is fully seated. If the screw plug is not fully seated, the threads still exert resistance and prevent the break-off of the lengthened portion.

5. Handling of the bone adjacent to the screw

If the superior facet is inappropriately handled, the movements of the screw head are limited, leading to difficulty in inserting the screw plug and uneven force distribution, thus readily damaging the screw plug. If the bone beneath the head of the screw is not smoothened, the head of the screw and the bone beneath will impact on one another.

6. Choice of screw entry angle

For fixation of L5–S1, if the entry angle of the screw is incorrectly chosen, it will cause the heads of the two screws to collide against each other, interfering with the placement of the system. The correct spatial relation between the screw plug and the rod should be known to achieve the optimal fixation results.

The rod should be bent; otherwise, it will result in uneven force distribution between the screw plug and the rod, affecting the outcome of fixation. There should be a gap between the screw and the bone surface; otherwise, the motion of the head of the screw will be limited, leading to uneven force distribution between the screw plug and rod, affecting the outcome of fixation.

7. The fracture is not fully reduced

Based on our clinical experience, for treatment of thoracolumbar fractures, we believe that the superior endplate of the adjacent lower vertebral body and the inferior endplate of the adjacent upper vertebral body of the fractured vertebral body should be kept parallel during reduction or in mild lordosis. Meanwhile, sufficient intervertebral disc height should be maintained, and if, with sufficient intervertebral disc height, the anterior vertebral body is still collapsed, indicating severe injury of the anterior longitudinal ligament and the intervertebral disc, no traction of the fractured end should be undertaken for reduction. This is the reason for unsatisfactory vertebral fracture reduction despite sufficient posterior and anterior distraction. In such cases, there is no need for multiple adjustments of the reduction devices so as to avoid screw loosening and pedicle fracture. To solve this problem, vertebroplasty can perform fracture reduction, that is, a balloon is advanced from the pedicle of the fractured vertebral body to achieve fracture reduction by dilatation, followed by placement of bone cement or cancellous bone, or a pedicle drill can enter the collapsed region of the fractured vertebral body to achieve reduction by prying, followed by filling of the cavity with cancellous bone via the pedicle trajectory. However, the effectiveness of the two methods is not definite.

8. The two extension rods cross each other after placement

For treatment of lumbar spondylolisthesis, if the two extension rods cross each other after their placement, reduction by the distractor will be affected. In this situation, the caudal nut is tightened first after screw placement so that there is enough space for the rostral offset holder to lift the screws for extension rod placement. Thus, distractor placement is not affected. After the intervertebral disc space is distracted, the screw nut is gradually lifted, reduction is done, and the screw is tightened. If lumbar lordosis is to be increased, the extension rod can be pushed caudally in the course of tightening.

9. Failure to achieve full reduction in spondylolisthesis

Full reduction can generally be achieved in the treatment of lumbar spondylolisthesis. Two steps are crucial for full reduction. First, the surgeon should accurately determine the severity of spondylolisthesis preoperatively and correctly estimate the lifting distance with appropriate lifting room preserved intraoperatively. Second, scar tissues, osteophytes, and entangled cords affecting reduction should be loosened completely intraoperatively.

The slip distance in the spondylolisthesis patient should be measured on lateral X-ray films before surgery. The patient is placed in the prone position during surgery for fluoroscopy to examine whether marked changes in the slip distance have occurred. If there are no apparent changes, the preoperative slip distance is used as the lifting distance. A lifting space for reduction that corresponds to the measured slip distance is preserved when a rod is used to lift the screws. Then, the caudal screw head is tightened to set the reduction space, followed by final tightening. As long as sufficient space is preserved for reduction, and the caudal screw head is firmly tightened without loosening, the reduction screws will not slip inside the bone. If the principle of caudal fixation and rostral lifting is followed, reduction can generally be achieved in spondylolisthesis patients.

In addition, the curvature of the rod should be appropriate. If the rod is bent at an excessive curvature, no sufficient lifting space is left. If the rod is bent at too small an angle, lumbar lordosis will decrease, even leading to flat back syndrome.

The presence of bony bridges in the anterior edge of the vertebral body affects reduction. A periosteum elevator can be inserted into the intervertebral disc space for prying and cutting off the bony bridge and loosening the vertebral bodies. Then, lifting reduction is done. If the bony bridge is not disrupted, reduction cannot be done, and the lifting screws will also be pulled out from the vertebral body.

10. Evaluation criteria for lumbar spondylolisthesis reduction

Radiological parameters for evaluation of spondylolisthesis reduction include the Taillard index, intervertebral disc space height, curvature of the lumbosacral spine, and height and width of the intervertebral foramen.

11. The use of offset holder

When more than three sets of pedicle screws are used for posterior fixation, pedicle screws should be best placed in a straight line. Otherwise, it will increase difficulty for rod placement. If the screws are not in a straight line, an offset can be used.

12. Management of crossed L5 and S1 pedicle screws

The two pedicle screws in L5 and S1 should be kept at an appropriate angle and distance. Otherwise, the two pedicle screws will cross each other and make it difficult for placing the offset holder. In such cases, the parallel distractor can be placed between the two sets of pedicle screws for gentle distraction. The lower blade of the parallel distractor is inserted, then the rod is placed, and finally the upper blade is inserted, and the screw is tightened.

13. Advantages of fixation of the injured spine

Fixation of the injured spine is consistent with bone biomechanical requirements, facilitates reduction of the injured spine, and reduces the breaking of internal fixation implants.

14. Indications of fixation of the injured spine fixation

The pedicle integrity of the injured spine should be determined via CT or CT 3D reconstruction (Fig. 9.78).

15. Length and angle of screws for the injured spine

The use of short screws is recommended for fixation, and the screw length is 2/3–3/4 of the length of a regular screw. The fixation angle is aimed in the direction of the solid portion of the bone. If the screw is advanced into the fractured portion of the bone, fixation strength will be markedly reduced (Fig. 9.79).

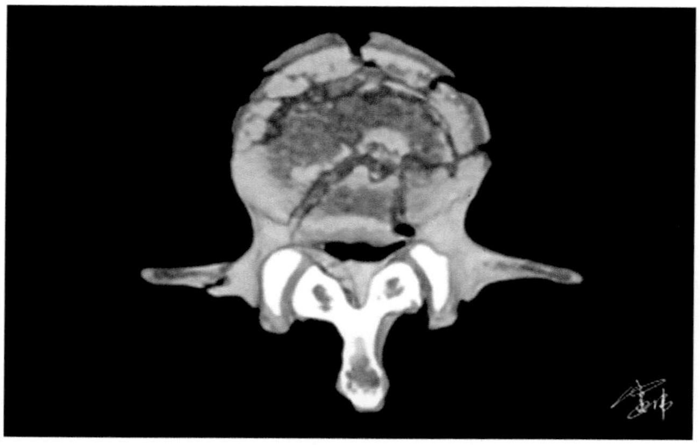

Fig. 9.78 The injured spine

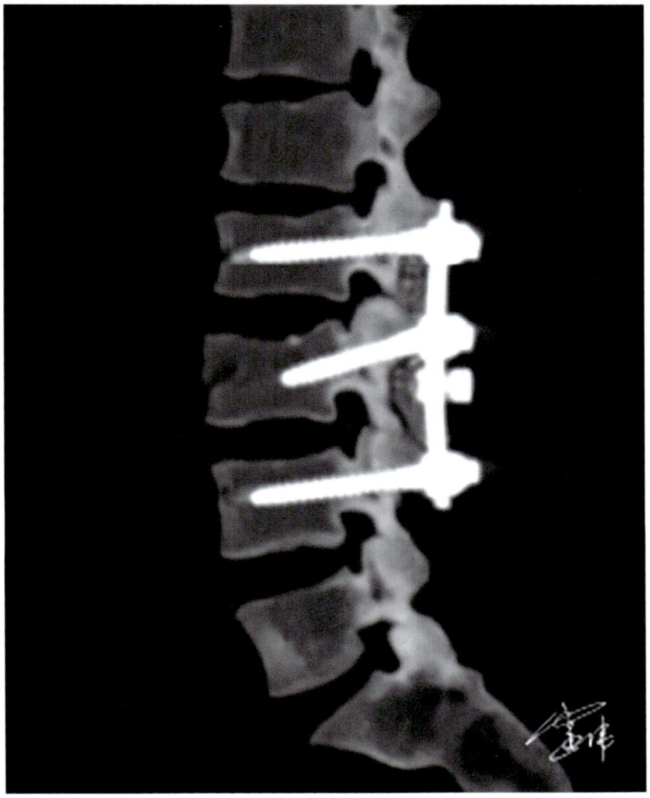

Fig. 9.79 Screw fixation of the injured spine

16. The diseased spine should not undergo pedicle screw fixation

Pedicle screws should be best avoided for diseased vertebral bodies such as with tuberculosis or tumor. On the one hand, the diseased bone has poor holding power for the screw. On the other hand, screw entry into the diseased bone region may facilitate spread of the disease.

17. Prevention of screw loosening in osteoporosis

Expansion pedicle screw fixation can be undertaken in cases of mild or moderate osteoporosis (Fig. 9.80). Partial reinforcement of the screw trajectory plus expansion screw fixation (Fig. 9.81) can be done in cases of severe osteoporosis (Fig. 9.82).

18. Implant fixation failure and principles of management

Common implant fixation failures include breaking of screws or rods, loosening of screws, and improper positioning of screws resulting in pedicle injury and screw entry into the spinal canal or intervertebral disc space. Late complications are mainly bone fusion failures, leading to pseudoarthrosis and breaking of screws or rods (Fig. 9.83).

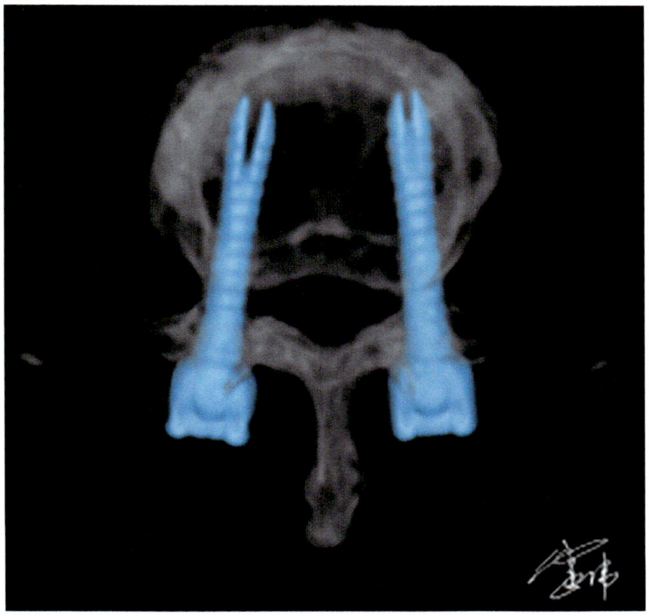

Fig. 9.80 Expansion pedicle screw fixation

For early postoperative complications, revision surgery should be undertaken as early as possible. For late (>3 months) postoperative complications, if bone fusion has been achieved, and the patient is asymptomatic, revision surgery can be postponed, and watchful observation can be undertaken. If the patient has implant-related clinical manifestations, revision surgery is carried out and the internal fixation can be removed. If bone fusion has not been achieved and pseudoarthrosis is formed, revision surgery can be postponed if the patient is asymptomatic and the patient can be closely watched. If symptoms occur, revision surgery is undertaken, and the implant is adjusted, or bone graft surgery is done.

Revision surgery should be immediately undertaken if implant-related neurologic symptoms have developed, regardless of whether they occur in the early or late stage (Fig. 9.84).

9.6 Postoperative Management

Patients should be cautioned to avoid any activities that may exert a pulling or shearing action on the implant or bone graft, thus impairing bone healing and leading to complications. When the spine is sufficiently stable and under support by external fixation, patients are encouraged to carry out appropriate, regular, and incrementally increasing activities to facilitate bone growth. Wearing durable external fixation devices until bone healing has been achieved by patients. Patients should receive proper guidance on activities from sitting to moving into and out of bed.

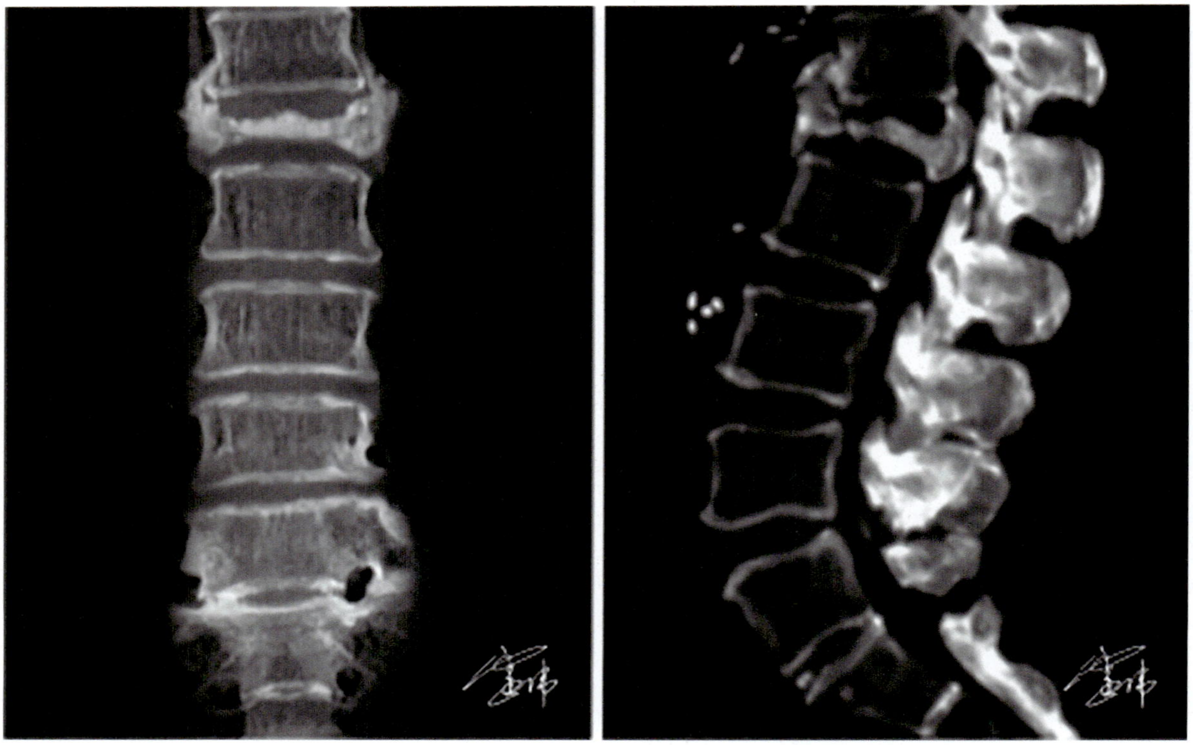

Fig. 9.81 Partial reinforcement of the screw trajectory plus expansion screw fixation

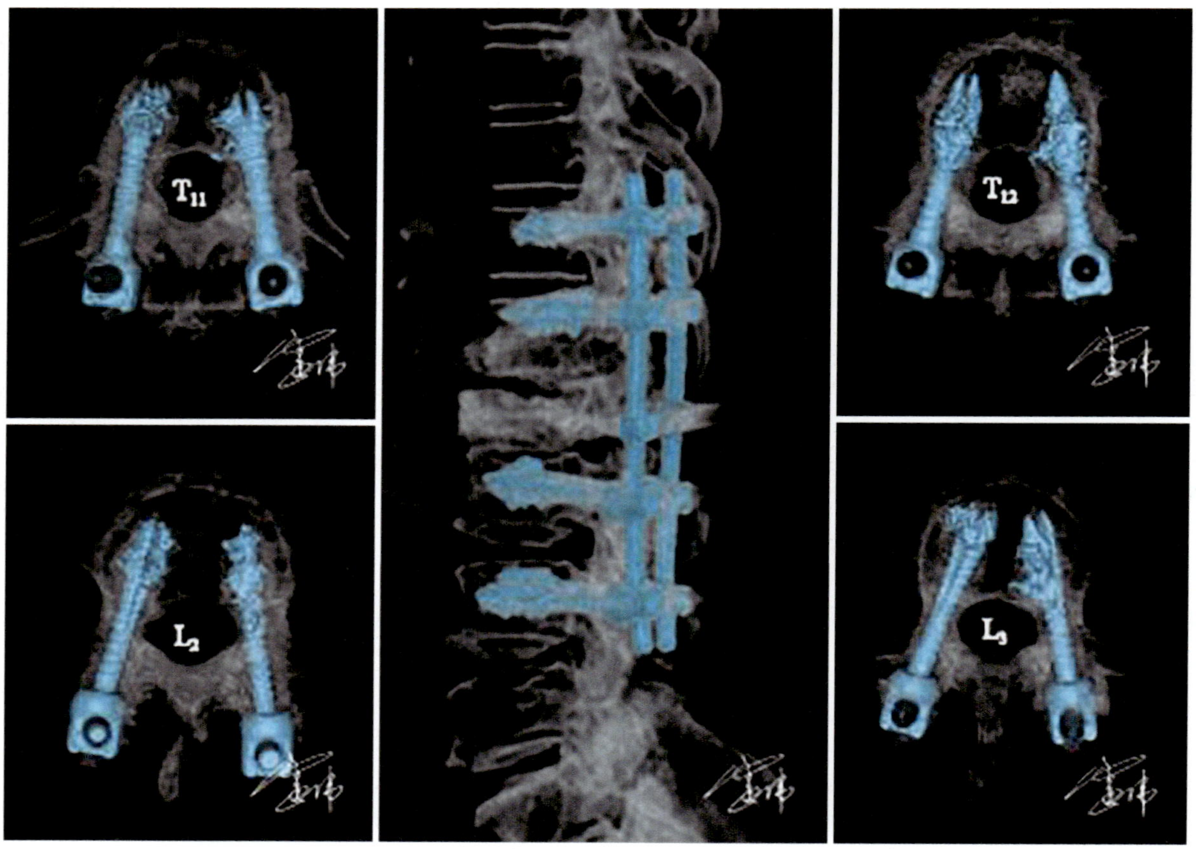

Fig. 9.82 L1 vertebral compression fracture (severe osteoporosis)

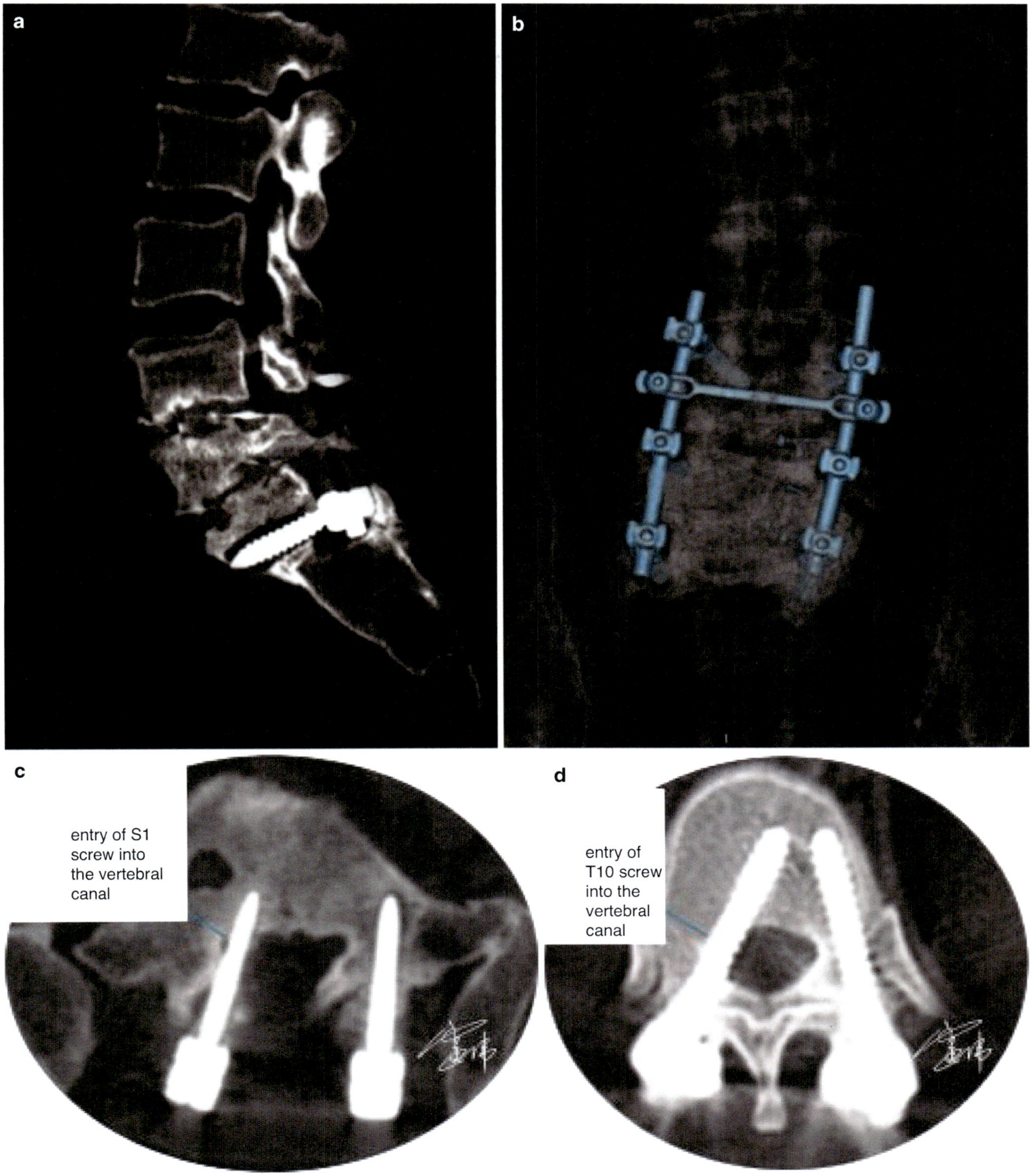

Fig. 9.83 Implant fixation failure. (**a**) CT 3D reconstruction (*sagittal view*); (**b**) CT 3D reconstruction (*posterior view*); (**c**) CT (*horizontal view*); (**d**) CT (*horizontal view*)

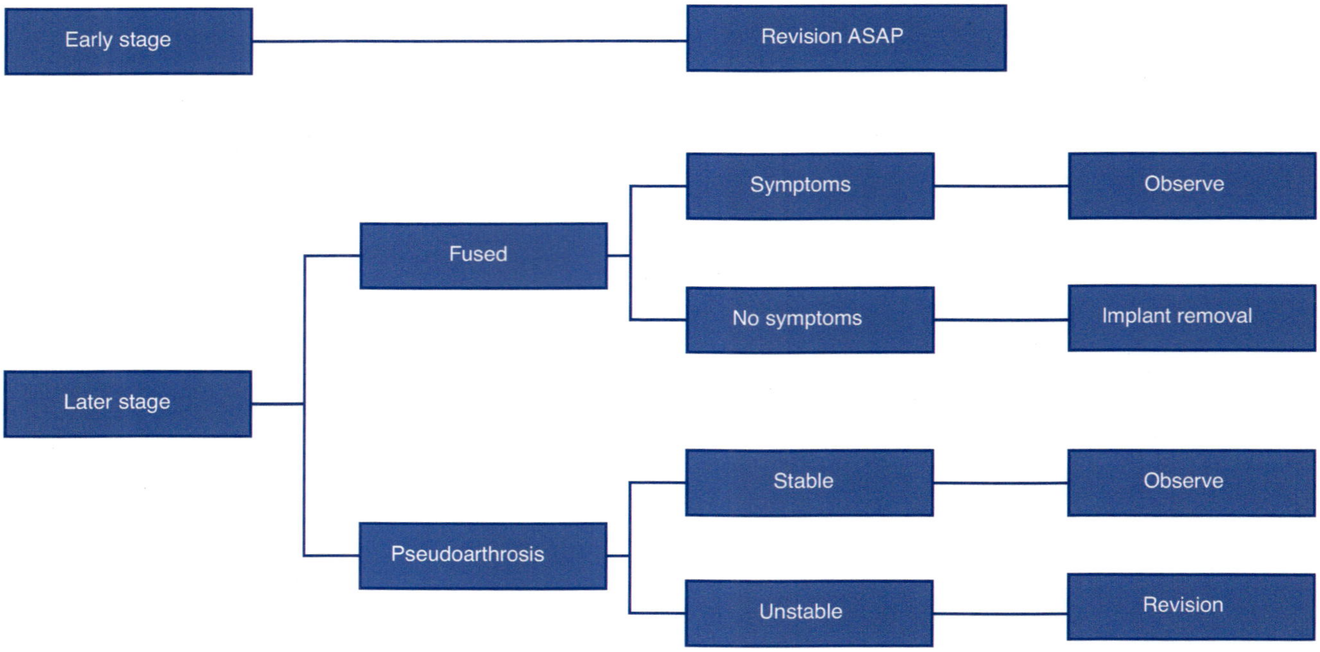

Fig. 9.84 Principles of management for failed implant fixations

Recommendation: Under the protection of external support, patients may start ambulation 1 week postoperatively, and the support can be removed 3–6 months postoperatively depending on bone healing.

References

1. Hadra BE. Wiring the spinous processes in pott's disease. J Bone Joint Surg. 1891;138(3564):1408.
2. Baker ADL. Treatment of scoliosis correction and internal fixation by spine instrumentation. London: Springer; 1962.
3. Michele AA, Krueger FJ. Surgical approach to the vertebral body. J Bone Joint Surg Am. 1949;31a(4):873–8.
4. Roy-Camille R, Saillant G, Mazel C. Plating of thoracic, thoracolumbar, and lumbar injuries with pedicle screw plates. Orthop Clin North Am. 1986;17(1):147–59.
5. Denis F. The three column spine and its significance in the classification of acute thoracolumbar spinal injuries. Spine. 1983;8(8):817–31.
6. Steffee AD, Biscup RS, Sitkowski DJ. Segmental spine plates with pedicle screw fixation. A new internal fixation device for disorders of the lumbar and thoracolumbar spine. Clin Orthop Relat Res. 1986;203:45–53.
7. Cotrel Y, Dubousset J. A new technic for segmental spinal osteosynthesis using the posterior approach. Revue de chirurgie orthopedique et reparatrice de l'appareil moteur. 1984;70(6):489–94.
8. Zindrick MR, Wiltse LL, Doornik A, Widell EH, Knight GW, Patwardhan AG, Thomas JC, Rothman SL, Fields BT. Analysis of the morphometric characteristics of the thoracic and lumbar pedicles. Spine. 1987;12(2):160–6.
9. Panjabi MM, Goel V, Oxland T, Takata K, Duranceau J, Krag M, Price M. Human lumbar vertebrae. Quantitative three-dimensional anatomy. Spine. 1992;17(3):299–306.
10. Ebraheim NA, Rollins JR Jr, Xu R, Yeasting RA. Projection of the lumbar pedicle and its morphometric analysis. Spine. 1996;21(11):1296–300.
11. Tan SH, Teo EC, Chua HC. Quantitative three-dimensional anatomy of lumbar vertebrae in Singaporean Asians. Eur Spine J. 2002;11(2):152–8.
12. Magerl FP. Stabilization of the lower thoracic and lumbar spine with external skeletal fixation. Clin Orthop Relat Res. 1984;189:125–41.

Surgical Techniques for Iliac Screws

10

Yabo Yan, Yi Huan, and Wei Lei

Abstract

The pelvic fixation technique can provide an additional pivot for the stabilization of the long fusion in lumbar fixation. This technique has been widely used in the treatment of lumbar spine deformity and sacral or lumbar tumor. Anatomic characteristics of the iliac bone, the entry point, entry angle, entry depth of the iliac screw, and operative details are demonstrated to guarantee the proper positioning of the screw. The characteristics, clinical indications and contraindications, and surgical technique of pelvic fixation system are described in detail. The applications of these techniques are presented in typical clinical cases. Pearls and pitfalls of the pelvic screw fixation are summarized at the end of this chapter.

Keywords

Iliac screw · Entry point · Entry angle

10.1 Iliac Screw Fixation Technique: A Historical Perspective

Lesions and diseases such as scoliosis in the lower lumbar spine and the iliac frequently require lumbosacral fixation involving the use of iliac fixation techniques. Iliac fixation methods have evolved over time:

In 1984, Allen and Ferguson [1] developed the iliac fixation technique, which is called the Galveston technique (Fig. 10.1).

In 1988, Cotrel-Dubousset [2] developed the internal fixation system and employed pedicle screws in the lumbosacral segment (Fig. 10.2).

In 2009, Sponseller [3] developed the sacral-alar-iliac fixation method (Fig. 10.3).

10.2 Data in Relation to the Ilium

The distance between the inner and outer tables of the ilium (the maximal diameter accommodating the iliac screw) varies between 5.5 and 7.0 mm and can accommodate a screw length of 52–68 mm. The iliac screw has an angle of approximately 13 degrees to the horizontal plane, 56 degrees to the coronal plane, and approximately 30 degrees to the sagittal plane (Table 10.1).

10.3 Iliac Screw Techniques

10.3.1 Determination of Screw Entry Points

Traditional iliac screw entry point is located at the bony protuberance superior to the posterior superior iliac spine, and the cortex is partially resected using a swing saw to expose the cancellous bone. The screw entry trajectory should be parallel to the posterior surface of the sacrum to facilitate iliac screw insertion (Fig. 10.4). Vaccaro proposed a new iliac screw placement method. The screw entry point is located lateral to the S2 pedicle (Fig. 10.5).

10.3.2 Screw Entry Angle

10.3.2.1 Entry Angle of a Single Iliac Screw

The entry trajectory is aimed toward the anterior inferior iliac spine from the posterior superior iliac spine (Trajectory C, Fig. 10.6).

Y. Yan · W. Lei (✉)
Department of Orthopedics, Xijing Hospital, Air Force Medical University, Xi'an, Shaanxi, China
e-mail: leiwei@fmmu.edu.cn

Y. Huan
Department of Radiology, Xijing Hospital, Airforce Military Medical University, Xi'an, China

W. Lei, Y. Yan (eds.), *Internal Fixation of the Spine*, https://doi.org/10.1007/978-981-16-1562-7_10

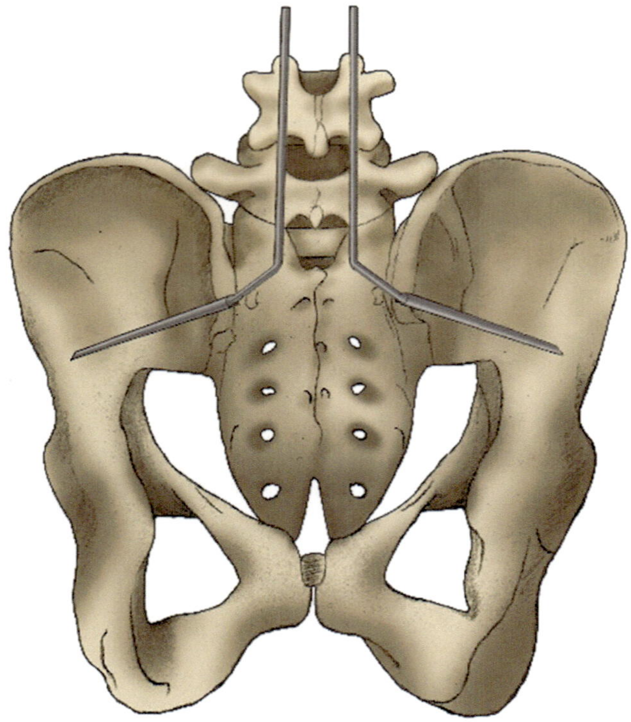

Fig. 10.1 The iliac fixation technique

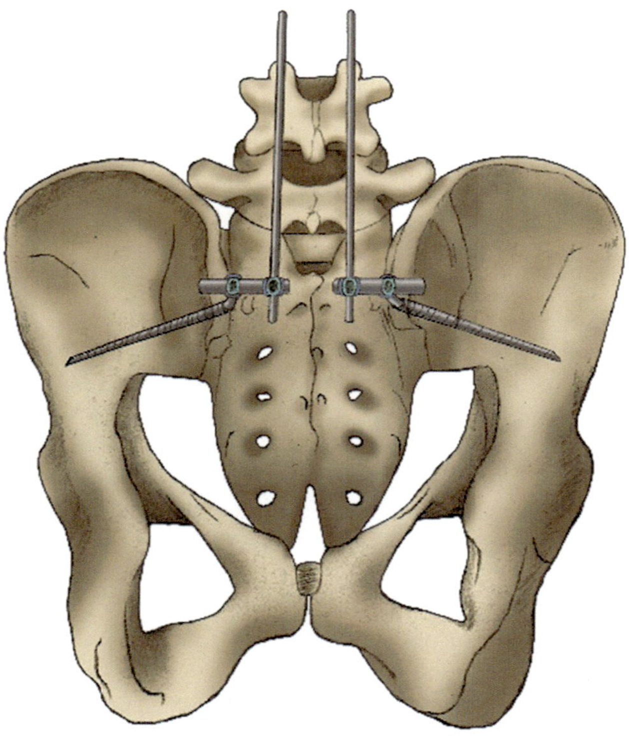

Fig. 10.2 Pedicle screws in the lumbosacral segment

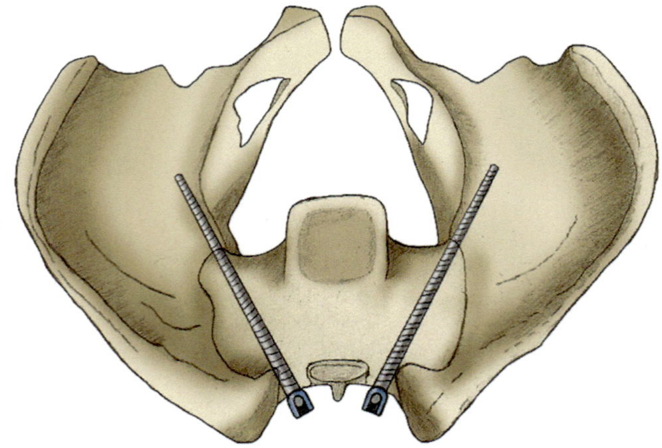

Fig. 10.3 Sacral-alar-iliac fixation method

10.3.2.2 Entry Angle of Double Iliac Screws

The entry angle of the first iliac screw is identical to that of a single iliac screw (Trajectory C, Fig. 10.6). The second iliac screw can be aimed toward the ipsilateral anterior inferior iliac spine, or toward 10 mm inferior to the highest point of the ipsilateral iliac crest (Trajectory B and A, Fig. 10.6). The iliac screw is inserted directly in the ipsilateral anterior inferior iliac spine; this trajectory has two narrow points, and caution should be exercised when inserting the screw in order to avoid penetrating the cortex and injuring adjacent nerves and vessels (Fig. 10.7).

10.3.3 Entry Depths of Iliac Screws

Conventional iliac screw dimensions are shown in Table 10.2. The most commonly used iliac screw dimension is 7.5 mm in diameter and 70 mm in length.

10.4 Surgical Procedures

10.4.1 Choosing the Iliac Screw Entry Point (Fig. 10.8)

10.4.2 Completing Iliac Screw Fixation (Fig. 10.9)

10.4.3 The Sectional View of the Iliac Screw Trajectory (Figs. 10.10, 10.11, 10.12, 10.13)

Table 10.1 Trajectory of iliac screws

Parameters	Iliac screw length	Iliac screw diameter	Angle between the iliac screw and the horizontal plane	Angle between the iliac screw and the coronal plane	Angle between the iliac screw and the sagittal plane
Posterior superior iliac spine to anterior inferior iliac spine	59.97 ± 7.99	6.00 ± 0.84	12.48 ± 7.16	56.41 ± 6.47	29.91 ± 5.55

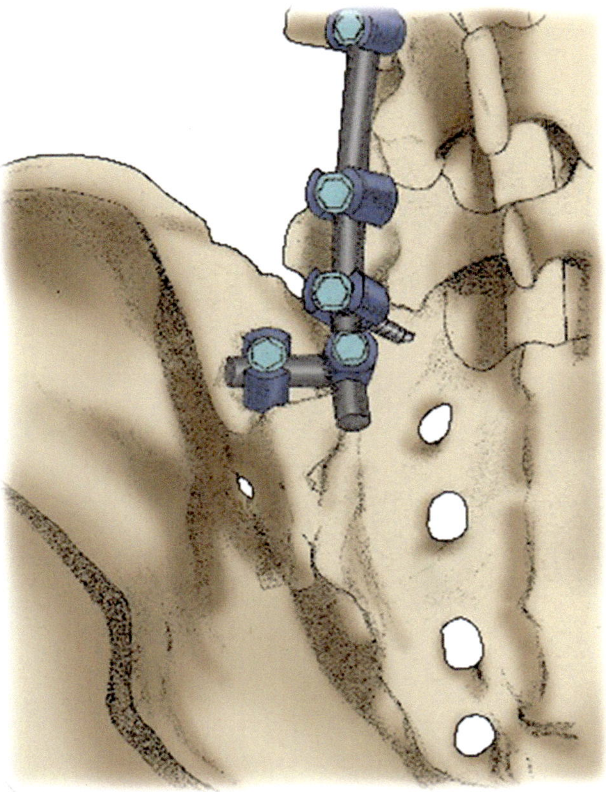

Fig. 10.4 Traditional screw entry path requires partial resection of the cortex

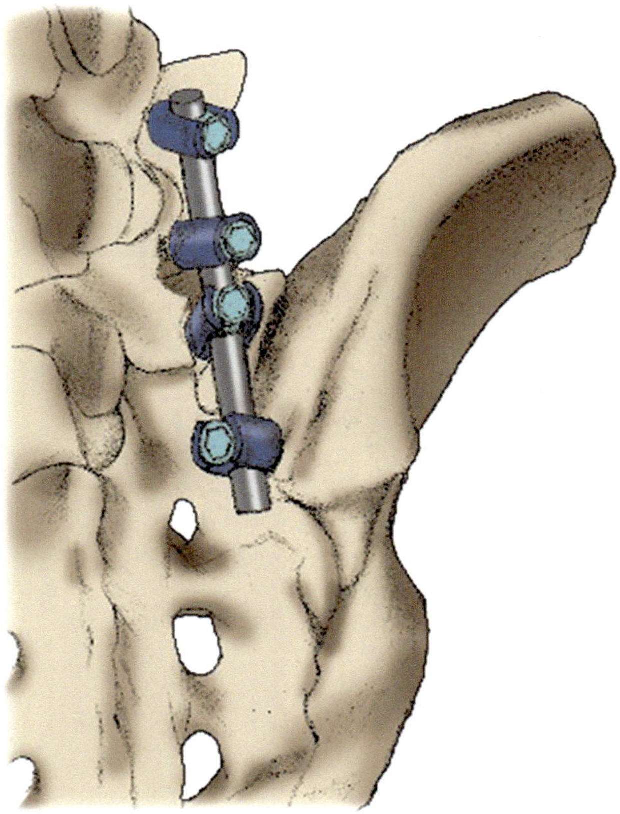

Fig. 10.5 Vaccaro proposed a new iliac screw placement method

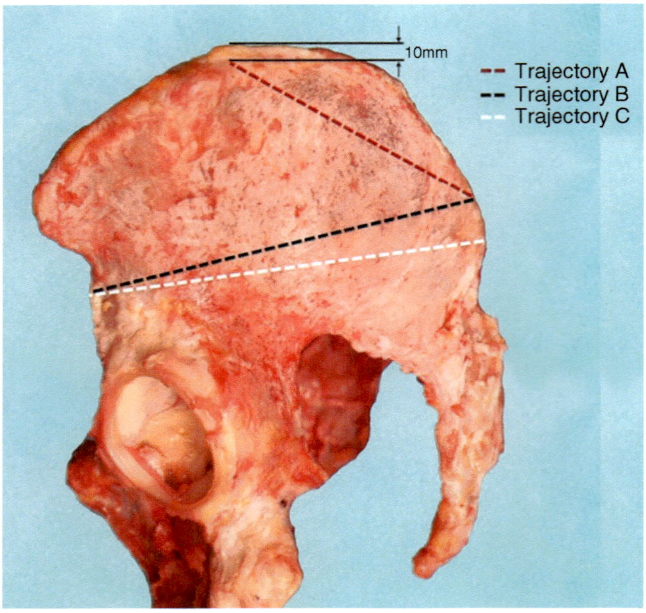

Fig. 10.6 Trajectory in iliac bone

Fig. 10.7 The sectional view of the iliac screw trajectory

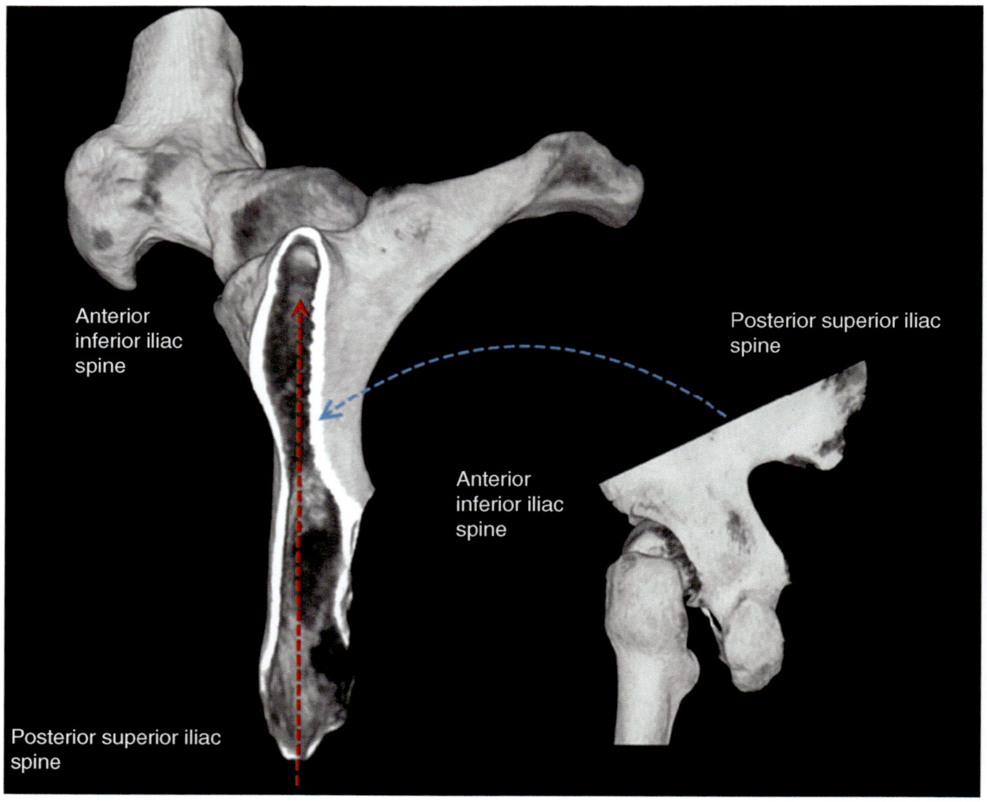

Table 10.2 Dimensions of commonly used iliac screws

Diameter, mm	Length, mm		
6.5	50	60	70
7.5	60	70	80
8.5	70	80	90

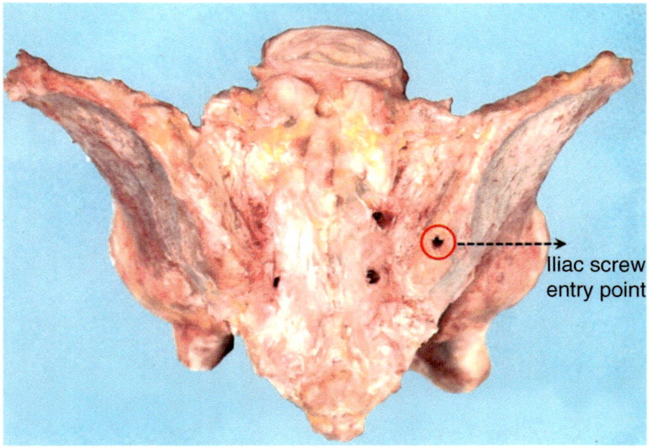

Fig. 10.8 Iliac screw entry point

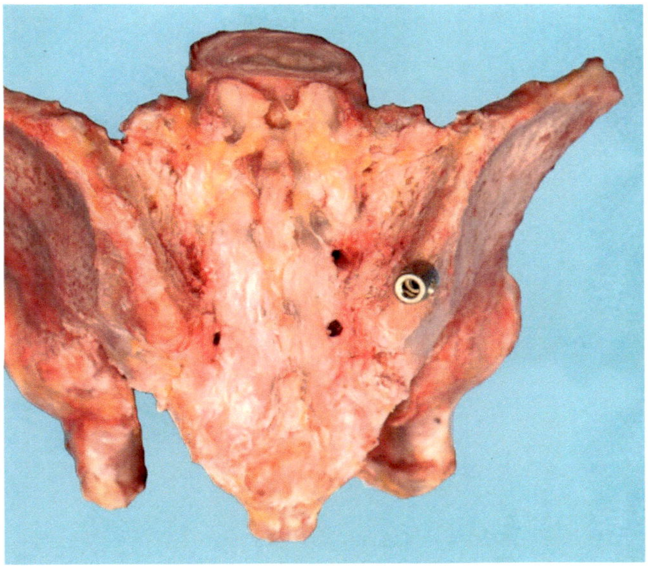

Fig. 10.9 The iliac screw is implanted

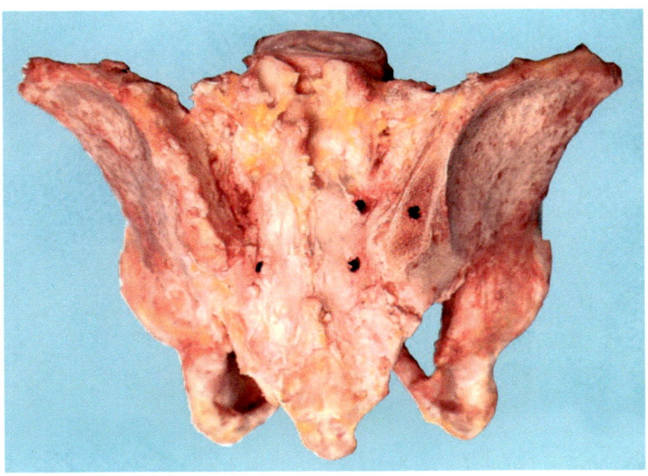

Fig. 10.10 The iliac screw trajectories

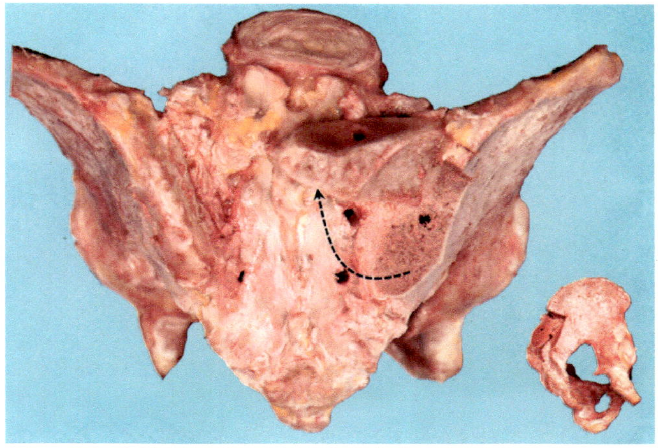

Fig. 10.11 The iliac screw trajectories

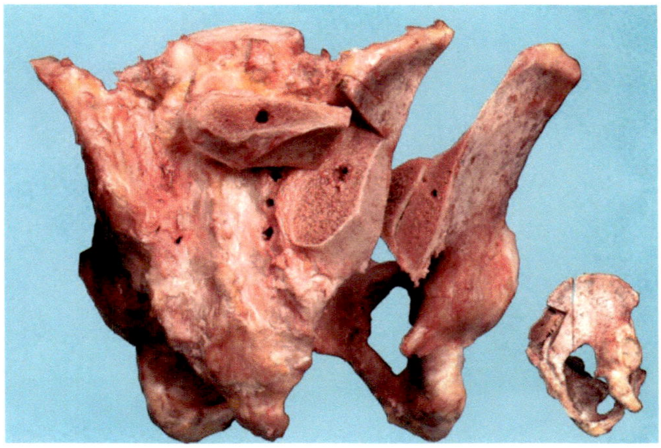

Fig. 10.12 The iliac screw trajectories

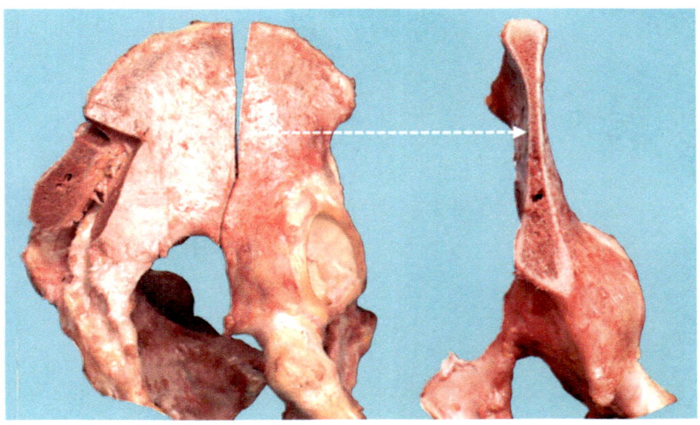

Fig. 10.13 The iliac screw trajectories

10.5 Imaging Features of Standard Iliac Screws (Fig. 10.14)

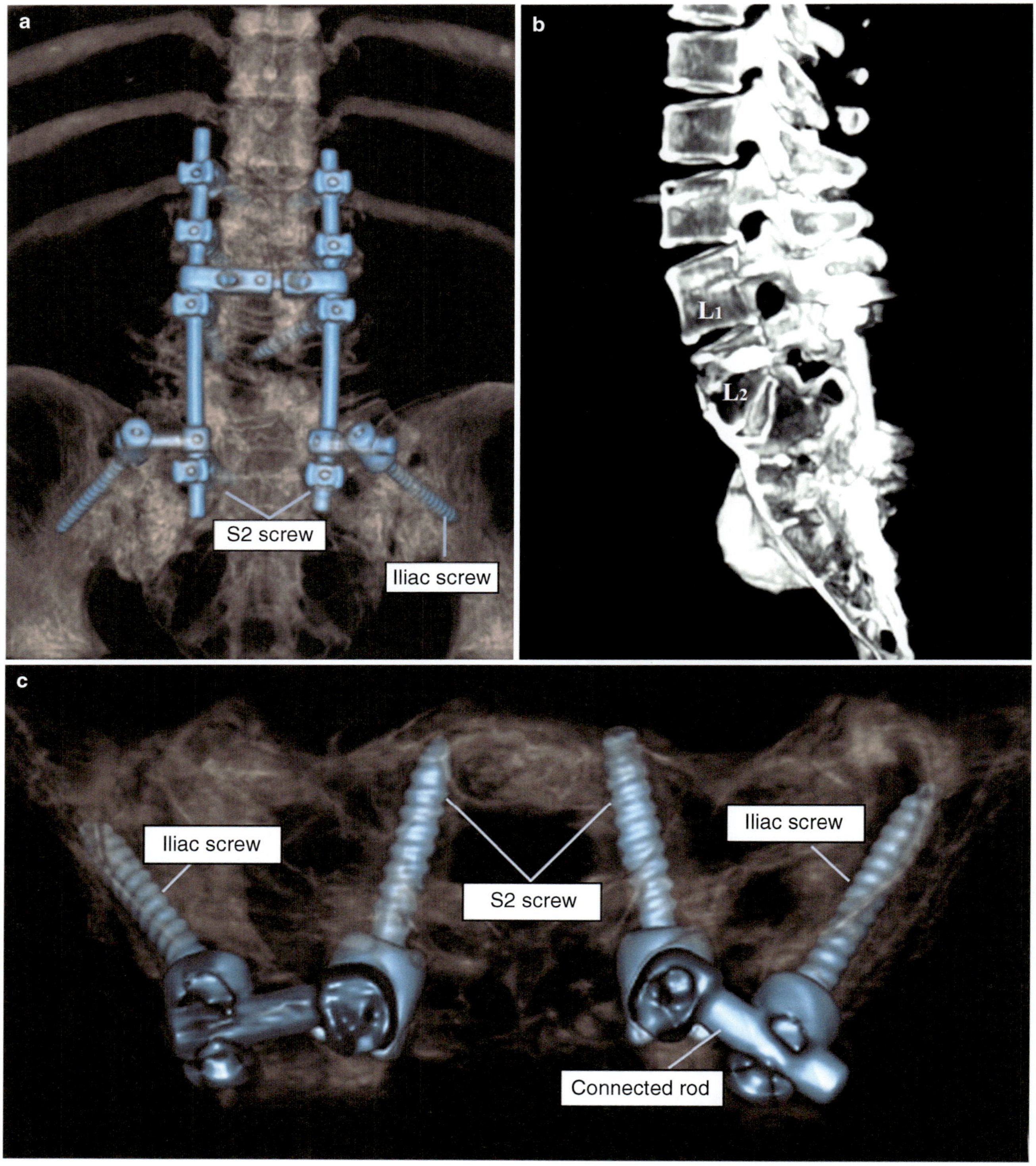

Fig. 10.14 3D CT image of iliac screw. (**a**) Posterior view of the construct; (**b**) Sagittal view of the construct; (**c**) Axial view of the construct

References

1. Allen BL Jr, Ferguson RL. The Galveston technique of pelvic fixation with L-rod instrumentation of the spine. Spine (Phila Pa 1976). 1984;9:388–94.
2. Cotrel Y, Dubousset J, Guillaumat M. New universal instrumentation in spinal surgery. Clin Orthop. 1988;227:10–23.
3. Sponseller PD, et al. Low profile pelvic fixation with the sacral alar iliac technique in the pediatric population improves results at two-year minimum follow-up. Spine (Phila Pa 1976). 2010;35(20):1887–92.

Surgical Techniques for Sacral Pedicle Screws

11

Wei Qi, Yabo Yan, and Wei Lei

Abstract

Sacral screw fixation is a commonly used procedure for lumbar spondylosis. This technique was first proposed by Roy-Camille in 1986 and has evolved over the decades. In this chapter, we thoroughly review the different sacral screw entry methods. Anatomic features of the sacral vertebral body, the entry point, entry angle, entry depth of sacral pedicle screw, and operative details are demonstrated to guarantee proper screw positioning. The characteristics, clinical indications and contraindications, and surgical technique of the sacral screw are introduced in detail. The applications of these techniques are illustrated in typical clinical cases.

Keywords

Sacral spine · Pedicle screw fixation · Surgical technique

11.1 Sacral Screw Fixation Technique: A Historical Perspective

In 1986, Roy-Camille et al. developed S1 screw entry method [1]. The sacral screw is entered on the lateral aspect of the S1 facet.

In 1992, Smith and Carlson et al. modified the Roy-Camille method [2], and the starting point of the screw was 2 mm lateral to and below the lower end of the S1 facet joint (Fig. 11.1).

In 1994, Morse et al. developed another S1 screw entry method [3]. The entry point is 5 mm inferior and 10 mm lateral to the inferior edge of the S1 facet (Fig. 11.2).

In 2014, Kubaszewski et al. developed a screw entry method through S1 articular process [4] (Fig. 11.3).

11.2 Anatomic Data in Relation to the Sacrum (Figs. 11.4, 11.5, 11.6, 11.7, and 11.8)

11.3 S1 Pedicles

For lateral sacral screw placement, it remains critical to prevent iatrogenic injury to the nerves and vessels. The average height of S1 pedicle is 2.26 ± 0.27 cm on the left and 2.22 ± 0.21 cm on the right, and the screw diameter is 0.7 cm [4]. The screw does not readily penetrate through the superior and inferior edge of the pedicle. Due to the anatomic features of nerves and vessels anterior to the sacrum and organs, the greatest risk is that S1 screw placement may cause inadvertent injury to the lumbosacral roots, the internal iliac vein, and the sacroiliac joint. The anterolateral region of S1 screw placement is the safest, and unless absolutely necessary, S2 fixation is not done. To ensure the safety of the sacral pedicel screw, four important angles should be measured (Fig. 11.9).

11.4 Determination of S1 Pedicle Screw Entry Points

S1 pedicle entry point is at the junction of the tangent line to the lateral margin of S1 articular process and the horizontal line of the inferior margin of the articular process (Fig. 11.10).

Due to anatomic variations of S1, screws can be entered from different points and in different directions, which mainly depend on instruments and bone quality.

W. Qi
Department of Surgery, Hospital of PLA Unit 63820, Mianyang, Sichuan Province, China

Department of Orthopedics, Xijing Hospital, Air Force Medical University, Xi'an, Shaanxi, China

Y. Yan · W. Lei (✉)
Department of Orthopedics, Xijing Hospital, Air Force Medical University, Xi'an, Shaanxi, China
e-mail: leiwei@fmmu.edu.cn

W. Lei, Y. Yan (eds.), *Internal Fixation of the Spine*, https://doi.org/10.1007/978-981-16-1562-7_11

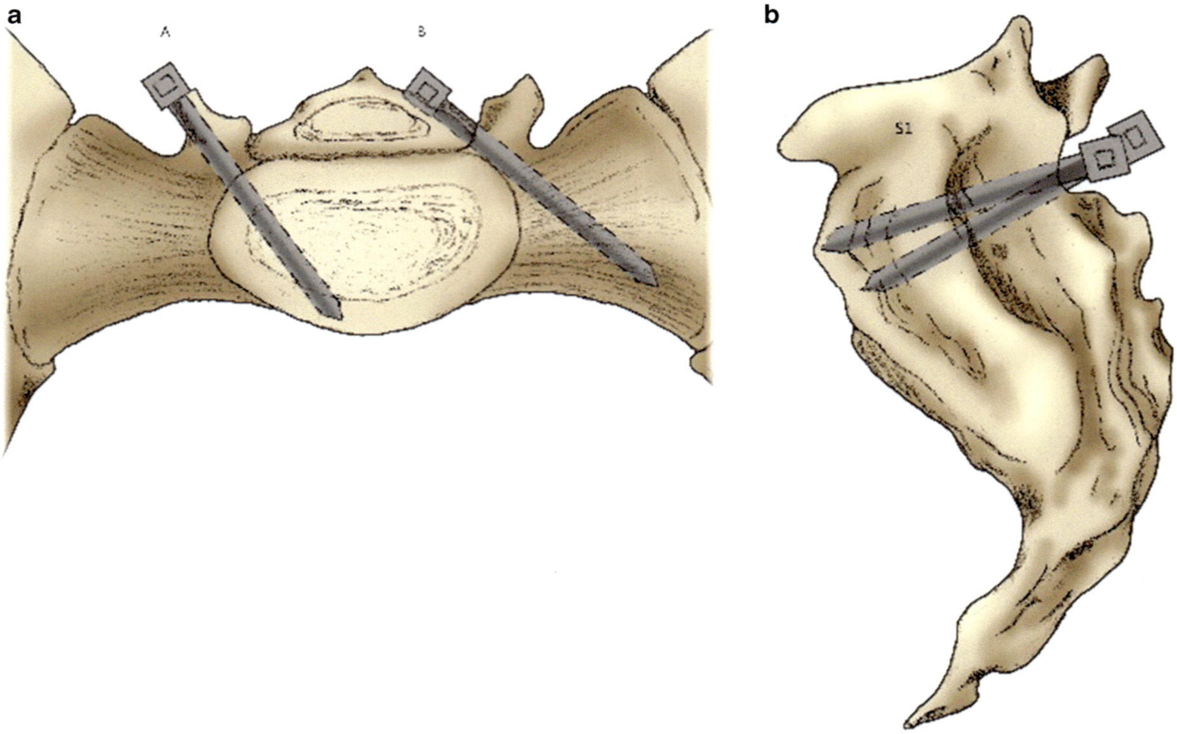

Fig. 11.1 Orientation of screws in the sacrum viewed in the transverse and sagittal planes: anteromedial orientation, 30° medial from sagittal and 20° caudal (**a**); and anterolateral orientation, 40°lateral and 30°caudal (**b**). Note that the screws were place through the anterior cortex of the sacrum

Determination of S2 screw entry points: The screw is entered at 1/2 to 1/3 of the distance between the inferior margin of S1 posterior foramen and the superior margin of S2 posterior foramen (Fig. 11.11).

11.5 Entry Angle of Sacral Pedicle Screws

11.5.1 Entry Angle of S1 Pedicle Screws

There are two methods for the entry angle of S1 pedicle screws (Fig. 11.12). Method 1: The entry angle is medially inclined 25°. Method 2: The entry angle is 35° lateral to the sacral ala. Method 1 is the most commonly used. The patient is placed in the prone position, and the screw is inclined 25–30° cephalad and aimed toward the sacral promontory and enters the subchondral bone. The sacrum is a flat bone, and the amount of bone is relatively scant in the sacral pedicle and the sacral ala. The sacral pedicle screw can be entered in the sacral body or sacral promontory anteromedially as the standard practice, or the sacral ala anterolaterally (Fig. 11.13). The sacral vertebrae vary widely in bone density: The subchondral bone has the highest density, while the sacral lateral mass is rather osteoporotic, even empty.

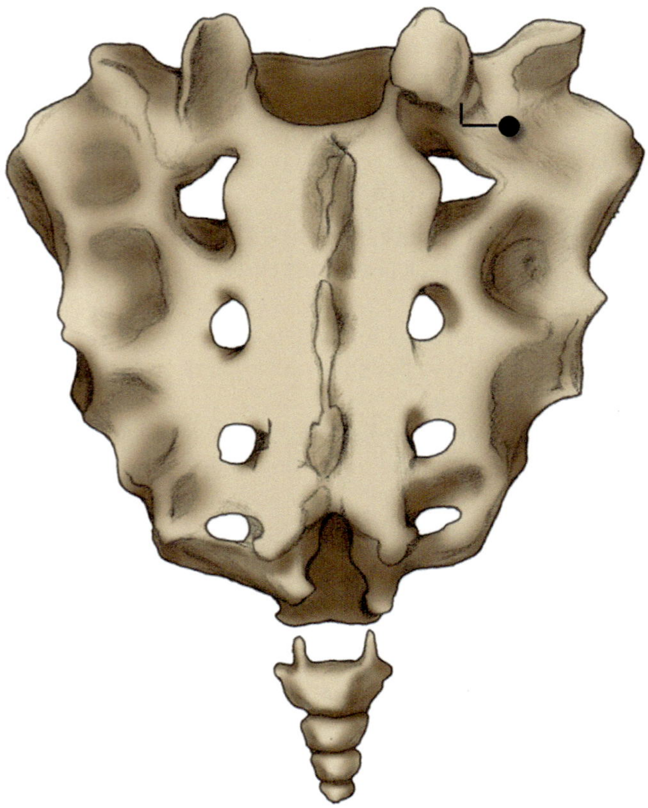

Fig. 11.2 Dorsal view of sacrum with location of the insertion site near S1 facet

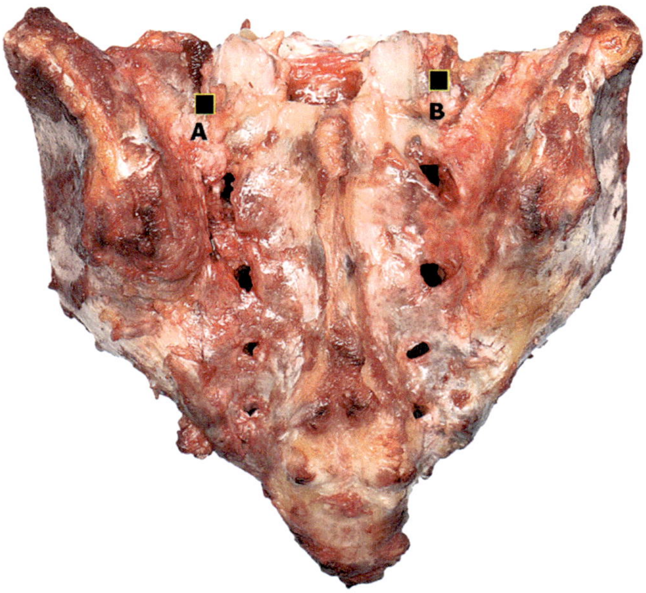

Fig. 11.3 Two different starting points for the classical (**a**) and modified (**b**) techniques

11.5.2 Entry Angles of S2 Screws

1. On the sagittal plane, the screw is entered with a medial inclination angle of 0°, and the trajectory is parallel to the S1 superior endplate (Fig. 11.14).
2. Method for pedicle screw placement: The screw is entered with a medial inclination angle of 40° and in parallel to the S1 superior endplate (Fig. 11.15).

Method for lateral mass screw placement: The screw is entered with a medial inclination angle of 28–30° and in parallel to the S1 superior endplate (Fig. 11.15).

11.6 Entry Depth of Sacral Pedicle Screws

In general, S1 pedicle screw is entered 30–40 mm, and S2 pedicle screw is entered 30 mm.

Fig. 11.4 The posterior view of the sacrum

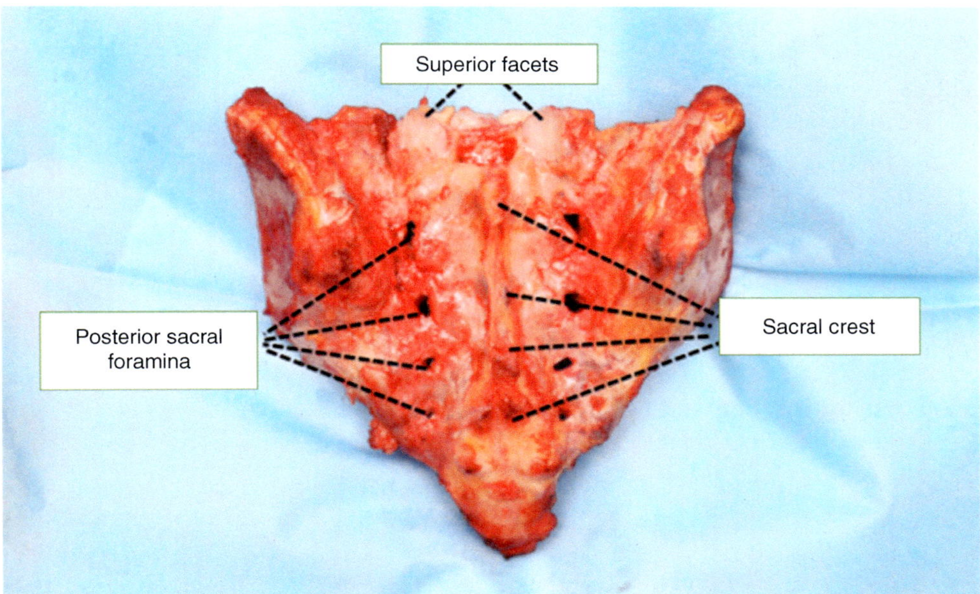

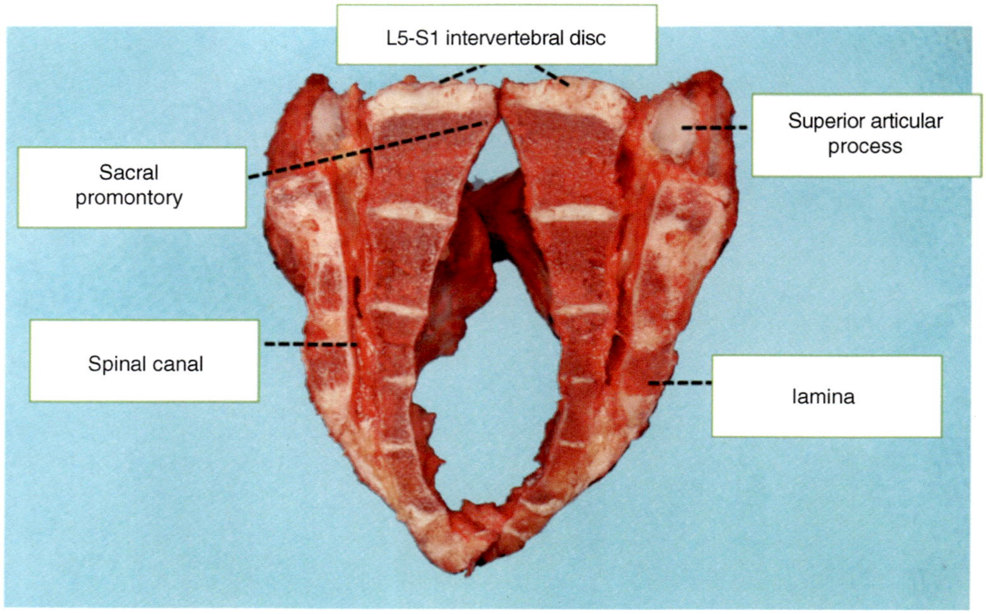

Fig. 11.5 The sectional view of the sacrum

11.7 Selection of Diameters of Sacral Pedicle Screws

The most commonly used screw diameters are 6.5–7.0 mm, and the diameter of S1 and S2 is kept identical (Fig. 11.16).

11.8 Surgical Procedures

For surgical steps and cautions, refer to the section on lumbar pedicle screw techniques

11.9 Imaging Features of Standard Sacral Pedicle Screws (Figs. 11.17, 11.18, 11.19, 11.20, 11.21, and 11.22)

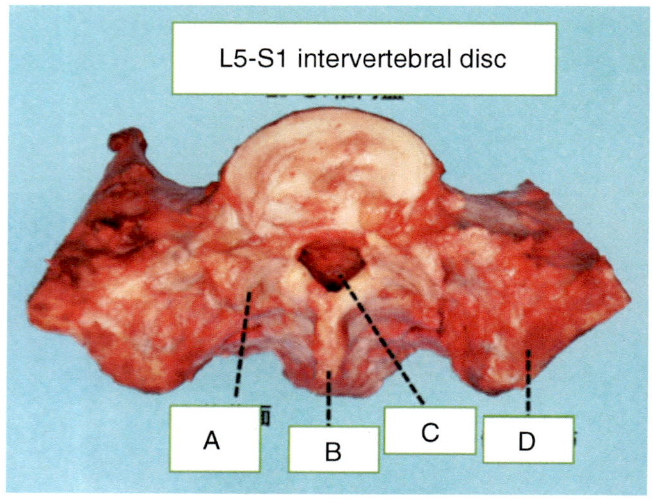

Fig. 11.6 The superior view of the sacrum. (**a**) Superior articular process; (**b**) Sacral crest; (**c**) Spinal canal; (**d**) Sacroiliac joint

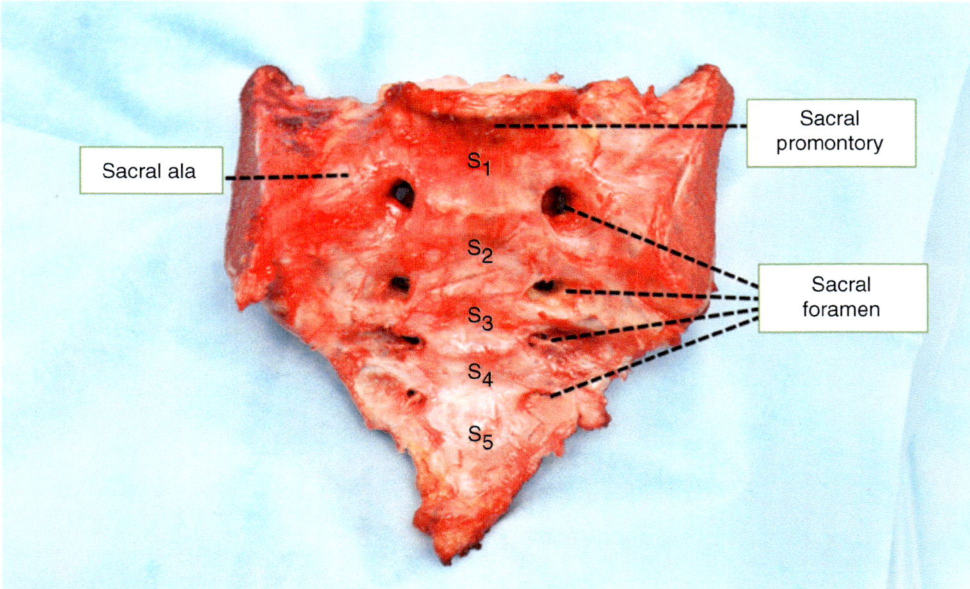

Fig. 11.7 The superior view of the anterior sacrum

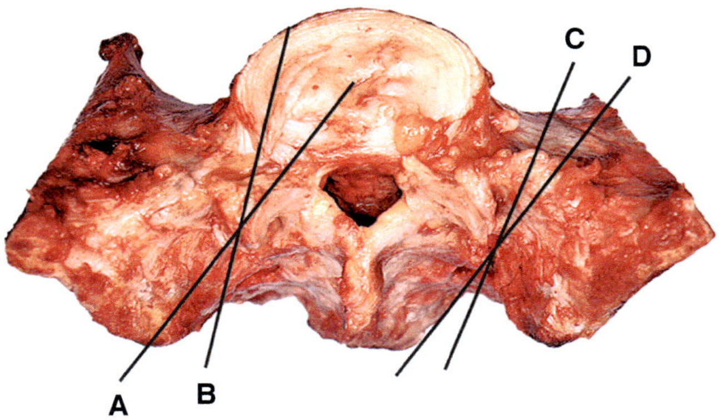

Fig. 11.9 Horizontal section of sacrum illustrated the four angles. The entry angle to the sacral sagittal plane of line A is 30.34° medially; the entry angle to the sacral sagittal plane of line B is 7.65° medially; the entry angle to the sacral sagittal plane of line C is 30.17° laterally; the entry angle to the sacral sagittal plane of line D is 48.67° laterally [3]

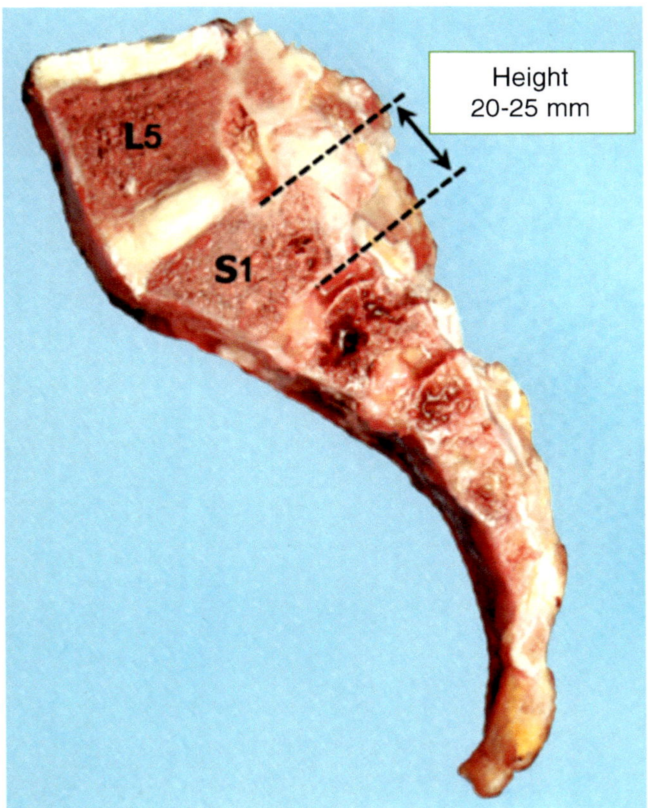

Fig. 11.8 Pedicle height

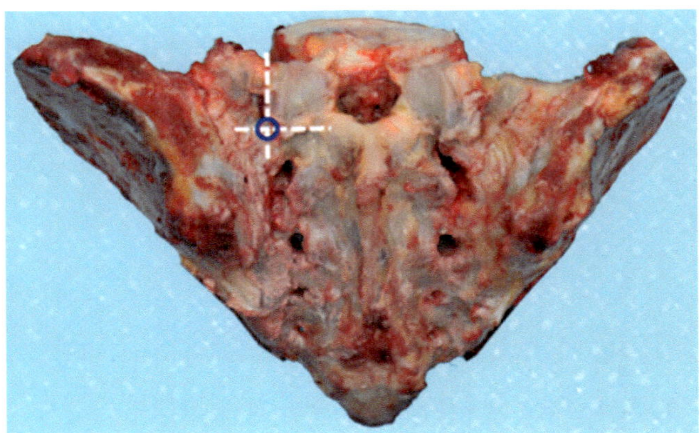

Fig. 11.10 S1 screw entry point

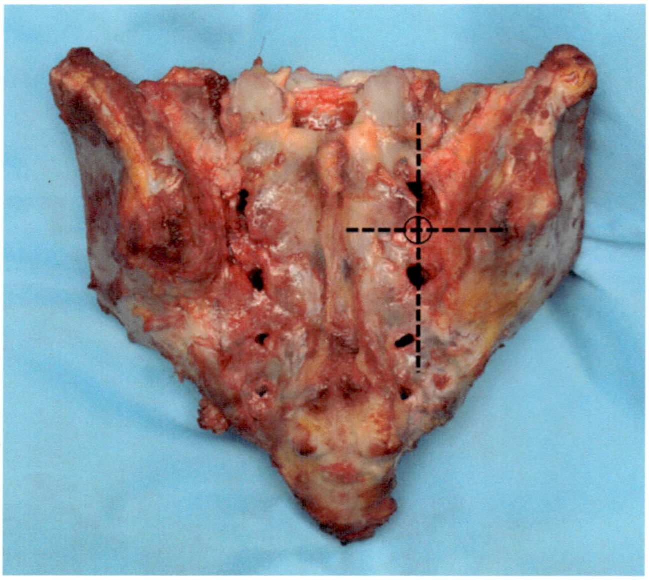

Fig. 11.11 S2 screw entry point

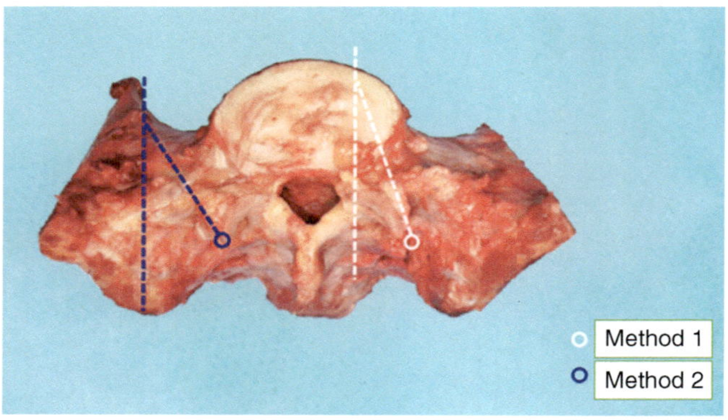

Fig. 11.12 The coronal view of S1 screw entry angle

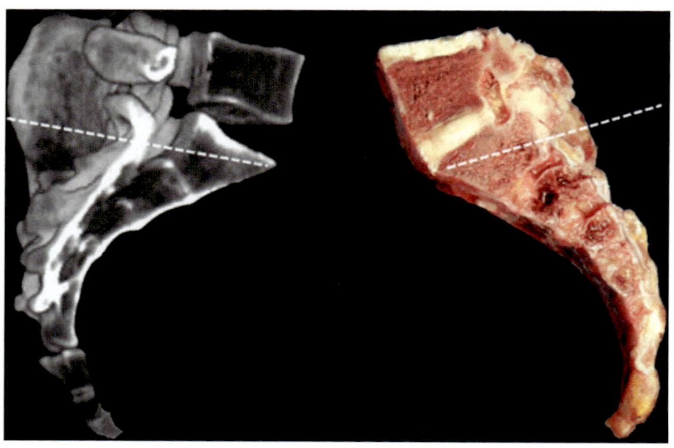

Fig. 11.13 The sagittal view of S1 screw entry angle

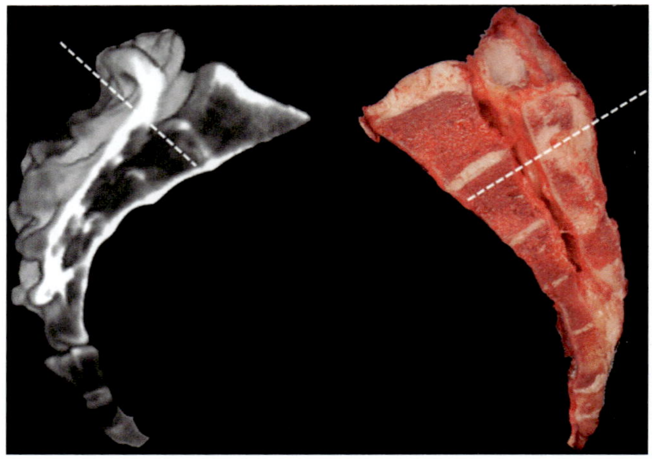

Fig. 11.14 The sagittal view of S2 screw entry angle. Left: 3D CT reconstruction; Right: anatomic section

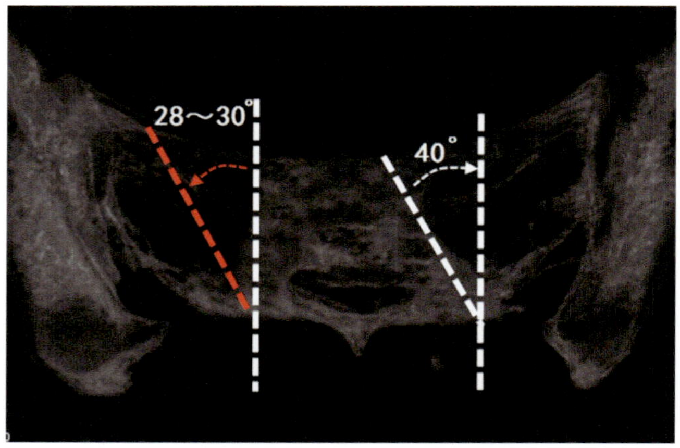

Fig. 11.15 The coronal view of S2 screw entry angle

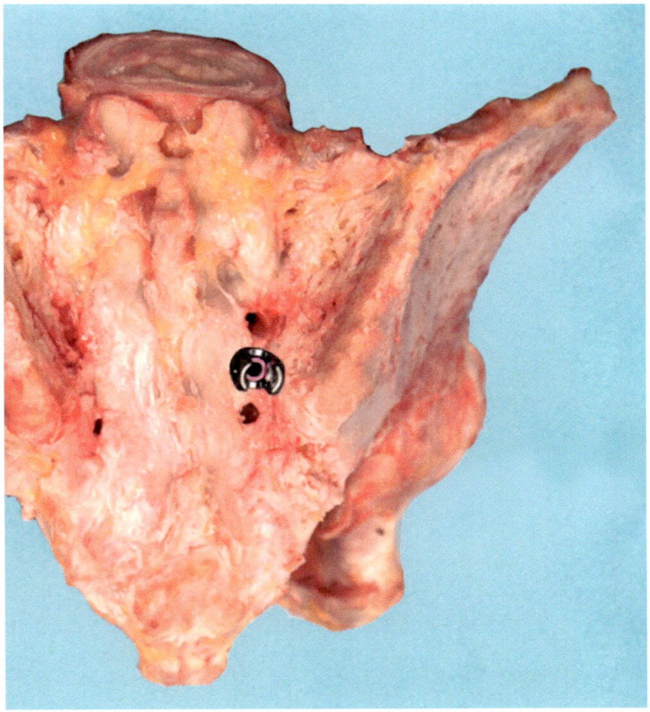

Fig. 11.16 S2 screw

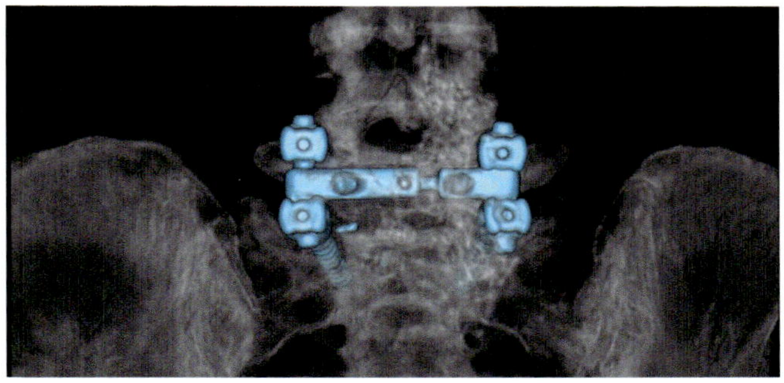

Fig. 11.17 The posterior view of L5–S1 screw fixation

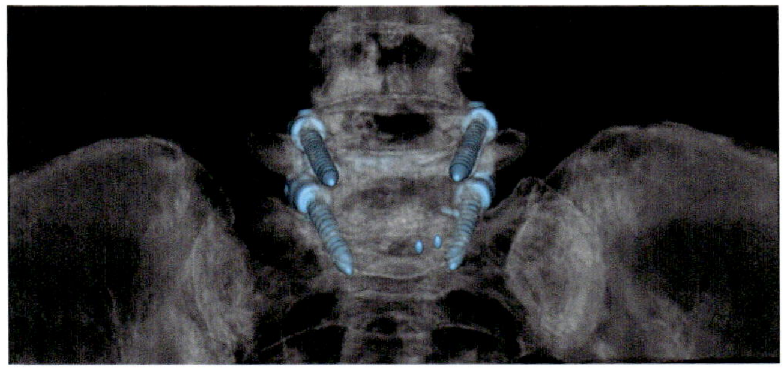

Fig. 11.18 The anterior view of L5–S1 screw fixation

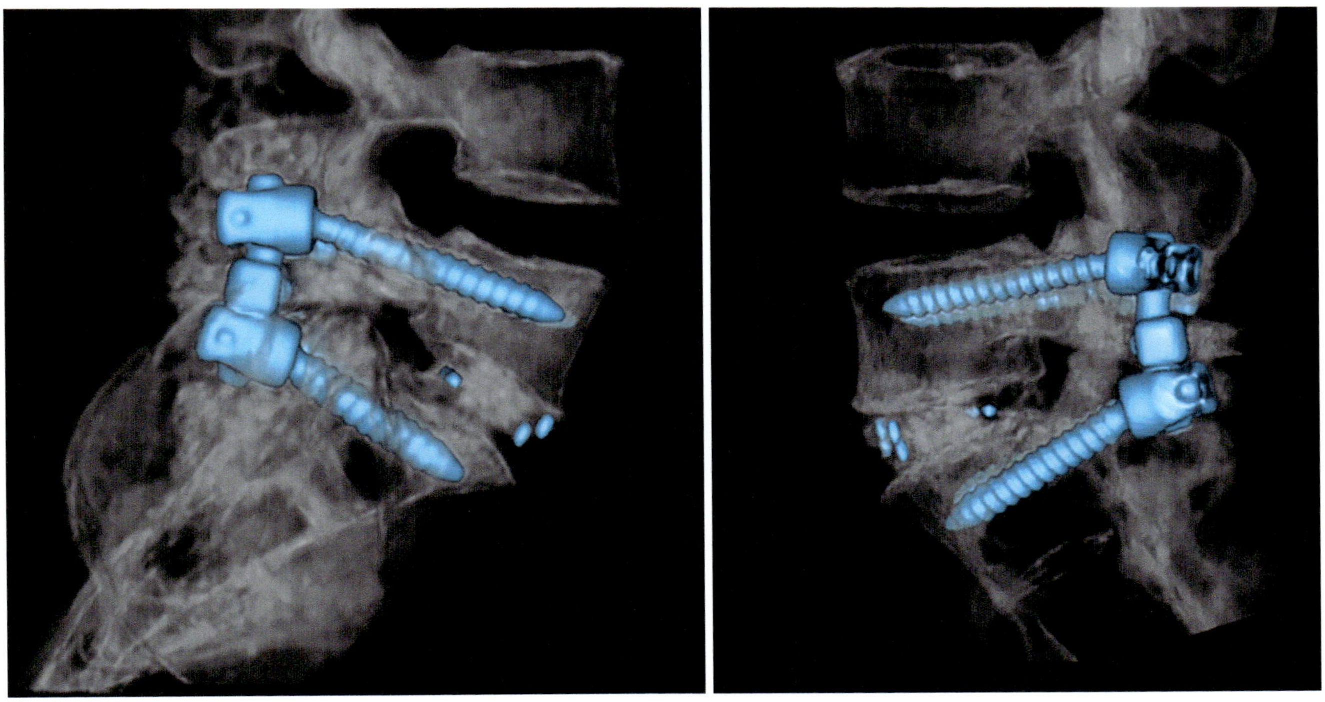

Fig. 11.19 The lateral view of L5–S1 screw fixation. Left: the lateral view of the sacral pedicle screw; Right: the lateral view of the sacral pedicle screw

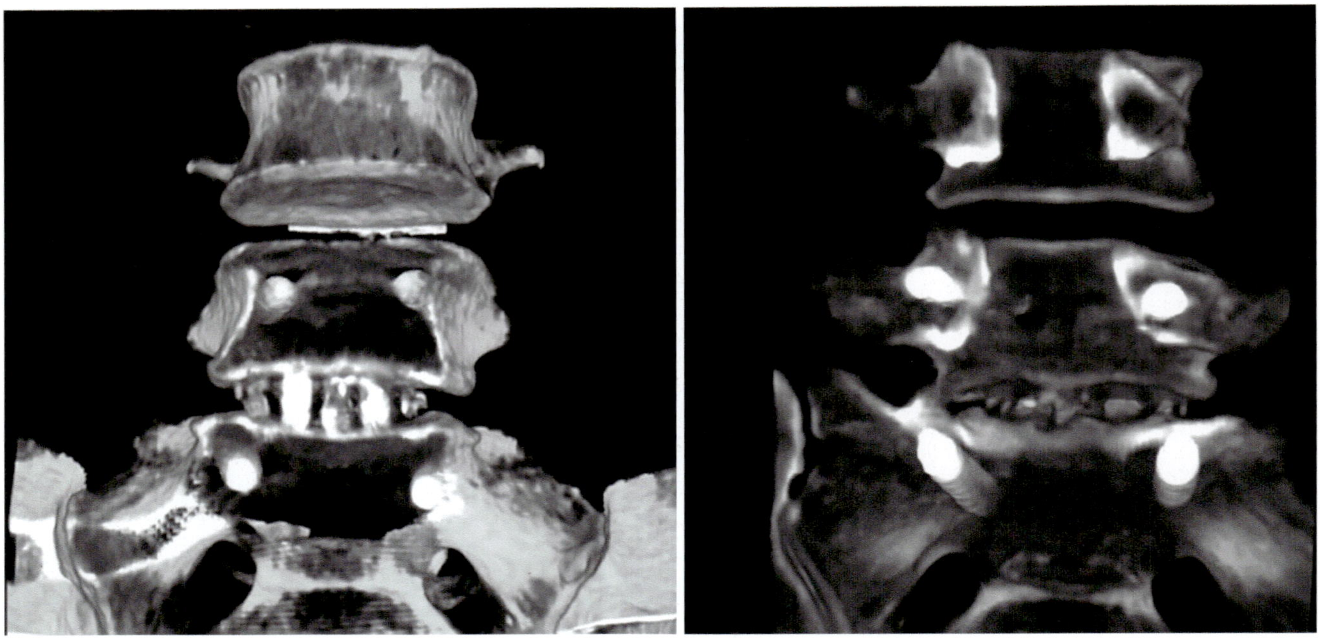

Fig. 11.20 L5–S1 screw fixation. Left: the anterior part of the vertebral body; Right: the posterior element

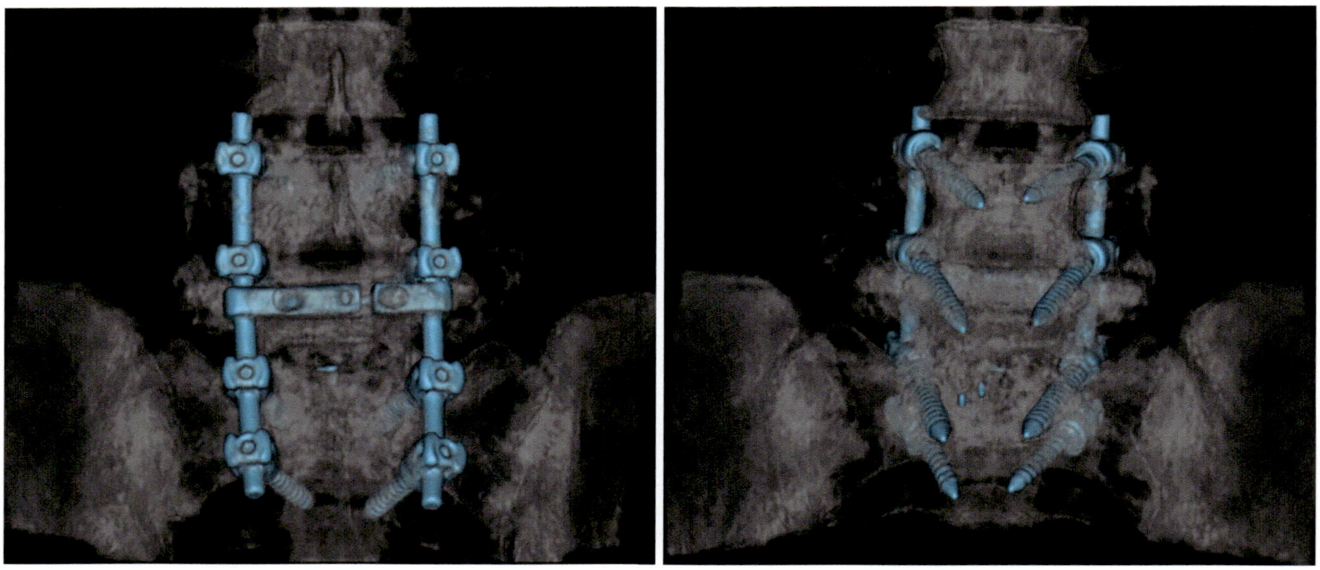

Fig. 11.21 L4–S2 screw fixation. Left: the posterior view; Right: the anterior view

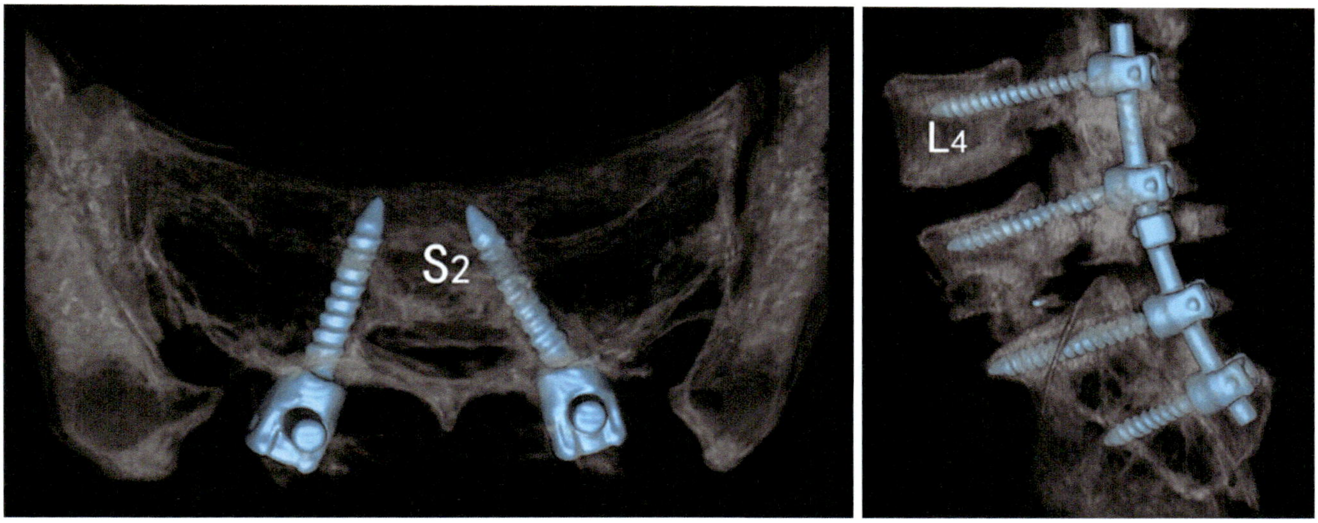

Fig. 11.22 L4–S2 screw fixation. Left: the axial view of the S2 pedicle screw; Right: the lateral view of the S1 and S2 pedicle screw

References

1. Roy-Camille R, Saillant G, Mazel C. Internal fixation of the lumbar spine with pedicle screw plating. Clin Orthop Relat Res. 1986;203:7–17.
2. Carlson GD, et al. Screw fixation in the human sacrum. An in vitro study of the biomechanics of fixation. Spine (Phila Pa 1976). 1992;17(6 Suppl):S196–203.
3. Morse BJ, Ebraheim NA, Jackson WT. Preoperative CT determination of angles for sacral screw placement. Spine (Phila Pa 1976). 1994;19(5):604–7.
4. Kubaszewski L, Nowakowski A, Kaczmarczyk J. Evidence-based support for S1 transpedicular screw entry point modification. J Orthop Surg Res. 2014;9:22.

Surgical Techniques for Thoracolumbar Anterior Internal Fixation

12

Pengchong Cao, Yabo Yan, and Wei Lei

Abstract

When a bone lesion is confined to the anterior column, the integrity of the posterior column should not be compromised; therefore, anterior internal fixation is an essential procedure in spine surgery. Thoracolumbar anterior internal fixation is used to reconstruct the anterior column after debridement of the anterior lesion, fracture reduction, and osteoporotic thoracolumbar vertebral collapse. In this chapter, the characteristics, clinical indications and contraindications, and surgical technique of the VANTAGE internal fixation system are introduced in detail. The applications of these techniques are further illustrated in representative clinical cases. Pearls and pitfalls of lumbar pedicle screw fixation are summarized at the end of this chapter.

Keywords

Thoracolumbar spine · Anterior internal fixation · Surgical technique

12.1 Thoracolumbar Anterior Internal Fixation Techniques: A Historical Perspective

Thoracolumbar anterior internal fixation techniques have evolved relatively recently, and mature anterior fixation instruments did not appear until the 1980s. The development milestones are summarized as follows:

P. Cao
Orthopedic Trauma Department of Tibet Military Region General Hospital, Tibet, China

Y. Yan · W. Lei (✉)
Department of Orthopedics, Xijing Hospital, Air Force Medical University, Xi'an, Shaanxi, China
e-mail: leiwei@fmmu.edu.cn

Hodgson and Stock first reported drainage of tuberculous abscess via a thoracolumbar anterior approach [1].

In 1953, Wenger et al. were instrumental in carrying out to correct scoliosis via an anterior approach. The fixation method involves the use of screws and connected steel wire or threaded rod in the lateral vertebral body.

Bohlman et al. were the first to carry out anterior instrumentation for thoracolumbar fracture [2], mainly in patients with late pain and paralysis after fracture of the thoracolumbar spine. As the technique is evolving, various anterior internal fixation instruments have emerged one after another, including the prominent work by Dwyer, Newton, Hall, and Zielke and other investigators [3]. Representative among them are the internal fixation instruments by Dunn et al. [4], followed by the anterior fixation method by Kostuick-Harrington, which greatly impact on vertebral body distraction and bone graft techniques.

The anterior fixation system developed by Kanedat et al. in the 1980s is so far the most extensively used [5].

12.2 Indications and Contraindications

12.2.1 Indications

The procedures are indicated for thoracolumbar anterior fixation, preferably for T10–L4 fixation.

1. Trauma
   (1) Burst fracture with anterior vertebral canal compression
   (2) Correction of fracture malunion
2. Degenerative changes

   Thoracic and thoracolumbar disc herniation

W. Lei, Y. Yan (eds.), *Internal Fixation of the Spine*, https://doi.org/10.1007/978-981-16-1562-7_12

3. Tumors

Anterior fixation and reconstruction after resection of benign or malignant tumors of the vertebral body or metastatic cancer

4. Infectious diseases

Anterior fixation and reconstruction after debridement of tuberculous lesions in the vertebral body

5. Congenital diseases and deformities
   (1) Anterior correction of congenital spine deformities
   (2) Anterior correction of idiosyncratic spine deformities

12.2.2 Contraindications

1. Lumbosacral fixation in general
2. Lateral displacement and fracture of the locked facet joint

12.3 Surgical Procedures (with the VANTAGE System)

12.3.1 Thoracolumbar Anterior Plate Fixation System: The Staple Method

12.3.1.1 Corpectomy

After the segments to be instrumented are determined, the associated vessels are dissected and ligated. Then, the fibrosus annulus is cut open, followed by the removal of the intervertebral disc. Corpectomy is performed in the diseased or compressed vertebral segments (Fig. 12.1) using the following steps:

(1) The rib head and pedicle are removed to expose the spinal canal.
(2) The intervertebral discs are then incised. In routine corpectomy, the cortex of the anterior and contralateral walls of the vertebral body is preserved.
(3) The vertebral bodies are removed with rongeurs, drills, and osteotomes.
(4) The spinal cord is decompressed with microsurgical curette.

The coronal diameter of the vertebral body above and below the corpectomized vertebral body is measured using a Depth/Screw Sizing Gauge to determine screw length. The screw length can also be determined by measuring the vertebral body width using the graduated scale on preoperative MRI/CT films.

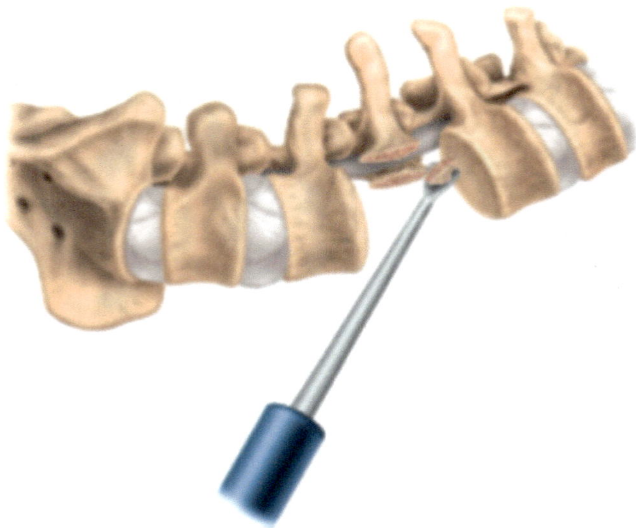

Fig. 12.1 Corpectomy

12.3.1.2 Staple Placement

The appropriate-sized staple is selected and positioned in place using the Staple Impactor Shaft (Fig. 12.2a). Staples, which are available in thoracic and lumbar sizes, are color-coded to indicate the orientation of the staples (dark green-caudal, light green-rostral, dark blue-caudal, and light blue-rostral). The staples are interchangeable and mirror images of each other. The largest staple that will fit within the confines of the vertebral body is used. The posterior margin of the staple should be as close to the posterior edge of the vertebral body as possible (Fig. 12.2b). Then, the staple is impacted in place using a mallet (Fig. 12.2c).

Slipping over the Staple Impactor Shaft, the drill guide is held firmly against the staple (Fig. 12.3a). The staple should be flush against the vertebral body. If the staple is not flushed, the protruding bone should be removed with a burr. With the drill guide over the staple, the drill or awl will create a trajectory for the posterior screw that is 10° anteriorly. Using the guide for the anterior position, it will create a pilot hole 10° posteriorly. The screws will converge at 20° (Fig. 12.3b). The drill guide is removed after creating both pilot holes. Until the staple is secured with the screws, it is held in place with the Staple Impactor. The screws are self-tapping. However, 4.5-mm and 5.5-mm taps are included in the surgical set (Fig. 12.3c) if tapping is preferred.

12.3.1.3 Screw Placement

The screws are then driven into the vertebral body until the head of each screw tightens against the staple (Fig. 12.4a). To ensure bicortical fixation, each screw should extend approximately 1 to 2 millimeters beyond the far cortex. The

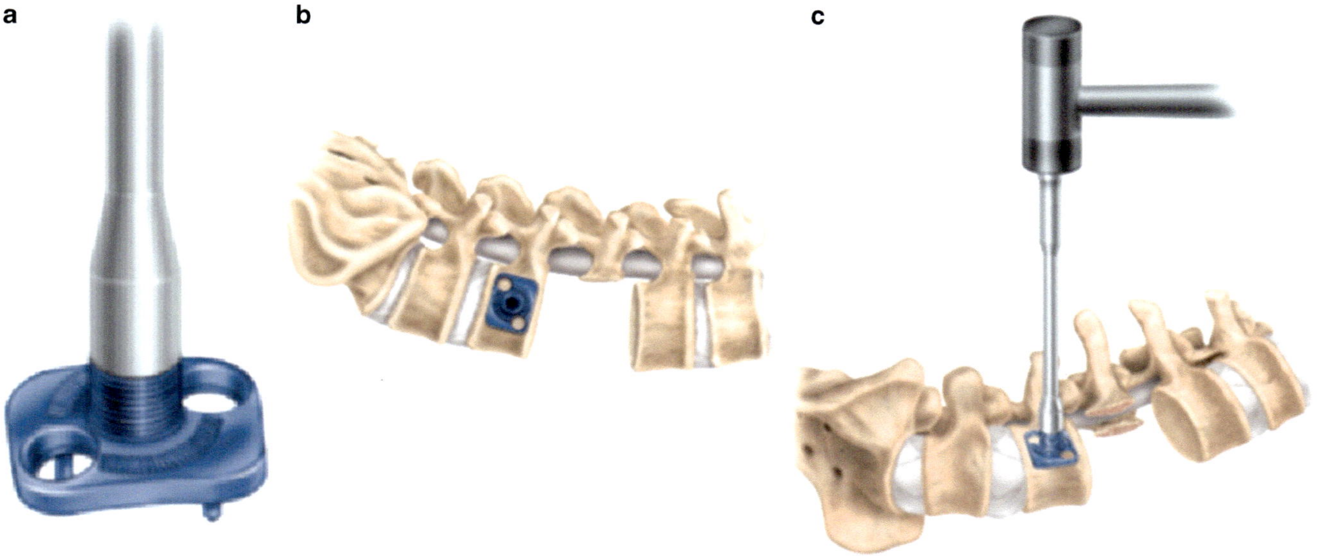

Fig. 12.2 Staple placement. (**a**) Connecting the staple. (**b**) Placing the staple. (**c**) The staple is impacted in place using a mallet

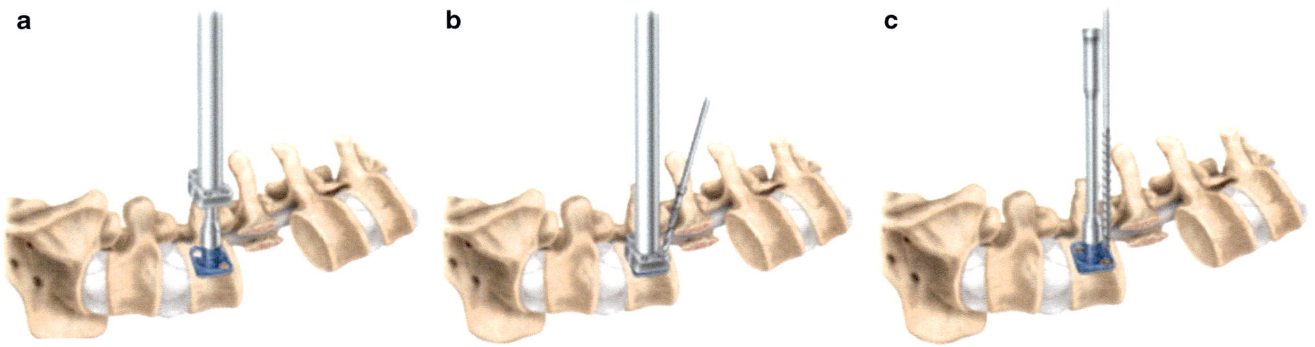

Fig. 12.3 Staple placement. (**a**) The drill guide is slipped over the Staple Impactor Shaft. (**b**) A hole is drilled. (**c**) After both pilot holes are created, the drill guide is removed

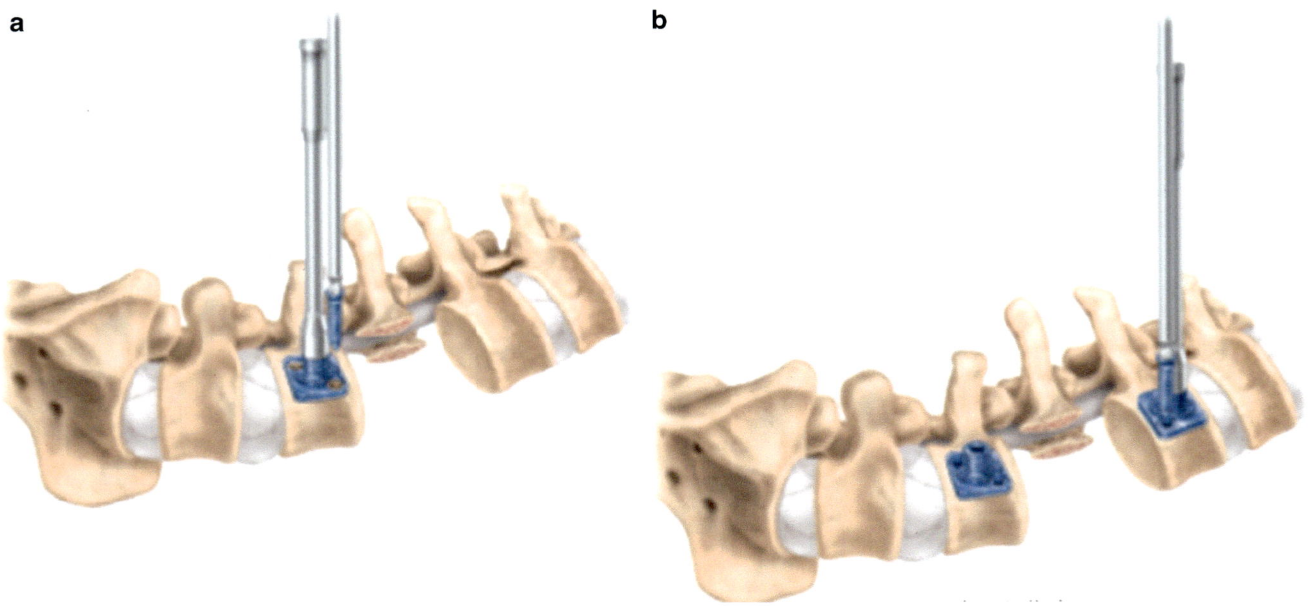

Fig. 12.4 Screw placement. The caudal staple is fixed (**a**) followed by fixation of the rostral staple (**b**)

staple/screw insertion process is repeated for the next staple (Fig. 12.4b).

12.3.1.4 Reduction, Graft Length Measurement, and Placement

The Quick Load Distractor may be used for simple or minimal reduction. The arm rings are loaded over the staple posts of the rostral and caudal staples (Fig. 12.5a). A distractive force is placed against the heads until the desired reduction is achieved. Then, the Measuring Caliper may be used to determine the required graft length (Fig. 12.5b). Distraction is released after careful selection, measurement, and placement of the graft into the corpectomy site. The ratchet lever is depressed on the Distractor until the graft comes into full contact with the superior and inferior endplates, and then the Distractor is removed from the surgical site (Fig. 12.5c).

12.3.1.5 Reduction Methods

The Modular Reduction Distractor should be used for more complex reduction. After the Modular Distractor Barrels are threaded onto the staple posts (Fig. 12.6a), the Modular Distractor Rack is applied onto the barrels, and the Quick Connect Ratcheting Handle is attached (Fig. 12.6b). Lordosis is restored by applying torque to the handles. Wing nuts are used to lock this position in place. Distraction and anterior/posterior rotation are applied using the butterfly nut until satisfactory reduction is achieved. Finally, the graft is placed as previously described.

12.3.1.6 Plate Measurement and Placement

Plate measurement can be taken from the scale located on the Modular Reduction Distractor. The Caliper can also be used for plate measurement. The plate size is measured from the center of the rostral staple post to the center of the caudal staple post, which will determine the appropriate length of the plate needed.

The Staple Impactor Shafts can be reattached to facilitate plate placement. This will allow the plate to be guided in place. The appropriate-sized plate is placed over the post of the staples with the slotted portion of the plate oriented superiorly (Fig. 12.7a). The shortest length plate should be chosen to minimize superior disc impingement and allow appropriate compression (Fig. 12.7b).

12.3.1.7 Loading the Nut

The Counter Torque Wrench is placed inside the T-Limiting Nut Driver, and the nut is then loaded onto the Counter Torque Wrench (Fig. 12.8a). The T-Limiting Nut Driver is used to start the nut on the fixed (caudal) end of the plate (Fig. 12.8b). The nut should not be completely tightened against the plate. The process is repeated for the slot (rostral) end of the plate (Fig. 12.8c).

12.3.1.8 Compression/Final Tightening

When osteoporosis is present, compression is optional and should be used with caution. If compression is deemed appropriate, the Parallel Compressor foot is loaded into one of the plate holes, and the other Compressor foot is loaded around the T-Limiting Nut Driver (Fig. 12.9a). The Compressor foot is compressed to the desired position, and final tightening is applied to the rostral nut. Then, the caudal nut is tightened (Fig. 12.9b). The T-Limiting Nut Driver is a limiting torque wrench driver that will click when it achieves 90 in./lb. The recommended torque should not be exceeded.

12.3.1.9 Closure/Postoperative Management

The construct is checked radiographically upon completion of instrumentation (Fig. 12.10). Closure is accomplished by first placing a chest tube and drain. The diaphragm is repaired using a running suture and stay sutures. As in the chest wall, muscles are closed in a layered fashion. A rigid brace is recommended for 8 weeks.

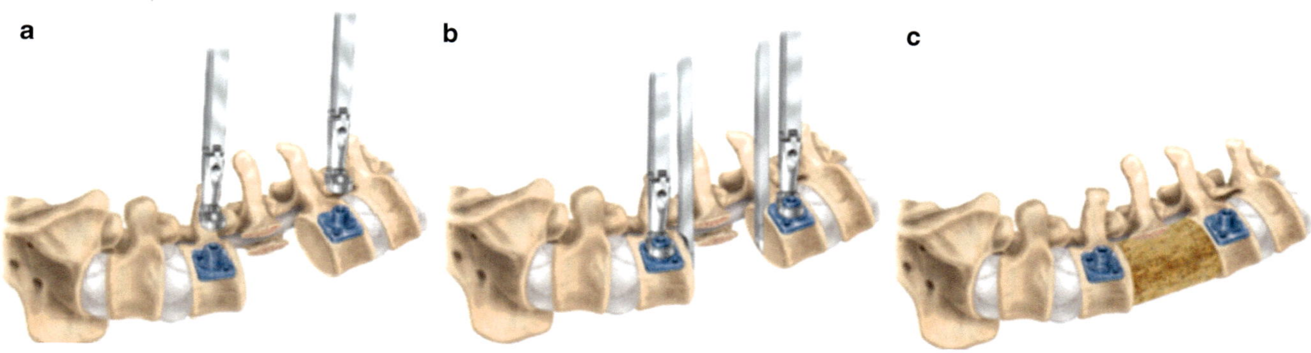

Fig. 12.5 Reduction, graft length measurement, and placement. (**a**) The distractor is connected. (**b**) The required graft length is measured. (**c**) The graft is implanted

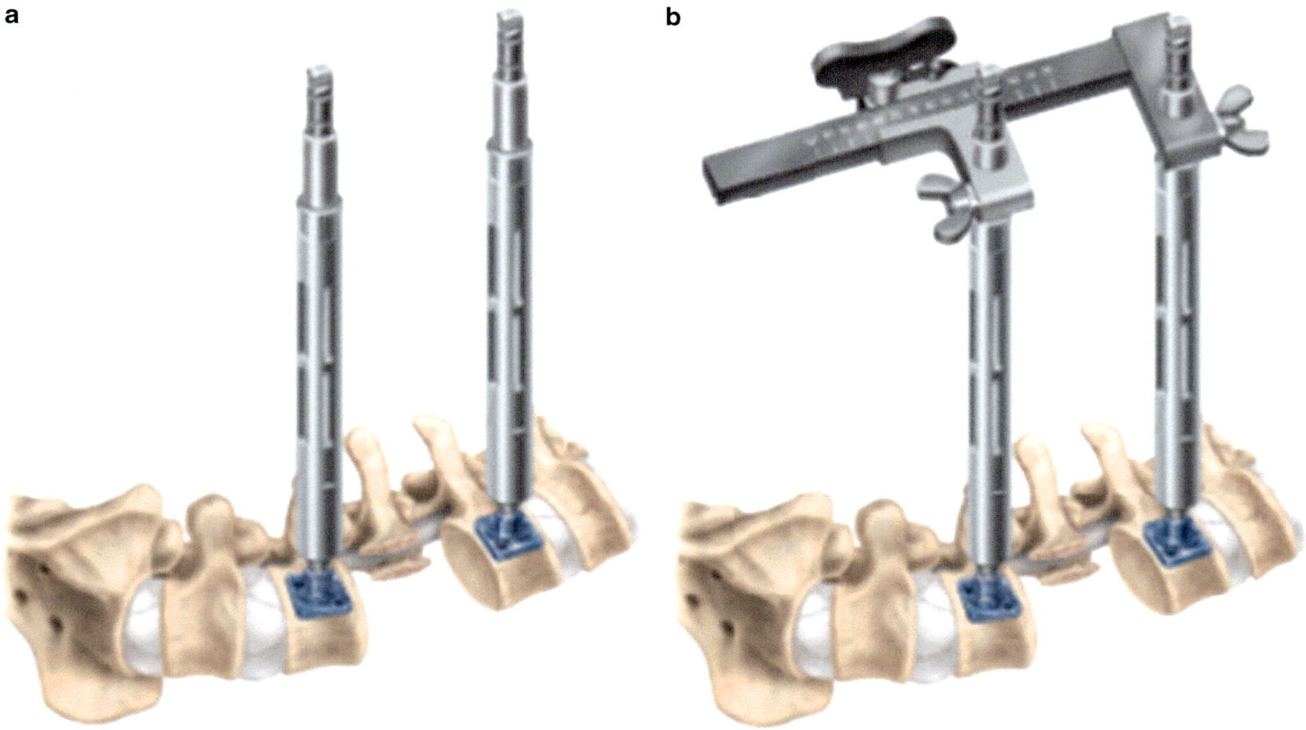

Fig. 12.6 Reduction. (**a**) The Modular Distractor Barrels are threaded onto the staple posts. (**b**) The Modular Distractor Rack is applied onto the barrels, and the Quick Connect Ratcheting Handle is attached

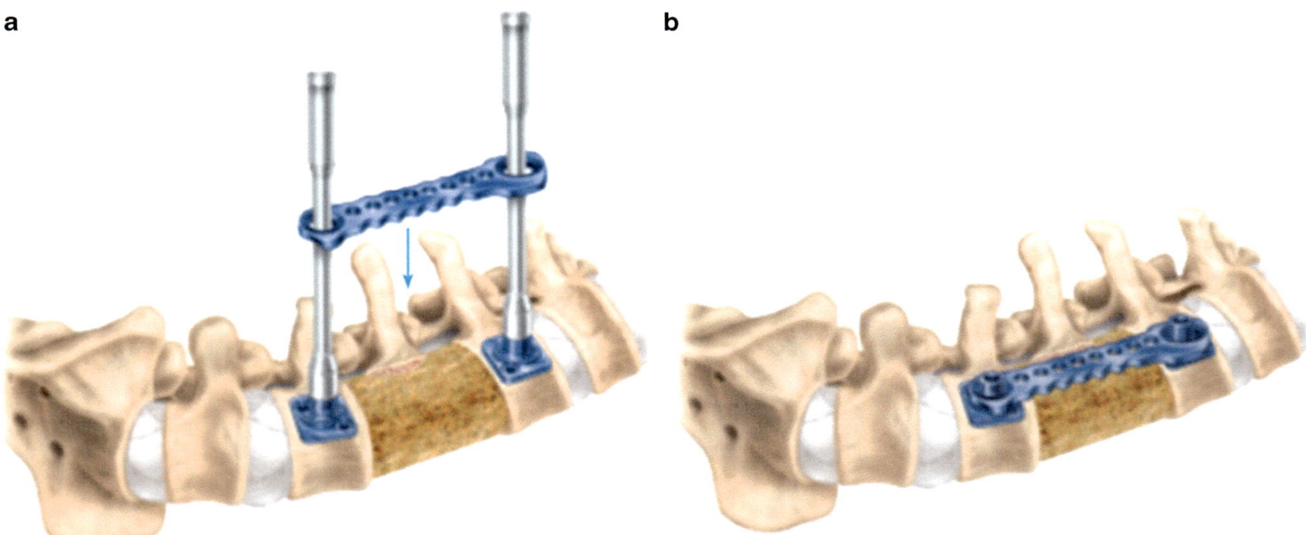

Fig. 12.7 Plate measurement and placement. (**a**) Plate placement. (**b**) The shafts are removed

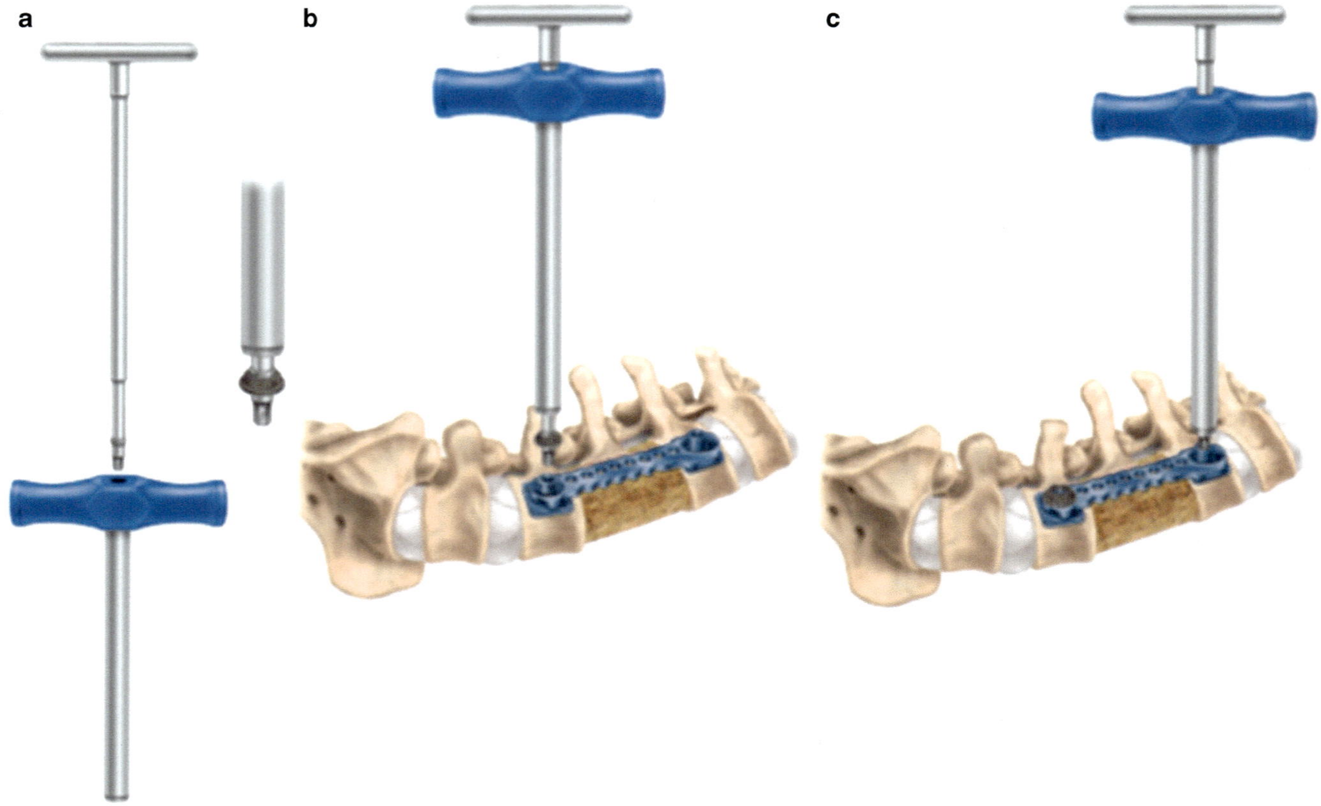

Fig. 12.8 Loading the nut. (**a**) The Counter Torque Wrench is placed. (**b**) The nut is loaded on the caudal end of the plate. (**c**) The nut on the rostral end of the plate is tightened

12.4 Thoracolumbar Anterior Plate Internal Fixation: The Single Bolt Option

12.4.1 Bolt Insertion

The bolt is positioned in a coronal plane with bicortical fixation. A pilot hole is created with an awl or drill and is tapped until its flared portion nests against the lateral surface of the vertebral body (Fig. 12.11). Then, the bolt is inserted in the center of the lateral surface of the vertebral body, which must be oriented to allow the plate to sit flush against the bone surfaces. When two bolts are used to fixate the distal ends of a corpectomy, their trajectory must be parallel.

12.4.2 Endoscopic Option

If desired, a Kirschner (K)-wire can be used to guide the bolt for endoscopic insertion. The K-wire is drilled into the vertebral body using a K-wire drill guide, whose trajectory and depth are monitored fluoroscopically. The K-wire is positioned in the intended bolt trajectory, and its proximal end must be anchored with a needle driver. The position of its tip is monitored by fluoroscopy in order to make sure it is not inadvertently advanced when the pilot hole is tapped and the bolt is inserted. The K-wire is removed after the bolt is inserted.

12.4.3 Reduction, Graft Length Measurement, and Placement

For simple or minimal reduction, the Quick Load Distractor may be used. The arm rings are loaded over the bolt posts (Fig. 12.12a). A distractive force is placed against the bolt posts until the desired reduction is achieved. Then, the Measuring Caliper may be used to determine the required graft length (Fig. 12.12b). Distraction is released after careful selection, measurement, and placement of the graft into the corpectomy site. The ratchet lever on the Distractor is depressed until the graft comes into full contact with the superior and inferior endplates. Then, the Distractor is removed from the surgical site (Fig. 12.12c).

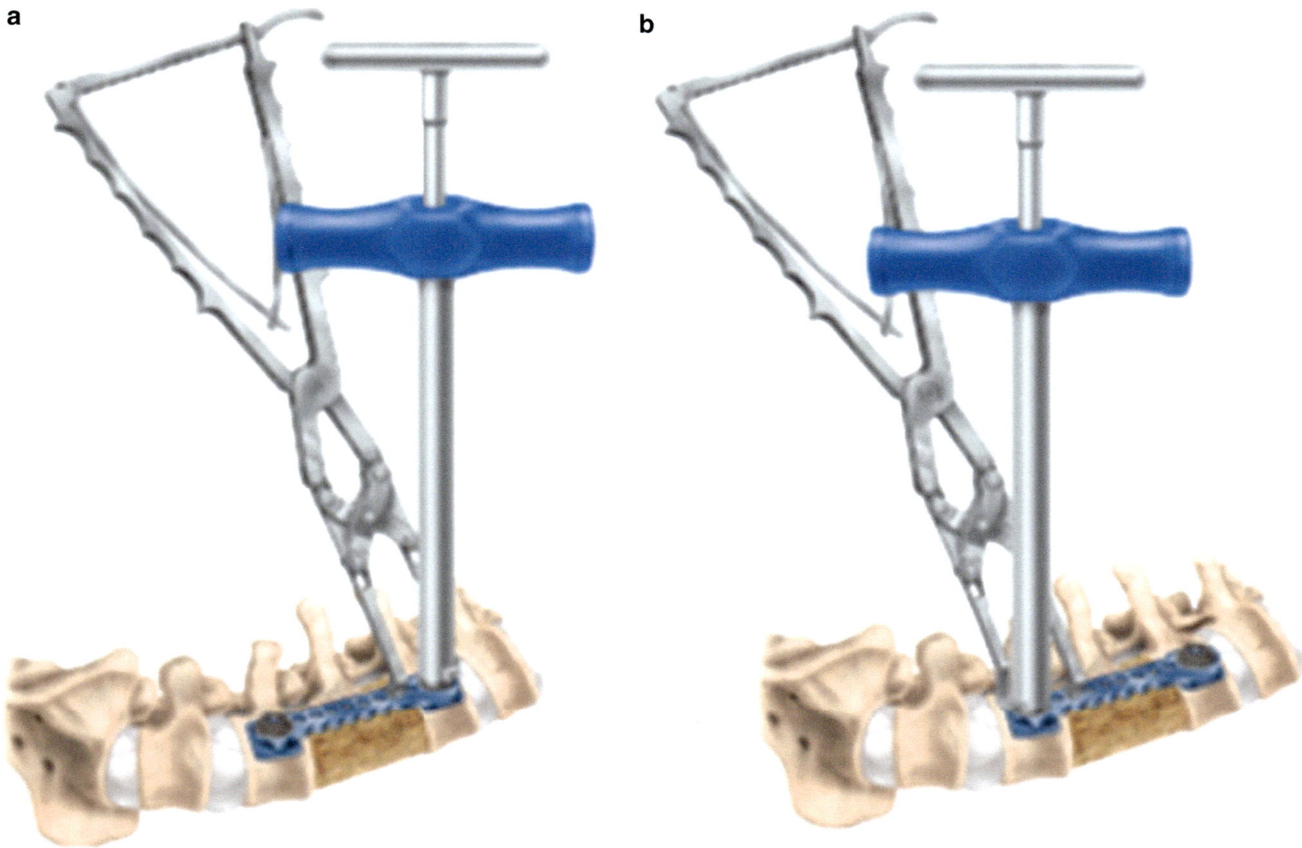

Fig. 12.9 Compression/final tightening. The Compressor foot is compressed to the desired position before final tightening of the rostral nut (**a**) and the caudal nut (**b**)

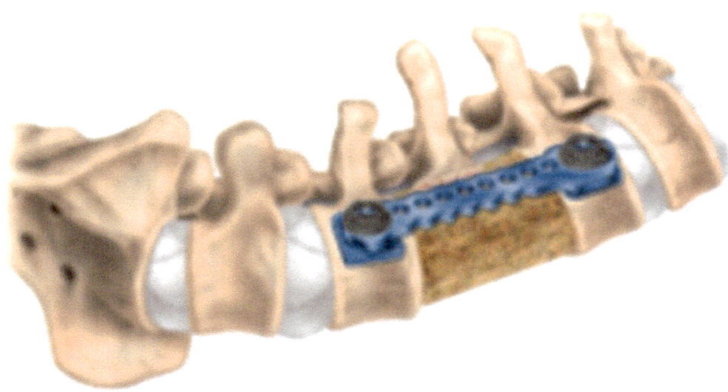

Fig. 12.10 Closure/postoperative management

12.4.4 Reduction Option

The Modular Reduction Distractor should be used for more complex reduction. The Modular Distractor Barrels are threaded onto the bolt posts (Fig. 12.13a). After the Modular Distractor Rack is applied onto the barrels (Fig. 12.13b) and the Quick Connect Ratcheting Handles are attached, torque is applied to the handles to restore lordosis. This position is locked in place using the wing nuts. Distraction and anterior/posterior rotation are applied using the butterfly nut until satisfactory reduction is achieved. The graft is placed as previously described.

12.4.5 Plate Measurement and Placement

The plate can be measured from the scale located on the Distractor or using the Caliper. The plate size is measured from the center of the rostral bolt post to the center of the caudal bolts post. This will determine the appropriate length of the plate needed.

The Staple Impactor Shafts can be attached to the bolt posts to facilitate plate placement, which will allow the plate to be guided in place. The appropriate-sized plate is placed over the post of the bolts with the slotted portion of the plate oriented superiorly (Fig. 12.14a). The shortest length plate is chosen to minimize impingement of the superior disc and allow appropriate compression (Fig. 12.14b).

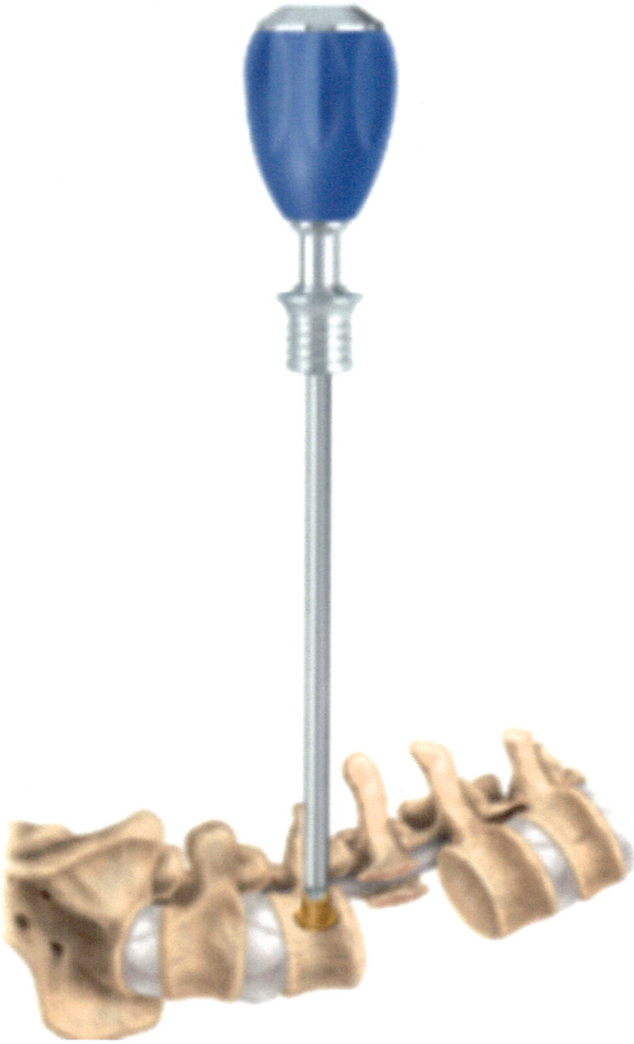

Fig. 12.11 Bolt insertion

12.4.6 Nut Placement

After the Counter Torque Wrench is placed inside the T-Limiting Nut Driver, the nut is loaded onto the Counter Torque Wrench (Fig. 12.15a). Then, the T-Limiting Nut Driver was used to start the nut on the fixed (caudal) end of the plate (Fig. 12.15b) and then the slot (rostral) end of the plate (Fig. 12.15c). The nut should not be completely tightened against the plate.

12.4.7 Compression/Final Tightening

Compression is optional, which should be used with caution in the presence of osteoporosis. If compression is deemed appropriate, the Parallel Compressor foot is loaded into one of the plate holes, and the other Compressor foot is loaded around the T-Limiting Nut Driver. The Compressor foot is compressed to the desired position before final tightening to the rostral nut (Fig. 12.16a) and the caudal nut (Fig. 12.16b). The T-Limiting Nut Driver is a limiting torque wrench driver that will click when it achieves 90 in./lb, and the recommended torque should not be exceeded.

12.4.8 Closure/Postoperative Care

The construct should be checked radiographically once instrumentation is complete (Fig. 12.17). Closure is accomplished by first placing a chest tube and drain. A running suture is used to repair the diaphragm and stay sutures. Same as that of the chest wall, muscles are closed in a layered fashion. A rigid brace is recommended for 8 weeks.

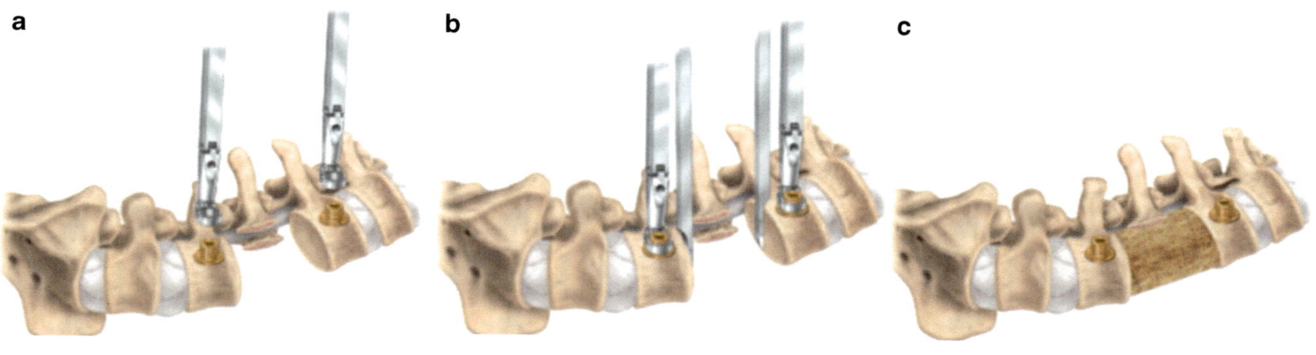

Fig. 12.12 Reduction, graft length measurement, and placement. (**a**) The Quick Load Distractor is connected. (**b**) The required graft length is determined. (**c**) The graft is placed

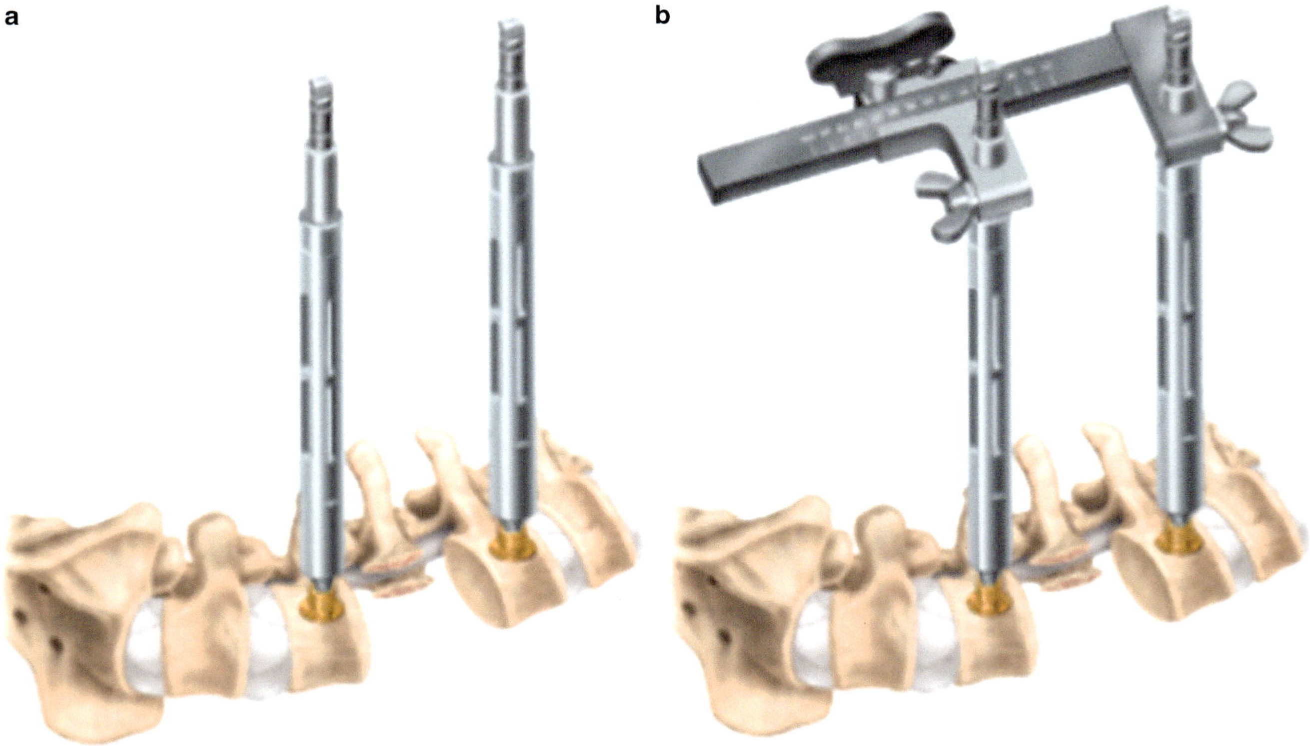

Fig. 12.13 Reduction. (**a**) The Modular Distractor Barrels are threaded into the bolt posts. (**b**) The Modular Reduction Distractor is then connected

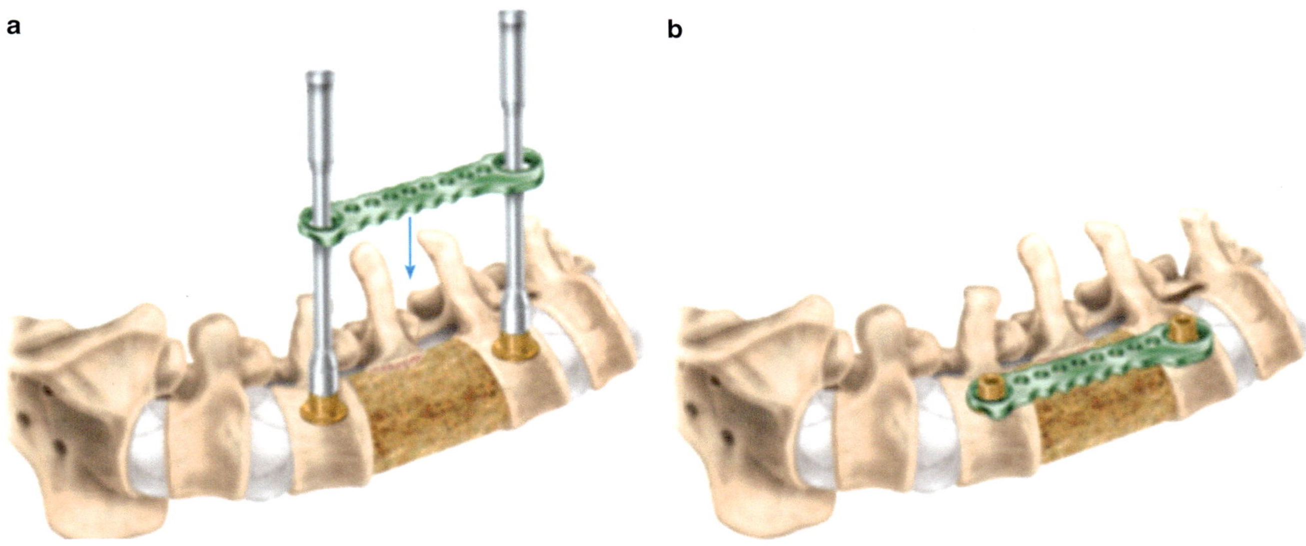

Fig. 12.14 Plate measurement and placement. (**a**) Plates are placed. (**b**) The Staple Impactor Shafts are removed

12.5 Clinical Cases

12.5.1 Case No. 1

Patient: A 27-year-old male complained of lumbar pain with bilateral lower limb sensorimotor impairment for 2 days after injury.

Diagnosis: T12 fracture with partial paralysis.

Surgery: Anterolateral spinal canal decompression and VANTAGE reduction and internal fixation.

Imaging data: Preoperative images are shown in Fig. 12.18, and postoperative images are shown in Fig. 12.19.

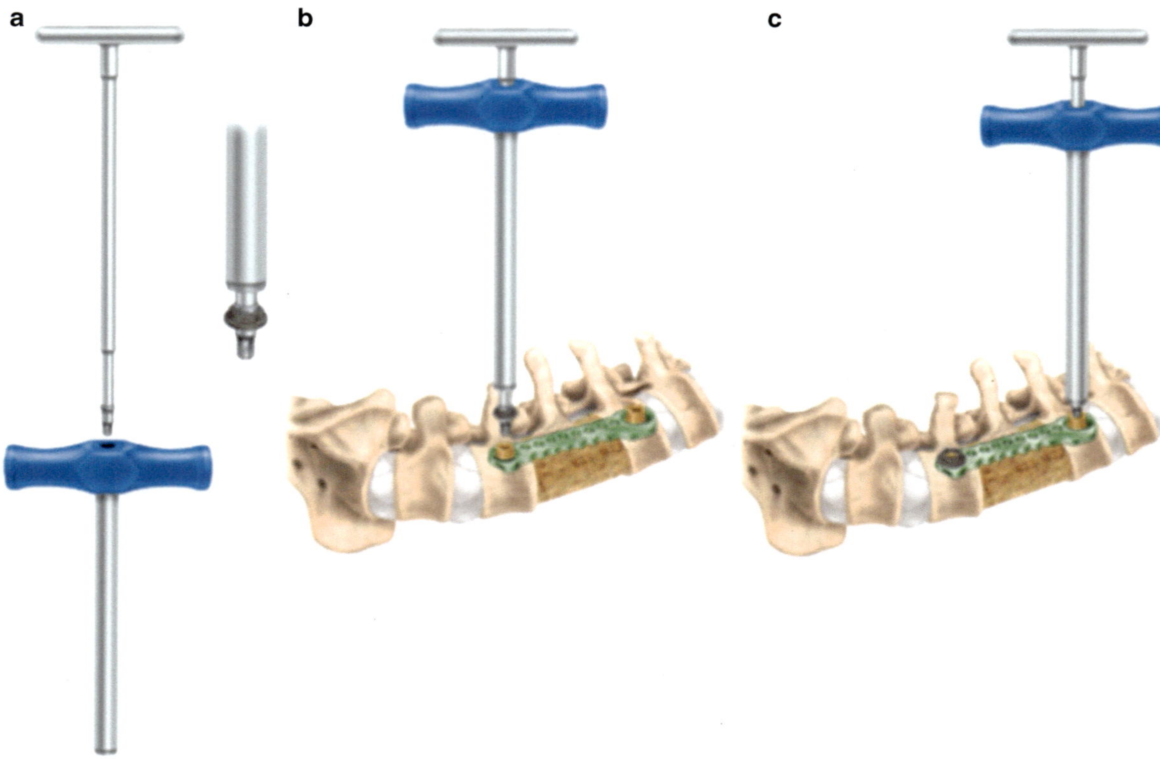

Fig. 12.15 Nut placement. (**a**) The Counter Torque Wrench is placed. The nut on the fixed (caudal) (**b**) and slot (rostral) end of the plate (**c**) is tightened

12.5.2 Case No. 2

Patient: A 38-year-old male complained of lumbar pain with bilateral lower limb sensorimotor impairment for 1 day after injury.

Diagnosis: L2 fracture with partial paralysis and lumbarization of the sacral vertebra.

Surgery: Anterolateral spinal canal decompression and CDH ANTARES reduction and internal fixation.

Imaging data: Preoperative images are shown in Fig. 12.20, an intraoperative image is shown in Fig. 12.21, and postoperative images are shown in Fig. 12.22.

12.6 Pearls and Pitfalls

1. Great caution should be exercised to avoid inadvertent injury to adjacent nerves and large vessels during the surgery.
2. Fixation should be done across the lesioned vertebral body, and screws should be placed in the vertebral body immediately above and below the diseased vertebral body even if parts of the diseased vertebral body appear normal grossly.
3. Screw insertion depth should be carefully measured to avoid injury to the contralateral structures due to excessively long screws.

12.7 Postoperative Care

Patients can start ambulation 1 week postoperatively. The support is worn for 8 weeks. In some patients, ambulation and activities depend on the condition of the patient and the surgical procedures.

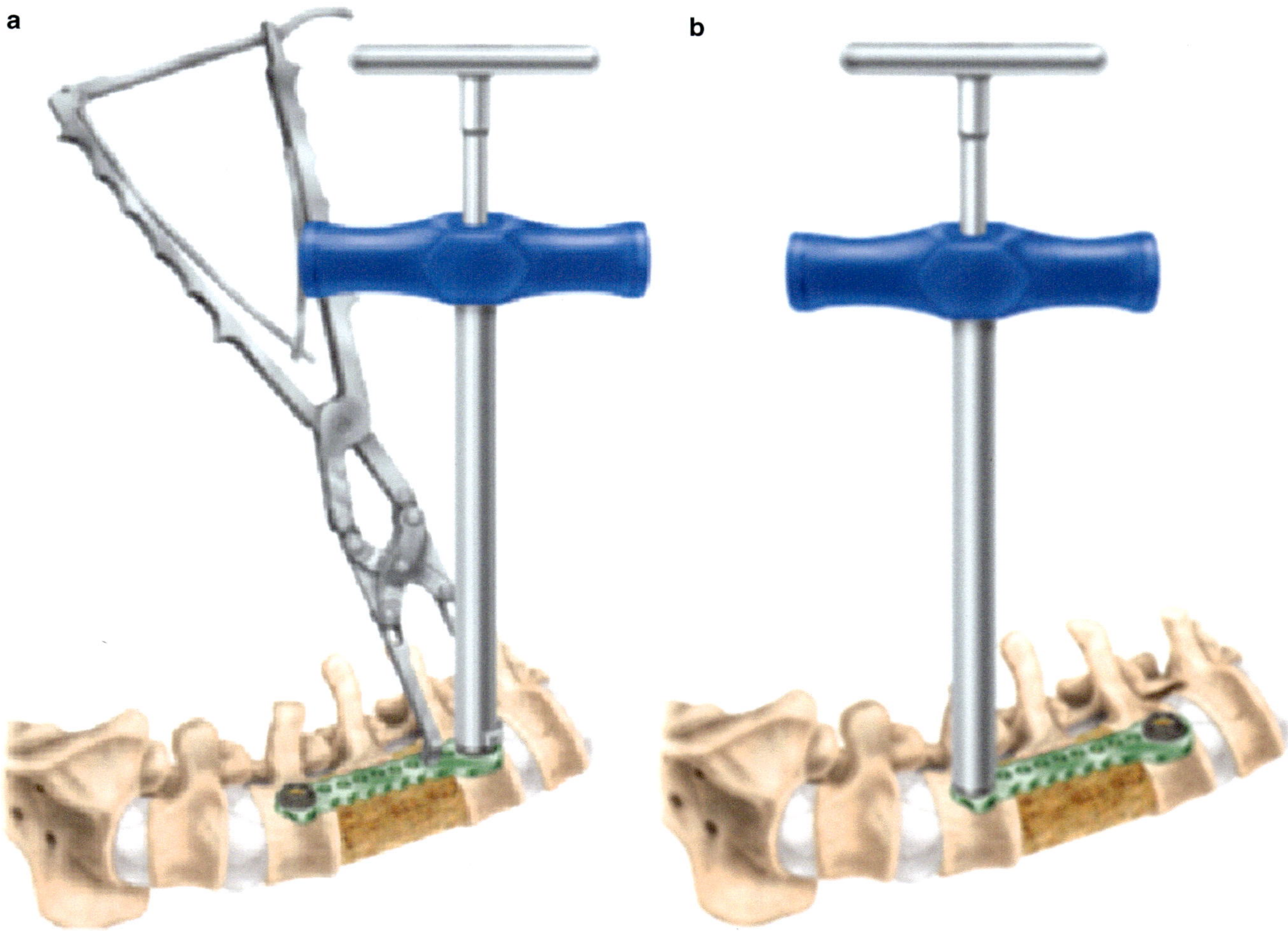

Fig. 12.16 Compression/final tightening. The Compressor foot is compressed to the desired position, and final tightening is applied to the rostral nut (**a**) and the caudal nut (**b**)

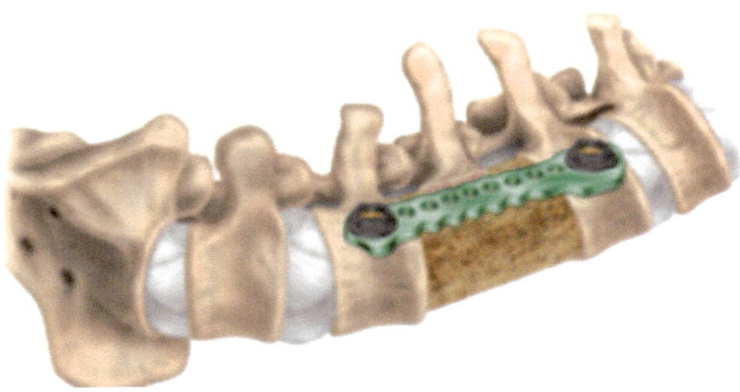

Fig. 12.17 Completion of placement

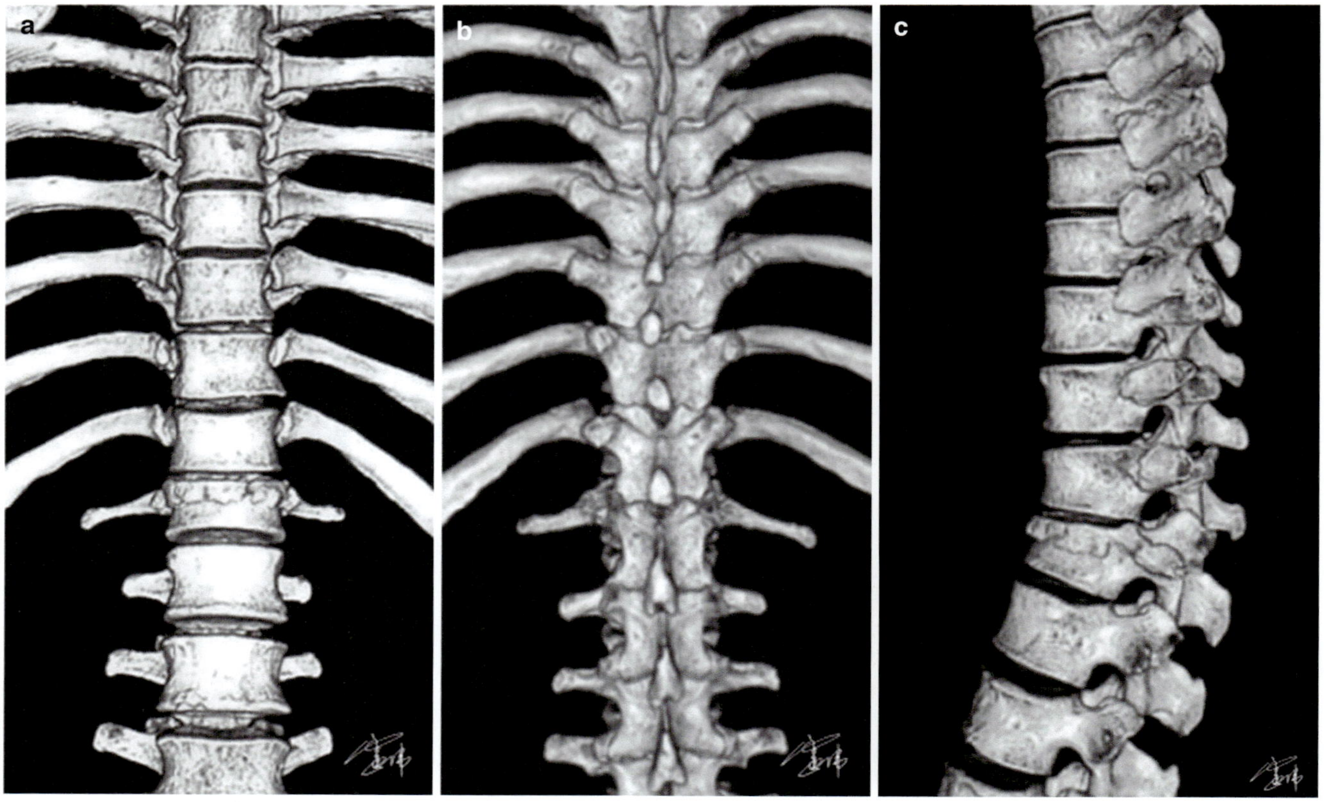

Fig. 12.18 Preoperative images. (**a**) CT 3D reconstruction (anterior view). (**b**) CT 3D reconstruction (posterior view). (**c**) CT 3D reconstruction (lateral view)

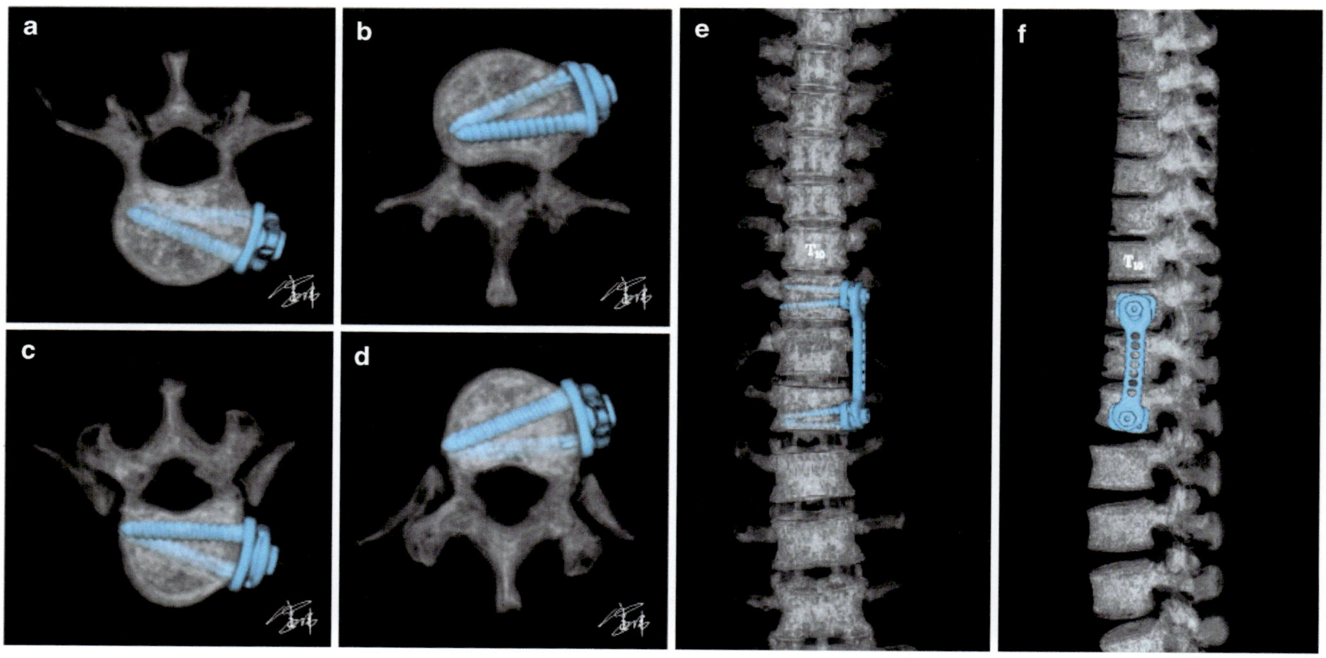

Fig. 12.19 Postoperative images. (**a**) L1 screw (superior view). (**b**) L1 screw (inferior view). (**c**) T11 screw (superior view). (**d**) T11 screw (inferior view). (**e**) CT 3D reconstruction (anterior view). (**f**) CT 3D reconstruction (lateral view)

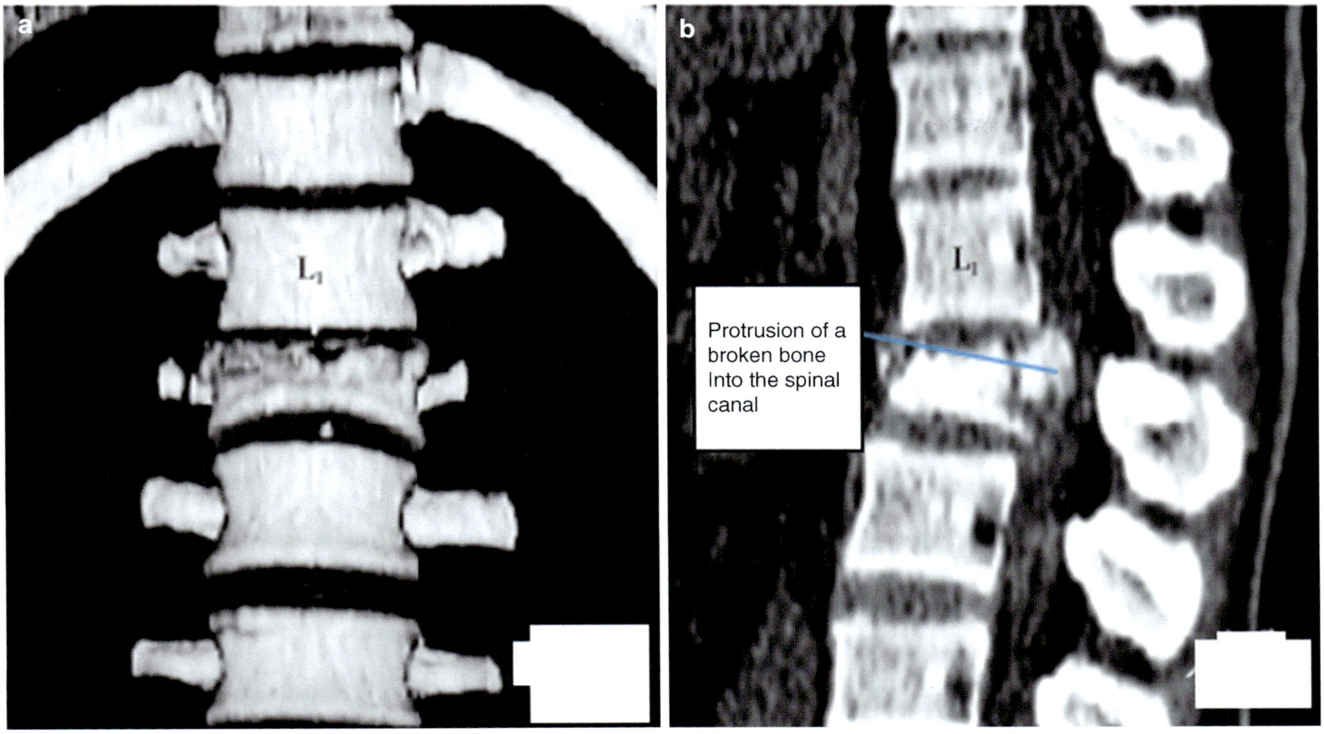

Fig. 12.20 Preoperative images. (**a**) CT 3D reconstruction (anteroposterior view). (**b**) CT 3D reconstruction (sagittal view)

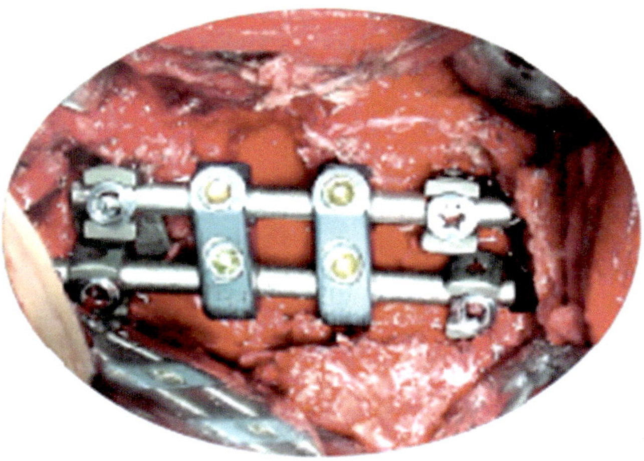

Fig. 12.21 Intraoperative image

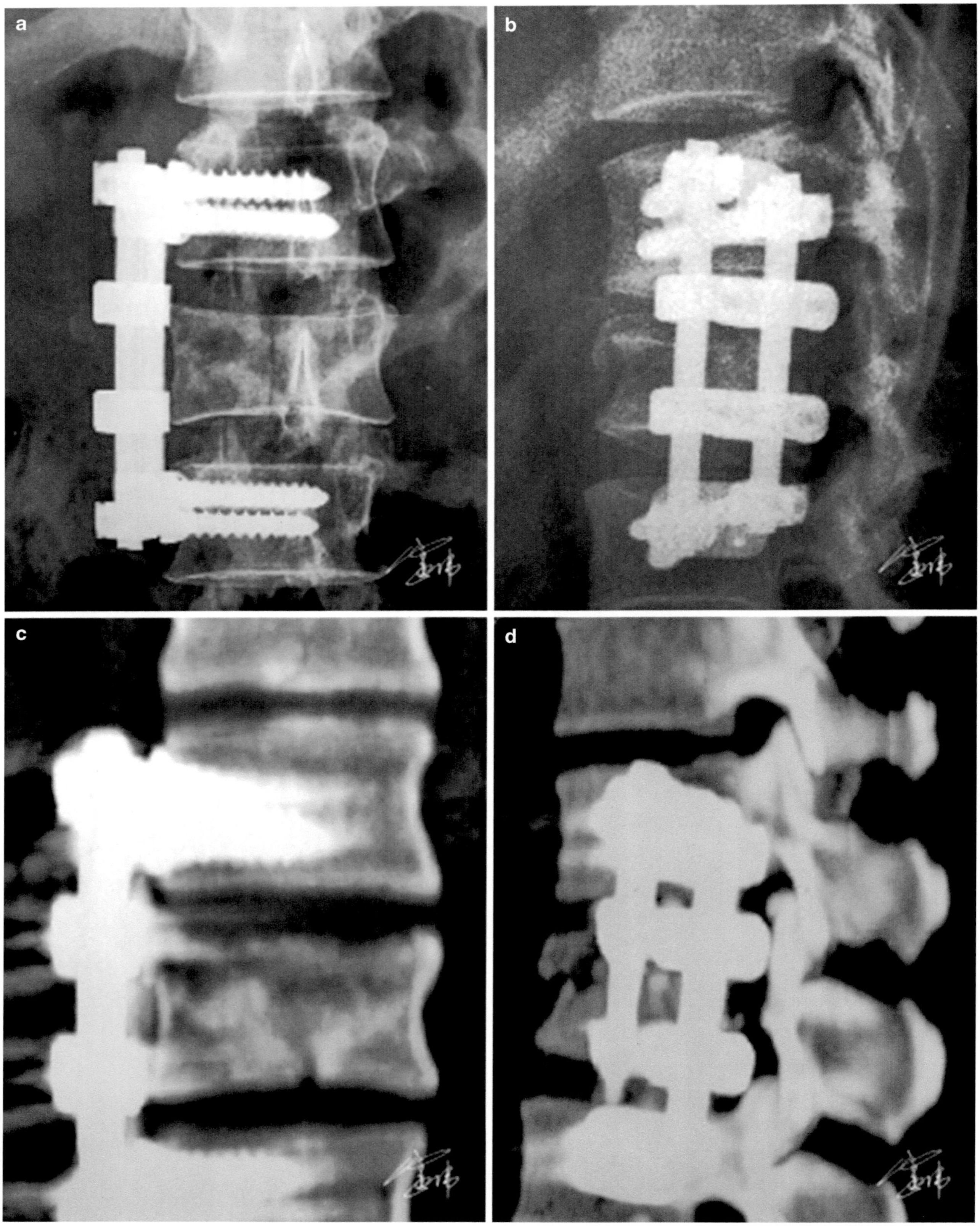

Fig. 12.22 Postoperative images. (**a**) CT 3D reconstruction (anteroposterior view). (**b**) CT 3D reconstruction (lateral view). (**c**) CT 3D reconstruction (coronal view). (**d**) CT 3D reconstruction (sagittal view)

References

1. Hodgson AR, Stock FE. Anterior spinal fusion a preliminary communication on the radical treatment of Pott's disease and Pott's paraplegia. Br J Surg. 1956 Nov;44(185):266–75.
2. Bohlman HH, Kirkpatrick JS, Delamarter RB, Leventhal M. Anterior decompression for late pain and paralysis after fractures of the thoracolumbar spine. Clin Orthop Relat Res. 1994 Mar;300:24–9.
3. Ghanayem AJ, Zdeblick TA. Anterior instrumentation in the management of thoracolumbar burst fractures. Clin Orthop Relat Res. 1997;335:89–100.
4. Dunn HK. Anterior stabilization of thoracolumbar injuries. Clin Orthop Relat Res. 1984;189:116–24.
5. Kaneda K, Taneichi H, Abumi K. Anterior decompression and stabilization with the kaneda device for thoracolumbar burst fractures associated with neurological deficits. J Bone Joint Surg. 1997;79(1):69–83.

13 Spine Minimally Invasive Internal Fixation Techniques and Their Applications

Zixiang Wu and Wei Lei

Abstract

Because of minimal invasion and the fast recovery, the spine minimally invasive internal fixation techniques are increasingly popular globally. There are various kinds of minimally invasive internal fixation instrumentation developed by many spine surgeons. In this chapter, we thoroughly reviewed the spine minimally invasive internal fixation procedure. Anatomic characters of the vertebral body, the entry point, entry angle, entry depth of sacral pedicle screw, and operational details were demonstrated to guarantee the proper position of screw. The characteristics, clinical indications and contraindications, and surgical technique of minimally invasive internal fixation techniques are introduced in details. The application of these techniques is presented in typical clinical cases.

Keywords

Minimally invasive internal fixation · Pedicle screw fixation · Surgical technique

In the history of spine surgery, with advancement of surgical concepts and internal fixation instruments, various minimally invasive internal fixation techniques have emerged. In 1977, Magerl [1] first proposed percutaneous pedicle screw fixation technique whose main purpose is to determine the safe distance for fixation before fusion surgery is undertaken. In 1982, on the basis of posterior lumbar interbody fusion (PLIF), Harms et al. [2] proposed the technique of transforaminal lumbar interbody fusion (TLIF). TLIF only disrupts the posterior structures of the lumbar spine unilaterally, and generally there is no intraoperative traction of the nerve roots. Because of these technical advantages, TLIF has rapidly gained popularity. In 1997, Foley and Smith [3] proposed a tubular distractor technique that solved the issue of minimally invasive surgery via a posterior approach and reduces traction and dissection of the paraspinal muscles by conventional posterior lumbar surgery. In 2001, Foley [3] put forward a brand new internal fixation system that allows percutaneous advancement of the curved rod over multi-axial screw and completed the first case of percutaneous fusion surgery (minimally invasive transforaminal lumbar interbody fusion, MIS TLIF) for fixation of the lumbar spine. Thereafter, percutaneous vertebra internal fixation techniques are widely applied in surgical treatment of thoracolumbar vertebra fractures, degeneration, and spinal tumors.

Spine minimally invasive internal fixation techniques mainly include thoracolumbar percutaneous pedicle screw internal fixation technique and direct or indirect vertebral canal decompression and fusion technique via various approaches, minimally invasive transforaminal lumbar interbody fusion technique (MIS TLIF), oblique lumbar interbody fusion (OLIF), direct lateral interbody fusion (DLIF), and anterior lumbar interbody fusion (ALIF).

The advantages of percutaneous spinal fixation techniques and various minimally invasive lumbar fusion surgeries include minimal invasiveness, less blood loss, low infection rate, mild postoperative pain, early ambulation, rapid recovery, no muscle stripping, reduced chronic pain in the spine due to multifidus muscle stripping, decreased muscle denervation, and disruption of blood supply, thus avoiding muscle atrophy [4].

This chapter mainly introduces thoracic percutaneous pedicle screw internal fixation technique (CD HORIZON SEXTANT II system and *LONGITUDE* system) and MIS TLIF.

Z. Wu · W. Lei (✉)
Department of Orthopedics, Xijing Hospital, Air Force Medical University, Xi'an, Shaanxi, China
e-mail: wuzixiang@fmmu.edu.cn; leiwei@fmmu.edu.cn

W. Lei, Y. Yan (eds.), *Internal Fixation of the Spine*, https://doi.org/10.1007/978-981-16-1562-7_13

13.1 Implants

The SEXTANT system family of percutaneous reduction products is the only percutaneous reduction system currently available. This system combines the LONGITUDE system and the SEXTANT II system for spondylolisthesis correction.

13.1.1 Multilevel Rod Inserter (Fig. 13.1)

13.1.2 Screw Retaining Sleeve (Fig. 13.2)

13.1.3 Screw Extenders (Fig. 13.3)

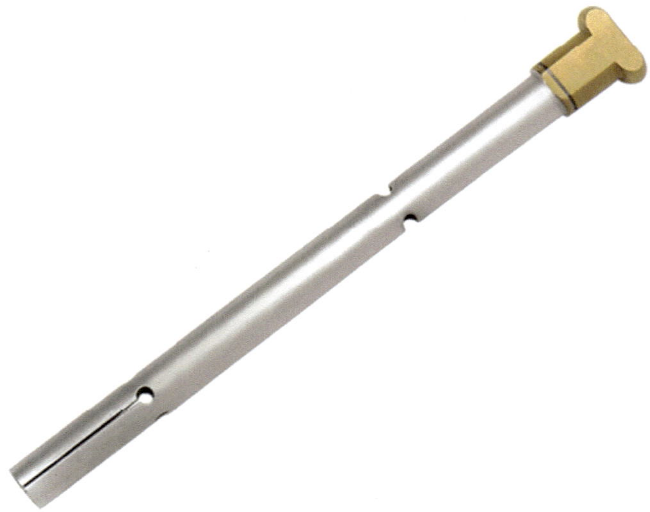

Fig. 13.2 Screw retaining sleeve

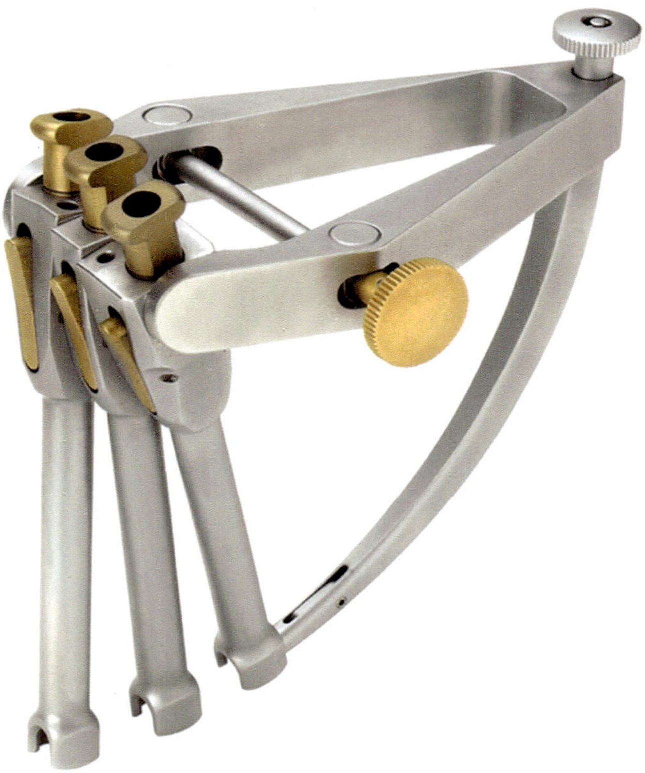

Fig. 13.1 Multilevel rod inserter

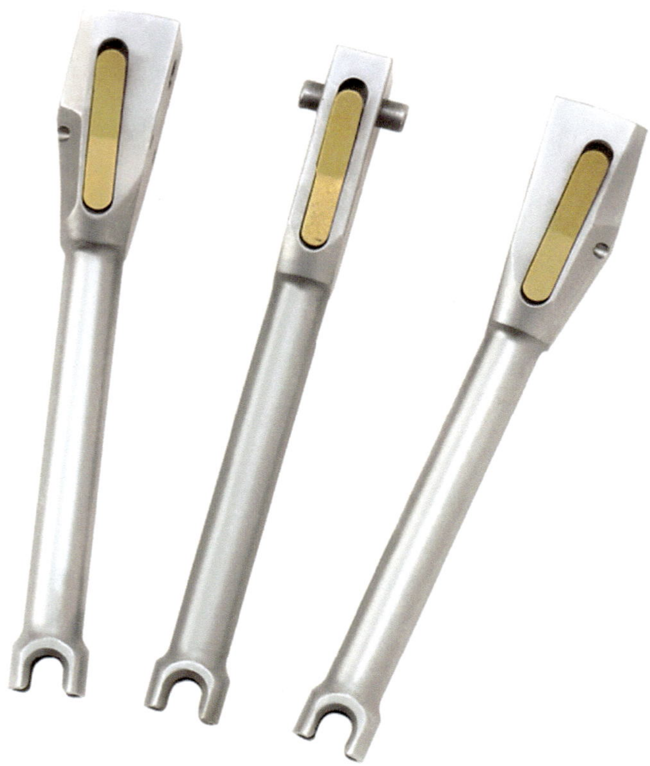

Fig. 13.3 Screw extenders

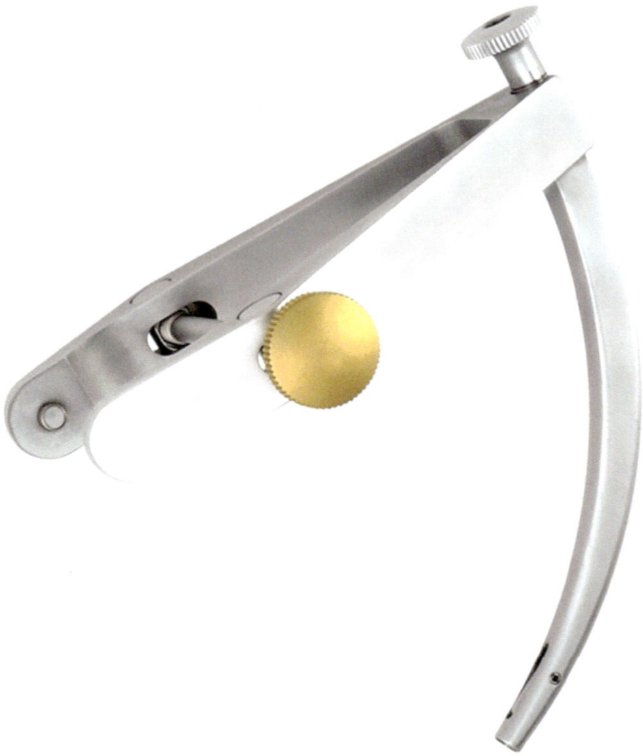

Fig. 13.4 The rod inserter arc arm

13.1.4 Rod Inserter Arc Arm (Fig. 13.4)

13.1.5 Multilevel Distractor Guide (Fig. 13.5)

13.1.6 Multilevel Stylet Guide (Fig. 13.6)

13.1.7 Rod Template (Fig. 13.7)

13.1.8 Rod Template Pointer (Fig. 13.8)

13.1.9 Multilevel Lucent Guide Clamp (Fig. 13.9)

13.1.10 Hollow Drill Bit (Fig. 13.10)

13.2 Features of the System

The arc arm is used to minimize puncture-induced bone-screw interface stress.

The reduction extender has a rod insertion window of 20 mm and is used to insert into the threaded inner sleeve.

The system can be used for spondylolisthesis reduction using a specific set of screws.

The LONGITUDE system and the SEXTANT II system are fully compatible.

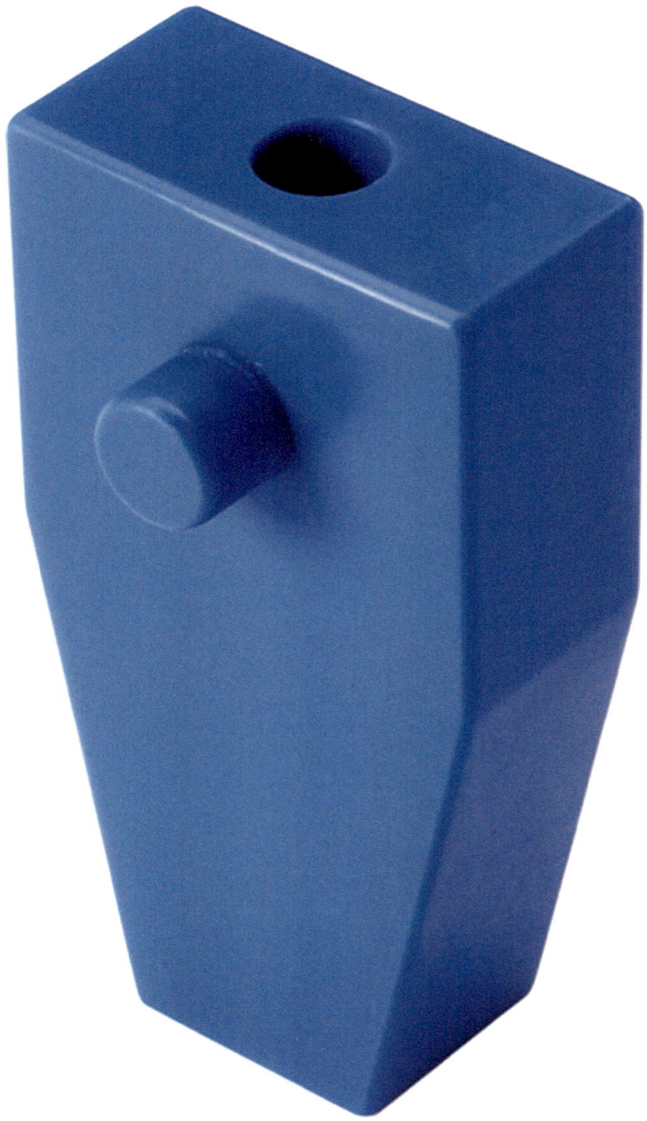

Fig. 13.5 Distractor guide

13.3 Clinical Indications and Contraindications

(1) Clinical Indications

- Fractures:

Single vertebra anterior column compression fracture; the height is compressed to less than 2/3, and the kyphotic angle is less than 30 degrees, and the vertebral canal sagittal diameter is reduced to less than 1/3.

No nervous system symptoms and no need for posterior decompression

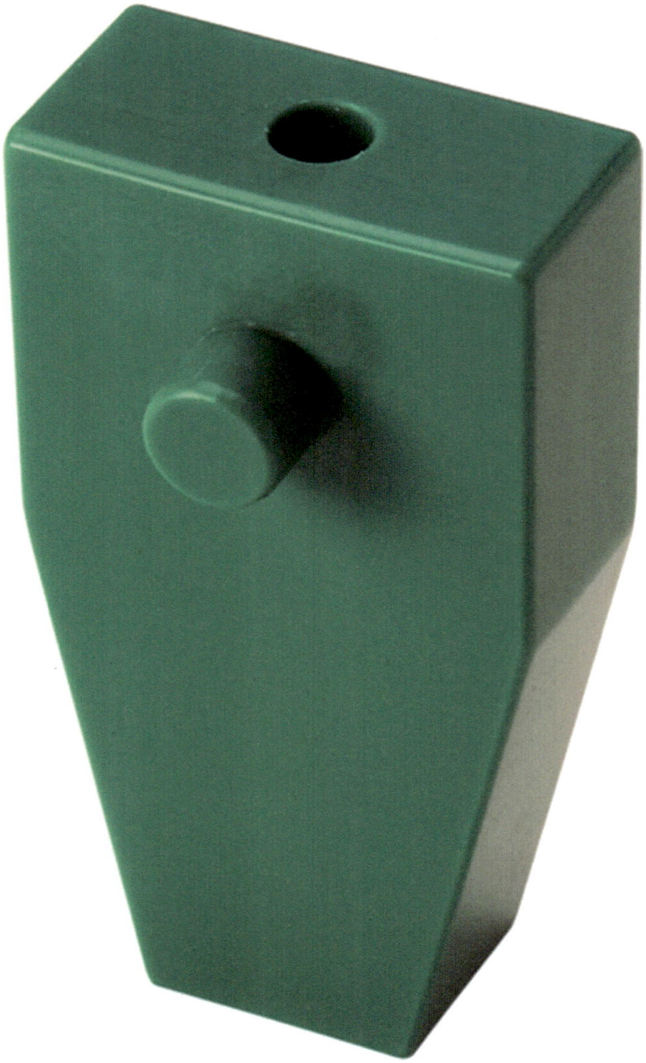

Fig. 13.6 Stylet guide

AO fracture classification: type A fracture

- Degeneration:

Intervertebral disc herniation, spinal stenosis, and mild (grade II and less) lumbar spondylolisthesis that can be managed by interlaminar fenestration decompression and which does not require extensive laminectomy decompression

(2) Contraindications

13.4 Surgical Procedures

13.4.1 Sextant Fixation Technique

13.4.1.1 Step 1: Preoperative Planning

Preoperative planning is very useful in selecting the proper entry starting point and screw direction. An axial view reveals the distance of the skin entry starting point from the body surface projection of the pedicle (Fig. 13.11). The starting point is rarely located above the pedicle.

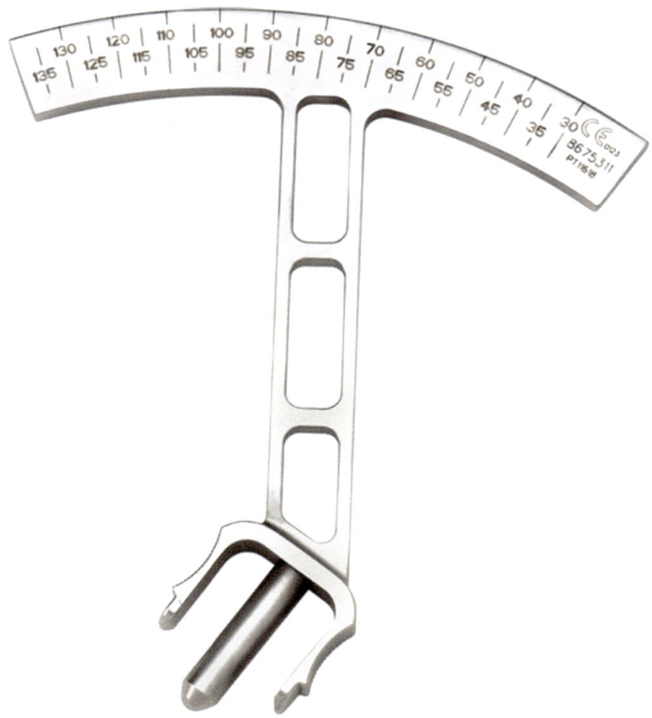

Fig. 13.7 Rod template

The patient is placed prone, and a radiolucent frame or chest rolls can be used. The knee-to-chest position should be avoided in surgery. The anteroposterior and lateral fluoroscopic images of the pedicle should be adequately obtained before proceeding to surgery (Fig. 13.12). Sometimes, the pedestals of the operating table make it difficult to obtain a true anteroposterior view of the pedicle, especially at the S1 level. Although patient positioning can be adjusted, operating tables that interfere with obtaining adequate anteroposterior fluoroscopic images should be avoided. The disinfection area should be as long as possible in the cephalocaudal direction as the rod inserted entry site may be far away from the actual surgically instrumented area.

13.4.1.2 Step 2: Selection of Screw Entry Site

A 22-gauge spinal needle is used to determine the skin entry site. The needle is placed directly over the pedicle guided by anteroposterior fluoroscopic images and then moved laterally 1–2 cm and inserted through the skin to reach the intersection of the facet and transverse process (Fig. 13.13). Accuracy of the starting site can be verified by both anteroposterior and lateral fluoroscopic images (Fig. 13.14a, b).

13.4.1.3 Step 3: Anatomic Considerations of the Pedicle

The pedicle can be considered to be a cylindrical structure. The intersection (the lateral edge of the cylinder) of the facet

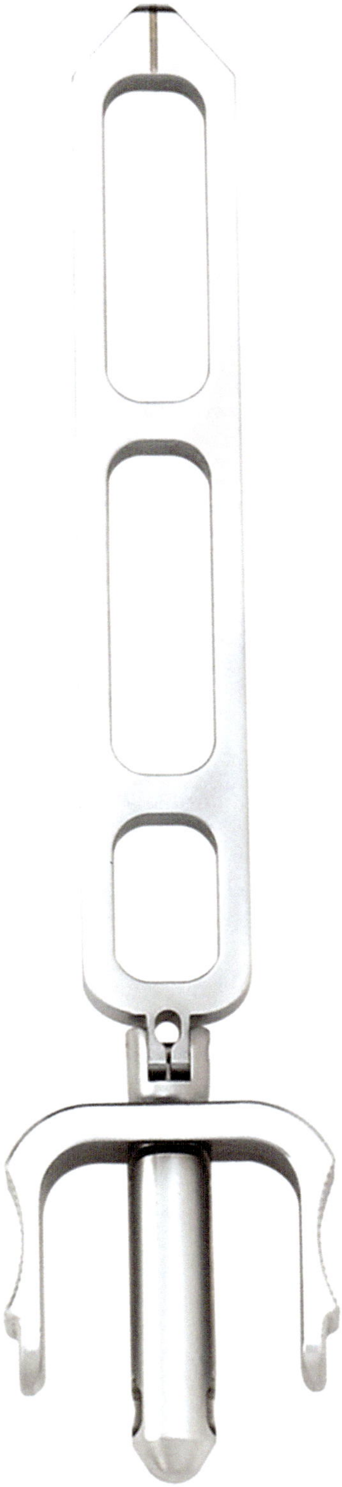

Fig. 13.8 Rod template pointer

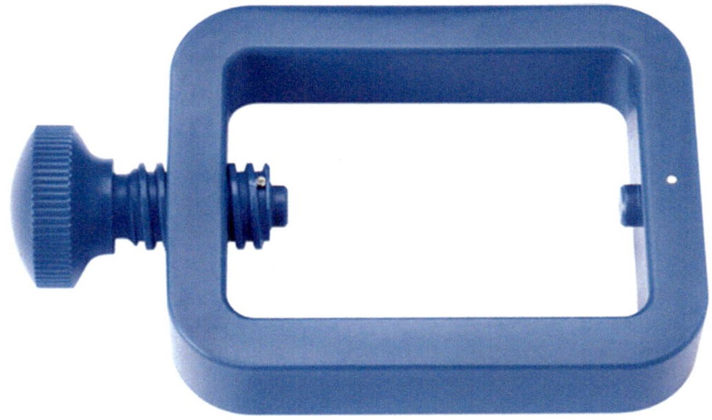

Fig. 13.9 Lucent guide clamp

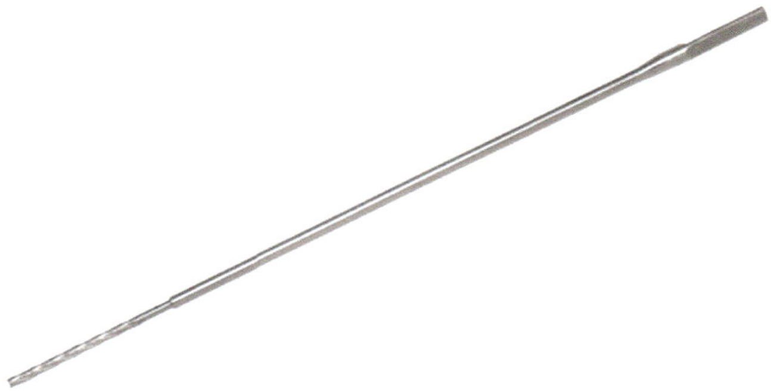

Fig. 13.10 Hollow drill bit

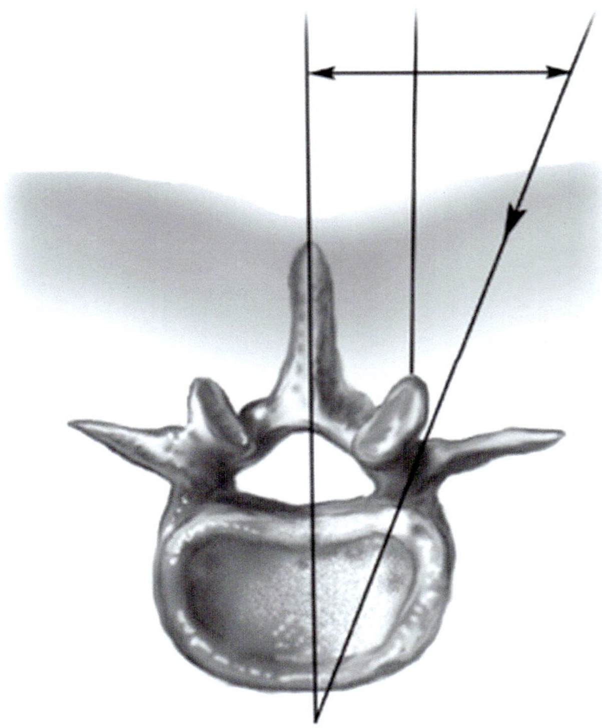

Fig. 13.11 Planning the entry starting point

and the transverse process is the ideal entry point for pedicle screw. The needle is aimed toward the medial wall of the cylinder, but should not get too close (Fig. 13.15).

13.4.1.4 Step 4: Using the Navigation System

If navigation instruments are available, the navigation system can be used to aid pedicle screw insertion. This step is skipped if a C-arm machine is used for navigation. The CD HORIZONTM SEXTANTTM instruments are designed to be fully compatible with the navigation system and have additional module with all the necessary attachments for use with the navigation system (Fig. 13.16). The advantage of using the navigation system is virtual demonstration of the safety of any proposed pedicle trajectory (Fig. 13.17), and the pedicle trajectory is known before navigating the pedicle. Another advantage is observation of the pedicle at multiple angles with less radiation exposure.

13.4.1.5 Step 5: Accessing the Pedicle (PAK Needle and Awl/Probe Option)

The PAK needle can be used to access the pedicle. After the PAK needle is placed at the intersection of the facet and the transverse process, it may partially enter the pedicle (Fig. 13.18). The anteroposterior image shows the needle tip at the lateral edge of the pedicle initially

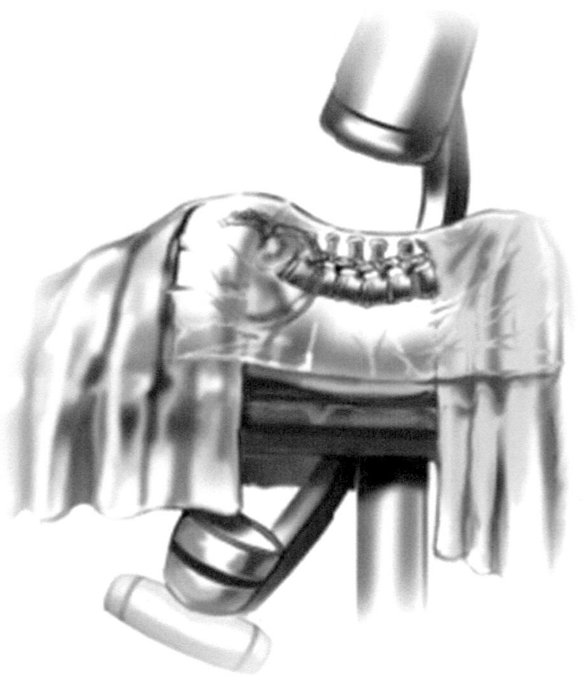

Fig. 13.12 Preoperative fluoroscopy

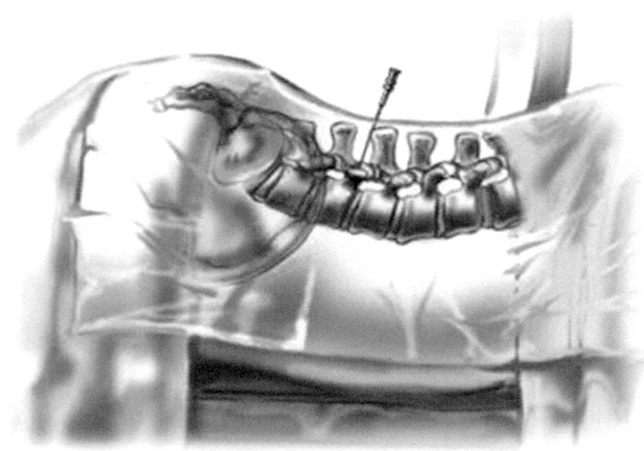

Fig. 13.13 Puncture

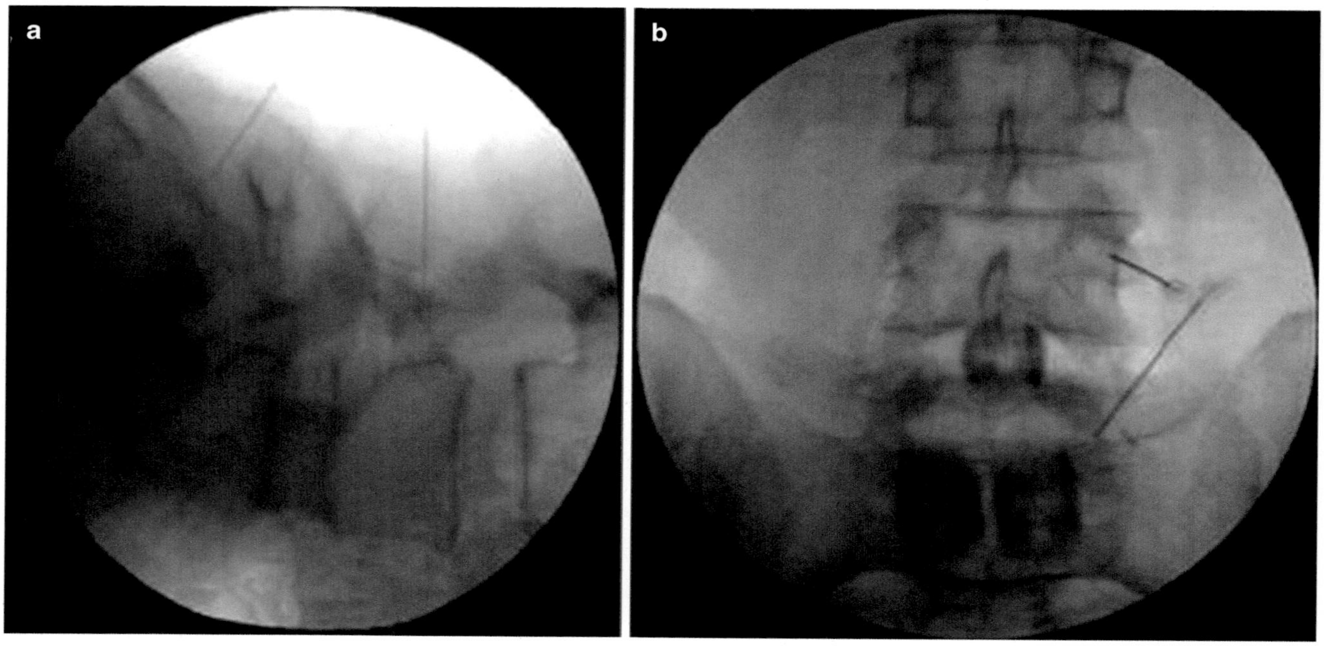

Fig. 13.14 Radiological confirmation. (**a**) Lateral image. (**b**) Orthogonal image

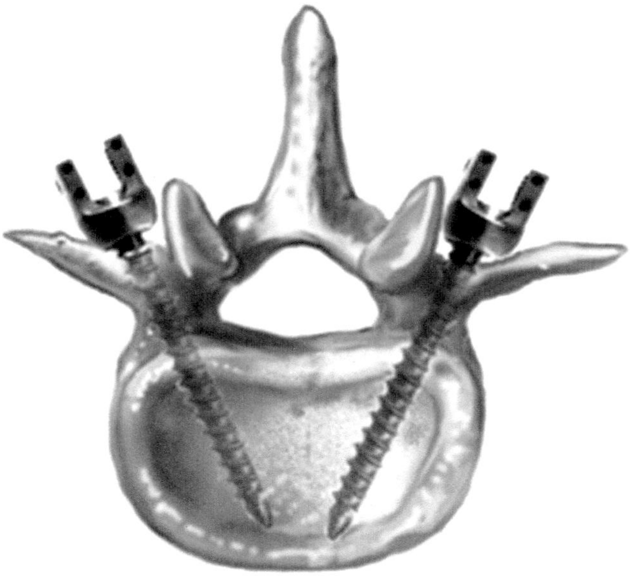

Fig. 13.15 Determination of the screw starting point

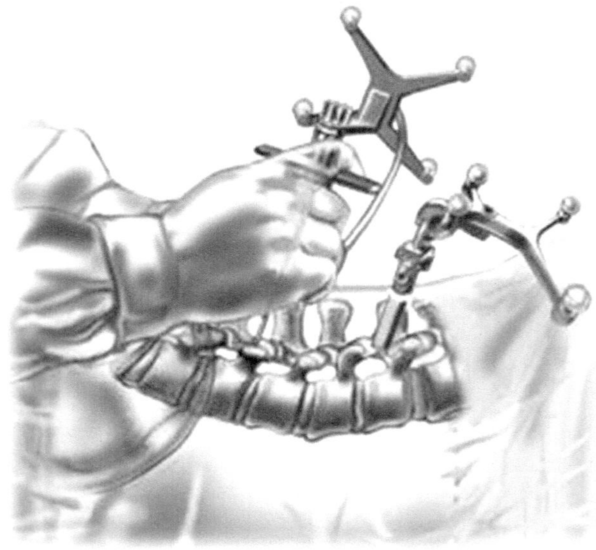

Fig. 13.16 Navigation-guided puncture

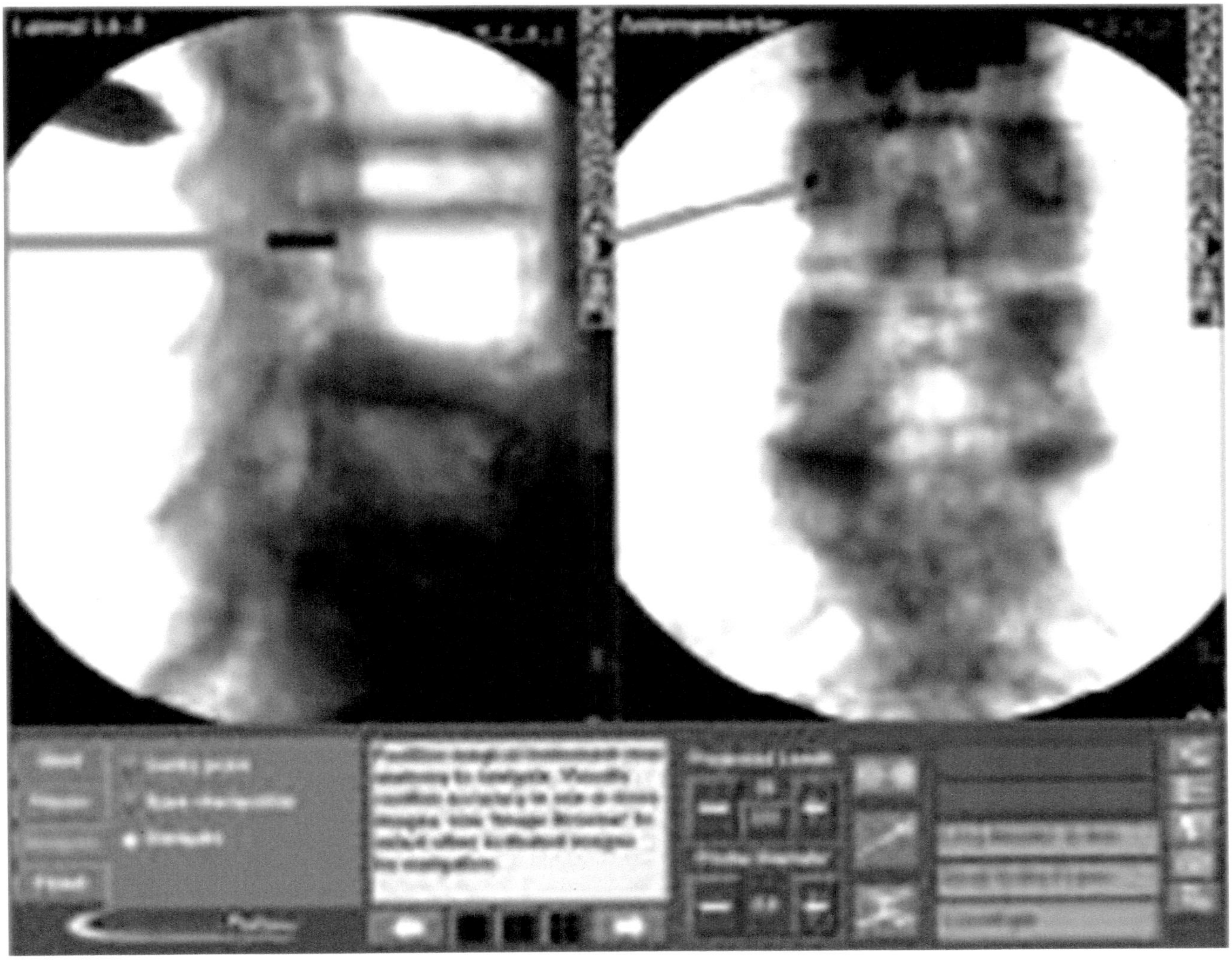

Fig. 13.17 Navigation-guided pedicle trajectory

(Fig. 13.19a and b) and is at the pedicle center on the anteroposterior image after the needle penetrates into the pedicle (which can be observed on the lateral image) (Fig. 13.19c and d).

The inner stylet is removed from the PAK needle, and then the guidewire is inserted into the pedicle (Figs. 13.20 and 13.21). Be extremely careful of the position of the guidewire. Random insertion of the guidewire causes severe consequences. Once the guidewire is inserted, the PAK needle can be removed.

- Awl Insertion

If no PAK needle is available, the "quick connect trocar (awl)" is used to gain access to the pedicle. The "quick connect awl" is first inserted into the "awl/probe sleeve." The awl is placed at the intersection of the facet and the transverse process, and then the pedicle is held at the "awl/probe sleeve" and the awl is partially advanced into

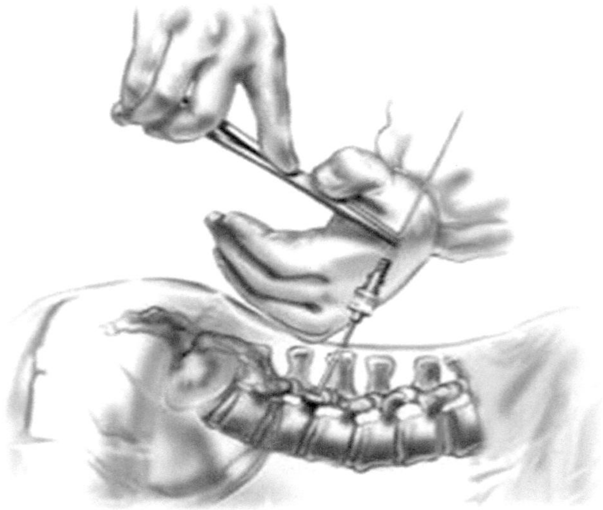

Fig. 13.20 Guidewire insertion

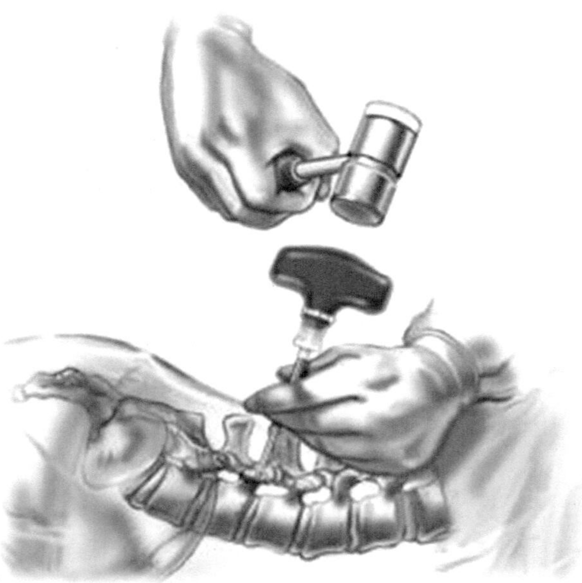

Fig. 13.18 PAK needle puncture

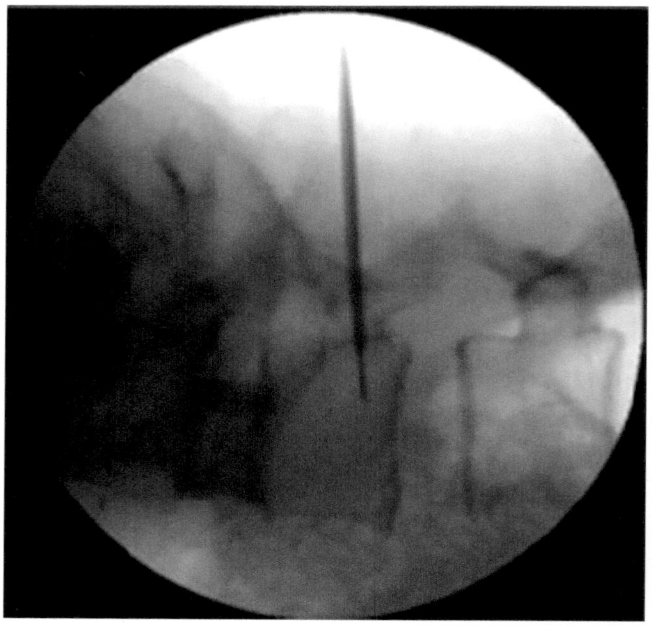

Fig. 13.21 Positioning confirmation

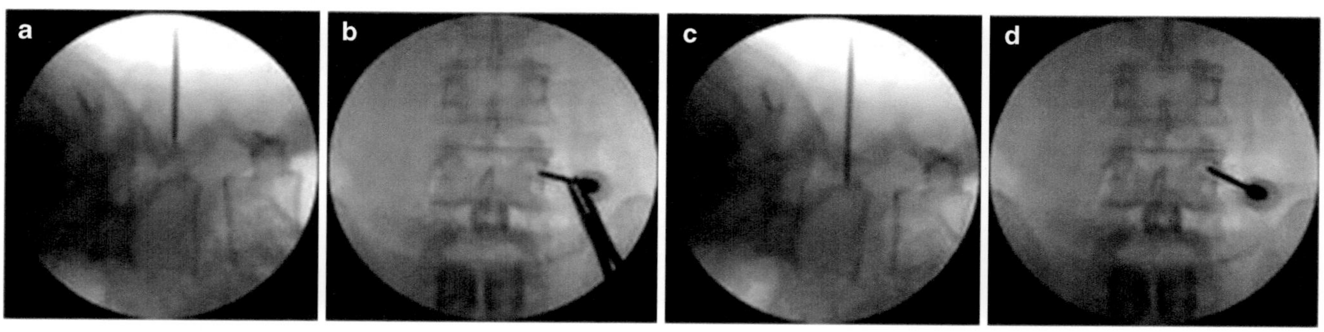

Fig. 13.19 Confirmation of accuracy of position. (**a**) Lateral image. (**b**) Orthogonal image. (**c**) Lateral image. (**d**) Orthogonal image

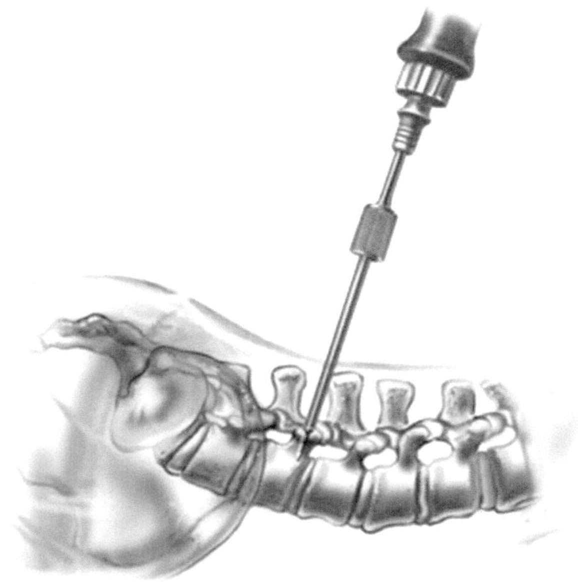

Fig. 13.22 Withdrawing the awl

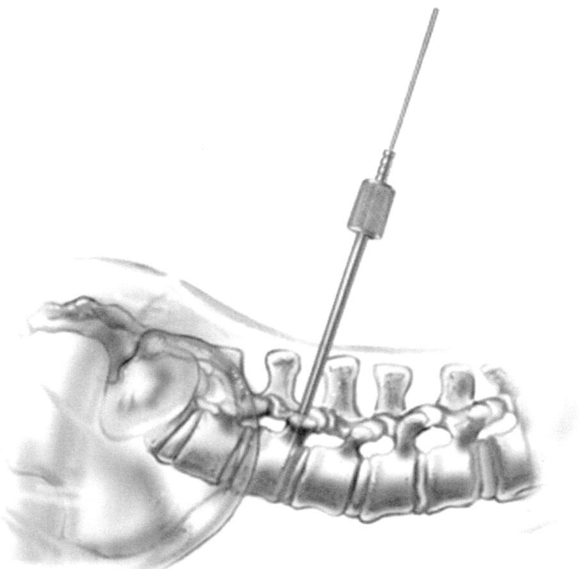

Fig. 13.23 Inserting the guidewire

the pedicle. The sleeve is maintained in place after withdrawal of the awl (Fig. 13.22). If further advances are desired, the quick connect probe can be inserted into the sleeve and into the pedicle. After removal of the probe, the guidewire centering sleeve is inserted into the awl (Fig. 13.23), and then the guidewire is advanced. Both sleeves are removed.

13.4.1.6 Step 6: Fascia Dilation

The muscle and fascia are dilated for screw placement. Three distractors are used and gently make an appropriate path

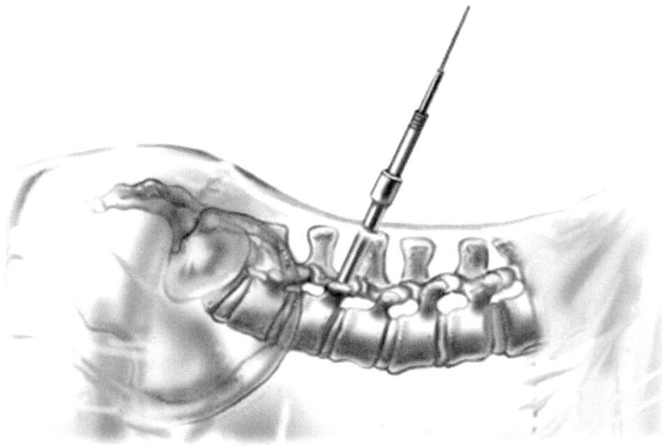

Fig. 13.24 Distractor dilation

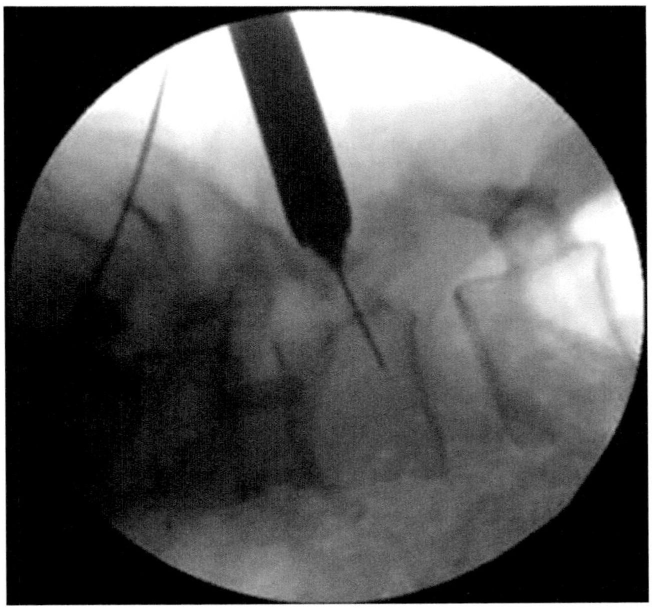

Fig. 13.25 Radiological confirmation

(Figs. 13.24 and 13.25). The first two distractors are removed, and the third distractor is left to act as a protection sleeve during tapping.

13.4.1.7 Step 7: Pedicle Preparation

The tap is placed over the guidewire through the third sleeve for tapping the pedicle (Fig. 13.26). In dense bone, it could be difficult to advance the screw; to prevent the screw from damage, a tap with the same diameter as that of the screw should be used. During tapping, fluoroscopy can be used to assure correct positioning of the guidewire and the tap (Fig. 13.27). Screw length can be determined by the calibration markings on the shaft of the tap. After completion of tapping, the guidewire is kept in place, while the distractor is removed

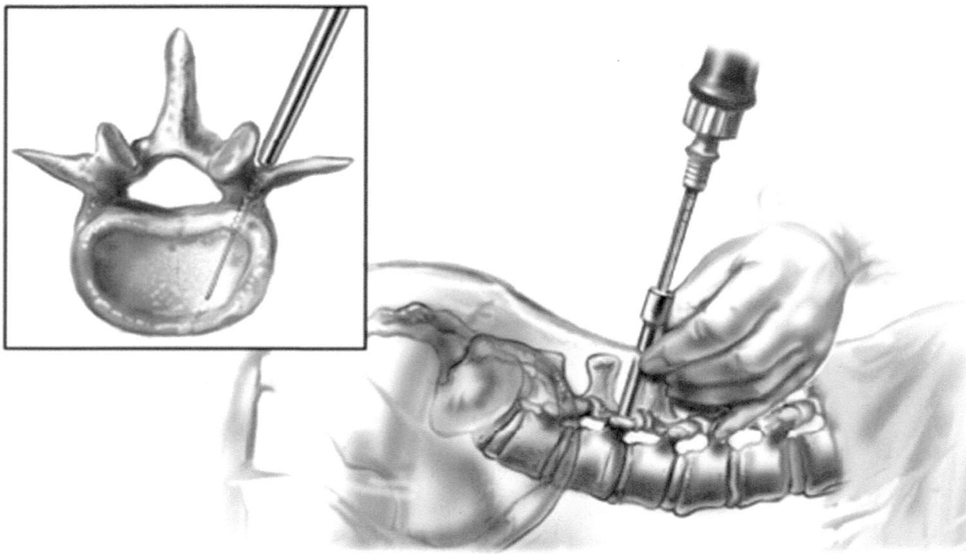

Fig. 13.26 The pedicle is tapped

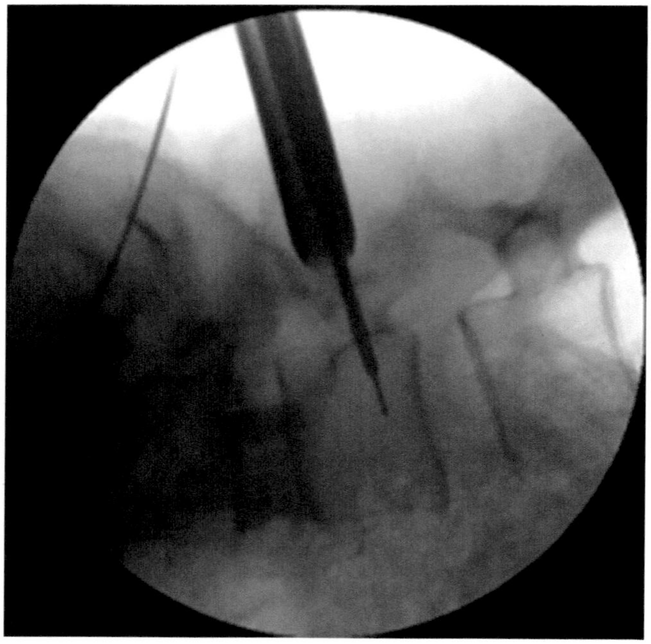

Fig. 13.27 Fluoroscopic confirmation

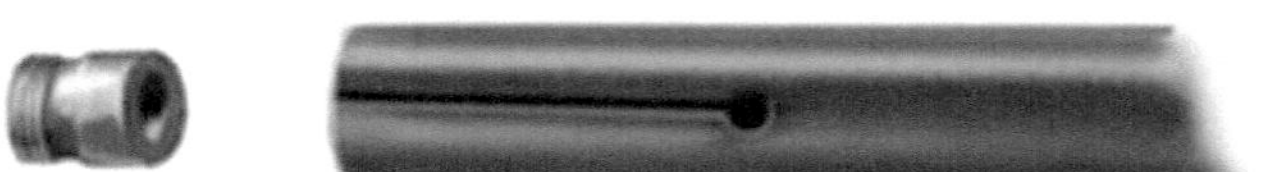

Fig. 13.28 Screw insertion

13.4.1.8 Step 8: Screw Extender Assembly

Before screw insertion into the pedicle screw, multi-axial screws must be assembled into the "screw extender." First, the smooth cap of the screw is pushed into the distal end of

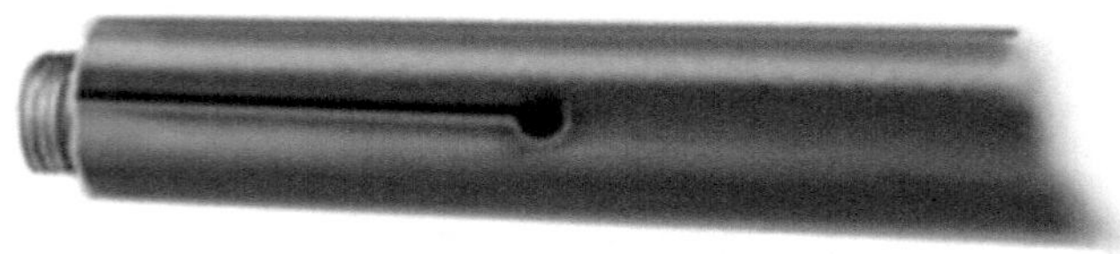

Fig. 13.29 The threaded end does not enter the sleeve

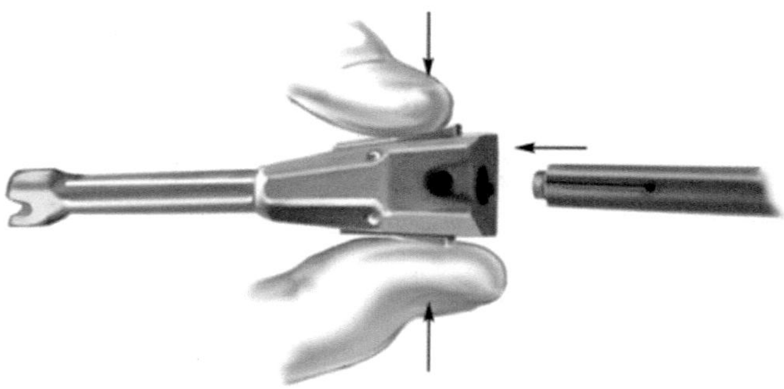

Fig. 13.30 Inserting the sleeve

the "screw retaining sleeve" (Fig. 13.28); the threaded end of the screw should not enter the sleeve (Fig. 13.29). Then, the "screw retaining sleeve" is inserted into the "screw extender" (Fig. 13.30). The two buttons on the distal end of the "screw extender" are initially depressed, and then released after the "screw retaining sleeve" is partially entered, with an audible click, indicating that the "screw retaining sleeve" is the appropriate position (Fig. 13.31).

Caution: Proper placement of the sleeve is very important, which assures correct rod engagement with the saddle of the screw.

A CDH M8 cannulated screw is assembled into the distal end of the "screw extender" (Fig. 13.32), and the "combina-

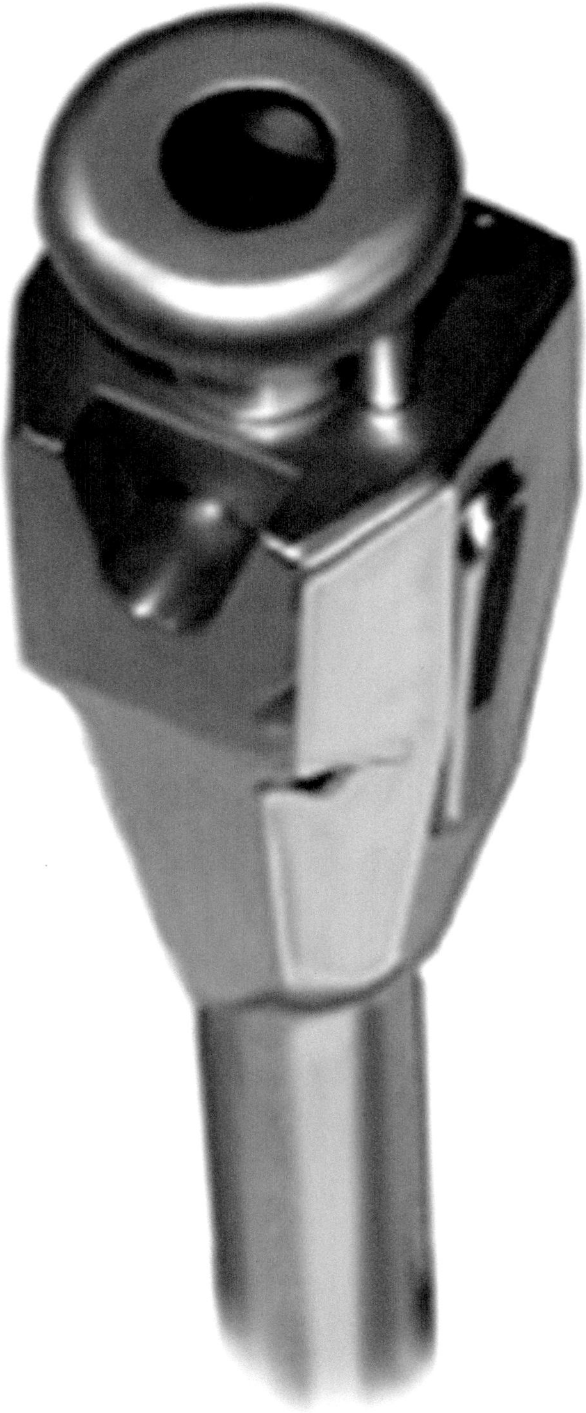

Fig. 13.31 Completion of the assembly

tion plug driver" is used to advance the screw (Fig. 13.33). The "screw retaining sleeve" can prevent the screw from traveling too far in the saddle of the M8 screw. Before implantation, visually inspect or manually insert the rod into the saddle of the screw for correct positioning.

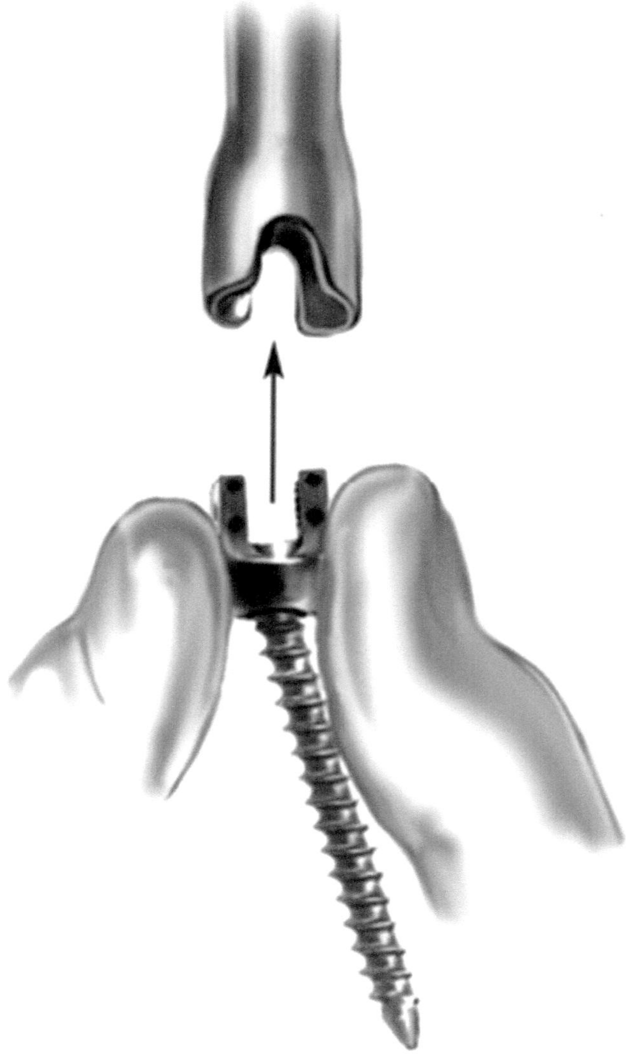

Fig. 13.32 Screw assembly

The screwdriver is placed from the top into the screw assembly of the screw extender and the screw retaining sleeve. The tip of the screwdriver is inserted into the head of the multi-axial cannulated screw via the set screw (Fig. 13.34). As the tip of the screwdriver passes through the set screw, extreme caution should be exercised during the maneuver not to change the position of the screw (Fig. 13.35).

13.4.1.9 Step 9: Screw Insertion

The entire screw set including the screw retaining sleeve and the screw extender, the set screw, and screw enters the pedicle via the guidewire. If there is difficulty in advancing the screw, the "screw assembly" can be removed while leaving the guidewire in place, and the tap with the same diameter as that of the screw is used to assure adequate preparation of the

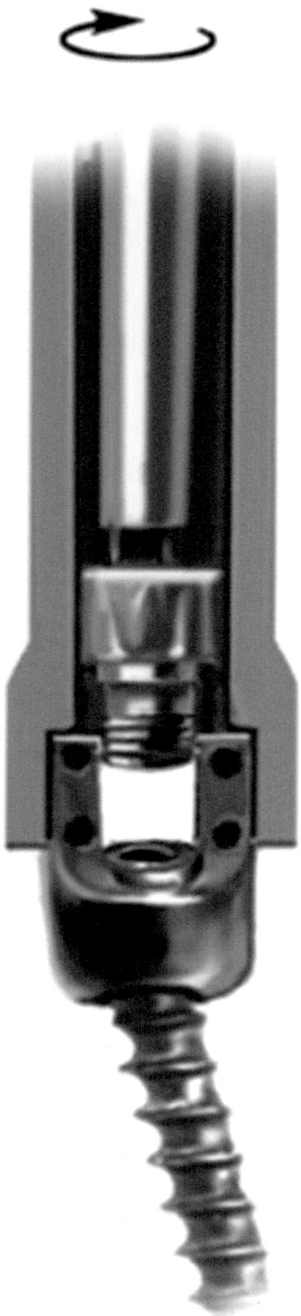

Fig. 13.33 Screw insertion

pedicle trajectory and prevent screwdriver damage. After advancing the "screw assembly" into the pedicle, the guidewire is removed to prevent its insertion into the pedicle. Make sure that the "screw assembly" is not inserted too far. If M8 multi-axial cannulated screw tail is flushed tightly against the bone, it will lose its multi-axial function, rendering subsequent steps difficult to perform (Figs. 13.36 and 13.37).

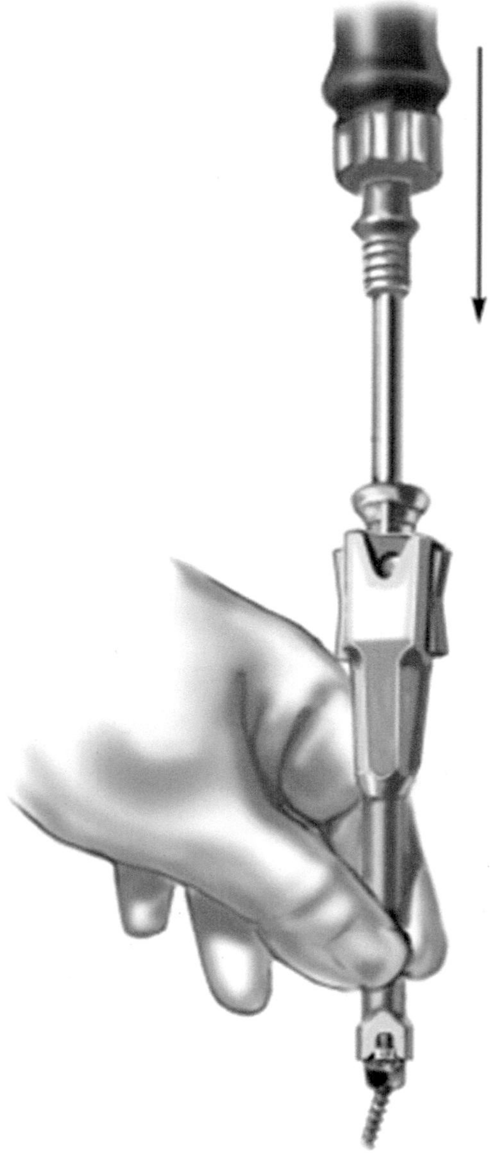

Fig. 13.34 Inserting the screwdriver

13.4.1.10 Step 10: Inserting the Second Screw

The second screw is placed on the same side using the above method (Fig. 13.38). After placement of the two screws, both "screw assemblies" should be of identical height outside of the skin and be freely movable.

13.4.1.11 Step 11: Connecting the Screw Extenders

The screw extender is rotated so that the distal two flat sides face each other (Fig. 13.39) and then attach each other via connectors on the surface with no gap between the two screw extenders. Once the two flat surfaces of the two screw extenders completely flush, the rod inserter can be connected.

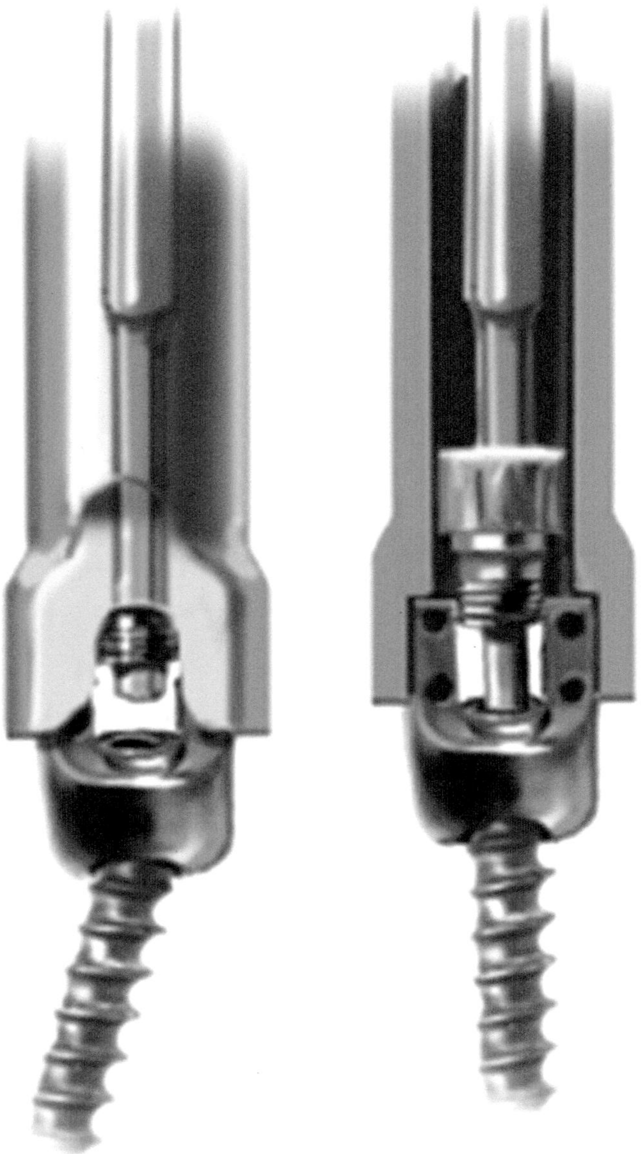

Fig. 13.35 Screw insertion

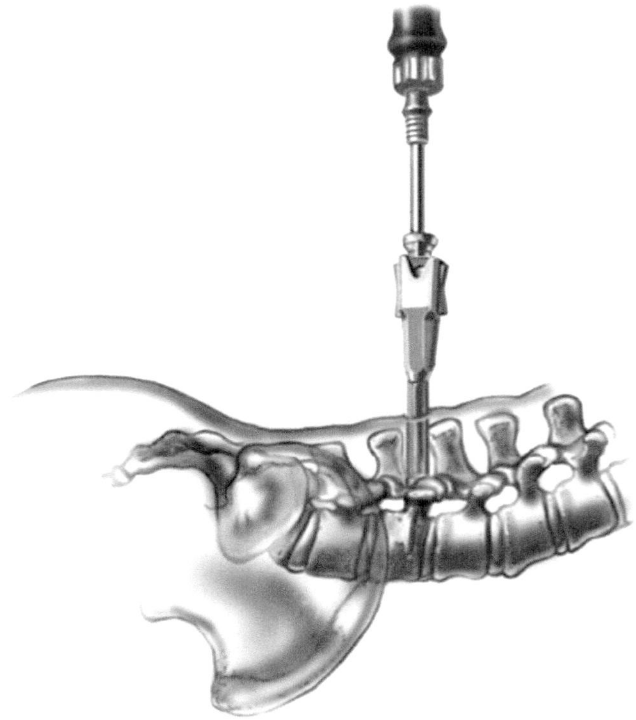

Fig. 13.36 Advancing the pedicle

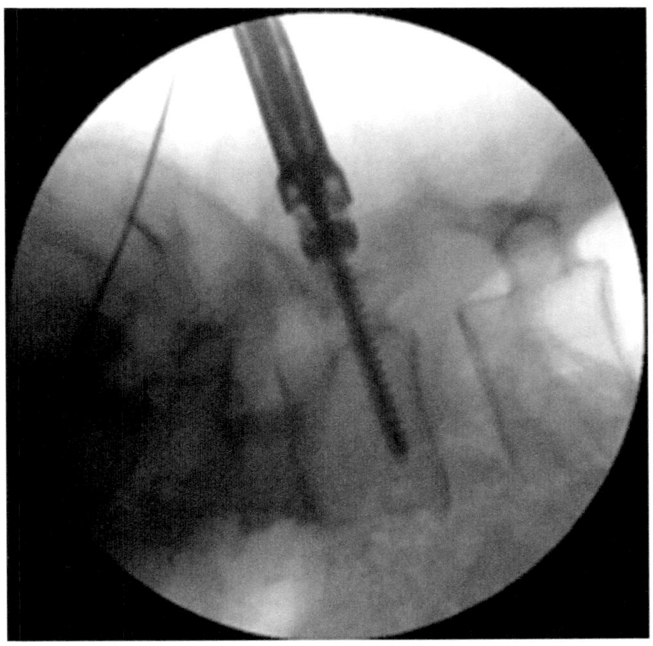

Fig. 13.37 Fluoroscopic confirmation

13.4.1.12 Step 12: Connecting the Rod Inserter and Trocar

The rod inserter is connected to the screw assembly by lining up the pegs of the rod inserter and the grooves of the screw assembly (Fig. 13.40). The screw on the "rod inserter" is rotated to ensure a secure fit. The thumb screw of the "rod inserter" is backed out and pushed down (Fig. 13.41) in order to push the "trocar" into the tip of the "rod inserter." Once the "trocar" is in place, the thumb screw is tightened to secure the "trocar tip."

13.4.1.13 Step 13: Inserting the Trocar

The "trocar" is used to make a path between the fascia and the muscles to reach the saddle (Fig. 13.42). A small skin incision is made, and under lateral fluoroscopy, the "trocar"

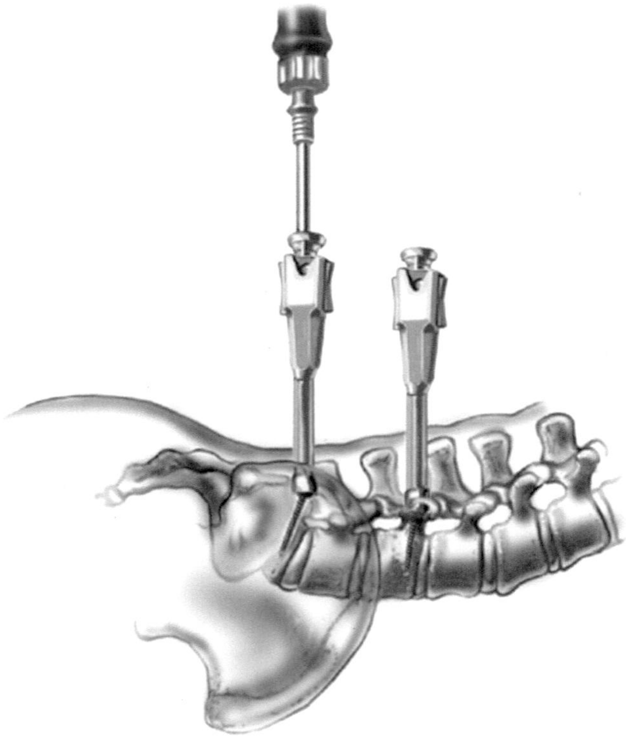

Fig. 13.38 Second screw placement

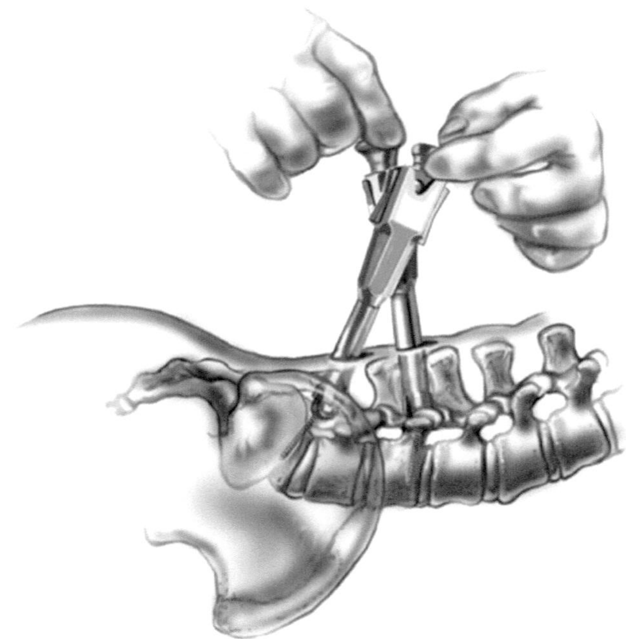

Fig. 13.39 Rotating the screw extenders

passes through the skin and the muscles to directly reach the saddle of the first screw.

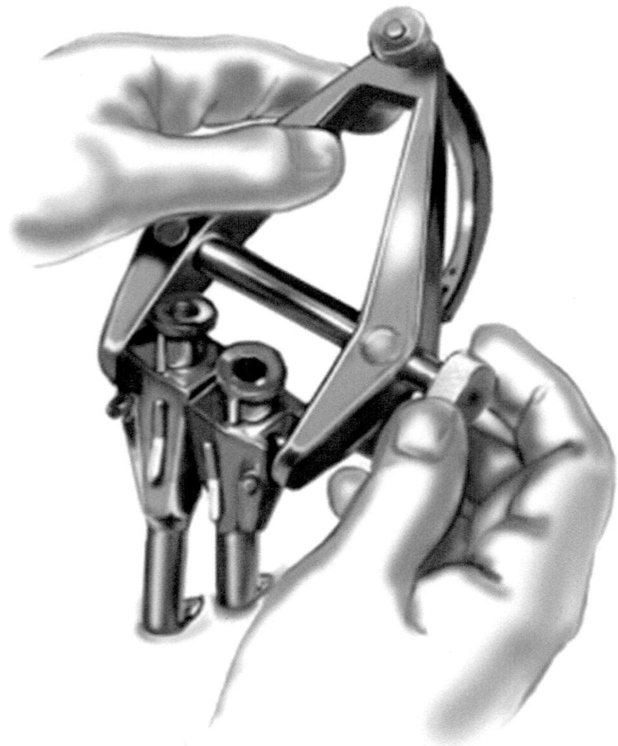

Fig. 13.40 Connecting the rod inserter

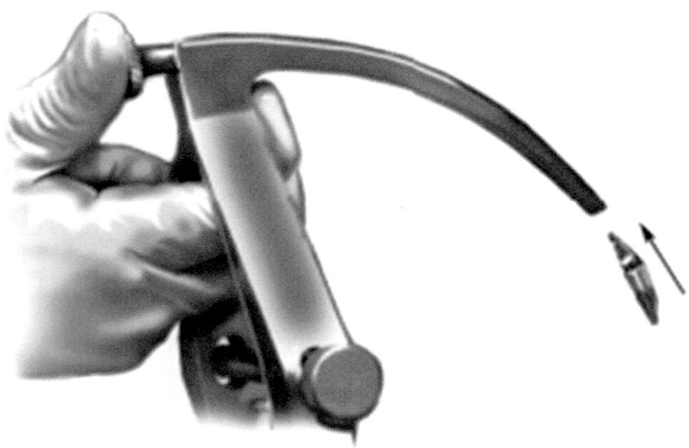

Fig. 13.41 Connecting the rod trocar tip

13.4.1.14 Step 14: Rod Measurements

The rod templates are separately connected to the distal screw extenders to measure rod length (Fig. 13.43). If the rod template exceeds the rod length, a larger size rod is chosen. After rods with appropriate length are determined, the rod templates are removed. As shown in the figure below, a rod length of 60 mm is chosen.

13.4.1.15 Step 15: Passing the Rod

The trocar is removed and replaced with the appropriately sized rod as determined above. The trocar is removed by reversing the steps for attachment. Under lateral fluoroscopy, the tip is inserted into the rod and passes in turn through the head of the first screw and the head of the second screw (Figs. 13.44 and 13.45).

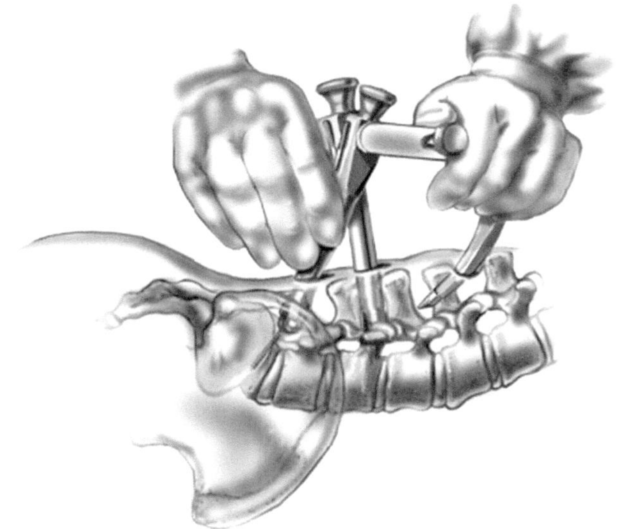

Fig. 13.42 Inserting trocar

13.4.1.16 Step 16: Final Tightening

After confirmation by anteroposterior, lateral, and oblique views that the rod is seated between the heads of the two screws, the set screw can be finally tightened. Caution should be exercised that before tightening the screw, the retaining screw sleeve must be lowered! Press the buttons on the screw extenders and lower the retaining screw sleeve. This step allows the tightened screw to engage the rod. The compressor handle may be used for provisional tightening (Fig. 13.46). Two compressor handles are assembled and used for compression, maintaining compression and provisional tightening. The final plug driver is used for final tightening until the tightened screw is sheared off (Fig. 13.47). The sheared-off portion of the screw remains inside the tightening screw sleeve.

13.4.1.17 Step 17: Removal of Screw Assembly

The "rod inserter" is taken from the "screw assembly." The "rod inserter" is detached from the rod so that the screw assembly can be pulled out of the patient (Fig. 13.48). The location of the final construct for internal fixation can be verified by anteroposterior and lateral fluoroscopy (Fig. 13.49a, b).

13.4.1.18 Step 18: Closure

Identical steps are done in the contralateral side. Closure is done with interrupted stitches for the fascia and subcuticular skin suture (Fig. 13.50).

Fig. 13.43 Measuring rod length

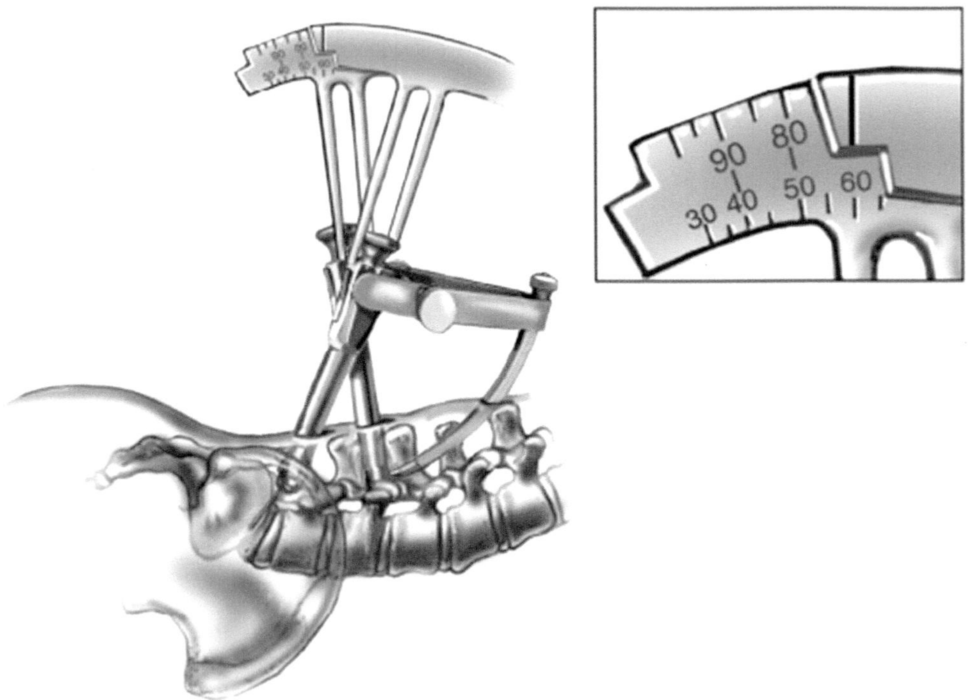

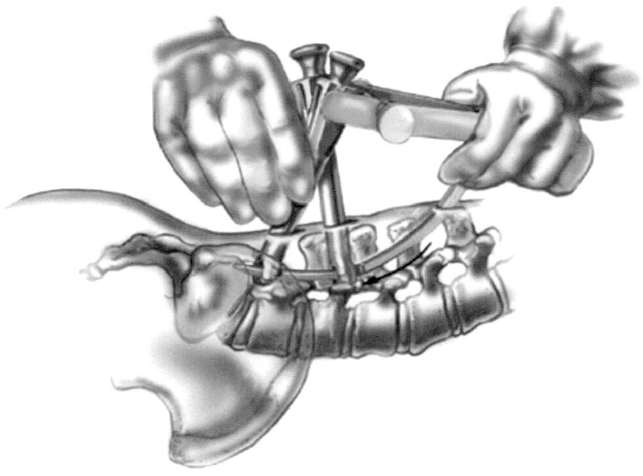

Fig. 13.44 Passing the rod

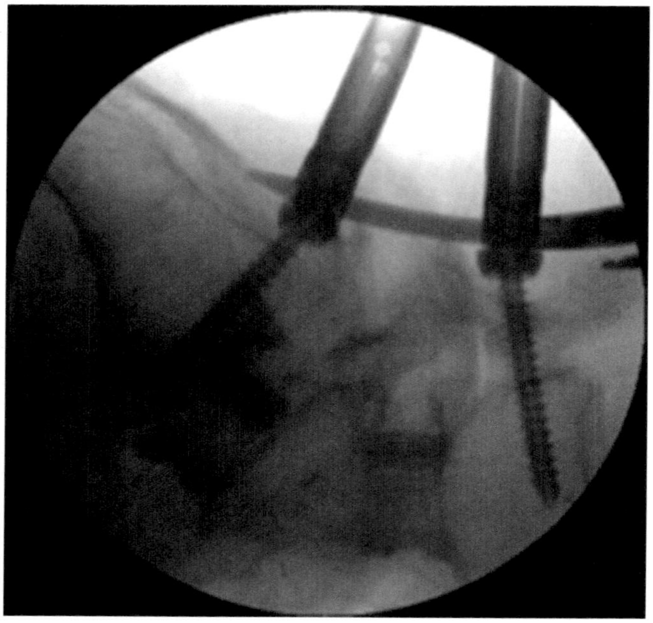

Fig. 13.45 Fluoroscopic confirmation

13.5 SEXTANT Percutaneous Pedicle Screw System

13.5.1 Alignment

For multilevel instrumentation, it is very critical to well align the three screws, which facilitate rod placement. Screw alignment can be done in a free-handed fashion, or using a mechanical targeting method. Multilevel CD HORIZON SEXTANT instrumentation gives surgeons a minimally invasive method for multilevel treatment of spinal diseases.

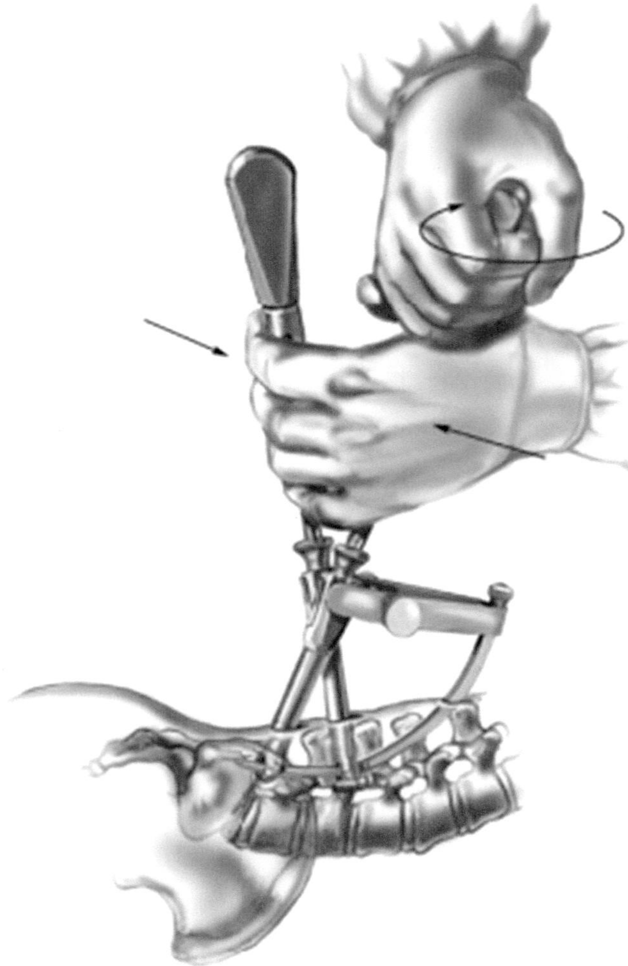

Fig. 13.46 Provisional tightening

13.5.1.1 Freehand Method for Pedicle Needle Insertion

Guided by orthogonal, lateral, and oblique fluoroscopy, three needles are inserted continuously so that the skin insertion and pedicle insertion points are aligned in the axial plane. Needle insertion is facilitated by drawing a line on the skin prior to needle advancement. The three screws and screw extenders are implanted. The two lateral extenders are placed for the most cephalad and caudal levels, while the middle extender is placed in the middle screw (Fig. 13.51) (skip to step 7).

13.5.1.2 Alignment Guide Method

The two outer extenders are implanted for the most cephalad and caudal levels (e.g., L4 and S1) (Fig. 13.52). Continue from step 2 to step 6.

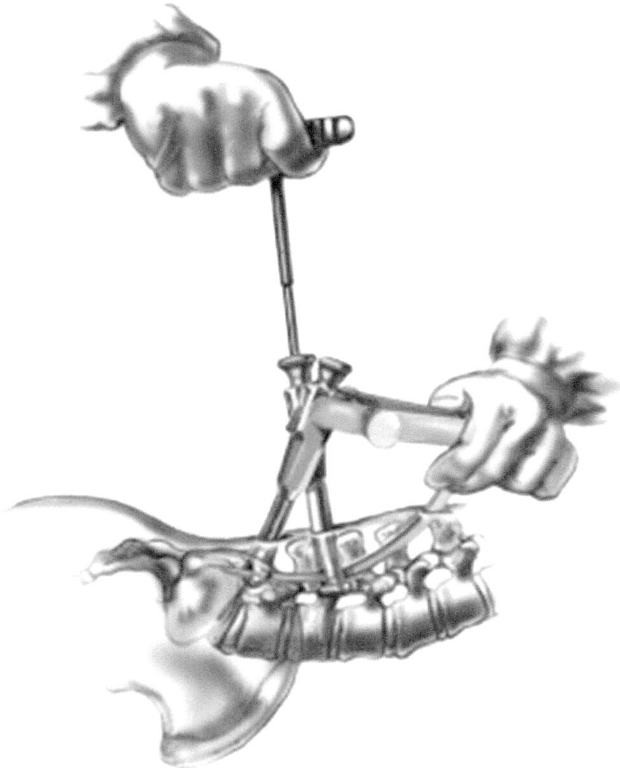

Fig. 13.47 Final tightening

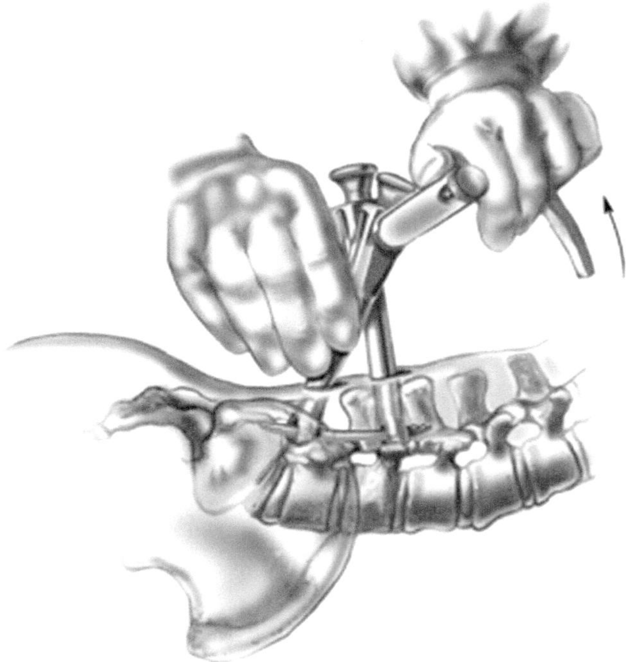

Fig. 13.48 Detached the rod inserter

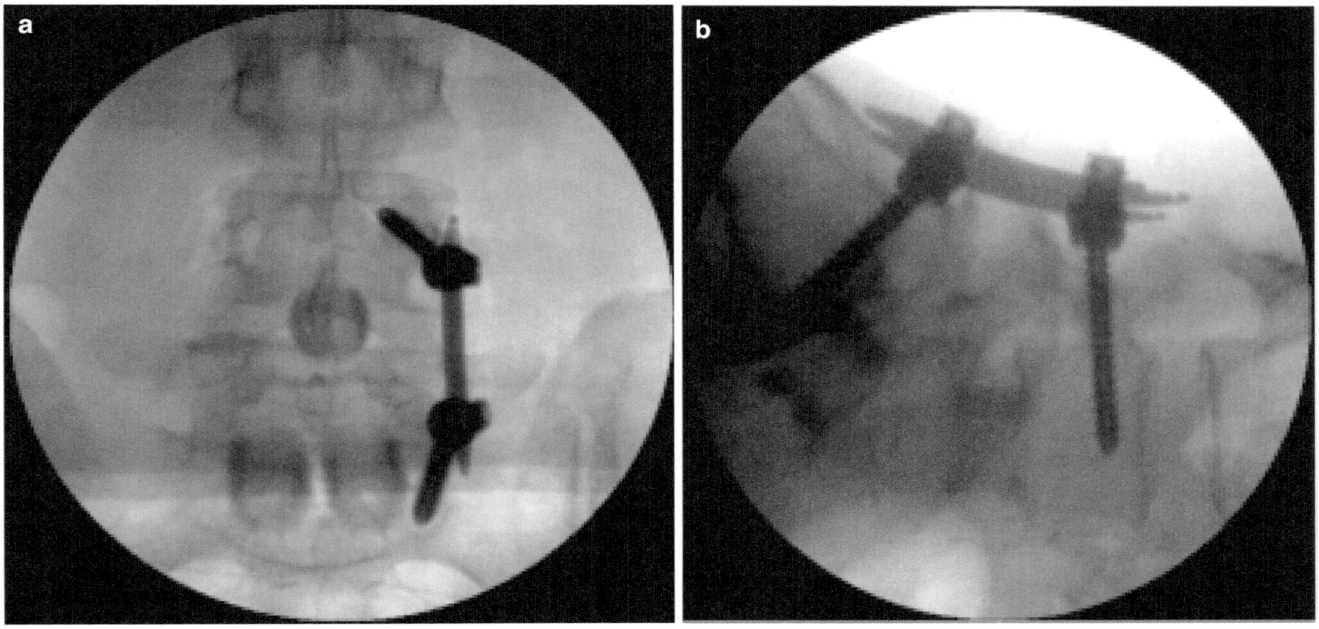

Fig. 13.49 Anteroposterior (a) and lateral (b) fluoroscopy

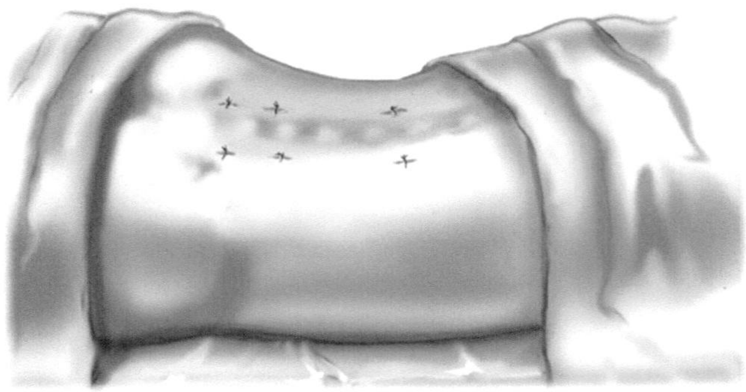

Fig. 13.50 Closure

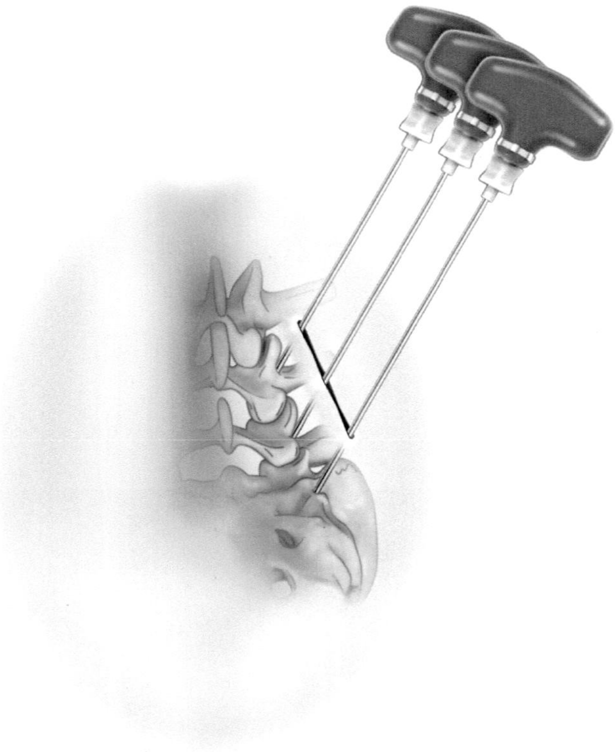

Fig. 13.51 Needle insertion

13.5.2 Connecting the Guide

The guide is connected with the two outer extenders and secured with a clamp. One guide is used for the distractor, while the other is used for the needle and drill (Fig. 13.53).

13.5.2.1 Step 1

The needle and distractor are inserted through the appropriate guide, and the middle pedicle is localized by fluoroscopy or a navigation system (Fig. 13.54).

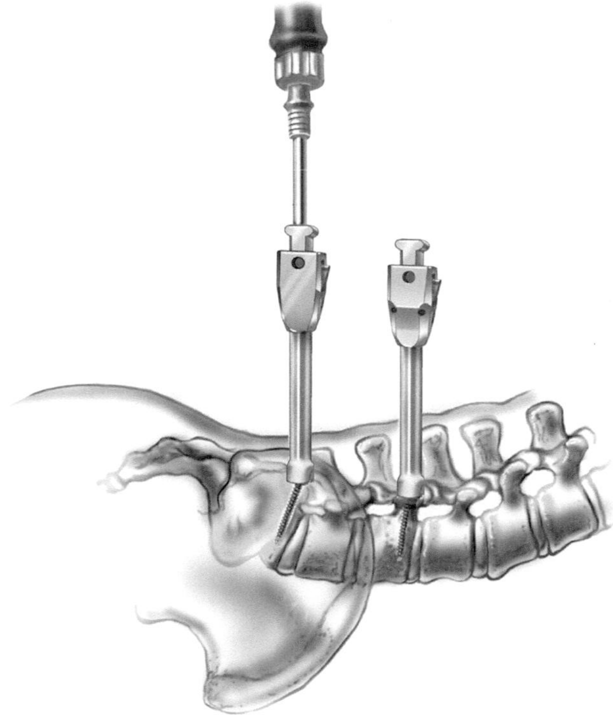

Fig. 13.52 Implant the outer extenders

13.5.2.2 Step 2

The needle and the distractor are inserted, and the guidewire is advanced through the needle and the distractor to enter the pedicle. The guide clamp and the guide are then removed followed by removal of the needle and the distractor. Only the guidewire is kept within the pedicle (Fig. 13.55).

13.5.2.3 Step 3

Dilation and tapping are done via the guidewire (Figs. 13.56 and 13.57).

13.5.2.4 Step 4

An appropriate-sized screw is assembled into the inner screw extenders and advanced into the pedicle over the guidewire (Fig. 13.58).

13.5.2.5 Step 5

The three screw extenders are rotated so that the caudal flat surfaces of the extenders are completely flushed through the pegs and grooves on the flat surfaces. Screw height may need to be adjusted to achieve proper connection. Once these steps are undertaken, the rod inserter is connected (Fig. 13.59).

13.5.2.6 Step 6

The trocar is assembled into the rod inserter, and the rod templates are placed on the outer extenders in order to determine the appropriate rod length (Fig. 13.60).

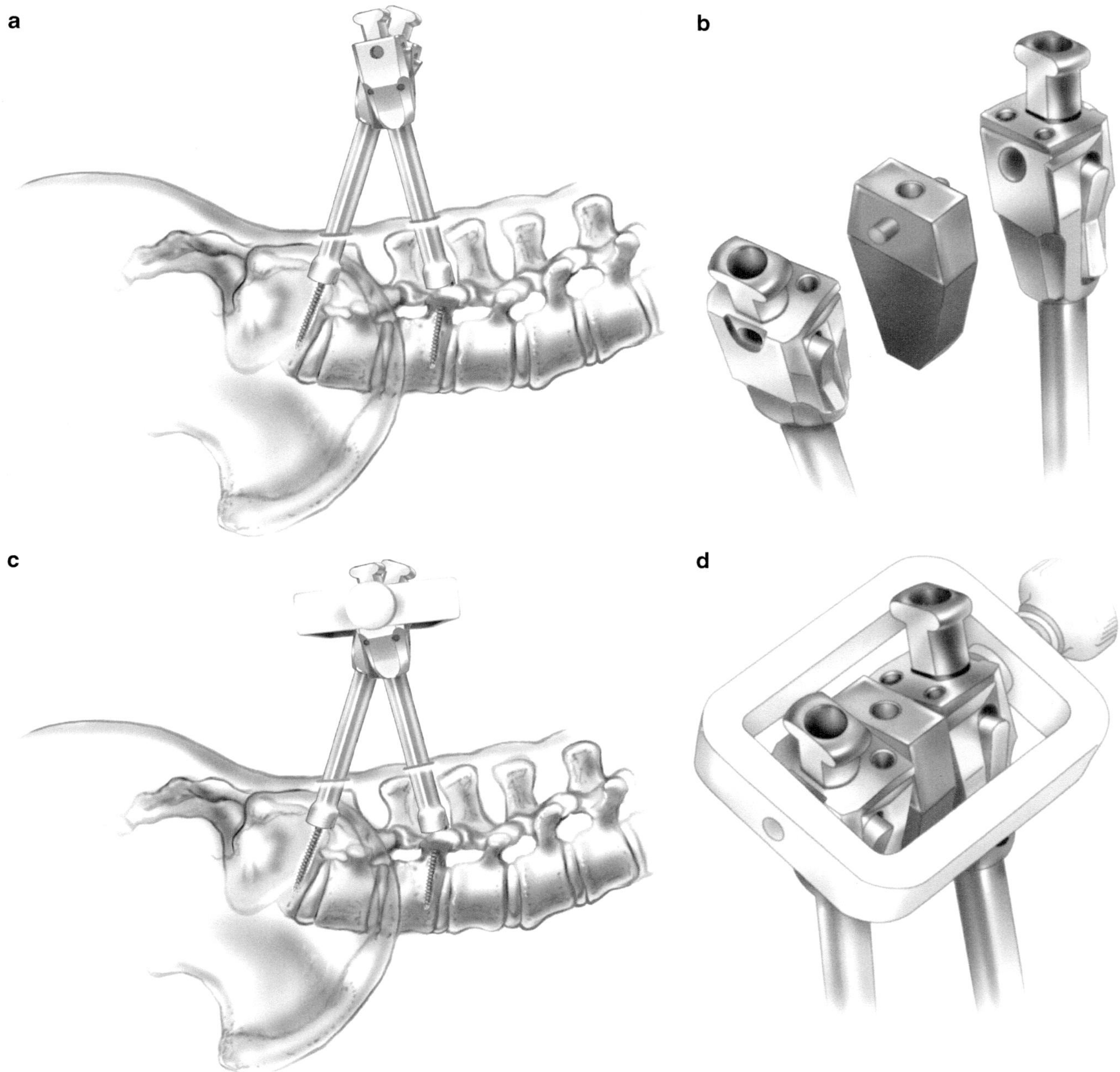

Fig. 13.53 Connect and secure the guide with the two outer extenders. (**a**) Align the two outer extenders. (**b**) Connect the two outer extenders. (**c**) Secure the two outer extenders with a clamp. (**d**) Outer extenders and clamp assembly

13.5.2.7 Step 7

The rod passes through the heads of the three screws (Fig. 13.61).

13.5.2.8 Step 8

After provisional tightening of the middle screw, compression is applied separately at the cephalad and caudal portion (Fig. 13.62). Thereafter, the screws on both sides are tightened. The three screws are sheared off separately. The rod inserter is detached and all assembly tools are removed.

13.6 CD HORIZON SEXTANT Spondylolisthesis Reduction Technique

13.6.1 Instruments and Implants

Before the screw is implanted in the pedicle, the reduction extenders should first be assembled (Fig. 13.63), which is facilitated by being done on the instrument table. The buttons on the two sides of the proximal outer sleeve of the

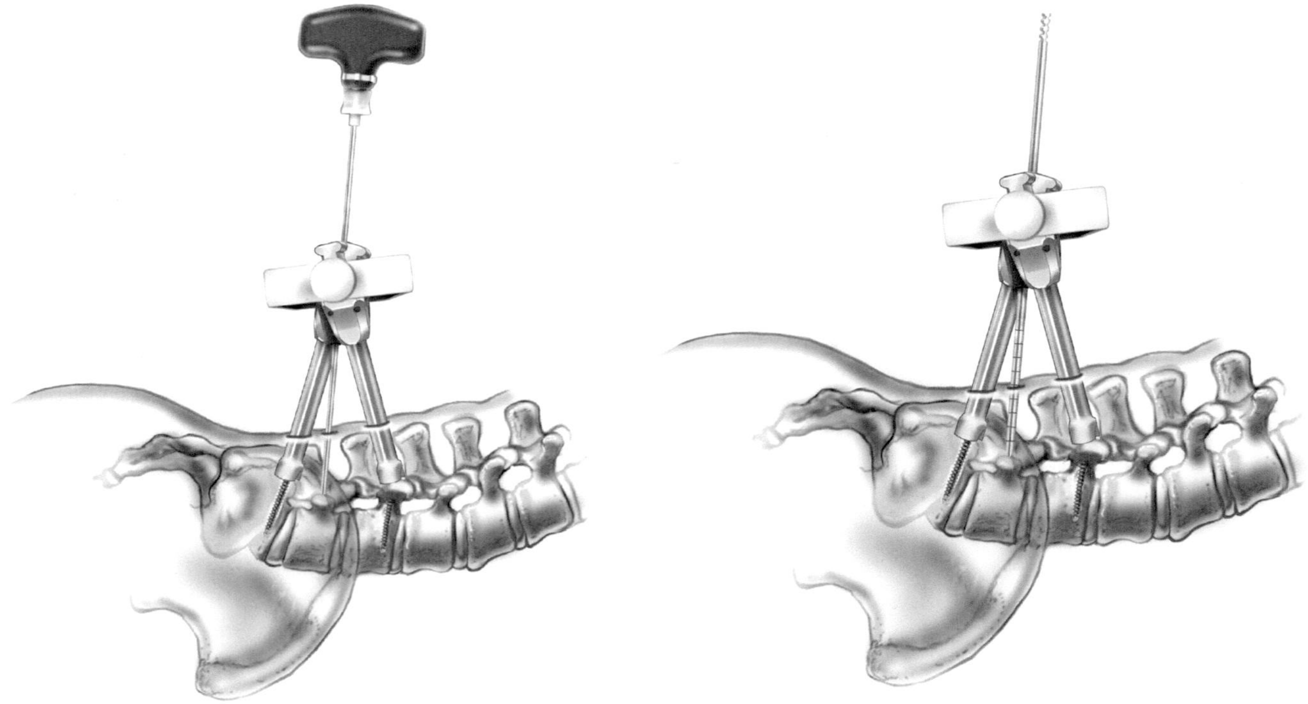

Fig. 13.54 Insert the needle and distractor

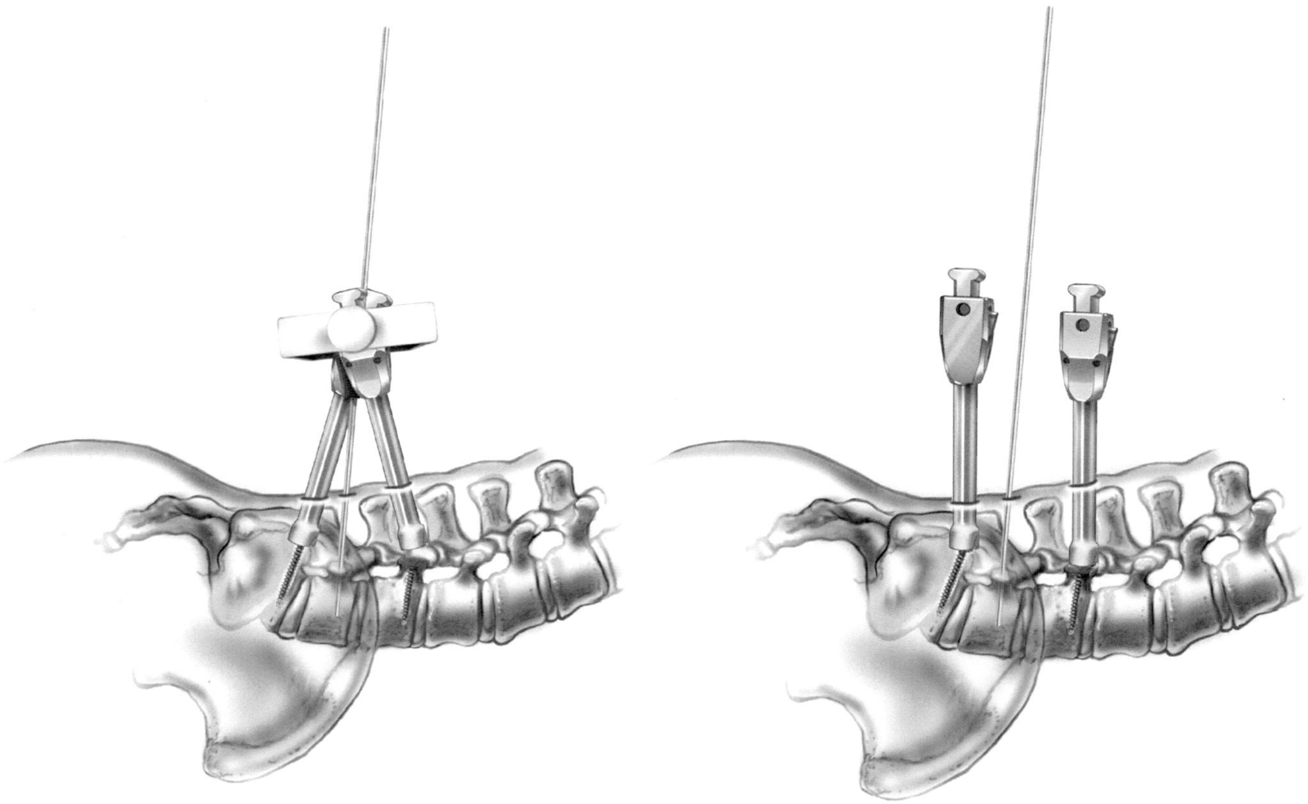

Fig. 13.55 Remove the guide clamp and keep the guidewire

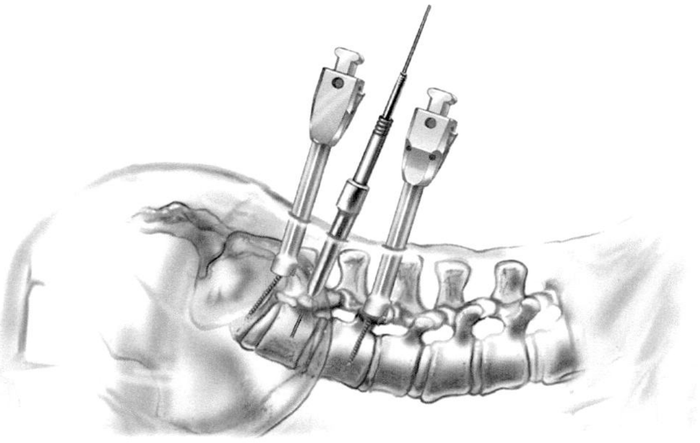

Fig. 13.56 Dilation

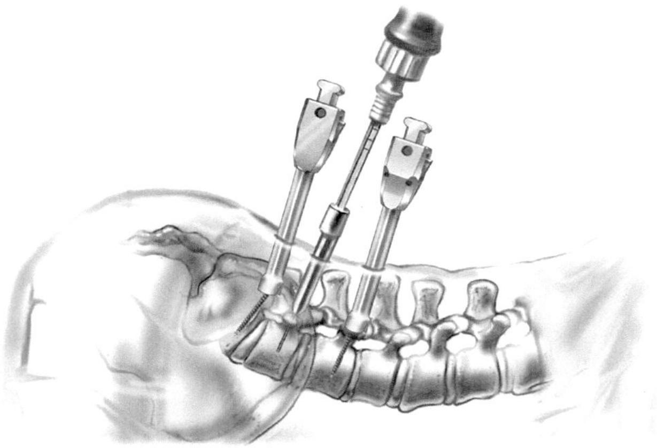

Fig. 13.57 Tapping

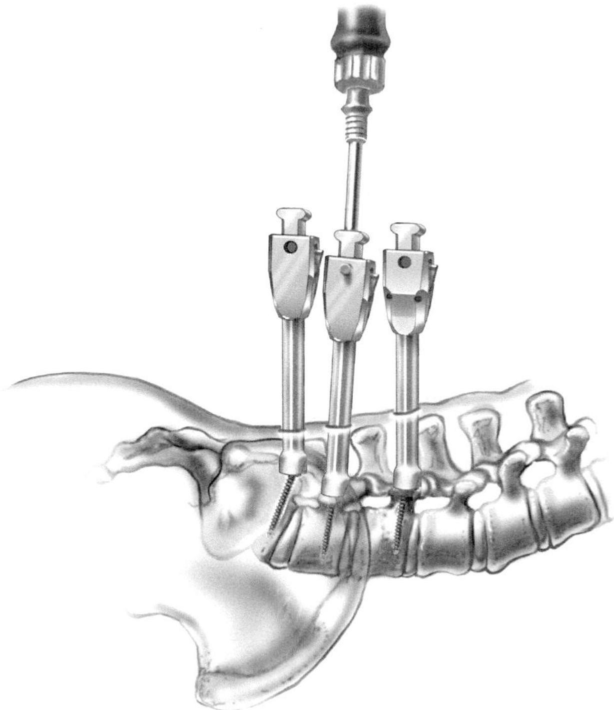

Fig. 13.58 Screw advancing

Fig. 13.59 Rotate the extenders

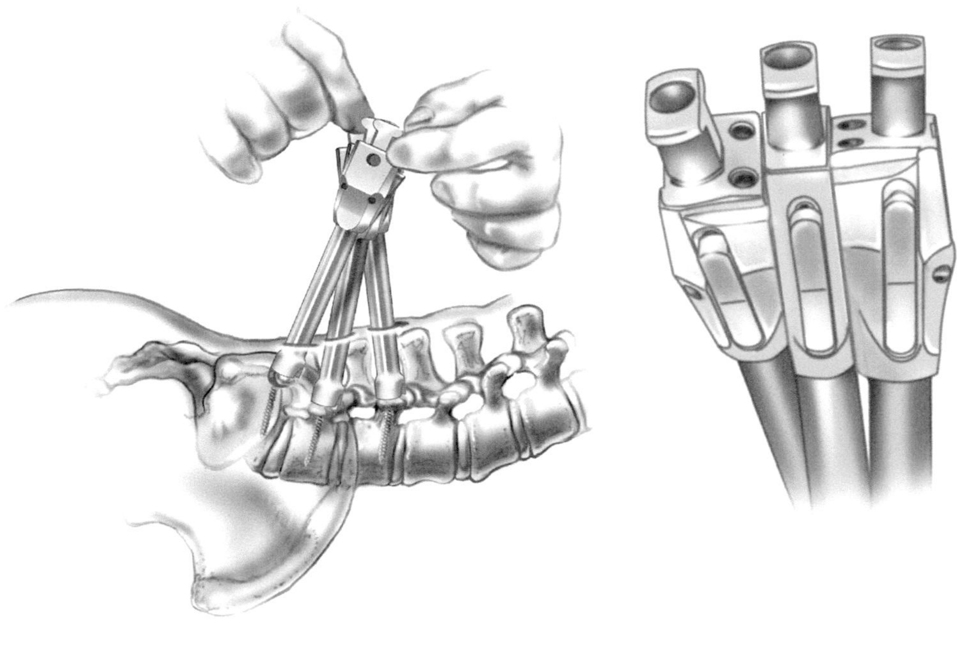

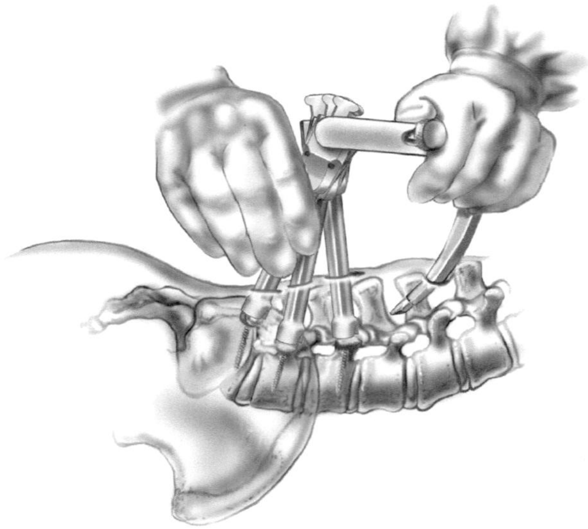

Fig. 13.60 Assemble the trocar

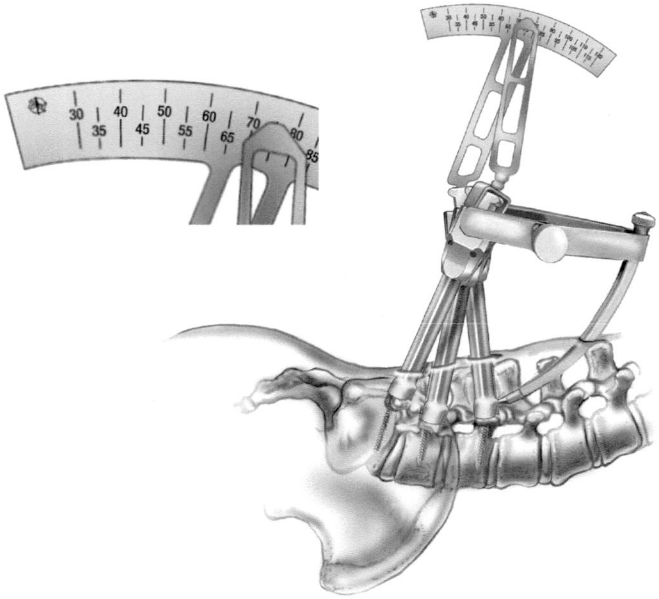

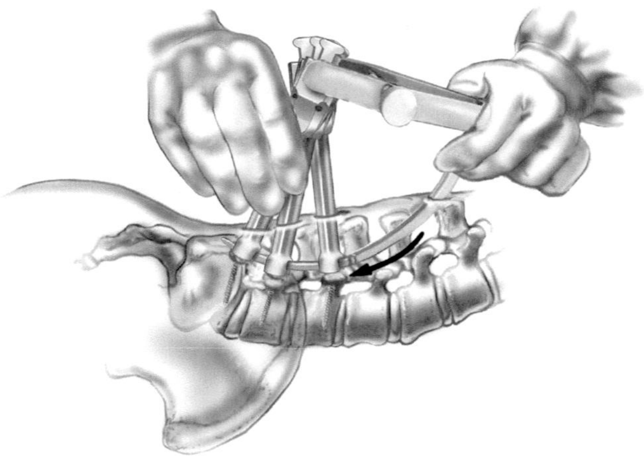

Fig. 13.61 Pass the rod

extender are depressed. The inner sleeve is inserted into the outer sleeve until resistance is encountered (Fig. 13.64a, b). The arrow on the inner sleeve should be visible through the window on the outer sleeve.

13.6.2 Screw and Extender Assembly

The extender assembly is placed on the instrument table, and the two buttons on the two sides of the extender are squeezed. The reduction nut on the top is rotated until a click is heard (Fig. 13.65), and the nut is continuously rotated until "LD" (load) appears in the reduction window on the extender (Fig. 13.66).

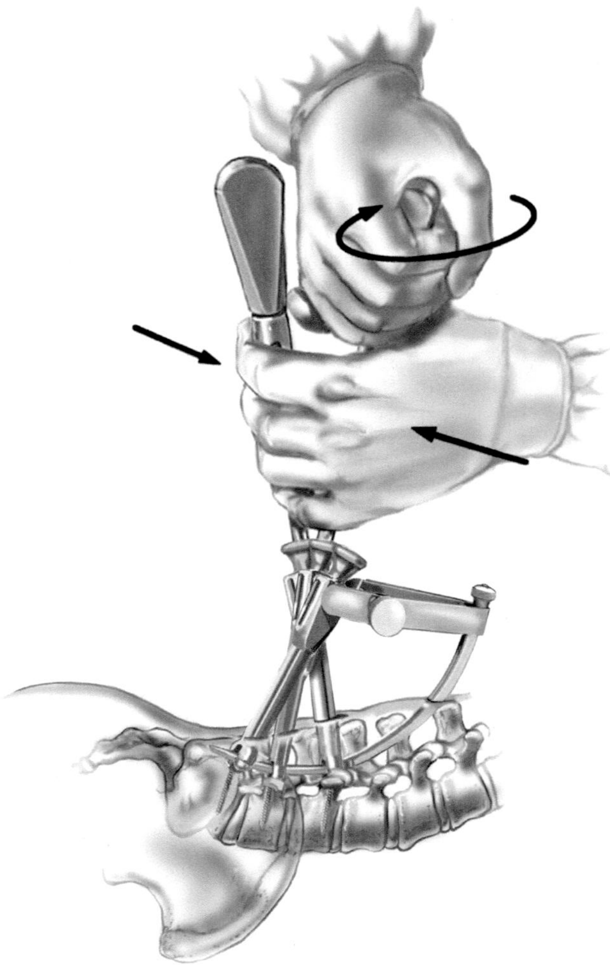

Fig. 13.62 Tighten the screws

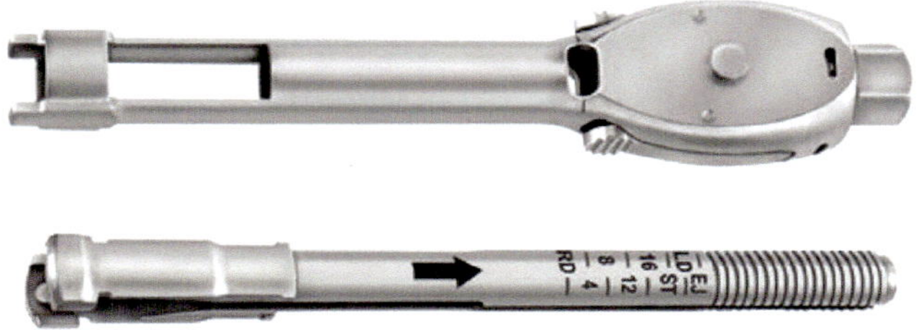

Fig. 13.63 Assemble the reduction extender

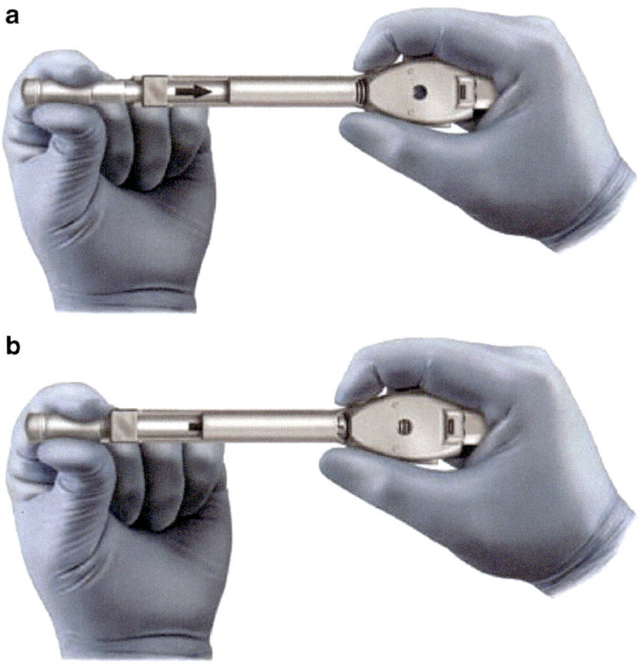

Fig. 13.64 (**a**): Insert the inner sleeve; (**b**): The inner sleeve should be visible through the window on the outer sleeve

13.6.3 Instruments and Implants

After the extender reduction window displays "LD," the LEGACY cannulated screw is inserted into the extender assembly (Fig. 13.67). After confirmation that the screw is correctly placed in the inner sleeve of the extender, the reduction nut is turned in a counterclockwise manner until "ST" (start) is displayed in the reduction window (Fig. 13.68a, b). At this moment, the screw should be securely locked in the extender (Fig. 13.69). The screw is pulled downward to make sure that the screw is securely connected to the extender. After the screw is secured onto the extender, if the screw is to be placed, the buttons on the two sides of the extender are squeezed, and the reduction nut is loosened and the screw is replaced. The new screw can be assembled into the extender by repeating the above procedures.

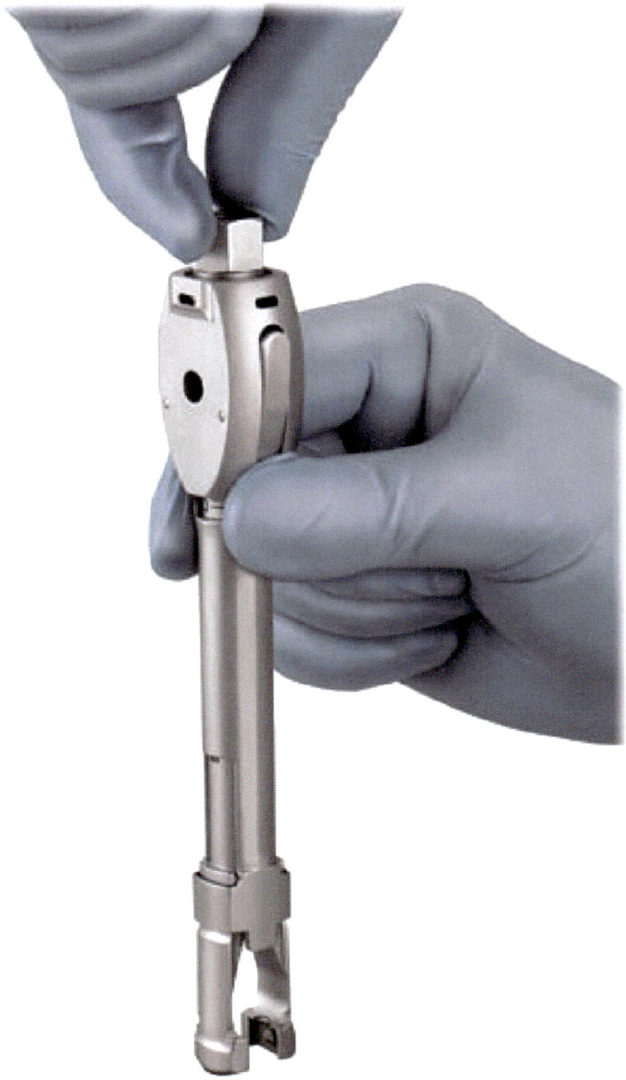

Fig. 13.65 Rotate the top nut

13.6.4 Measuring Reduction Amount

Before spondylolisthesis reduction, under monitoring by intraoperative lateral fluoroscopy, the spondylolisthesis depth gauge instrument is used to determine the amount of reduction of spondylolisthesis. The card slot of the depth gauge instrument is placed on the posterior edge of the spondylolisthetic vertebral body, and the calibrated side is placed on the posterior edge of the neutral vertebral body, which is adjacent to the spondylolisthetic vertebral body (Fig. 13.70a). The spondylolisthesis distance can be read from the scale above the arrow in the card slot (Fig. 13.70b). For accuracy of measurement, the depth gauge instrument should be placed in the same position on the posterior edge of the two vertebral bodies as much as possible. Before the screw and the extender assembly are placed over the guidewire, the

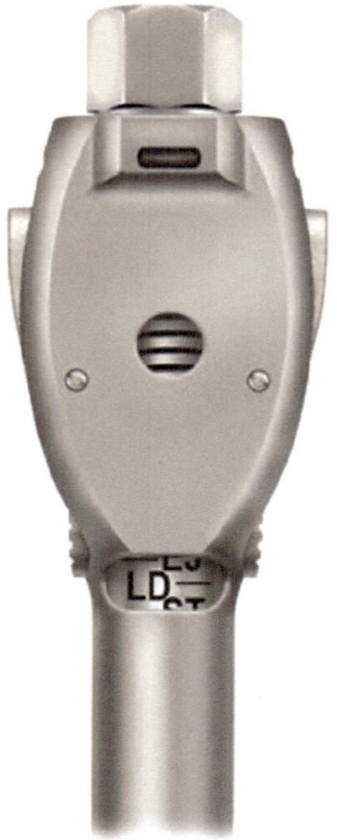

Fig. 13.66 "LD" appears

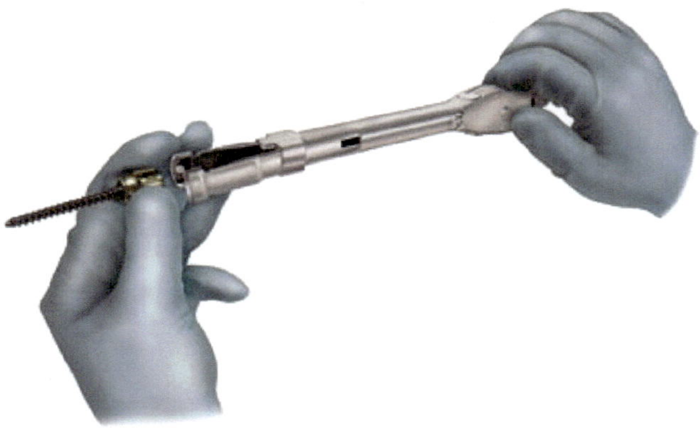

Fig. 13.67 Insert the cannulated screw

amount of reduction should be first set. The extender for the non-spondylolisthetic vertebral body should be in the neutral position, with the number "4" displayed in the reduction window (Fig. 13.70c). The extender for the vertebral body requiring reduction should be set at the estimated amount of reduction needed. For example, to achieve 8 mm of reduction, the extender should be adjusted so the number "8" is displayed in the window.

13.6.5 Screw Insertion

The retaining screwdriver is inserted into the screw extender assembly (Fig. 13.71a). The tip of the driver should pass into the U-shaped groove of the CD HORIZON® LEGACY™ cannulated multi-axial screw until the driver fully engages

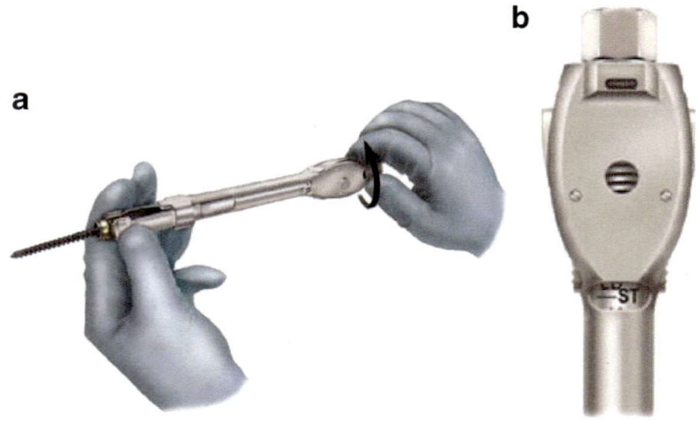

Fig. 13.68 (**a**): Turn the nut; (**b**): ST appears

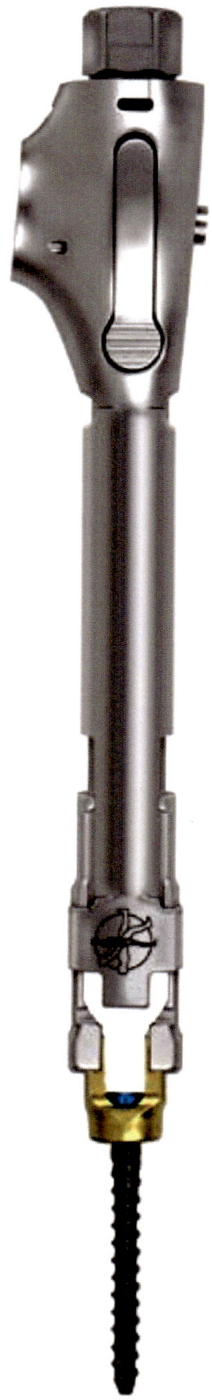

Fig. 13.69 Secure the cannulated screw

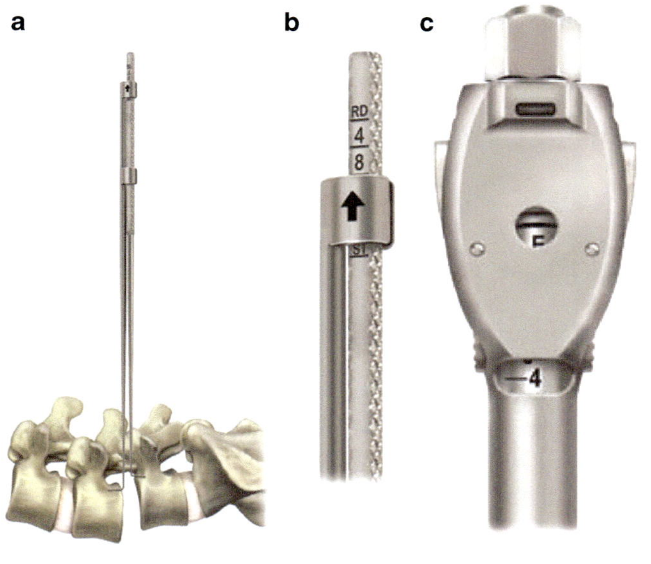

Fig. 13.70 (a): The depth gauge; (b): Read the scale; (c): "4" displays

the screw (Fig. 13.71b). The cannulated screwdriver may be used as an alternative to the retaining screw.

The extender assembly in the neutral position is inserted into the non-spondylolisthetic vertebral body. If the screw is difficult to advance, the assembly is removed while leaving the guidewire in place. If there is any movement of the guidewire during removal of the screw assembly, the guidewire position is confirmed by anteroposterior and lateral fluoroscopy. A tap with the same diameter as the inserted screw is chosen for pedicle tapping, and then the screw extender assembly is reinserted.

Caution: During tapping, it is important to keep the tap and the guidewire in the same axis. If a change in trajectory is required, the outer sleeve of the PAK needle is placed along the guidewire. Then, the guidewire is removed and replaced with the inner stylet. After the screw is advanced into the vertebral body, the guidewire is removed.

The screw should not be inserted too far. If the multi-axial screw is inserted too far, the multi-axial head of the screw will lose its multi-axial capabilities, rendering it difficult for

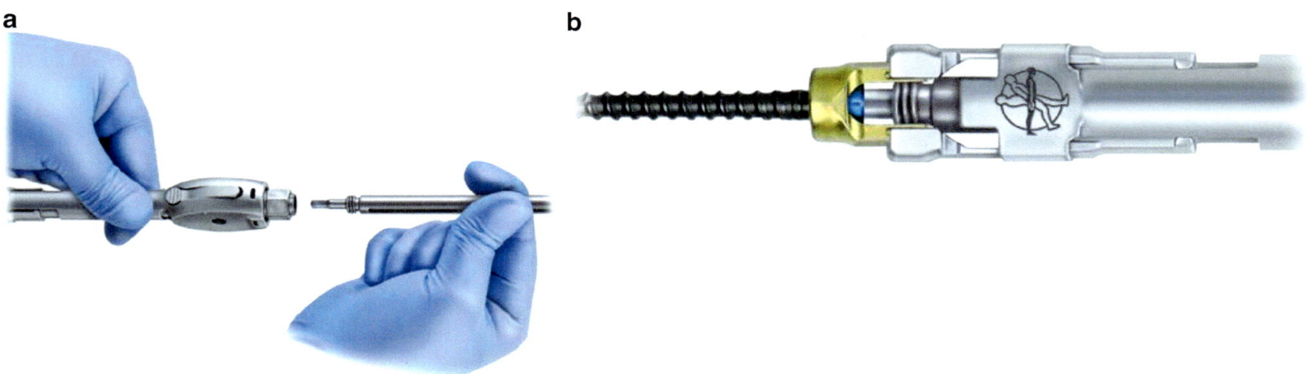

Fig. 13.71 (**a**): Insert the screwdriver; (**b**): Engaging the screw

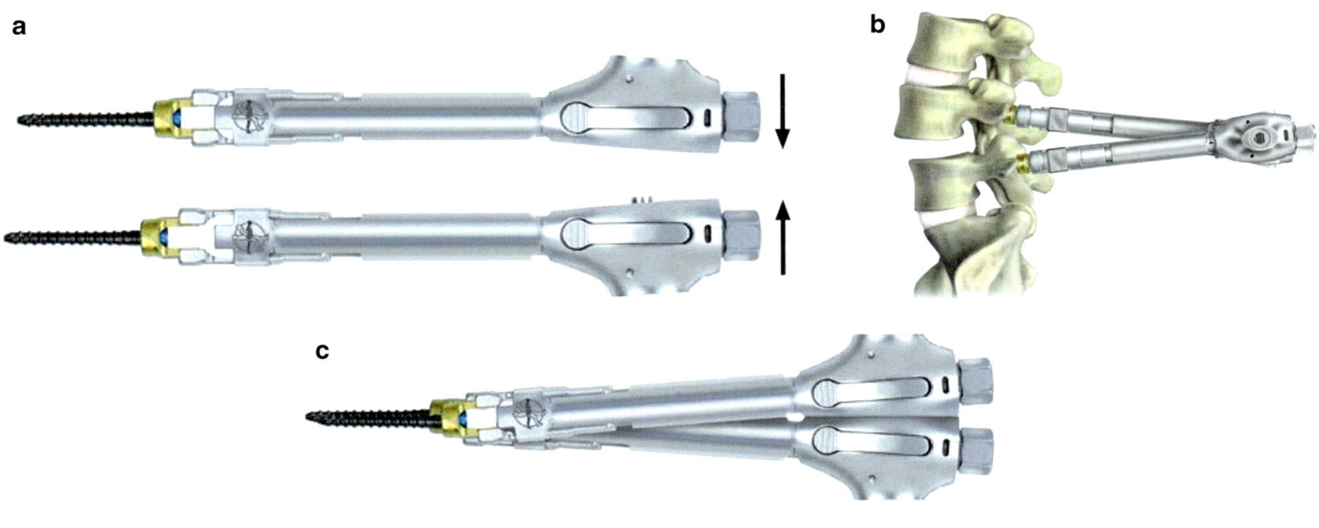

Fig. 13.72 (**a**): Rotate the extenders; (**b**): Mate the extenders; (**c**): No gap between the extenders

subsequent steps. The screw is inserted onto the vertebral body requiring reduction using the extender set for the amount of reduction required.

13.6.6 Connecting the Extenders

The extenders are rotated so that the flat sides are facing each other (Fig. 13.72a). The male and female parts are then mated together and rotated so that there is no gap between the extenders (Fig. 13.72b, c). If there is difficulty in connecting the extenders, adjust the amount of reduction by the extenders using the reduction nut driver so that the extenders are connected. To facilitate rod insertion, the number displayed on any extender reduction window should be greater than 4, which is the minimal distance for inserting the screw into the fixation rod.

13.6.7 Trocar Assembly

Before the rod inserter is connected to the extenders, the latch on the side of the rod inserter is opened, and the trocar is assembled onto the rod inserter. The latch is then closed (Fig. 13.73a, b). The trocar is pulled on to make sure that it is firmly secured.

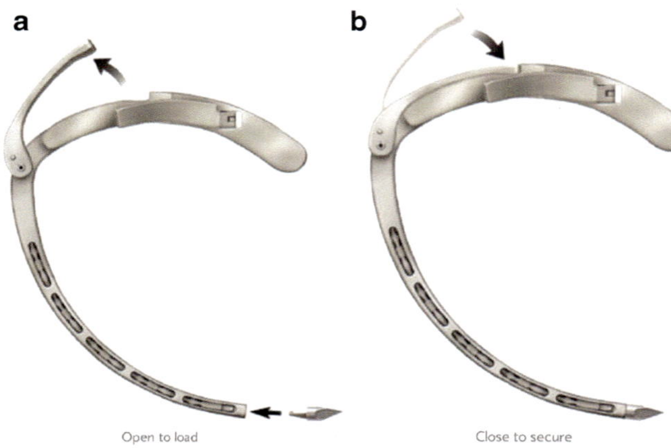

Fig. 13.73 (**a**): Open to load; (**b**): Close to secure

13.6.8 Connecting the Rod Inserter

Open the latch on the side of the rod inserter. Then, one arm of the rod inserter holding the extender is opened and is connected to the tip of one extender (Fig. 13.74a). Thereafter, the other arm is secured to the other extender (Fig. 13.74b). After confirmation that the extenders are securely fit in the arc, the latch is restored to its original position (Fig. 13.74c). Successful connection of the rod inserter with the extenders assures proper passage of the fixation rod through the U-shaped screw saddle (Fig. 13.74d).

13.6.9 Preparation of the Soft Tissue Trajectory

The trocar tip is used to help make a path through the fascia and muscle down to the saddle of the first screw. A small skin incision is then made, and then the trocar tip is advanced through the muscle until it hits the U-shaped saddle of the first screw (Fig. 13.75a, b). The trocar tip position should be confirmed by lateral fluoroscopy.

Caution: The trocar tip should not be inserted too far. It is fine when it reaches the U-shaped saddle of the screw.

13.6.10 Connecting the Rod Inserter

The rod template is inserted into the cephalad extender, and the rod inserter pointer is placed into the caudal extender. The rod template pointer is placed on the stationary rod template to determine the rod length (Fig. 13.76).

After rod placement, the rod template is removed. Then, the rod inserter is withdrawn and the trocar tip is removed. The fixation rod is then assembled.

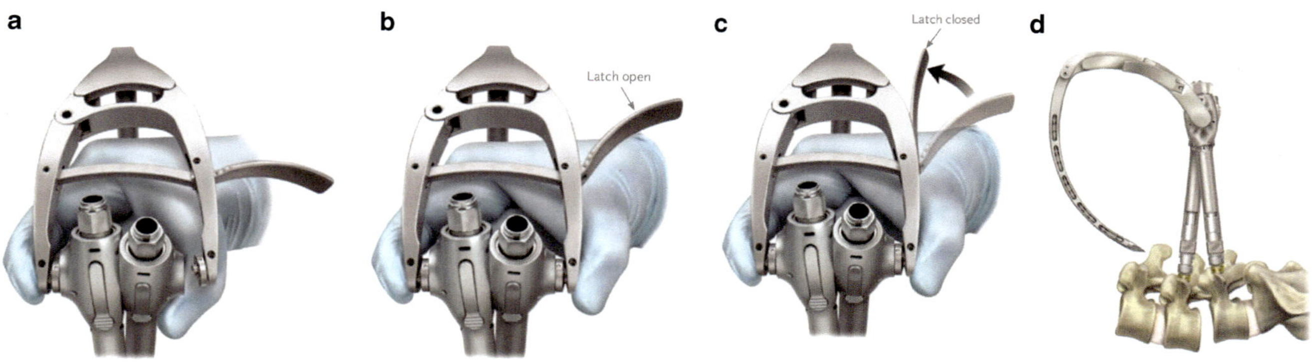

Fig. 13.74 (**a**): Connect one arm to the extender; (**b**): Connect the other arm. (**c**): Close the latch; (**d**): Successful connection

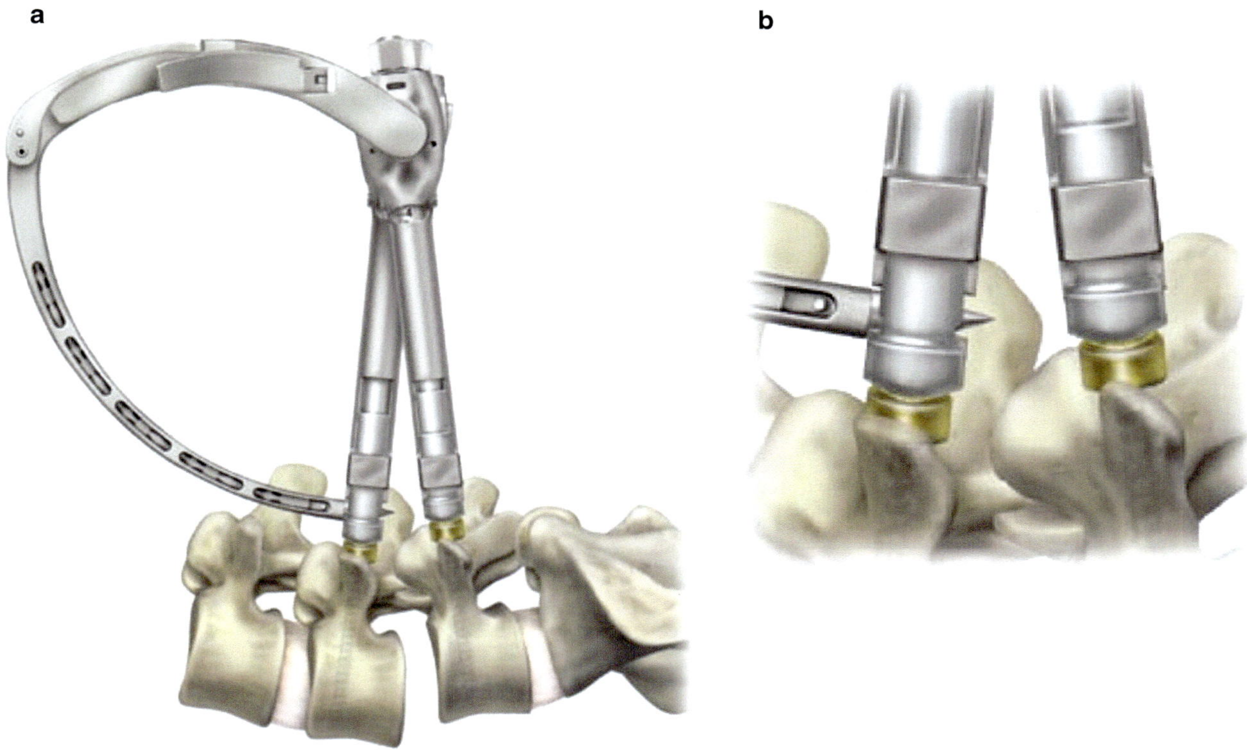

Fig. 13.75 (**a**): Advanced the trocar tip; (**b**): The trocar tip position

Fig. 13.76 Determine the rod length

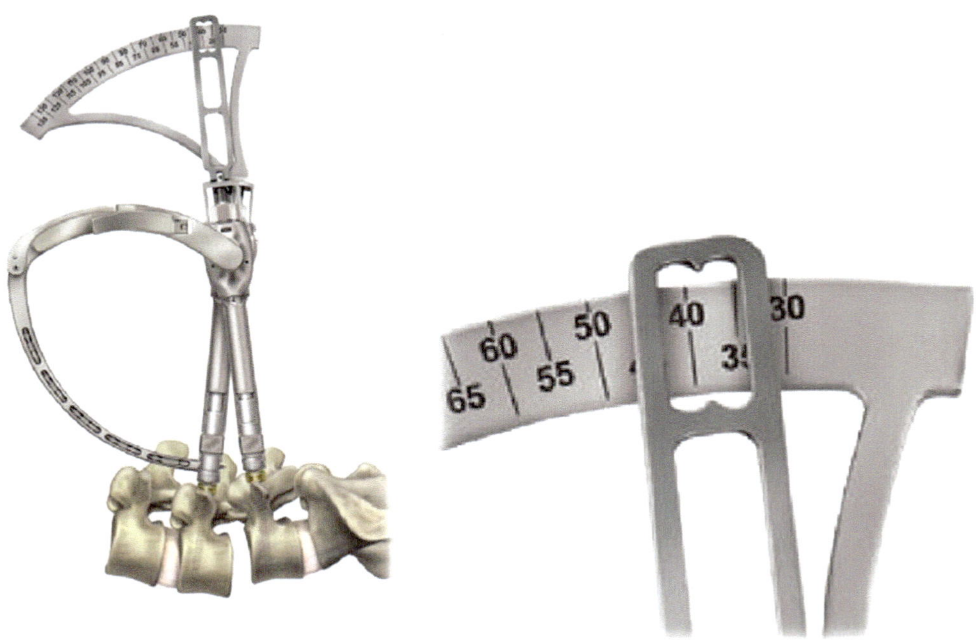

13.6.11 Verification of Rod Passage

To confirm that the rod is through all the screw heads, the bone screwdriver can be used for visual verification whether the rod has successfully reached the U-shaped screw saddle. Push the button on the slider and let it slide to the tip of the driver. The verification driver is placed into the extender in the first screw (Fig. 13.77a). Move the slider to the tip of the extender (Fig. 13.77b) and remove the driver.

13.6.12 Passing the Rod

After the trocar tip is withdrawn, the rod collet is opened and the trocar tip is replaced with an appropriately sized fixation rod. The collet is closed and the fixation rod is tightened.

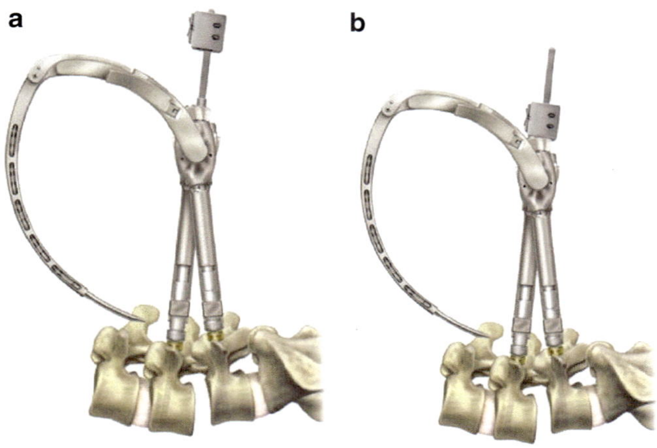

Fig. 13.77 (**a**): Place the verification driver. (**b**): Move the slider

Confirm that the rod is aligned with the axis of the arc by sighting both the side and top-down views. The rod inserter is advanced so that the fixation rod enters the U-shaped saddle of the first screw (Fig. 13.78a). Insert the verification driver into the extender. The presence of a definite distance between the slider of the verification driver and the tip of the extender confirms accurate entry into the U-shaped saddle of the screw (Fig. 13.78b). Rod position can also be verified by fluoroscopy.

Continue advancing the rod inserter so that the fixation rod enters the U-shaped saddle of the second screw. Then, the verification driver is used for confirmation. The rod passage is complete when the trocar is exposed outside of the U-shaped saddle of the distal screw.

After passage of the rod, the extender of the non-spondylolisthetic vertebra is set as "RD" (reduction) (Fig. 13.78c), that is, providing leverage for spondylolisthesis reduction.

13.6.13 Screw Insertion

The Set Screw Retaining Compressor is used to assemble the screw. Push the button on the Compressor handle and insert the screw on the distal tip of the Compressor (Fig. 13.79a, b). Release the button and tug on the screw to ensure a secure connection.

Before screw assembly, adjust the orientation of the rod inserter in the sagittal plane so that the head of the multi-axial screw is positioned for spondylolisthesis reduction (Fig. 13.80a). The screw is assembled first for the neutral vertebral body and provisionally tightened (Fig. 13.80b).

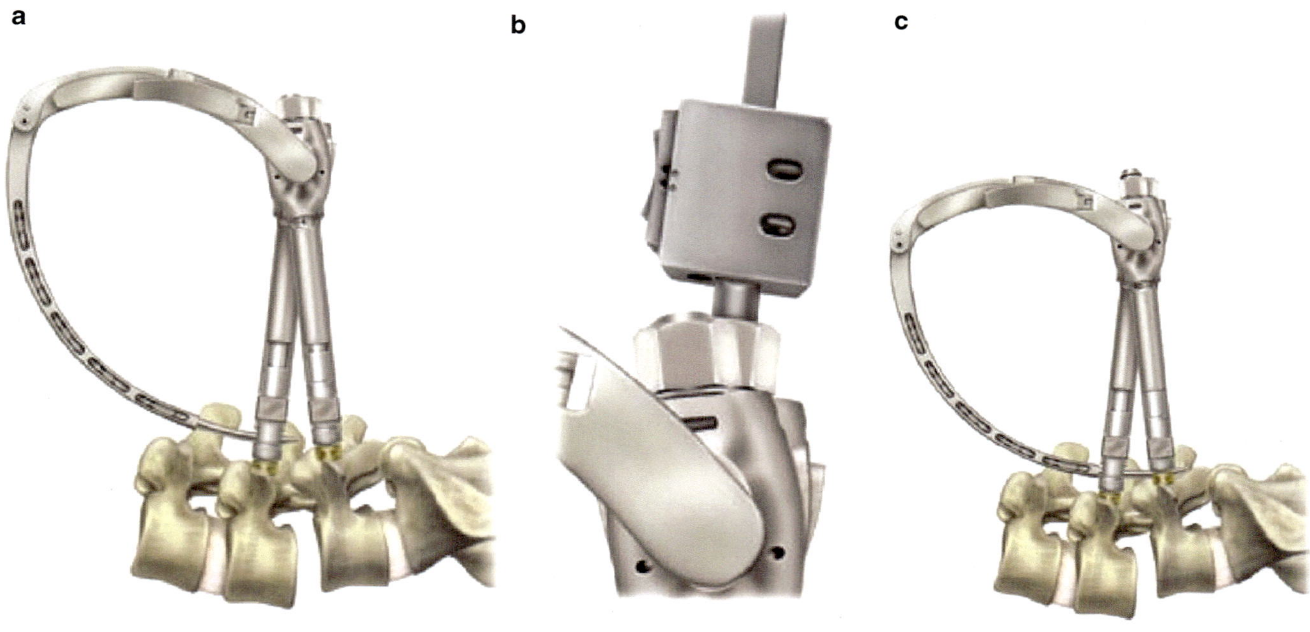

Fig. 13.78 (**a**): The rod enters the U-shaped saddle of the screw. (**b**): Confirm the entry; (**c**): Passage of the rod

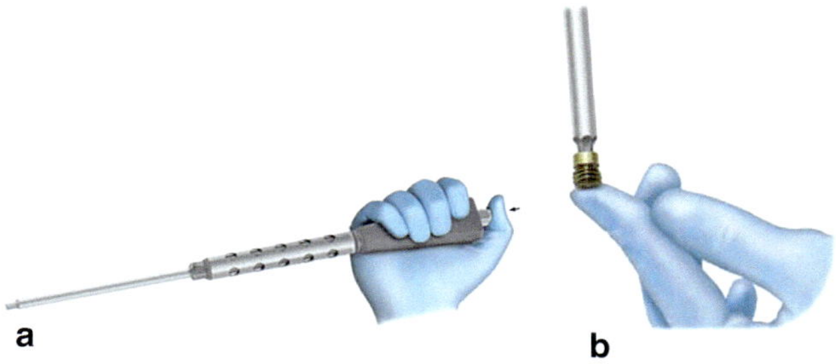

Fig. 13.79 (**a**): The compressor handle; (**b**): Insert the screw

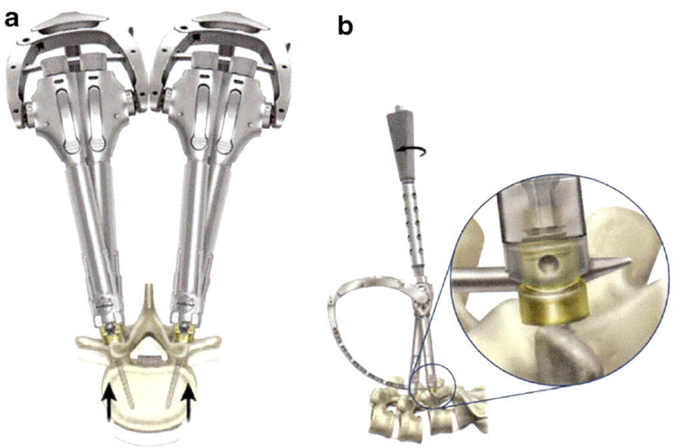

Fig. 13.80 (**a**): Adjust the orientation of the rod inserter; (**b**): Assemble the screw for the neutral vertebral body

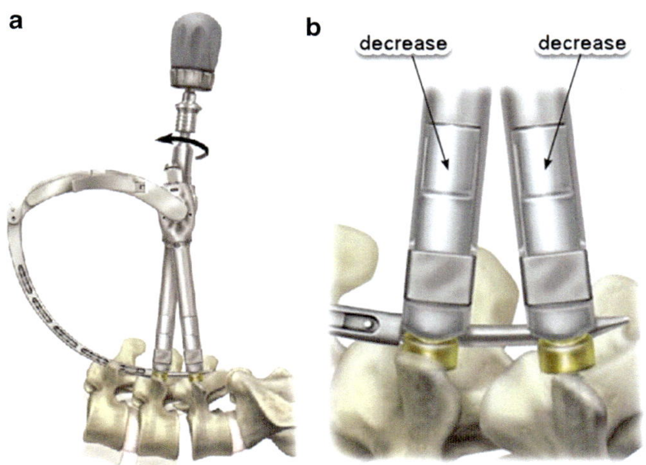

Fig. 13.81 (**a**): Assemble the reduction nut driver; (**b**): Achieve the reduction

13.6.14 Spondylolisthesis Reduction

After the reduction nut driver is assembled onto the quick connect handle, it is connected with reduction nut on the tip of the extender (Fig. 13.81a). The handle is slowly turned to achieve spondylolisthesis reduction (Fig. 13.81b). The process of spondylolisthesis reduction is monitored by fluoroscopy to assure that the screw is not pulled out of the vertebral body. After successful reduction, the screw is inserted using a break-off driver.

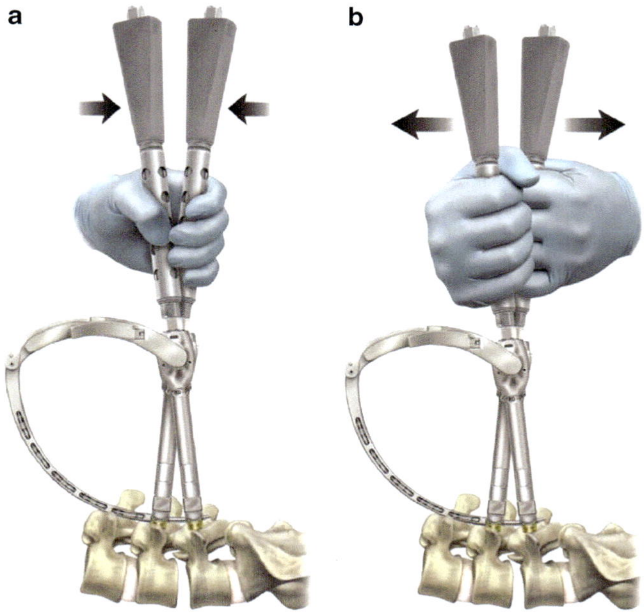

Fig. 13.82 (**a**): Compression; (**b**): Distraction

13.6.15 Compression and Distraction

Before compression or distraction, the screw in the neutral vertebra is loosened, while the screw for the vertebra to be reduced should not be loosened. Tightly hold the two compressor drivers to apply compression. Then, tighten the screw (Fig. 13.82a). Distraction can be achieved by pulling apart the two drivers. Then, the screw is tightened (Fig. 13.82b).

13.6.16 Breaking-Off the Tip of the Screw

The rod inserter can serve as the counter-torque device during screw break-off. After the screw is tightened, the break-off handle is connected to the compressor driver to complete final tightening and breaking-off the tail portion of the screw (Fig. 13.83). The sheared-off portion of the screw is retained in the compressor driver and is removed together with the driver. Do not push the button on the top of the Compressor handle until it is completely removed from the extender shaft as this will release the screw prematurely and the sheared-off portion of the screw becomes detached from the driver and falls into the extender shaft.

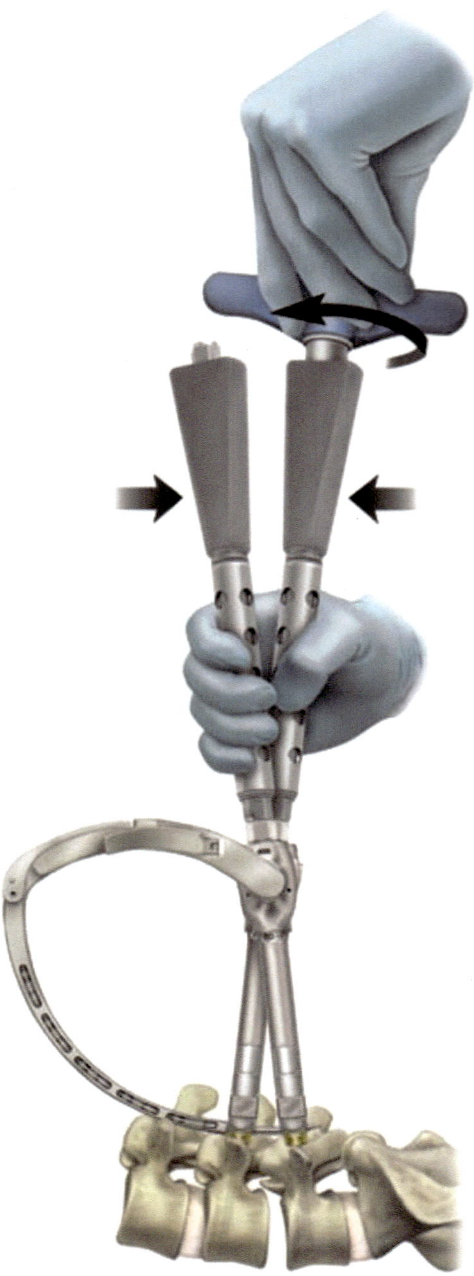

Fig. 13.83 Breaking-off the tip of the screw

13.6.17 Removing the Assembly

The latch on the tip of the rod inserter is opened to release the fixation rod from the rod inserter. Then, the rod-holding arm of the rod inserter is withdrawn (Fig. 13.84a). Then, open the rod inserter with the side lever and remove the rod inserter from the extender (Fig. 13.84b).

The reduction nut on the tip of the extender is loosened in a counterclockwise direction. When the inner sleeve of the head of the extender reaches "ST" (start), depressing buttons on the extender and the extender will release the screw. When it reaches "EJ" (eject), the extender can be removed. Gentle side-to-side rocking may assist in removal of the extenders. The final construct can be verified with anteroposterior and lateral fluoroscopy.

13.6.18 Connecting the Extenders

When performing a two-level procedure, the multilevel reduction extender assembly is used, including two multilevel outer reduction extenders and one multilevel middle reduction extender. Extender placement depends on the type of spondylolisthesis.

13.6.19 Screw Implantation

Screw attachment should be performed as previously described in the one-level procedure section (P9) for assembling the screw and extenders. The screw extender assembly is set in the corresponding vertebral body based on the number and position of listhesed vertebral bodies.

The screw extender assembly is placed over the guidewire, and mate the extenders together (Fig. 13.85a, b). If the extenders are at different heights, the cannulated Ratcheting Egg Handle and the reduction nut driver are used to adjust the height of the middle extender (Fig. 13.85c, d). The Rod Trocar Tip is attached to the inserter and the assembly is attached to the extenders as previously described.

13.6.20 Spondylolisthesis Reduction

As previously described, prior to performing the reduction, prepare the trajectory in the soft tissue, measure the rod length, insert the rod, and verify rod placement using the verification driver and fluoroscopy. When measuring the rod length during a two-level procedure, be sure to use the rod measurement tools in the top and bottom extenders and not the center one. Once the rod is in place, use the cannulated Ratcheting Egg Handle and the reduction nut driver to adjust the height of the outer extenders until "RD" (reduced) appears in the window of the extenders. Place and provisionally tighten the screws in the screws in the cephalad and caudal vertebral bodies to hold the rod in place during the reduction maneuver using the screw retaining compressor.

Begin reducing the listhesed vertebral body by turning the cannulated Ratcheting Egg Handle and the reduction nut driver clockwise (Fig. 13.86a). The reduction process should be gradual and verified frequently with fluoroscopy. When the reduction is complete, insert a screw in the screw head to hold the correction (Fig. 13.86b).

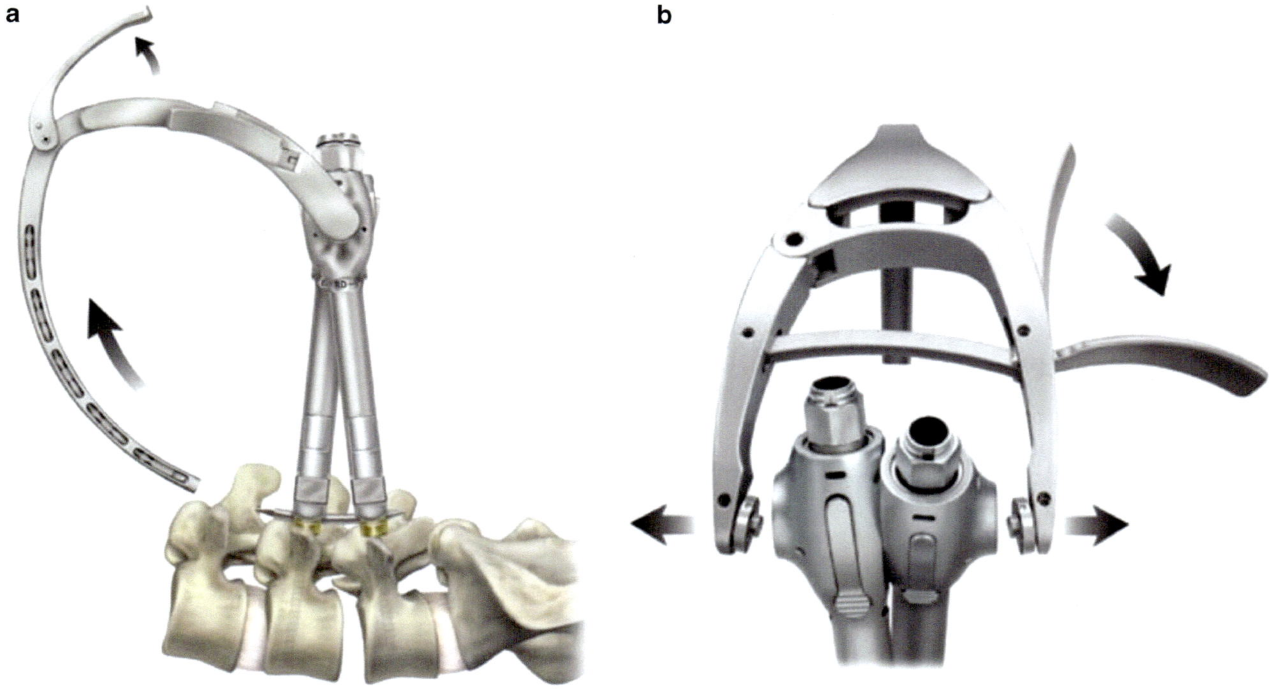

Fig. 13.84 (**a**): Open and unload; (**b**): Open and remove

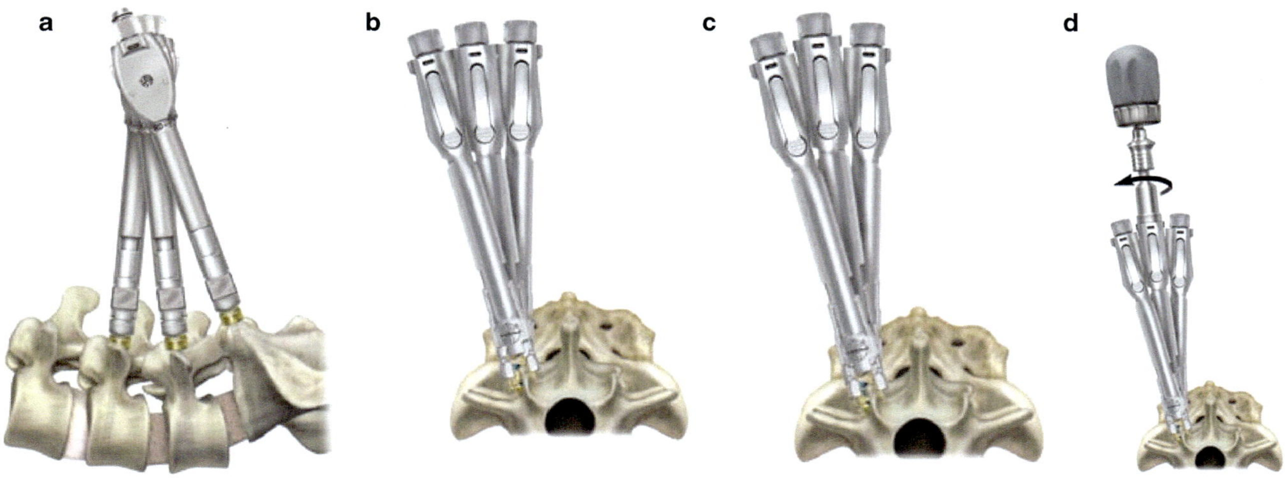

Fig. 13.85 (**a**): Lateral view of the mated extenders; (**b**): Anterior view of the mated extenders; (**c**): Extenders at different heights; (**d**): Adjust the height of the extender

13.6.21 Internal Fixation

If compression or distraction is performed, it should be performed against the middle vertebral body. Do not loosen the screw on the reduced vertebral body once correction has been achieved. The screws should be broken off, as previously described. The final construct should be verified with fluoroscopy (Fig. 13.87).

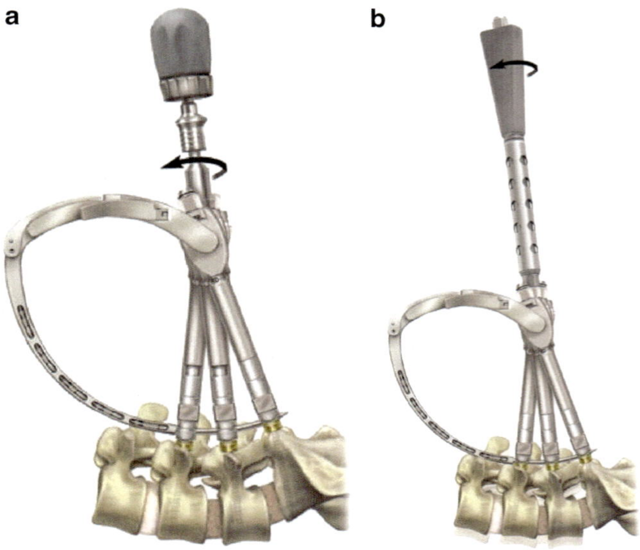

Fig. 13.86 (**a**): Turn the handle clockwise; (**b**): Insert a screw

13.6.22 Unilateral Reduction Technique

When performing a unilateral reduction procedure, the interbody graft may be placed before or after rod insertion and vertebral body reduction, depending upon surgeon preference. Some surgeons choose to insert an interbody trial into the disc space to serve as a fulcrum during the reduction step (Fig. 13.88a). By using this method, the interbody graft is placed after reduction is achieved, which eliminates the possibility of interbody graft shifting during the reduction step (Fig. 13.88b). Once the reduction is complete, the contralateral side is instrumented using the standard percutaneous technique.

13.6.23 Bilateral Reduction Technique

When performing a bilateral procedure, adequate vertebral body release and interbody graft placement must be performed prior to rod insertion (Fig. 13.89a).

Once the rod is passed, the extenders on the non-listhesed vertebral bodies should be adjusted to show "RD" (reduced) in the extender window. Reduction can be achieved bilaterally using a cannulated Ratcheting Egg Handle and reduction nut driver on each side of the listhesed vertebral body (Fig. 13.89b). Reduction can also be achieved by moving from one side to the other making one turn on each side until reduction is complete (Fig. 13.89c).

The T27 Removal Driver is used to remove the CD HORIZON® LEGACY™ cannulated multi-axial screws, set screws, and rods may be removed by applying set screw and turning counterclockwise.

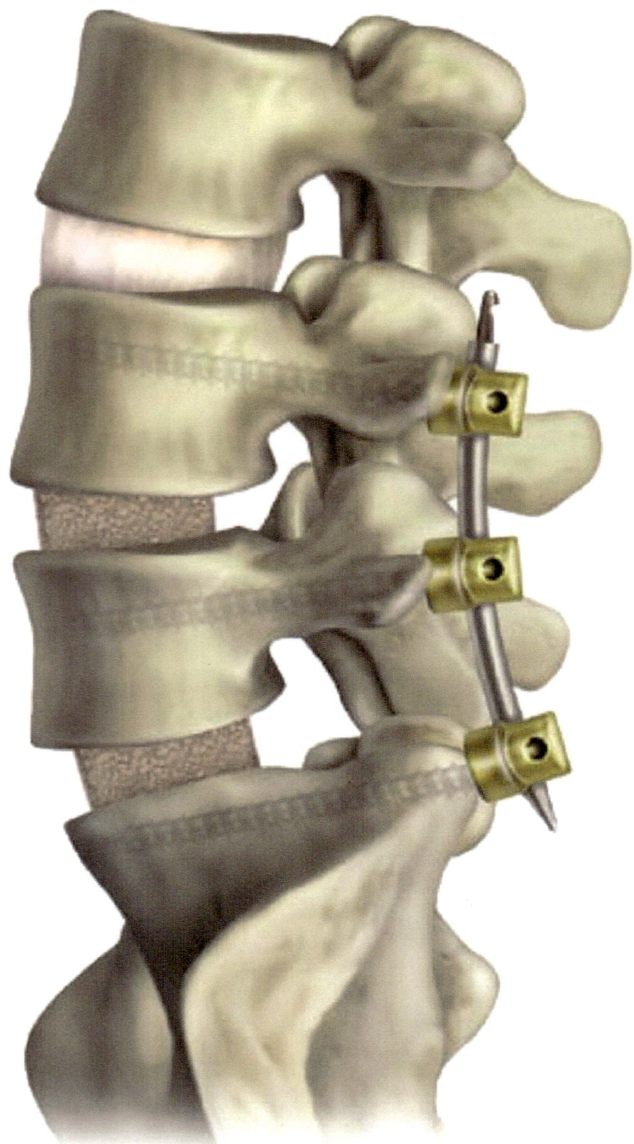

Fig. 13.87 Final construct

13.7 The Multilevel Percutaneous Internal Fixation System

13.7.1 Preoperative Plan

Preoperative plan can be made to determine screw entry site and direction. The anteroposterior and axial films show the approximate location angle of thoracic pedicle screws (Fig. 13.90). Apart from the steps described below, bone graft is required when implants are used.

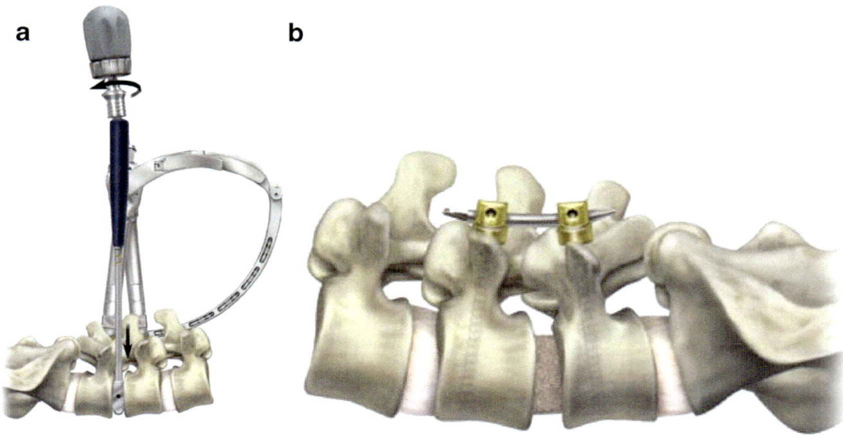

Fig. 13.88 (**a**): Interbody trial reduction; (**b**): Position of the interbody graft

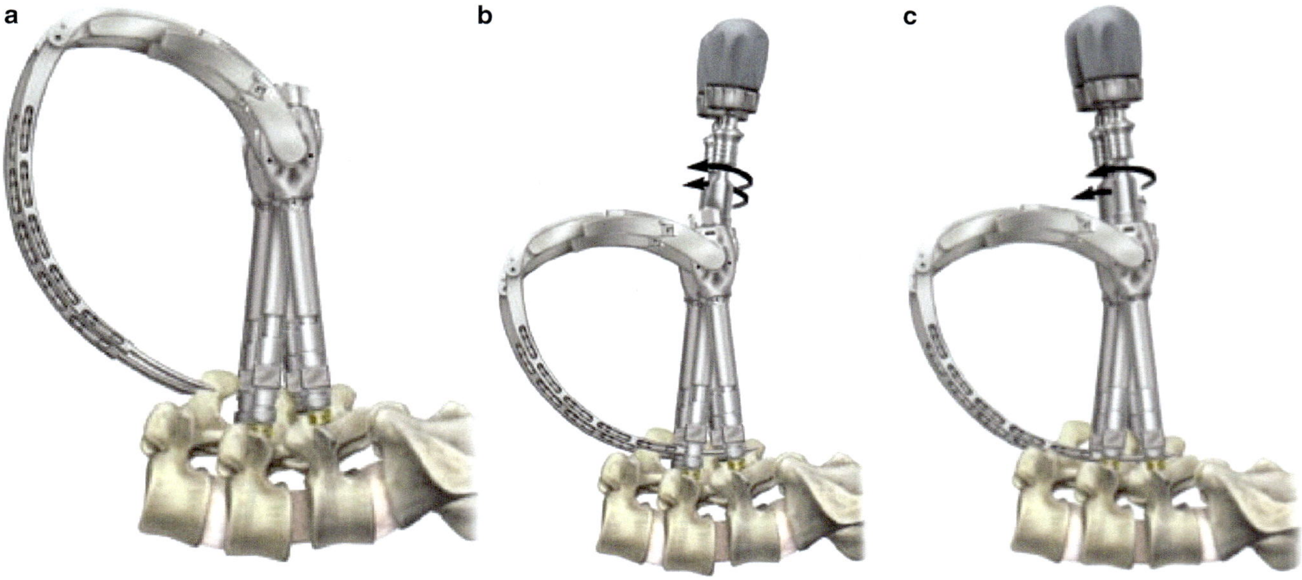

Fig. 13.89 (**a**) Vertebral body release and interbody graft placement; (**b**): Using the cannulated Ratcheting Egg Handle and reduction nut driver to reduce; (**c**): Reduction from one side to the other

13.7.2 Patient Position

Patients are placed in the prone position. Radiolucent frames or chest pad towel can be used. Knee-to-chest position should be avoided. Make sure that anteroposterior and lateral fluoroscopic images of the pedicles can be obtained before proceeding to the next step (Fig. 13.91).

13.7.3 Skin Incision

A 22-gauge spinal needle is used to determine the proper location of skin incision (Fig. 13.92a). By the anteroposterior images, the puncture needle is placed in the skin area directly superior to the pedicle and then moves laterally 1–2 cm and enters the skin at the intersection of the facet and the transverse process (Fig. 13.92b).

Anteroposterior and lateral images should be used to determine proper needle entry site (Fig. 13.93a, b). Once the entry site is set, an incision, approximately 18 mm in length, is made in the skin and fascia.

13.7.4 Entering the Pedicle

A PAK needle connected to a nerve integrity monitor is used to puncture the pedicle using the entry site determined as described above (Fig. 13.94a). The PAK needle enters the pedicle via the intersection of the facet and the transverse process. The trajectory of the needle is con-

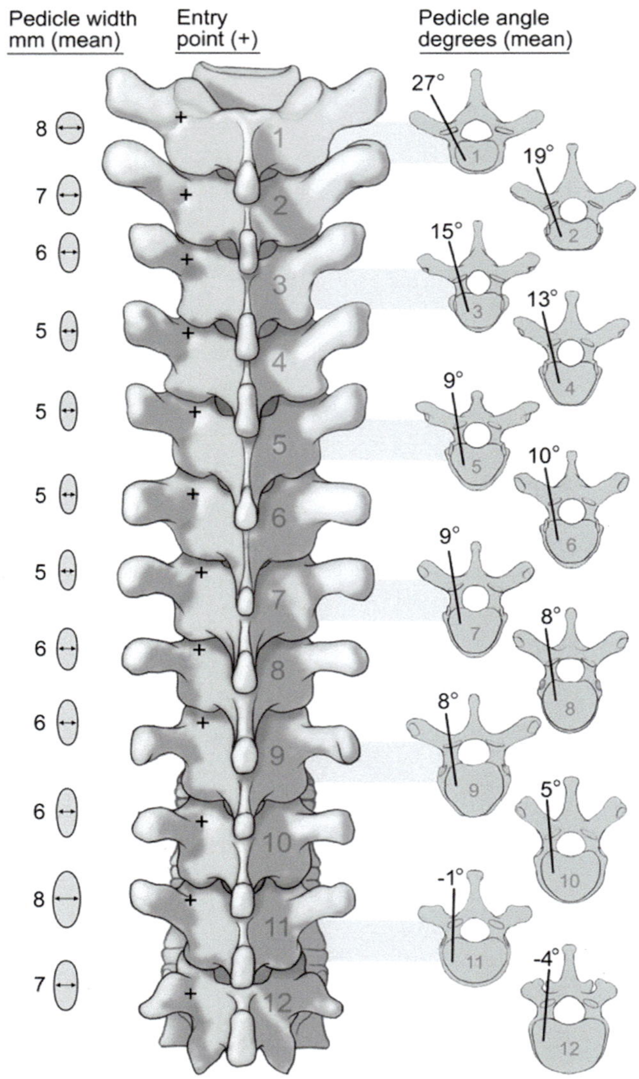

Fig. 13.90 Screw entry site and direction

trolled under anteroposterior and lateral fluoroscopy intermittently. On the anteroposterior images, the needle tip starts from the lateral border of the pedicle; when the needle reaches the pedicle base, the images show that the needle tip has reached the center of the pedicle (Fig. 13.94b, c, d).

Pearls: If at the base of the pedicle the needle is inside the pedicle while the sleeve enters the vertebral body obliquely, the oblique needle may be shown to penetrate the inner wall of the pedicle (Fig. 13.95).

Pearls: NIM PAK needle is advanced until it passes beyond the junction of the pedicle and the vertebral body facilitates guidewire placement. When the NIM PAK needle reaches the base of the pedicle on lateral fluoroscopy, anteroposterior and lateral fluoroscopy is undertaken to make sure that the needle is placed in the pedicle center.

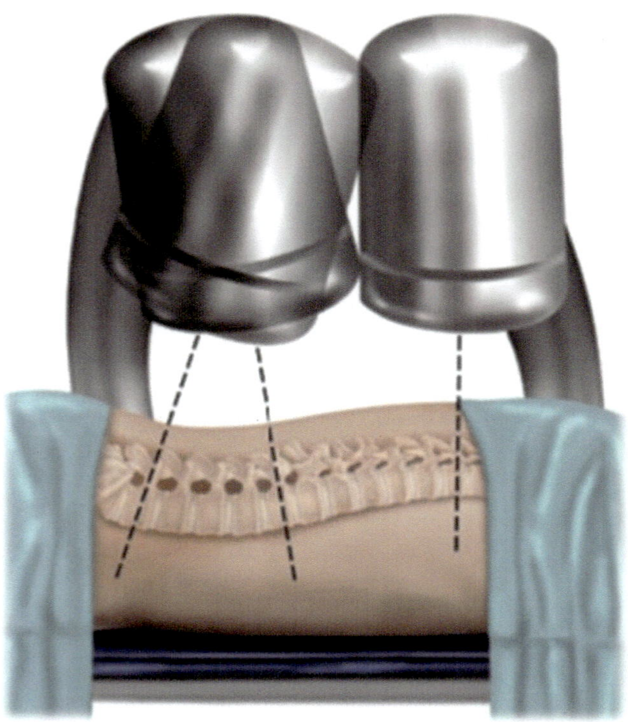

Fig. 13.91 Patient position

13.7.5 Neuromonitoring of Nerve Integrity

For neuromonitoring, a NIM PAK needle may be used to access the pedicle. Triggered EMG monitoring can be performed during advancement of the needle into the pedicle to ensure proper placement. The trigger EMG can monitor any stimulation of the nerve roots during needle advancement (Fig. 13.96a, b, c).

13.7.6 Removal of Handle and Needle Stylet

To remove the NIM PAK needle handle, rotate the tightening device to the unlock position and gently pull up the handle. Make sure that the cannula is not removed from the pedicle (Fig. 13.97). If a PAK needle is used, the needle style should then be removed.

13.7.7 Guidewire Insertion

The guidewire is inserted into the cannula and advanced into the pedicle (Fig. 13.98a). The cannula of the NIM PAK needle is removed using the rotation technique and leave the guidewire in place (Fig. 13.98b).

Pearls: The guidewire should be advanced 50–70% into the vertebral body to facilitate screw placement (Fig. 13.98a).

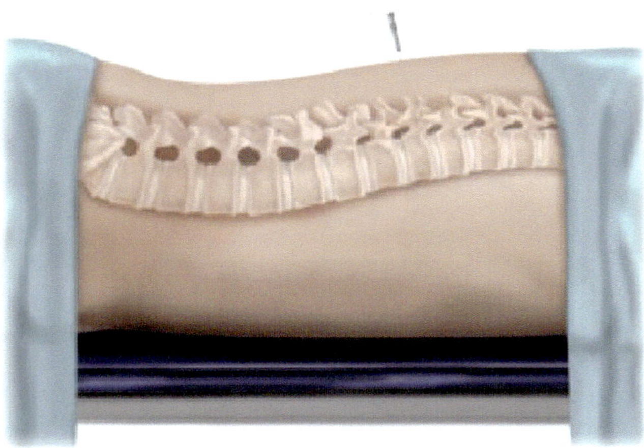

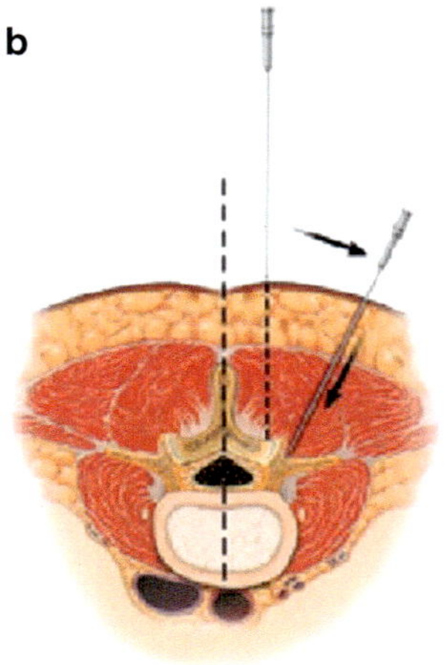

Fig. 13.92 (**a**): Determine the proper location of skin incision; (**b**): Enter the needle at the intersection of the facet and the transverse process

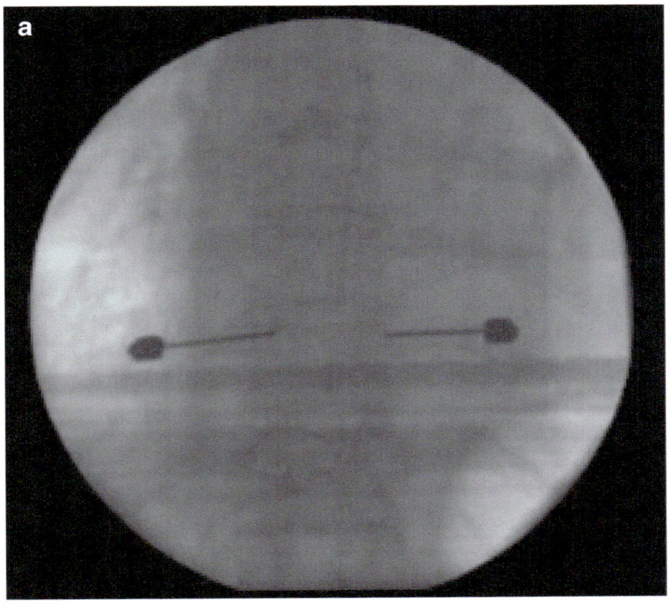

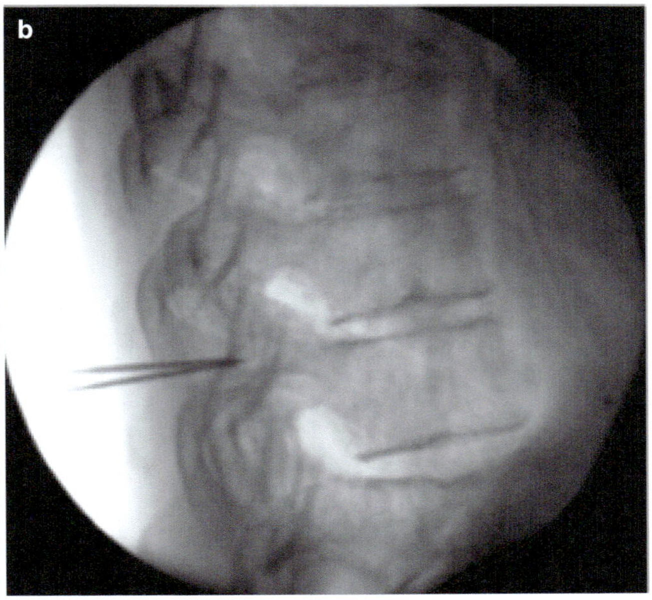

Fig. 13.93 Anteroposterior (**a**) and lateral images (**b**)

Be careful when removing the cannula so that the guidewire is not taken out at the same time. The guidewire should be held firmly when the cannula is removed (Fig. 13.98b).

13.7.8 Advancing the Remaining Guidewire

Repeat steps 2 to 6 to insert the remaining guidewire (Fig. 13.99). Please note, for the sake of simplicity, placement of the guidewire, screw extenders, and rod is shown only on one side.

13.7.9 Dilation of the Muscles

The fascia and muscle should be dilated before screw placement (Fig. 13.100a). Three ordered dilators are used to gently make a path of the appropriate dimension (Fig. 13.100b). When the NIM-SPINE system is used, the large size blue disposable dilator should be used.

Pearls: The dilator should be flushed against the bony structure to maximally prevent soft tissue creepage into the trajectory.

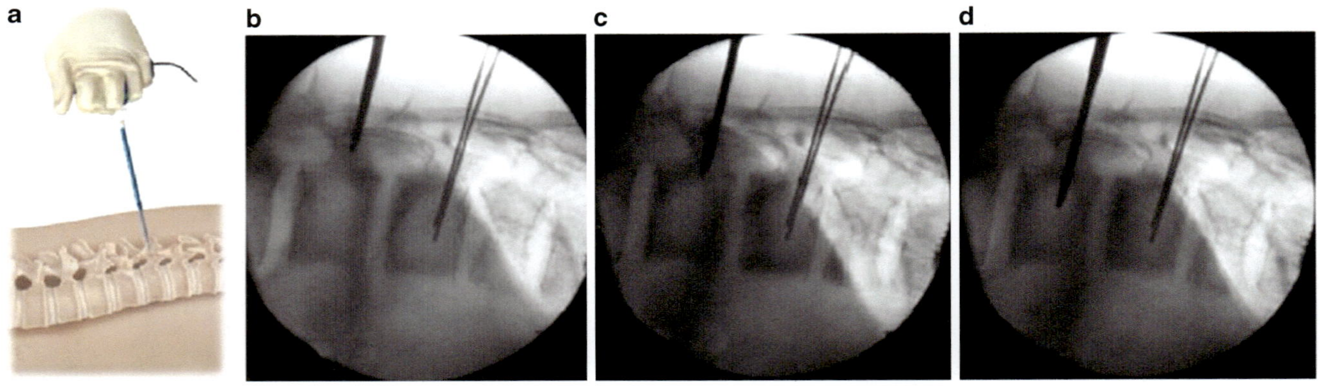

Fig. 13.94 (**a**): PAK needle; (**b**, **c**, **d**): The needle tip enters the pedicle

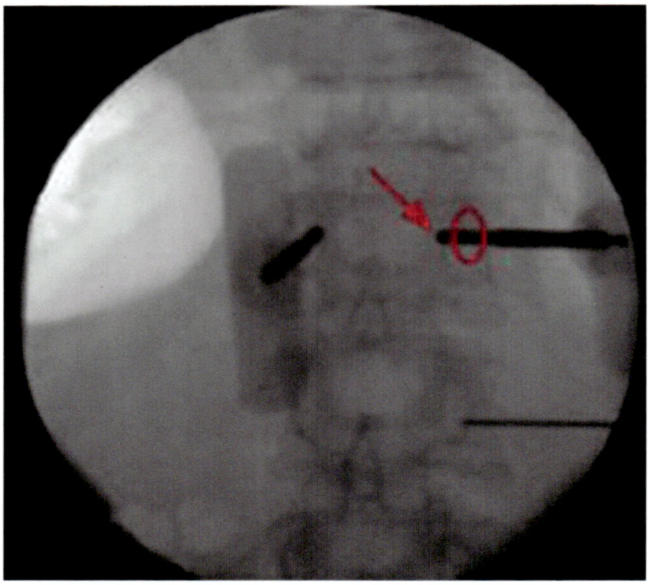

Fig. 13.95 Penetrate the inner wall of the pedicle

13.7.10 Removal of the Dilators

The first two dilators are removed, leaving the third dilator to serve as a tissue protection sleeve during tapping (Fig. 13.101).

Pearls: When removing the first two dilators, be careful that the guidewire is not removed at the same time.

13.7.11 Pedicle Tapping

The pedicle is prepared by placing the tap over the guidewire and through the third dilation sleeve (Fig. 13.102a). The tapped pedicle is further evaluated using the NIM-SPINE system, and the tap is stimulated using a surgeon-directed ball tip probe (Fig. 13.102b).

13.7.12 Tap Removal

The tap is removed, but the guidewire should be left in place (Fig. 13.103).

Pearls: If you tap beyond the tip of the guidewire, bone within the end of the tap may cause the guidewire to pull out as you remove the tap. To avoid this, advance the guidewire through the tap before you remove the tap from the vertebral body.

13.7.13 Removal of the Last Dilator

Remove the last dilator and keep the guidewire in place (Fig. 13.104). Repeat steps 9–13 for other vertebral segments.

13.7.14 Inserting the Inner Sleeve

Before screw insertion in the pedicle screw, the screw extenders should be assembled with appropriate screws. The inner sleeve is inserted into the extender, and make sure that the marks in the window on the extender can be seen (Fig. 13.105). The inner sleeve is inserted until the arrow on the inner sleeve becomes invisible through the window on the outer sleeve.

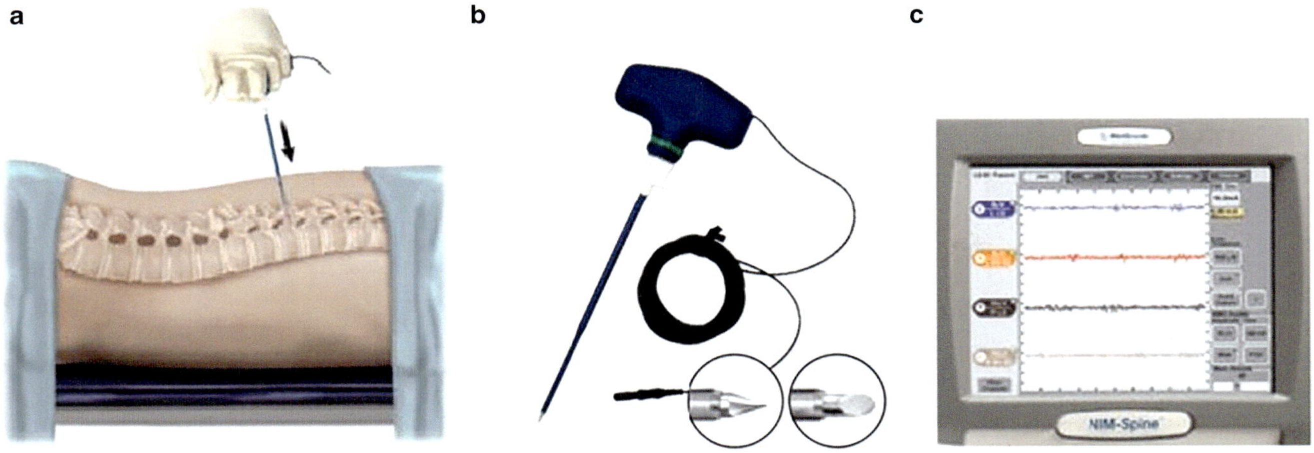

Fig. 13.96 (**a**): The PAK needle, (**b**): Needle connected to the neuromonitoring device, (**c**): The neuromonitoring device

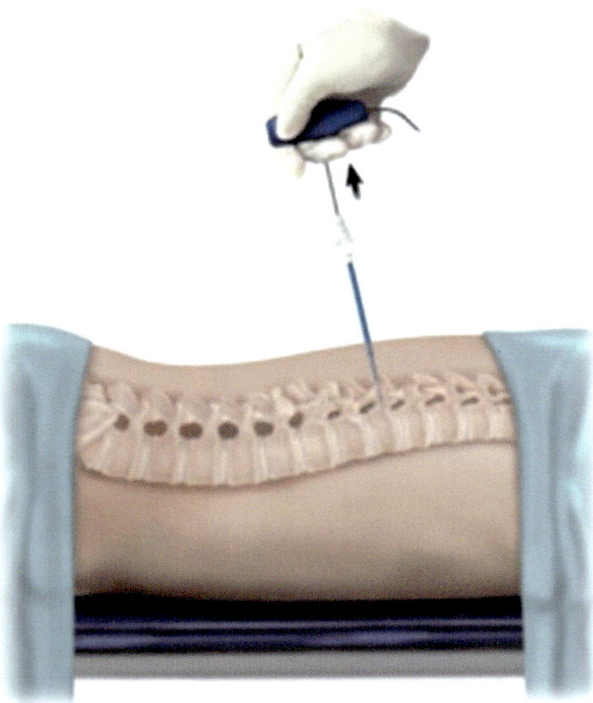

Fig. 13.97 Remove the handle and keep the cannula

13.7.15 The Inner Sleeve Is Adjusted to "LD"

Rotate the proximal hexagon screw on the inner sleeve. A click can be heard when "EJ" (ejection) reaches the window. Let the marker pass through the window until "LD" (load) is aligned with the window (Fig. 13.106a, b). There is no click sound when the inner sleeve stops at "LD."

Pearls: If at the beginning the hexagon screw can rotate freely but the inner sleeve does not advance, gently pull up the inner sleeve to make the thread fit.

Pearls: If there is difficulty in tightening the hexagon screw manually, a handle with a hexagon connector can be used to increase leverage (Fig. 13.107).

13.7.16 Assembling and Tightening the Screw

An appropriate screw is inserted into the distal inner sleeve after the "LD" is aligned. Make sure that the head of the screw closely matches the inner sleeve (Fig. 13.108a). Rotate cephalad hexagon screw on the outer extender until the inner sleeve is at "ST" (start) and clicks. The marker can be seen on the window and the top of the hexagon knob (Fig. 13.108b, c).

Pearls: If there is difficulty in rotating the hexagon screw, examine screw alignment and make sure that the screw is not slightly rotated.

13.7.17 Screwdriver Insertion

The retaining bone screwdriver is inserted into the screw extender assembly. The tip of the driver passes into the multiaxial screw until the driver fully engages the bone screw. Thread the sleeve of the retaining driver into the head of the screw until it is finally tightened.

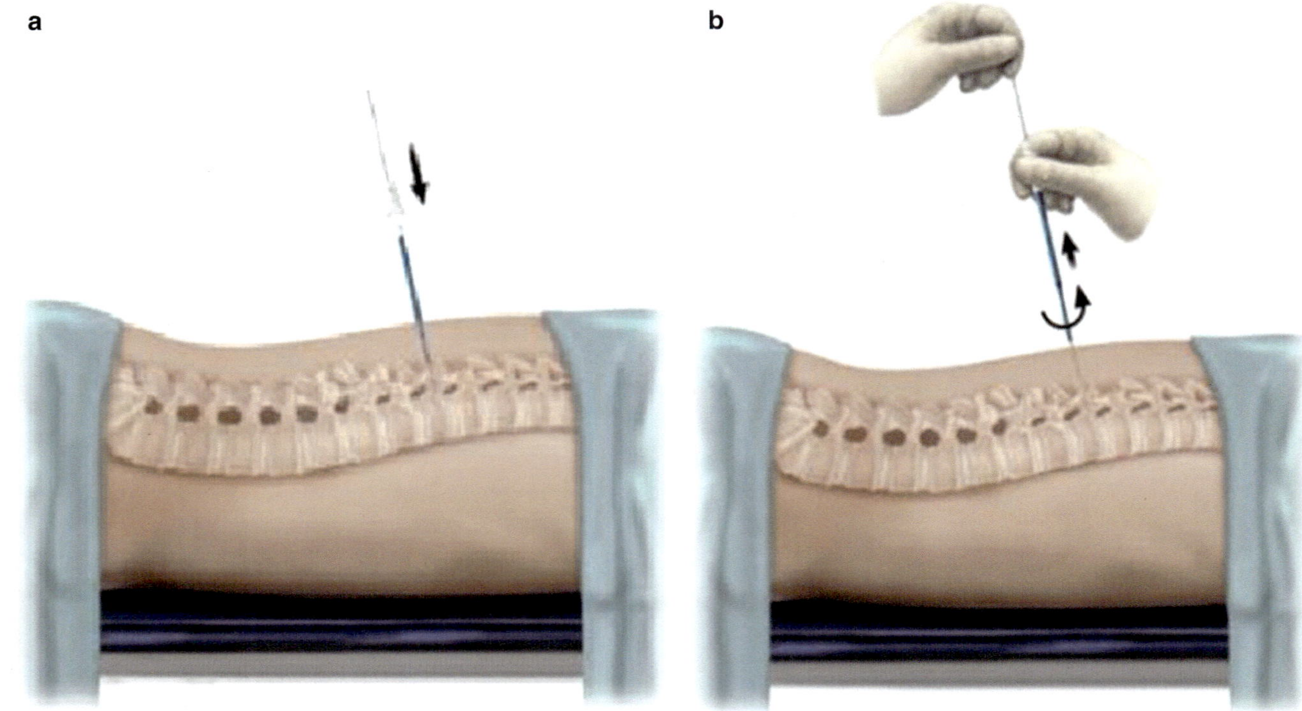

Fig. 13.98 (a): Insert the guidewire; (b): Remove the cannula

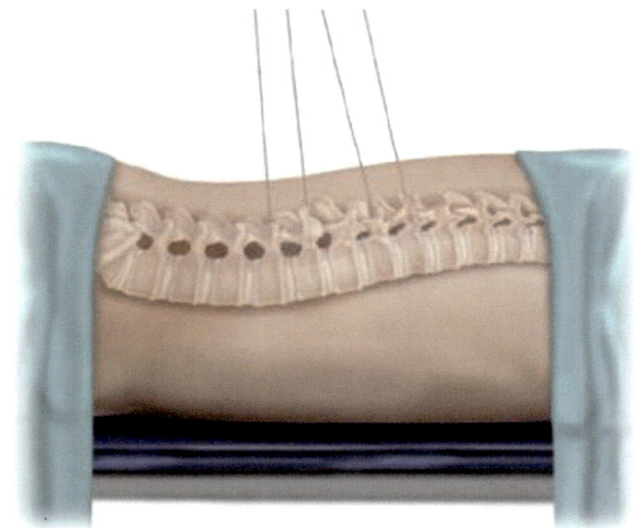

Fig. 13.99 Insert the remaining guidewire

Pearls: If desired, the non-retaining bonescrew driver can be used.

13.7.18 Insertion of the Screw Extender Assembly into the Pedicle

The entire screw extender assembly is inserted over the guidewire and into the pedicle (Fig. 13.109a, b). If the multi-axial head of the LEGACY cannulated screw is driven too forcefully against the bone, it will lose its multi-axial capabilities.

Pearls: The guidewire can be removed after the screw assembly retains the pedicle in order to avoid the guidewire to be inadvertently brought in.

Pearls: Extreme caution should be exercised to avoid pulling out the guidewire inadvertently by inserting the screw without guide.

Pearls: Once the screw is in place, screw extenders push away the fascia and skin surrounding the screw extender using a nerve hook.

13.7.19 Placement of the Remaining Screw Extenders

Steps 7–19 are repeated and additional screw extenders are placed (Fig. 13.110).

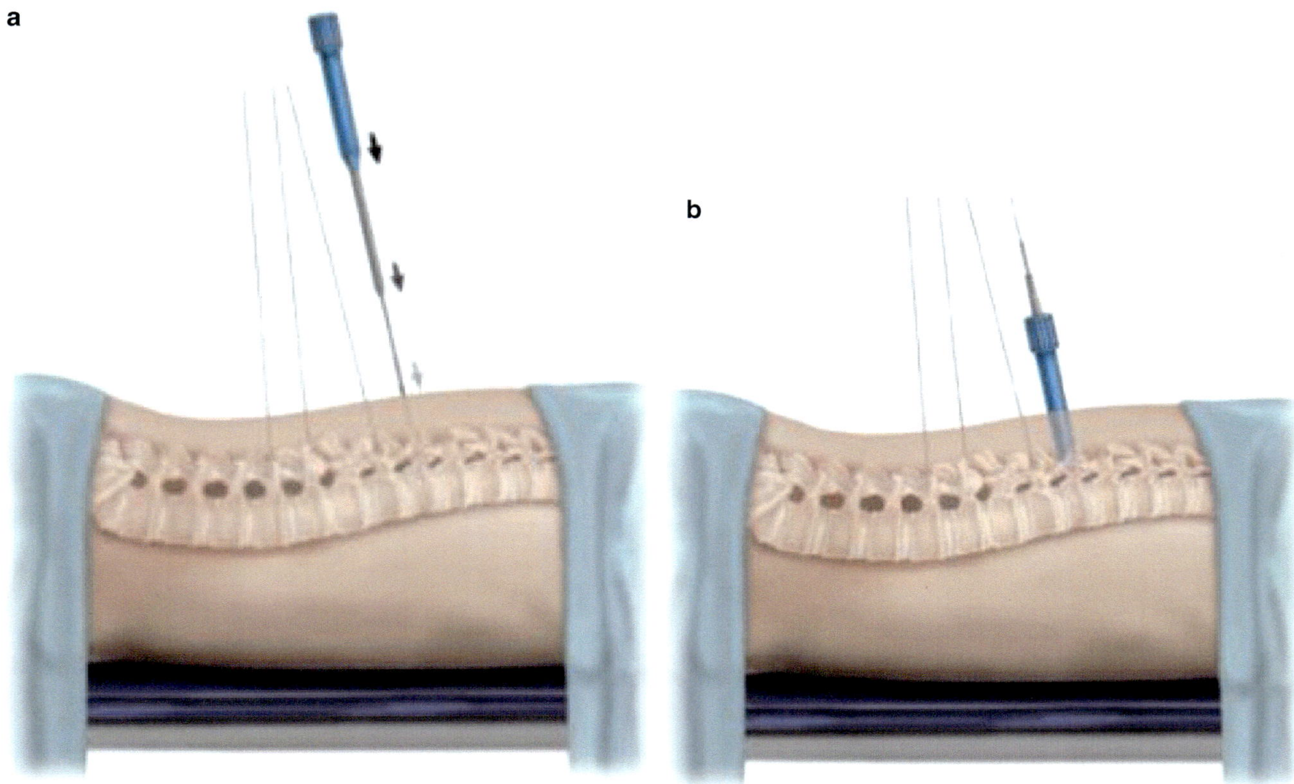

Fig. 13.100 (**a**): Dilate the fascia and muscle; (**b**): Three ordered dilators

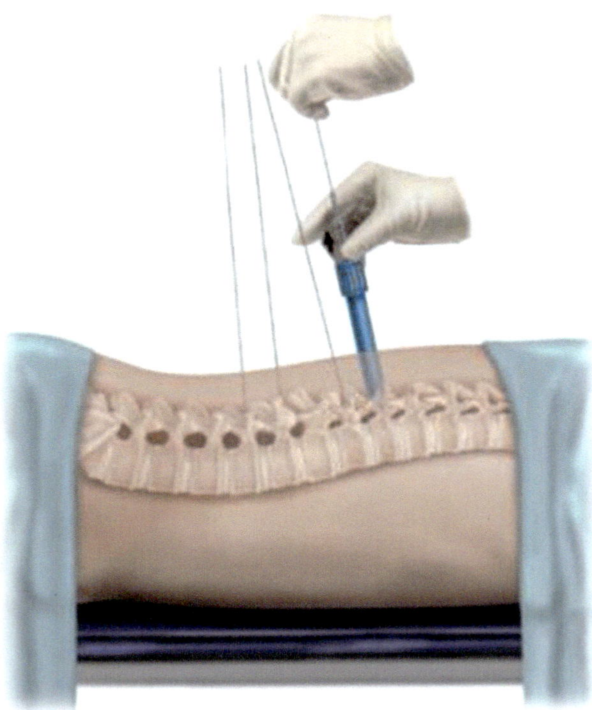

Fig. 13.101 Remove the first two dilators

13.7.20 Extender Alignment for Passing the Rod

Once all the extenders are assembled in place, rotate the extenders so that the button and the window face inward/outward (Fig. 13.111).This makes the distal rod window in the extender in the same line, allowing the rod to pass through.

13.7.21 Measuring the Rod Length

The rod template is flushed against the extender and placed on the skin. The rod template should completely fit the skin based on the body surface curvature (Fig. 13.112). The rod length is calculated by reading the length from the rod template.

13.7.22 Attaching the Rod to the Rod Inserter

An appropriately sized rod is inserted by opening and lifting the latch on the top of the rod inserter through pushing back the latch on the back. Then, the latch on the top is closed until

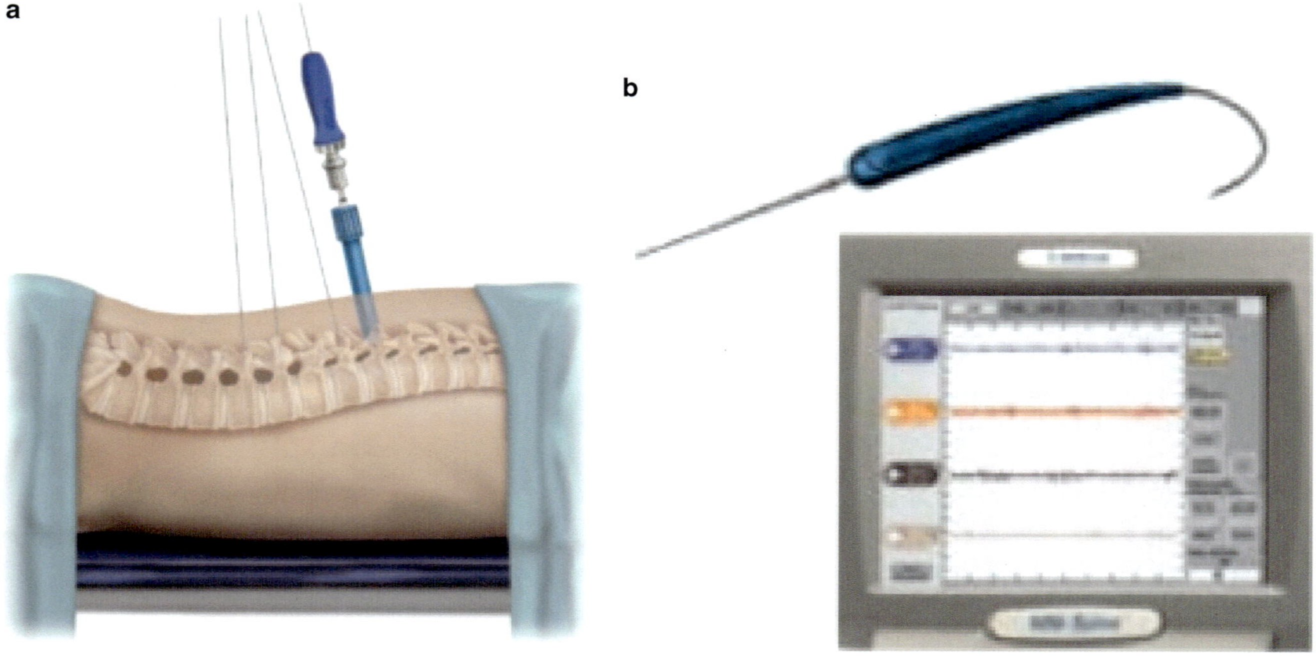

Fig. 13.102 (**a**): Tap the pedicle; (**b**): NIM-SPINE system

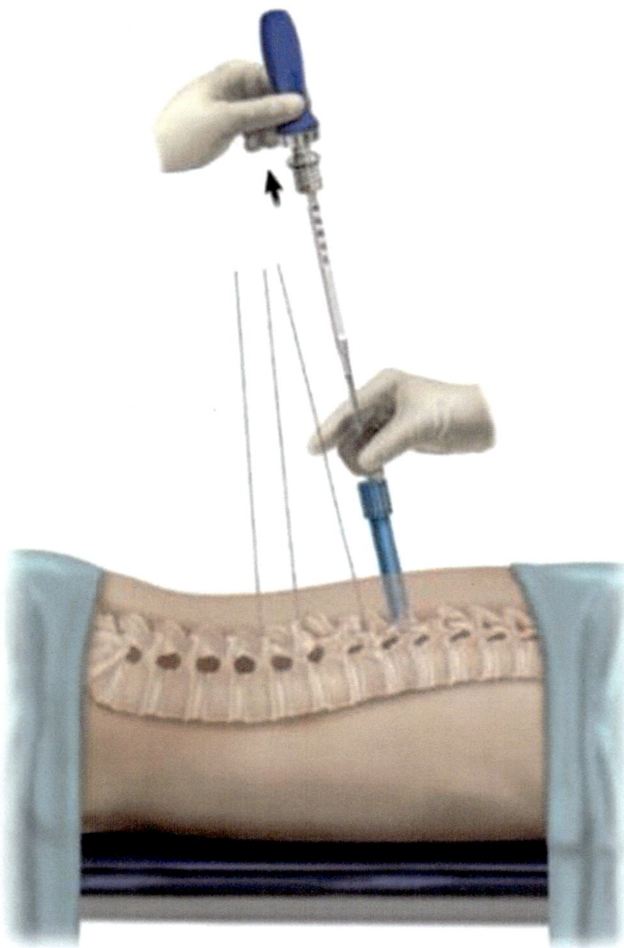

Fig. 13.103 Remove the tap

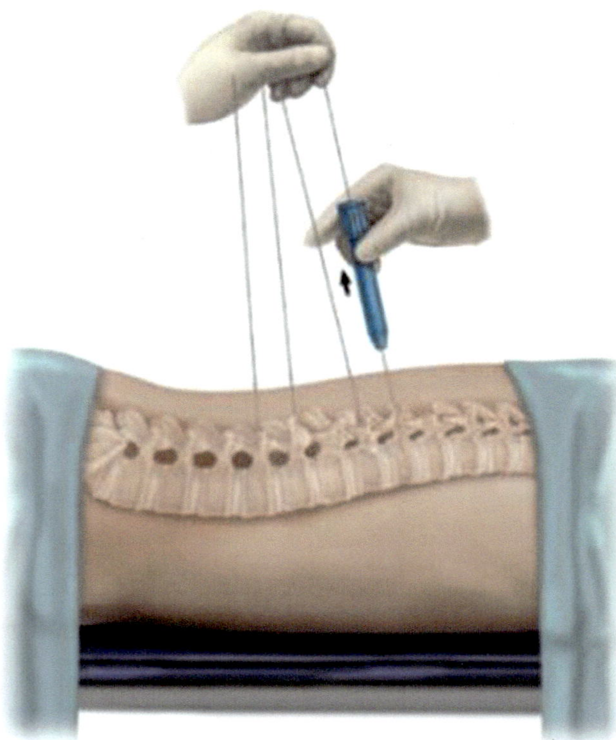

Fig. 13.104 Remove the last dilator

a click is heard, indicating that the rod is locked (Fig. 13.113a, b). If necessary, a rod bender can be used to bend the rod according to the physiological curvature of the spine.

Pearls: Do not bend the rod before attaching the rod to the rod inserter.

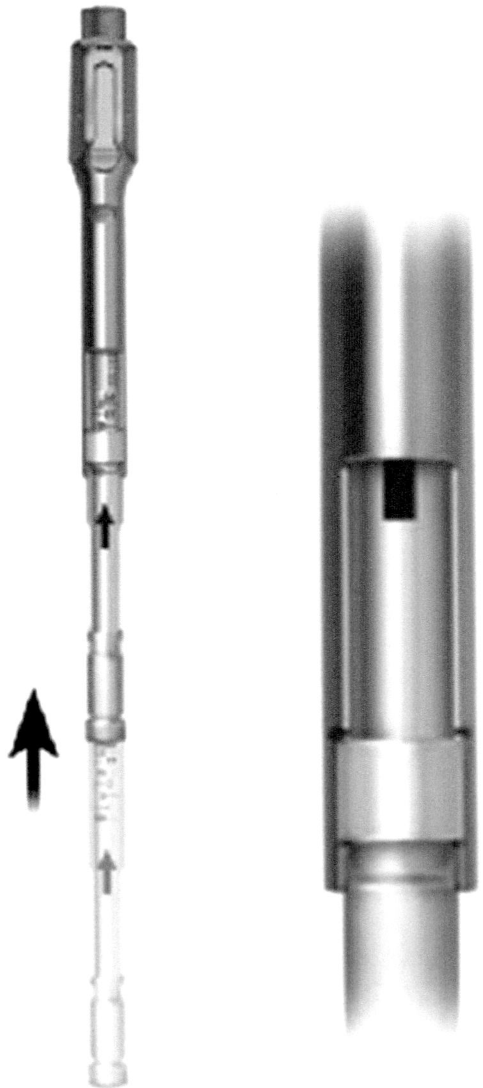

Fig. 13.105 Insert the inner sleeve

Pearls: To estimate the rod curvature, the rod inserter can be placed lateral to the patient, and at the same time lateral fluoroscopy is taken. Then, the bent rod is compared to the trajectory of the screw and necessary adjustment can be made.

13.7.23 Estimating Rod Entry Site

Attach the rod entry locator to the most cephalad extender and adjust the extenders so that they are vertical to the skin surface or slightly oriented toward the caudal extenders (Fig. 13.114). Let the rod entry locator freely fall to the skin and make a vertical incision appropriately 1 cm in length.

Warning: If the most cephalad extender is not vertical to the skin surface or oriented slightly toward the caudal extender, the estimated rod entry site may be more cephalad than it should be.

13.7.24 Passing the Rod Through the First Extender Cephalocaudally

Pass the rod through the skin incision and the fascia until the opening of the first extender (Fig. 13.115a). Under anteroposterior and lateral fluoroscopy, search manually for the window in the first extender that allows the rod to pass (Fig. 13.115b).

Warning: It is very important to pass the rod in a cephalocaudal direction along the overlapping vertebral laminas, which is another measure for protecting the vertebral canal from injury.

13.7.25 Confirmation of Rod Passing

Once the rod is believed to have passed the first (or several) extender(s), the following method can be used for confirmation:

1. Place the rod confirmation device inside the extender. If the black line is visible superiorly, it indicates that the rod has passed the extenders (Fig. 13.116). If the black line is not visible, it indicates that the rod has passed the extenders yet.
2. If a *multi-axial screw is used*, rotate the extenders manually (Fig. 13.117). If any of the extenders rotates freely, it indicates that the rod has not passed through that extender.

13.7.26 Passing the Rod Through the Remaining Extenders

After the rod passes through the first extender, the handle for passing the rod can be guided manually, which can also be guided by anteroposterior and lateral fluoroscopy, rod confirmation device, and rotation technique. The rod is then passed through the remaining extenders (Fig. 13.118a, b and c).

Pearls: When passing a rod with a kyphotic arc, the surgeon can rotate the handle to pass the rod into the body. For example, the rod is attached to the handle via the arc on the coronal plane, and the handle is kept lateral to the rod. Pass the rod through the two cephalad extenders in the lordotic arc, and thereafter turn the handle 180 degrees and the rod becomes kyphotic. Then, pass the rod through the remaining two extenders (Fig. 13.119).

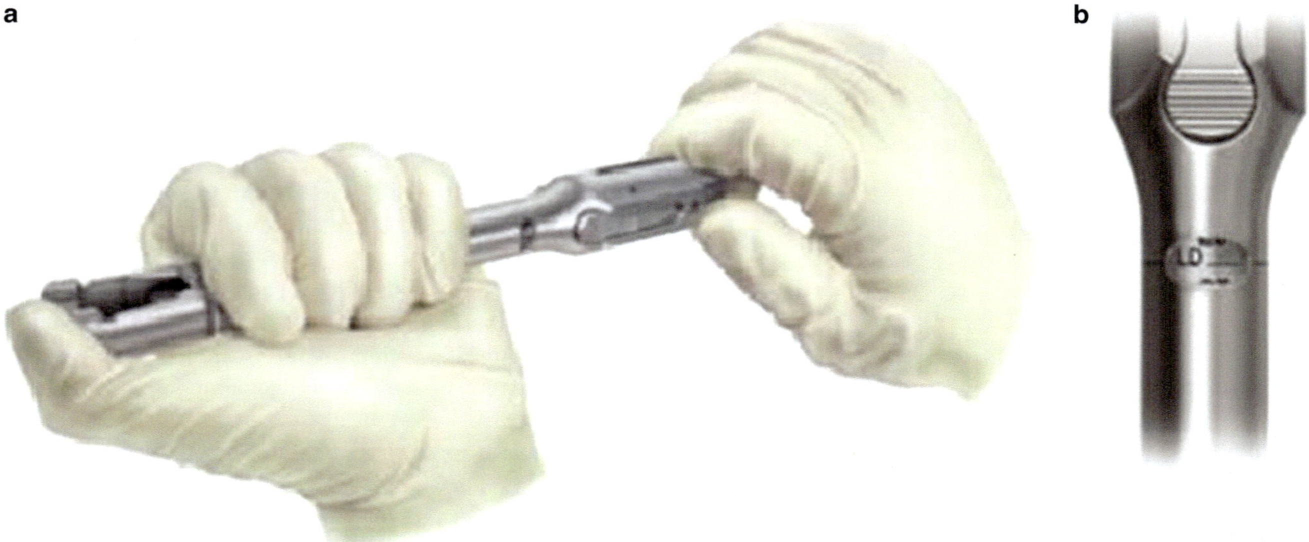

Fig. 13.106 (**a**): Adjust the inner sleeve; (**b**): "LD" is aligned with the window

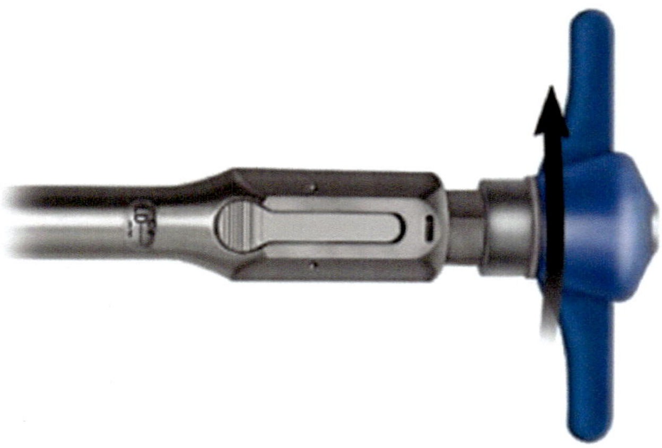

Fig. 13.107 Use a handle to tighten the screw

13.7.27 Verification of Hanging Rod

After verification that the rod has passed through all the extenders, lateral fluoroscopy is undertaken to make sure that the rod inserter does not enter the first extender. It is acceptable that the rod hangs on the cephalad and caudal extenders (Fig. 13.120a, b).

Pearls: The rod inserter may pass through the first extender. It is important to verify by fluoroscopy that only the rod passes through the extender. A small segment of the rod should be seen between the extender and the ball-shaped rod inserter under fluoroscopy.

13.7.28 Gradual Reduction of Extenders

The rod inserter is kept immobile, and reduction nut and ratchet handle are used to gradually reduce each extender to "RD" (reduction) (Fig. 13.121).

Pearls: Gradual reduction of the extenders is very important (Fig. 13.122). Complete reduction of an extender before reduction of other extenders will exert great rod pressure on the remaining extenders, rendering their subsequent reduction difficult.

Warning: When the extenders show "RD," do not excessively rotate the reduction nut; otherwise, undue pressure will be exerted on the screw head.

13.7.29 Passing the Contralateral Rod and Reduction of Extenders

Repeat steps 20–28 to pass the contralateral rod (Fig. 13.123).

13.7.30 Assembling the Screw

Pull up the T-shaped handle of the screw retaining compressor and assemble the screw on the distal tip of the compressor (Fig. 13.124).

Pearls: Before final breaking of the screw, proper rod position should be confirmed by fluoroscopy.

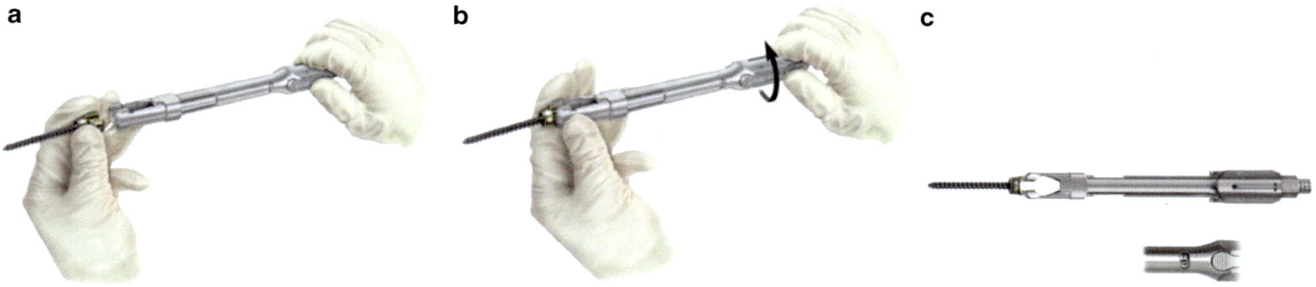

Fig. 13.108 (**a**): Match the screw; (**b**): Rotate the cephalad hexagon screw; (**c**): Assemble the screw

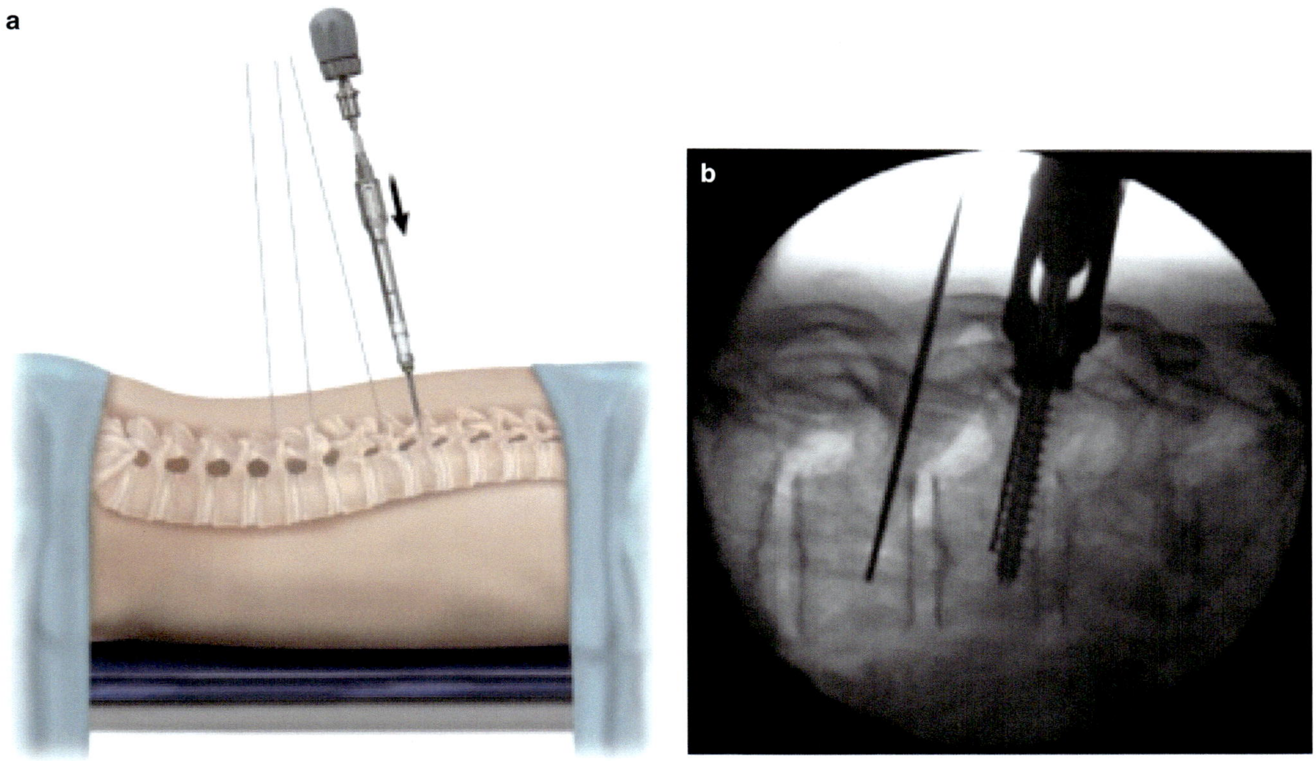

Fig. 13.109 (**a**): Insert the screw extender assembly into the pedicle; (**b**): Lateral image to assure the screw position

13.7.31 Assembling the Counter Torque Wrench and Break-Off

Put the counter torque wrench into the first extender to maintain extender position (Fig. 13.125a). Insert the screw compressor with an assembled screw into the extender. Rotate the screw compressor until the screw breaks off while retaining the counter torque wrench (Fig. 13.125b). Remove the counter torque wrench and the screw compressor and also remove the break-off portion of the screw by pulling up the T-shaped handle.

Pearls: If there is difficulty in inserting the screw, the following can be attempted:

1. Assemble the suction ring trephine to the break-off handle and connect the suction device. Pass the trephine downward into the rod. Remove blood clots and soft tissue that block screw entry by rotating the trephine (Fig. 13.126).
2. The reduced extender is withdrawn for half a circle to reduce pressure on the screw head.

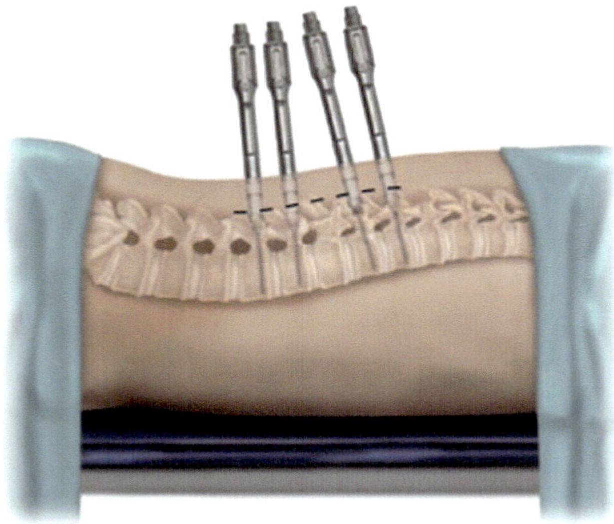

Fig. 13.110 Place the remaining screw extenders

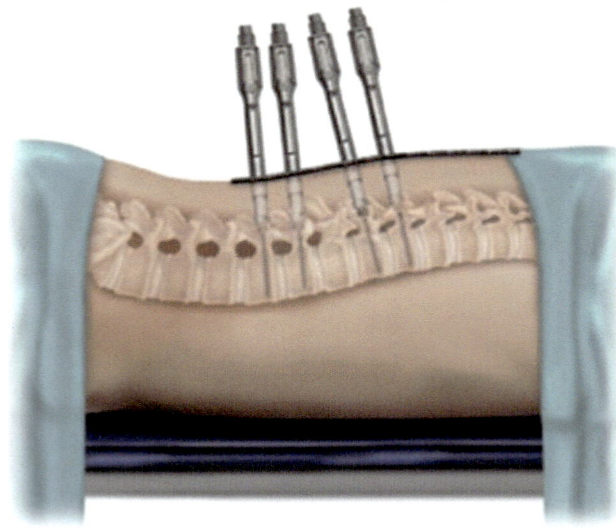

Fig. 13.112 Measure the rod length

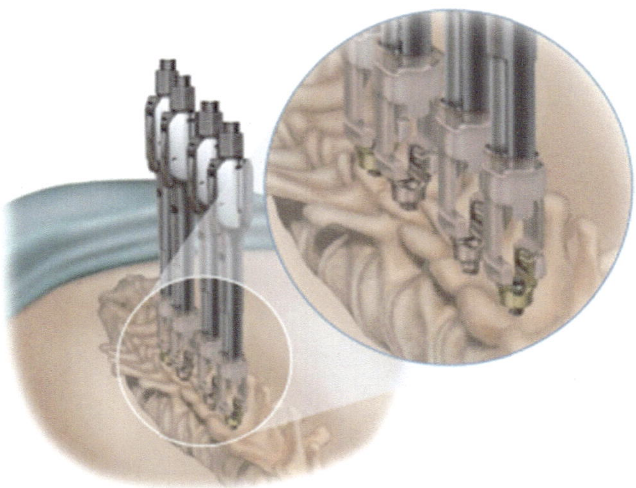

Fig. 13.111 Extender alignment for passing the rod

Warning: If the rod is bent, make sure that the rod inserter is held steady, and do not deviate in any direction to avoid rod rotation before breaking off the screw.

13.7.32 Compression/Distraction

Provisionally tighten one of the screws in the extenders as a pivot for compression or distraction. Do not break the screw. Pull up the T-shaped handle to remove the screw compressor while keeping the screw in place (Fig. 13.127). Furthermore, the handle and the reduced extender are withdrawn half a circle to allow the extender to slide along the rod.

Put compressor/distractor in the extenders in a cephalo-caudal order as close to the skin as possible. Rotate the clip on the compressor/distractor for compression or distraction.

Once compression/distraction is complete, assemble the counter torque wrench onto the extender without any screw. Use the screw compressor to hold and insert the screw and then finally break off the screw (Fig. 13.128). Connect the provisionally tightened screw and use the T-shaped handle to connect the screw compressor. After insertion into the extender, retain and then break off the screw.

13.7.33 Compression/Distraction of the Remaining Segments and Final Break-Off of the Screw

Repeat steps 30 to 32 for compression/distraction of the extenders in the remaining vertebral segments (Fig. 13.129).

13.7.34 Removal of Rod Inserter

Push back the latch on the tip of the rod inserter and open the latch to release the rod and then remove the rod inserter (Fig. 13.130).

13.7.35 Removal of Extenders

After breaking-off of all the screws, turn the reduction nut and move back the first extender to "ST" until it clicks. Then, continue moving back the extenders by depressing the but-

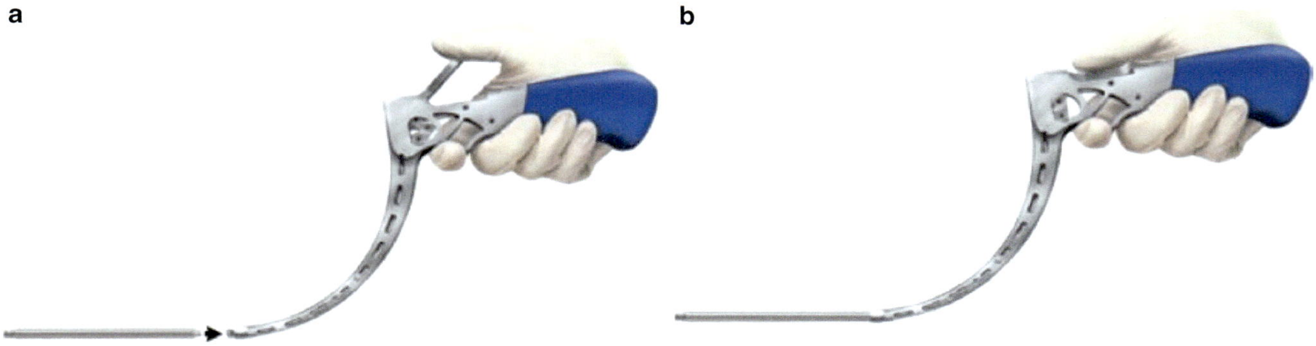

Fig. 13.113 (**a**): Insert the rod; (**b**): Close the latch

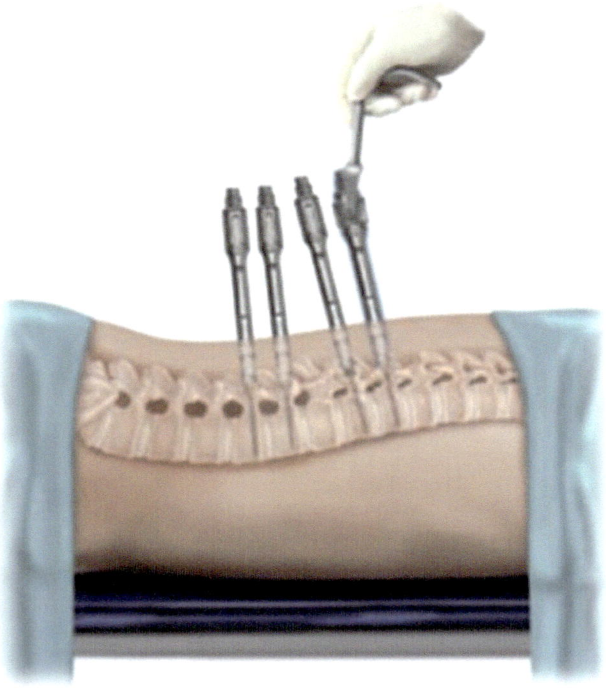

Fig. 13.114 Estimate the rod entry site

tons on the sides of the extenders. Release the buttons once the extender moves back. When the extender reaches "EJ," a click is heard. Gentle side-to-side rocking may assist in removal of the extenders.

13.7.36 Removal of the Remaining Extenders and Wound Closure

Repeat step 35 until all the remaining extenders are removed. Closure is accomplished with a few interrupted stitches in the fascia, a subcuticular skin suture, and Steri-Strips (Fig. 13.131).

13.7.37 Disassembly of Screw Extenders

When disassembling screw extenders, maintain the extenders in the "EJ" position. Depress the buttons on the sides of the extender and turn the reduction nut in a counterclockwise manner (Fig. 13.132a) until the reduction nut is completely loosened (Fig. 13.132b). Tightly hold the inner sleeve and pull out the extender assemblies individually. Avoid extruding on the distal extenders. After the reduction nut is completely loosened, use force to pull out the inner sleeve (Fig. 13.132c).

13.7.38 Implant Explantation

If required, the CD HORIZON LEGACY cannulated multi-*axial* screw and CD HORIZON LONGITUDE rod may be removed. For exposure of screw head, use the stripping technique or better the METRx system dilation technique (Fig. 13.133a). The driver retaining screw may be removed by applying the T27 Removal Driver to the set screw and turning counterclockwise until the set screw is removed. Use the Cochlear clamp to retain the cephalad trocar of the first screw and remove the rod through the most cephalad incision (Fig. 13.133b). A retaining or non-retaining screwdriver can be used to remove all the screws.

Pearls: If there is difficulty in inserting the screwdriver, a spherical screwdriver can be used to align the screw head and the rod for removal.

Pearls: The CD HORIZON LEGACY counter torque wrench can be used to retain and then insert the screw.

Pearls: Removing the tubular distractor first may facilitate rod removal.

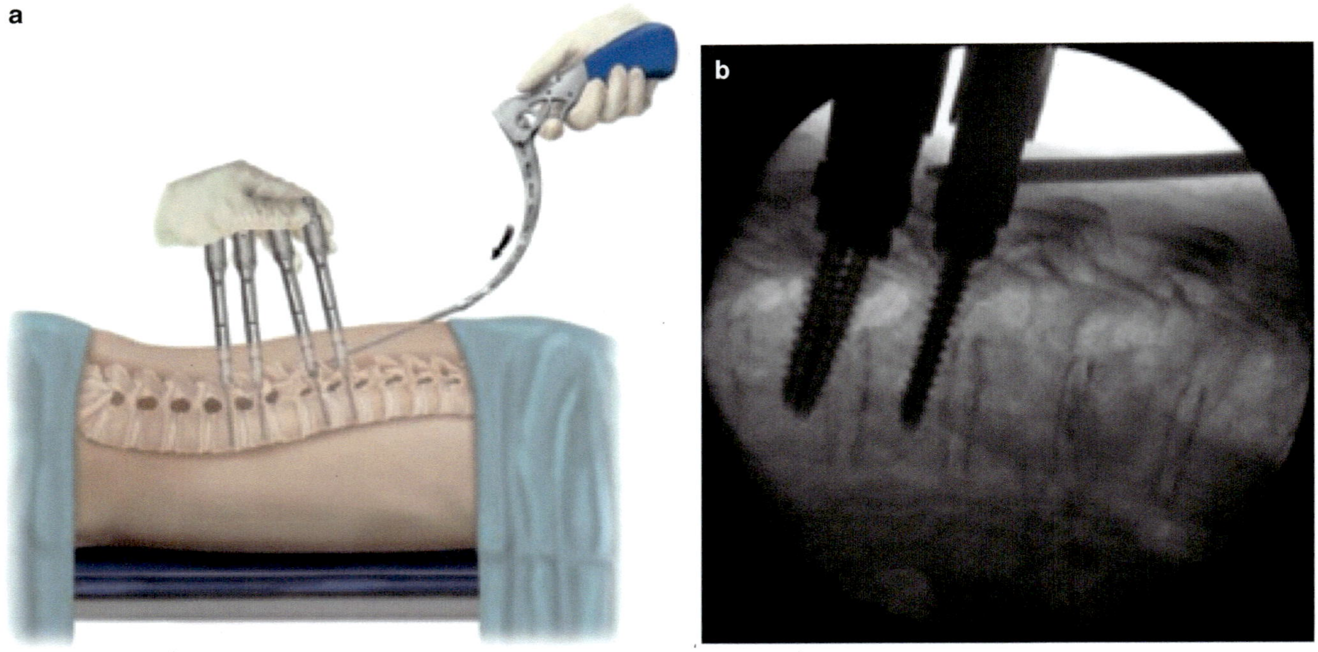

Fig. 13.115 (**a**): Pass the rod through the first extender; (**b**): Under the fluoroscopic guidance

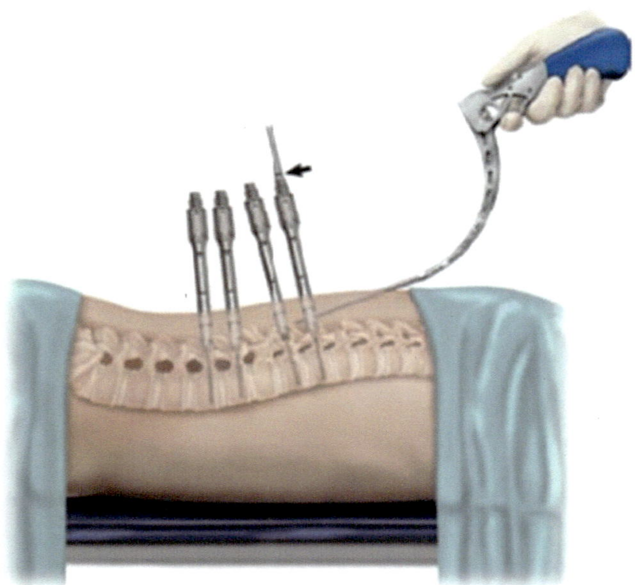

Fig. 13.116 Confirm the rod passing by device

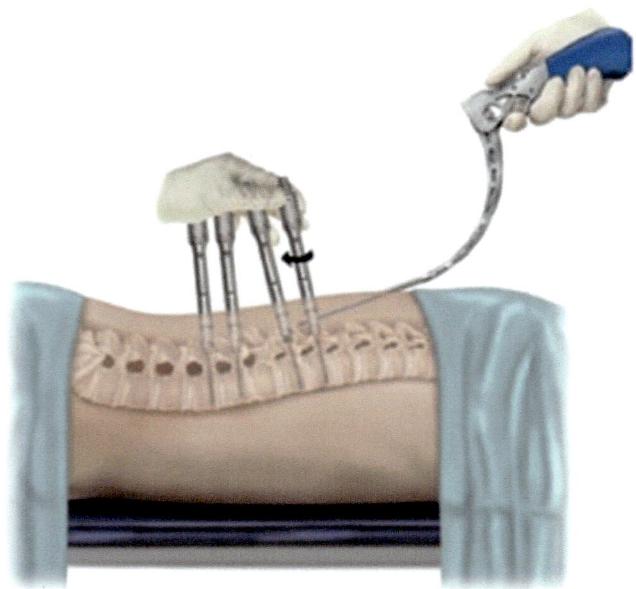

Fig. 13.117 Confirm the rod passing by rotating the extenders

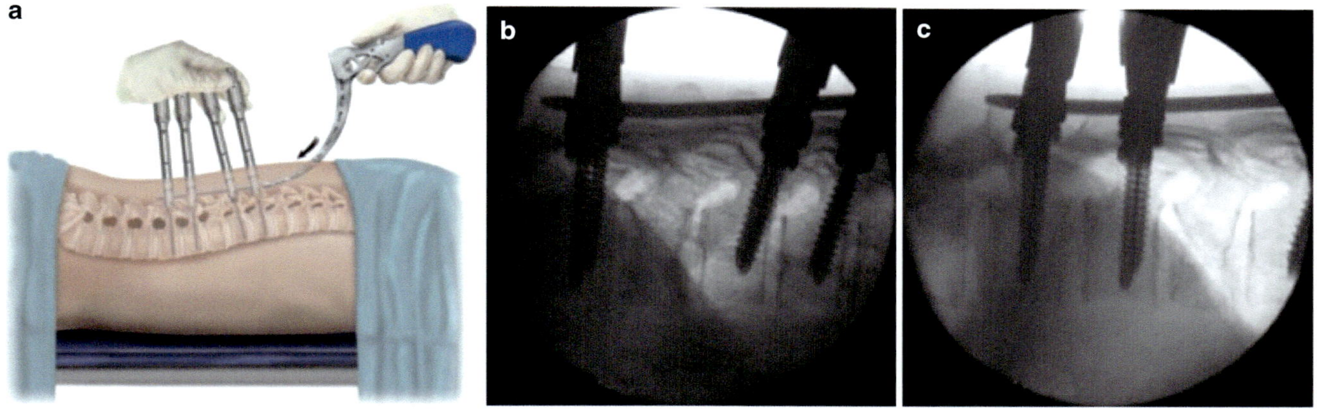

Fig. 13.118 (**a**): Pass the rod through the remaining extenders; (**b**): Pass the third screw; (**c**): Pass the fourth screw

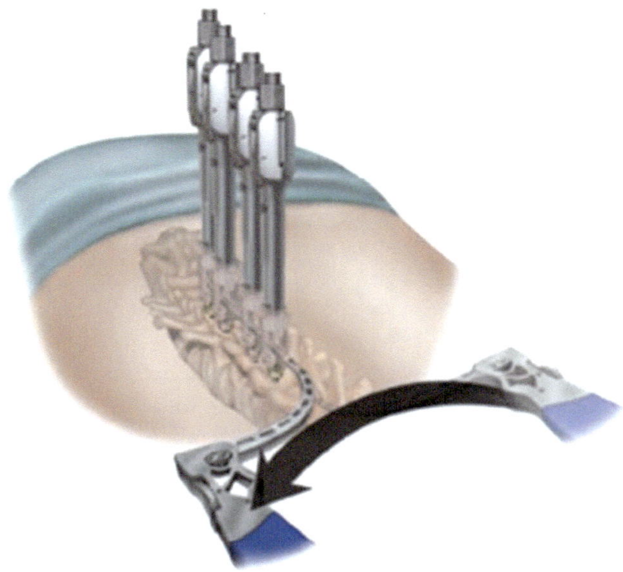

Fig. 13.119 Rotate the handle

13.8 Clinical Cases

13.8.1 Case No. 1

Patient: A 39-year-old man with back pain and radiating pain of the right lower extremity for 10 days and worsening for 8 days.

Diagnosis: L5–S1 intervertebral disc herniation.

Surgery: Sextant technique, L5–S1 right intervertebral fenestration with removal of nucleus pulposus from the intervertebral disc, L5 and S1 pedicle screw internal fixation.

Imaging data: Preoperative (Fig. 13.134), intraoperative (Fig. 13.135), and postoperative (Fig. 13.136) images are shown below.

13.8.2 Case No. 2

Patient: A 32-year-old man with back pain for 1 day due to trauma.

Diagnosis: L1 vertebral body fracture.

Surgery: Sextant technique, T12 and L1 pedicle screw reduction and internal fixation.

Imaging data: Preoperative (Fig. 13.137), intraoperative (Fig. 13.138), and postoperative (Fig. 13.139, Fig. 13.140) images are shown below.

13.8.3 Case No. 3

Patient: A 31-year-old man with back pain for 2 days after trauma.

Diagnosis: L1 vertebral body fracture.

Surgery: Sextant technique for T12, L1 and L2 pedicle screw reduction and internal fixation.

Imaging data: Preoperative intraoperative (Fig. 13.141) and postoperative (Figs. 13.142, 13.143) images are shown below.

13.8.4 Case No. 4

Patient: A 48-year-old man with back pain for 2 days after trauma.

Diagnosis: T10–T11 vertebral fracture.

Surgery: Navigation-guided LONGITUDE technique T9–12 percutaneous pedicle screw implantation and fracture reduction.

Imaging data: Preoperative (Figs. 13.144, 13.145, and 13.146), intraoperative (Figs. 13.147, 13.148, and 13.149), and postoperative (Figs. 13.150, 13.151) images are shown below.

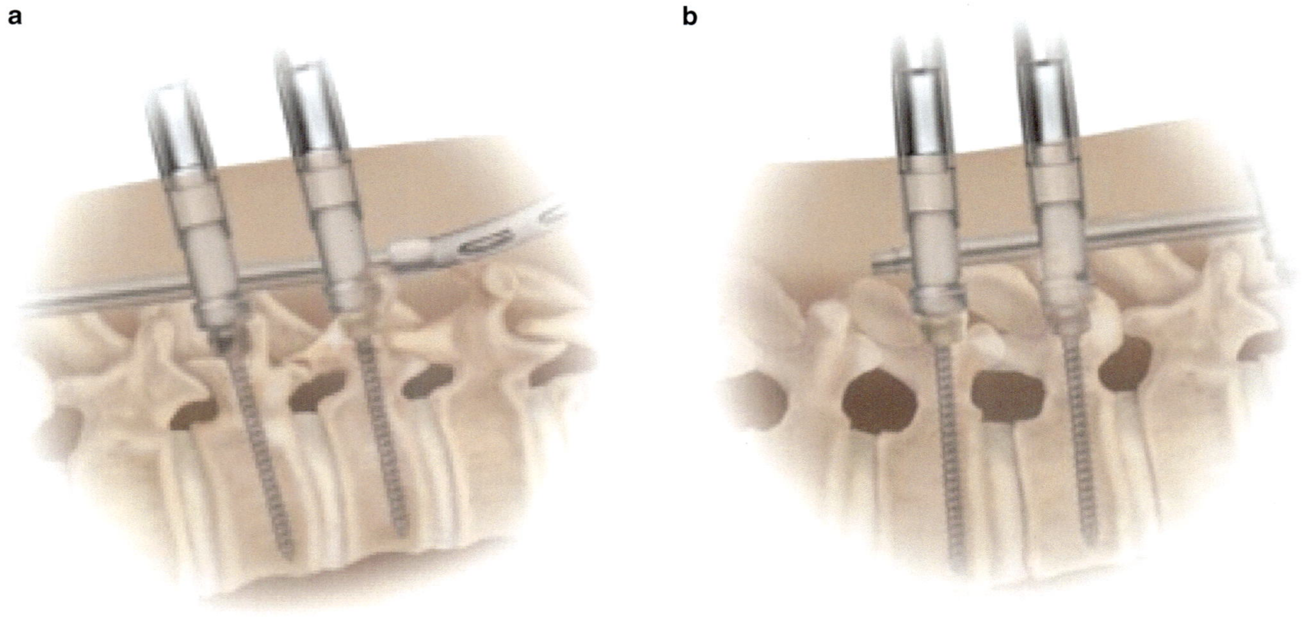

Fig. 13.120 (**a**): The rod beyond the cephalad extender; (**b**): The rod beyond the caudal extender

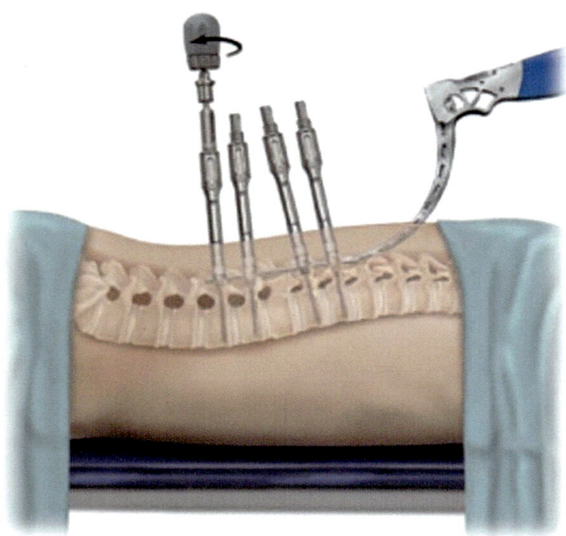

Fig. 13.121 Reduction

13.9 Caveats and Lessons

1. The surgical indications of percutaneous pedicle screw internal fixation of vertebral fractures are thoracic/lumbar vertebral stable fractures that do not need decompression. Percutaneous pedicle screw internal fixation could achieve reduction of the injured spine and establish immediate spine stability.
2. Posterior percutaneous pedicle screw internal fixation can be done for single segment thoracolumbar vertebral body fracture. Single segment fixation only needs to stabilize one spinal motor unit and minimize loss of motor abilities. However, vertebral injury and collapse of the intervertebral body space between the injured segment and the superior vertebral body. As a result, fixation and long-term outcome are poor.
3. Pedicle screw internal fixation of the segments spanning the injured vertebra as well as the superior and inferior adjacent vertebral bodies increase spine stability and reduce the incidence of postoperative vertebral injuries and collapse of the intervertebral body space; however, two motor units are sacrificed with this approach.
4. Early fracture union is very important in patients who have received percutaneous pedicle screws for simple thoracolumbar fracture as no bone graft fusion is undertaken. The patient should wear lumbar support for external fixation for 3 months postoperatively, which promotes fracture healing and prevents collapse of the intervertebral body space. Case No. 2 started ambulation 1 month postoperatively without lumbar support, and follow-up visit at 3 months postoperatively showed vertebra injuries

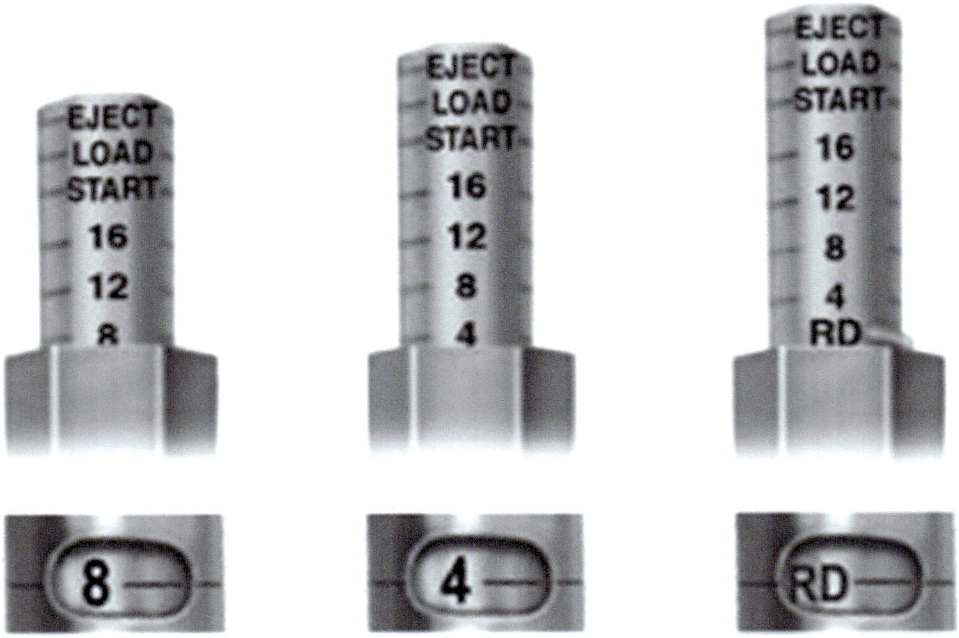

Fig. 13.122 Figure gradual reduction

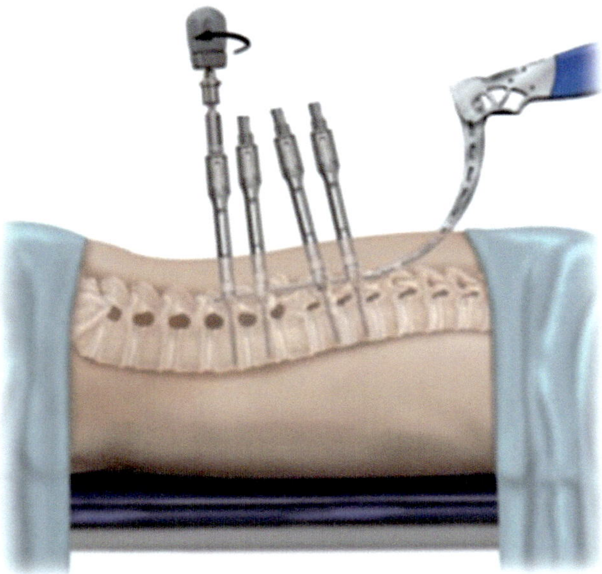

Fig. 13.123 Passing the contralateral rod and reduction of extenders

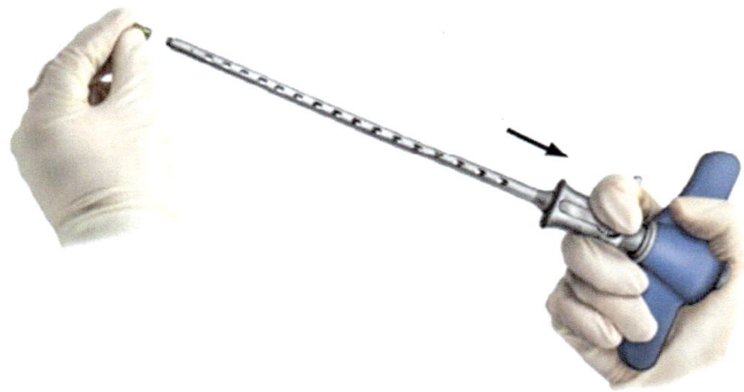

Fig. 13.124 Assemble the screw

and prevents collapse of the intervertebral body space (Fig. 13.152a, b).

5. Under assistance by C-arm fluoroscopy, the percutaneous pedicle screw entry site can be more lateral than open surgery to have a larger inner angle and increase the anti-pullout strength of the screw. The entry site of the lumbar screw can be at the intersection of the base of the transverse process and the line connecting the base of the superior articular process. The entry site of the thoracic screw can be at 2–3 o'clock or 9–10 o'clock on orthogonal fluoroscopy of the pedicle.

13.9.1 Postoperative Management

Readers can refer to the CDH LEGACY system for postoperative management.

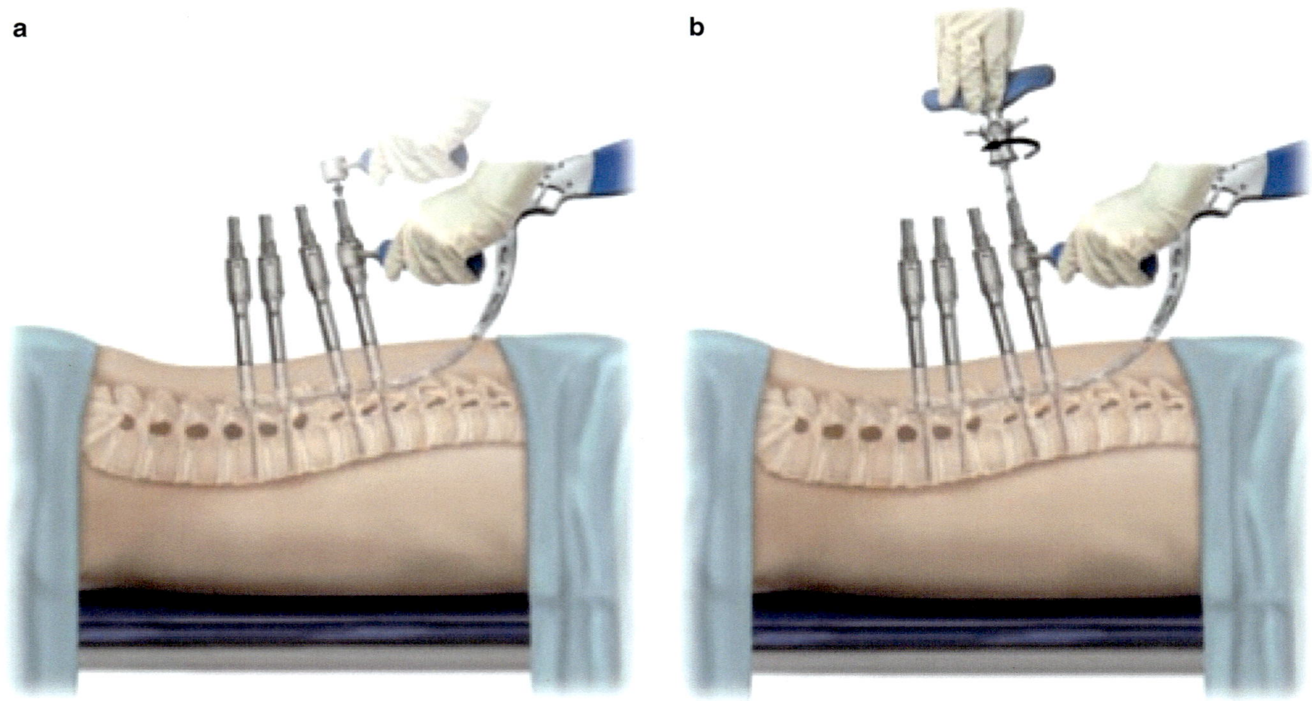

Fig. 13.125 (**a**): Assembling the counter torque wrench; (**b**): Break-off

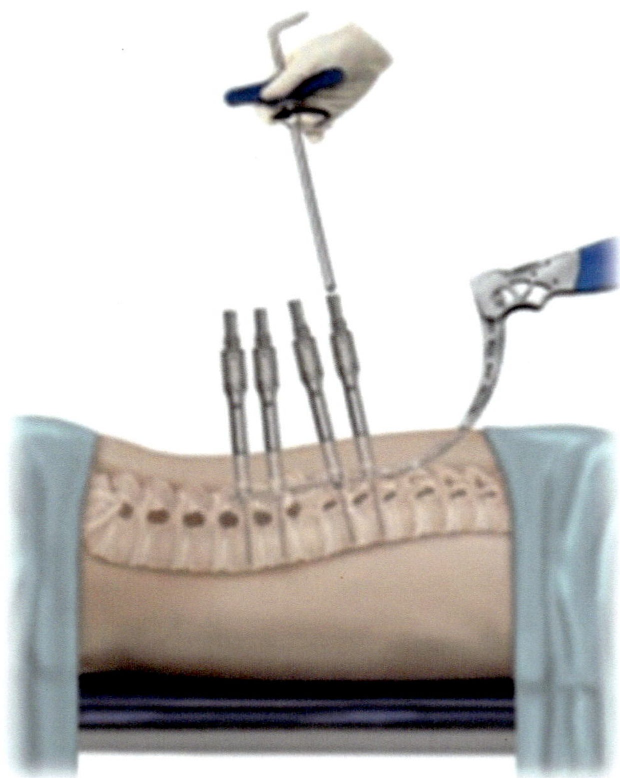

Fig. 13.126 Assemble the suction ring trephine

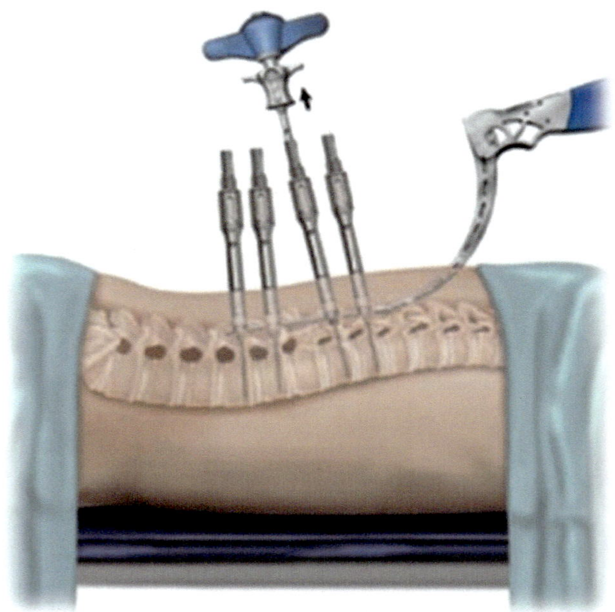

Fig. 13.127 Remove the screw compressor

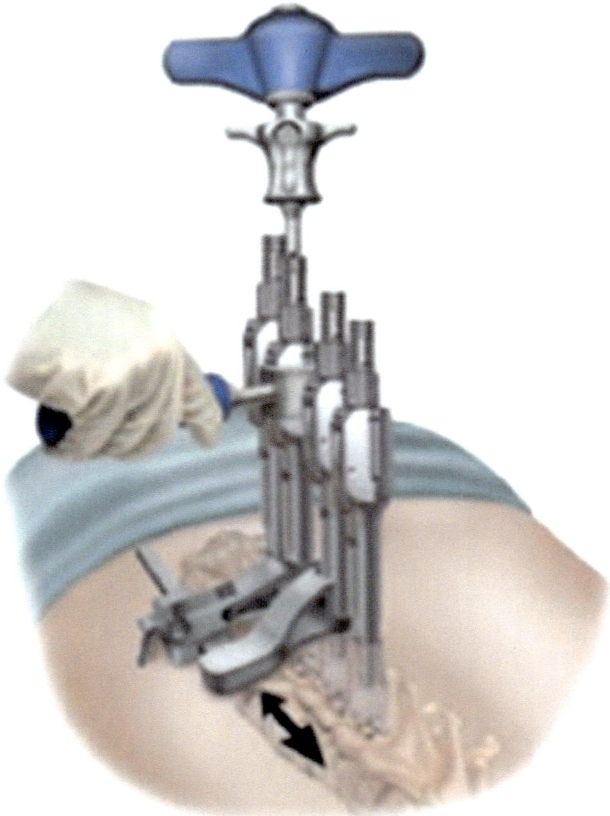

Fig. 13.128 Break-off

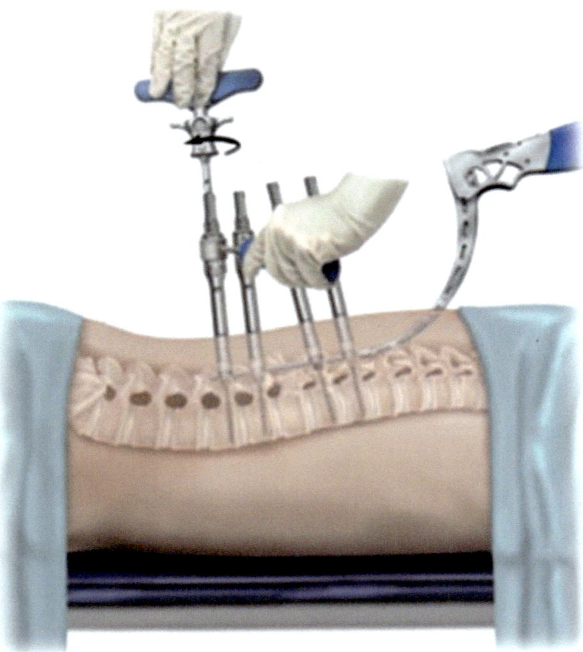

Fig. 13.129 Final break-off

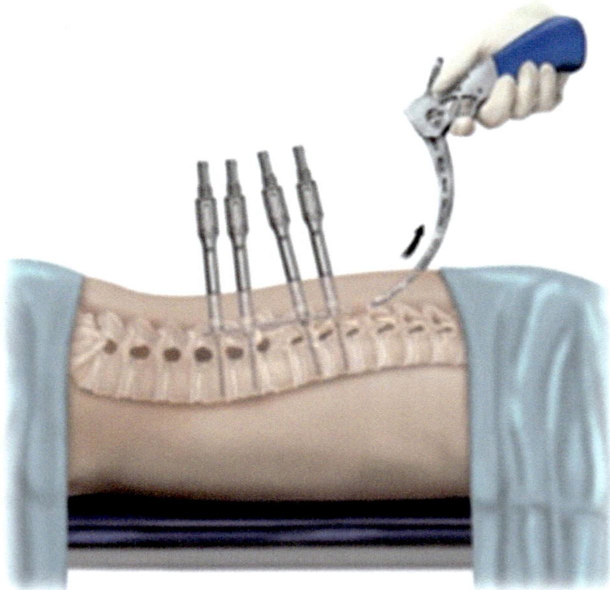

Fig. 13.130 Remove the road inserter

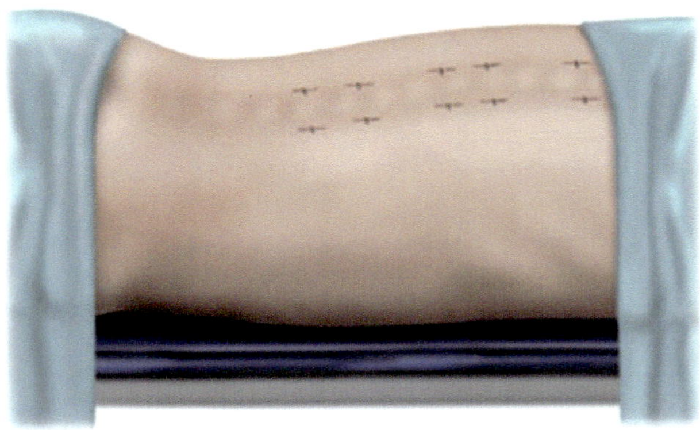

Fig. 13.131 Closure

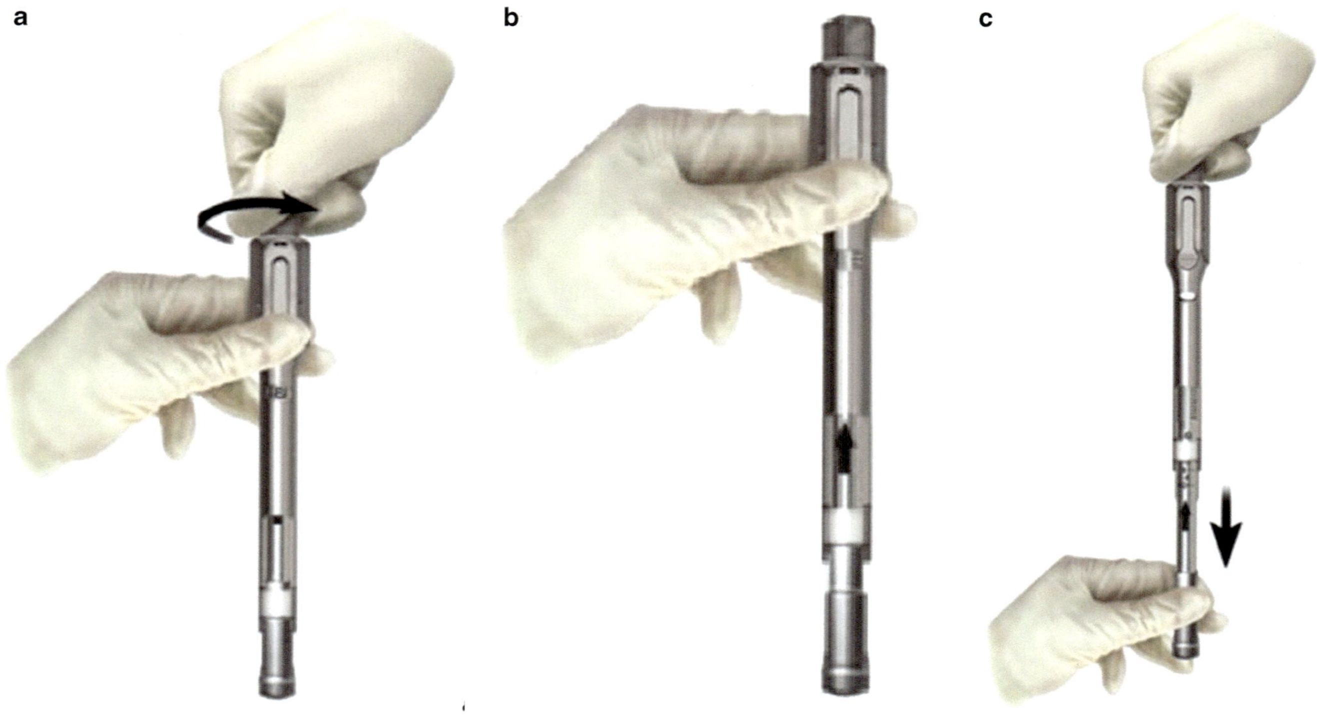

Fig. 13.132 (**a**): Turn the reduction nut; (**b**): The reduction nut is completely loosened; (**c**): Pull out the inner sleeve

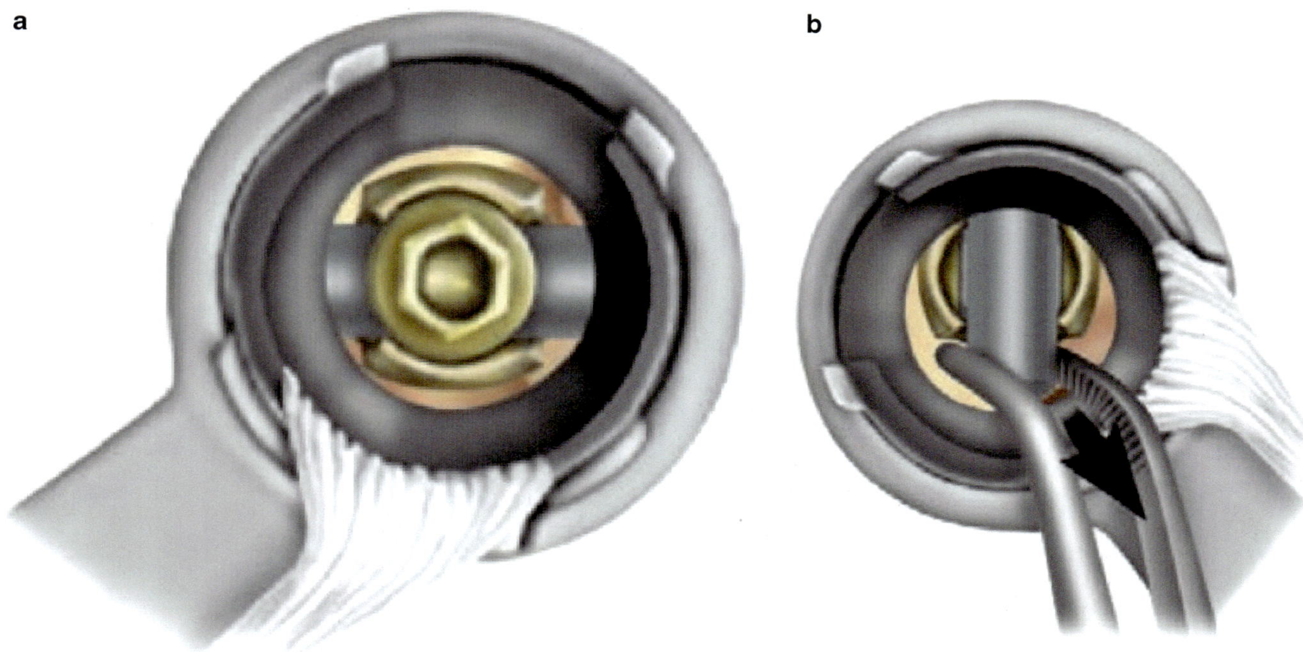

Fig. 13.133 (**a**): The METRx system dilation technique; (**b**): Remove the rod

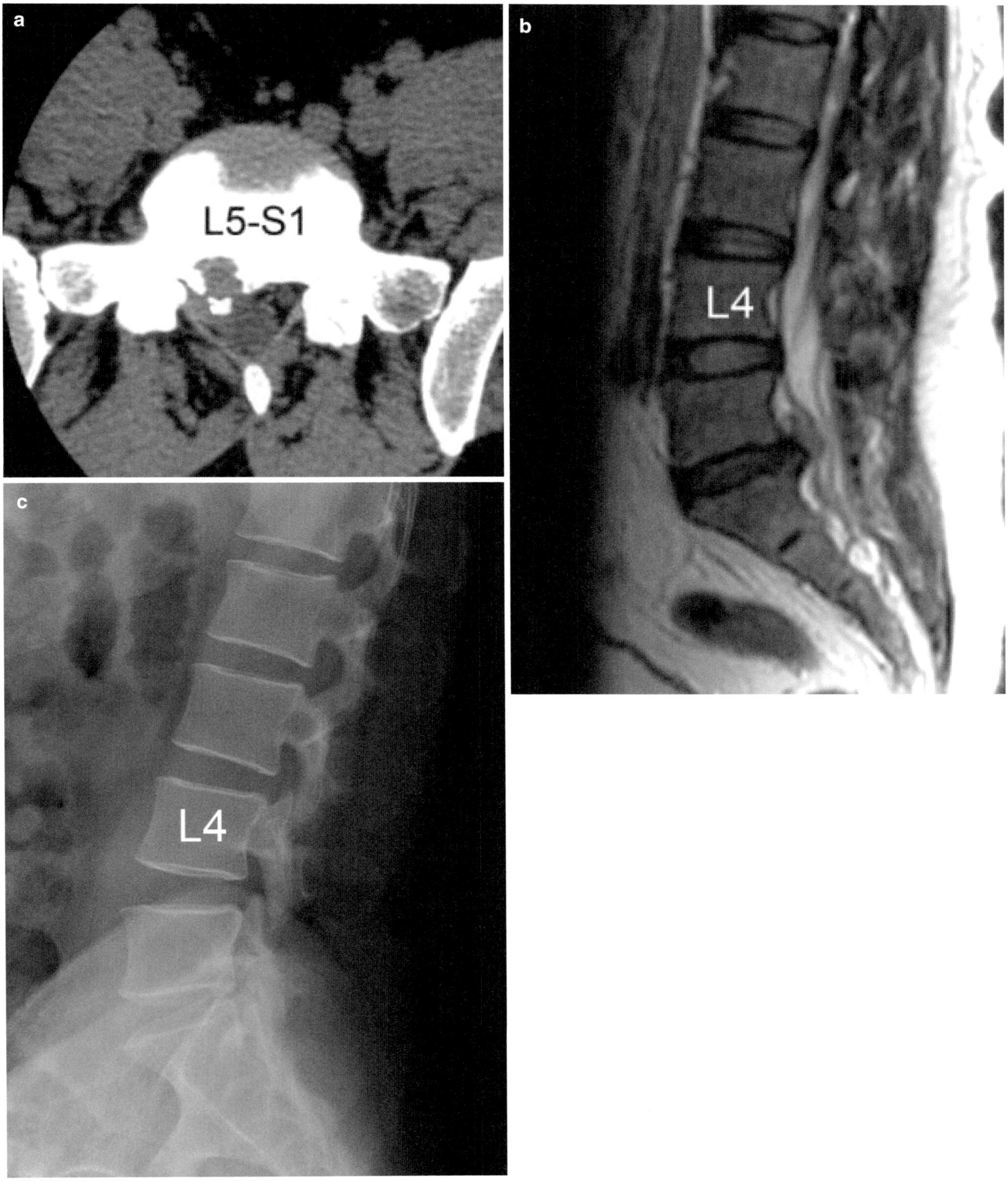

Fig. 13.134 (**a**): Preoperative CT (horizontal view). (**b**): Preoperative MRI (sagittal view). (**c**): Preoperative radiograph (lateral view)

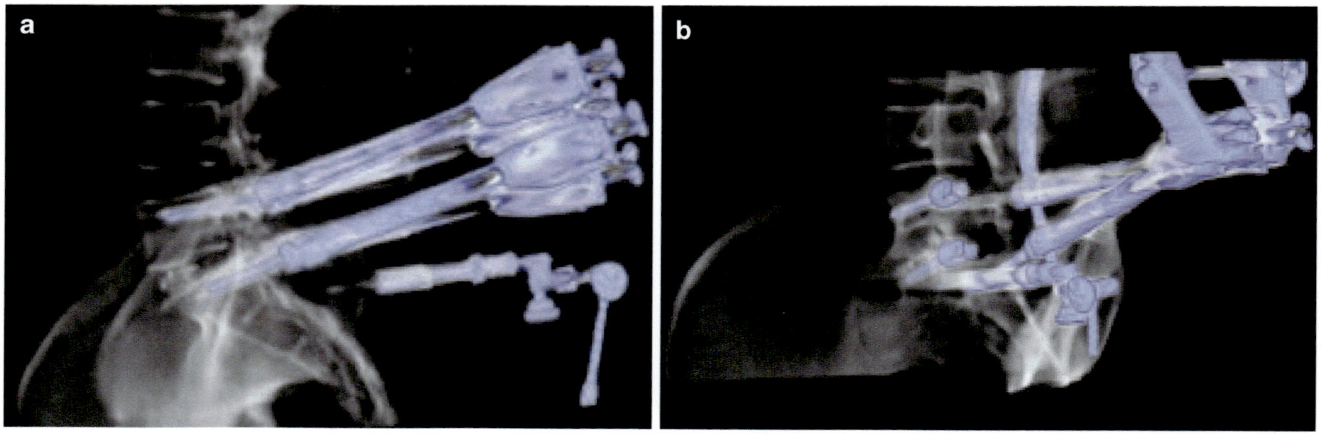

Fig. 13.135 (**a**): Intraoperative fluoroscopy (lateral view); (**b**): Intraoperative fluoroscopy (oblique view)

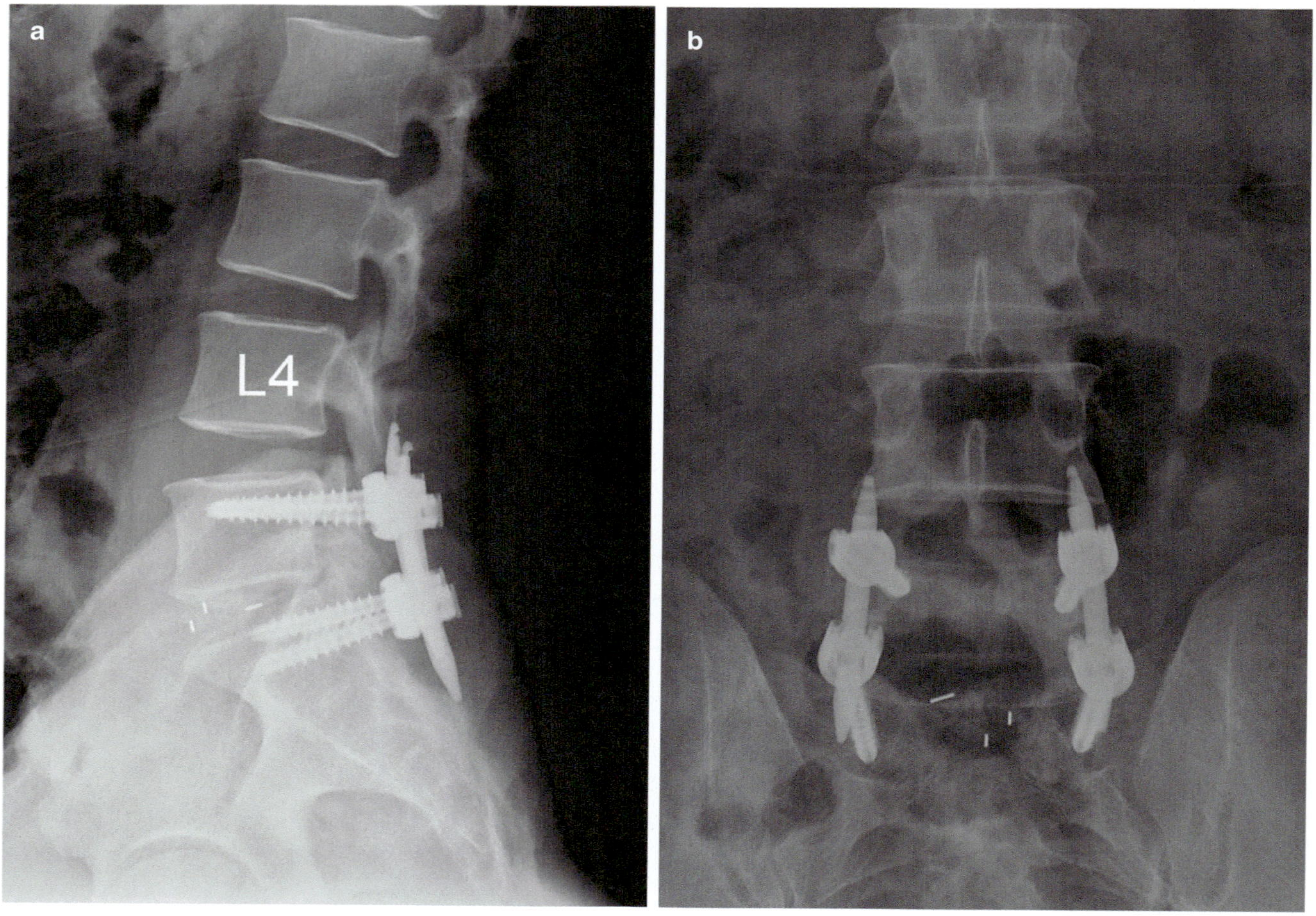

Fig. 13.136 (**a**): Postoperative radiograph (lateral view); (**b**): Postoperative radiograph (anteroposterior view)

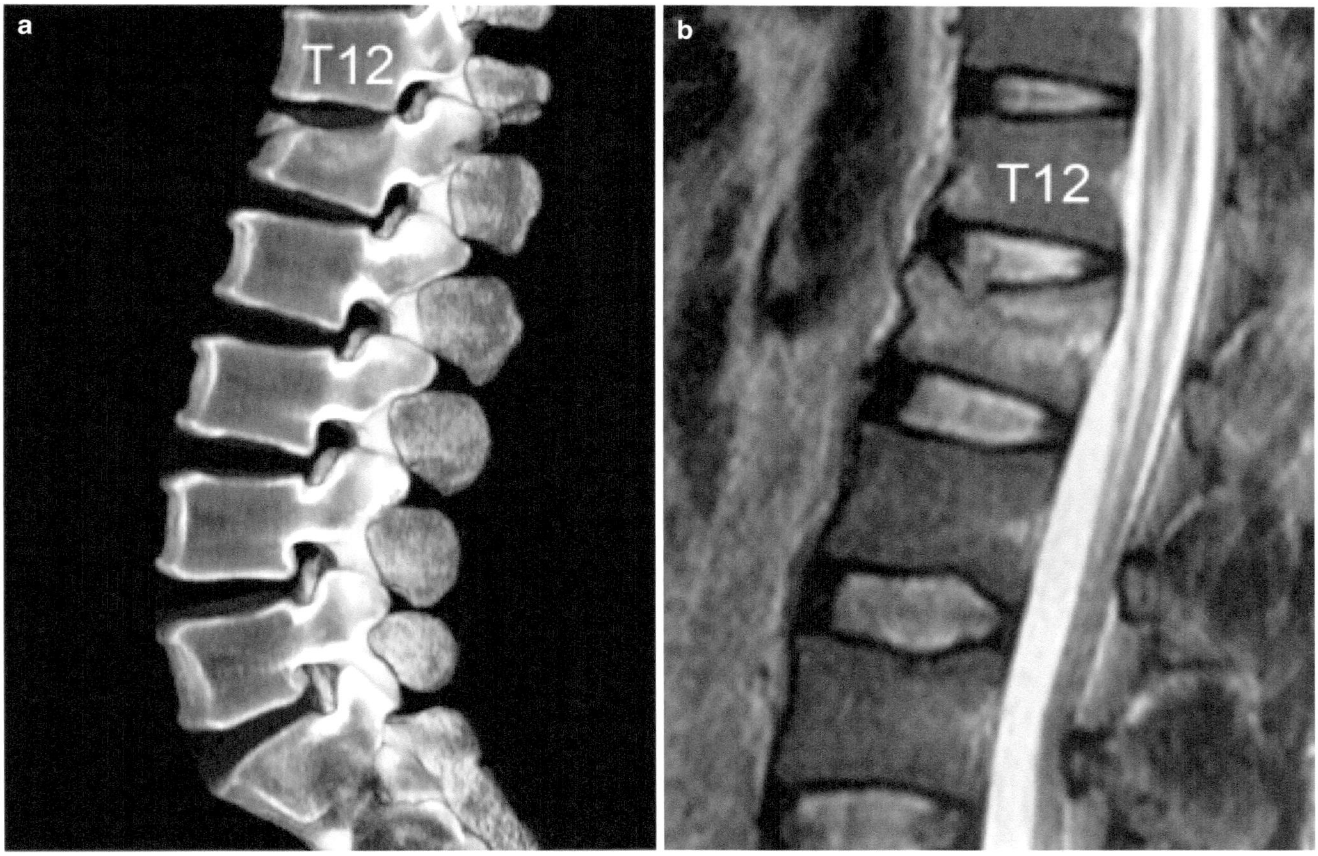

Fig. 13.137 (**a**): Preoperative 3D CT (sagittal view); (**b**):Preoperative MRI (sagittal view)

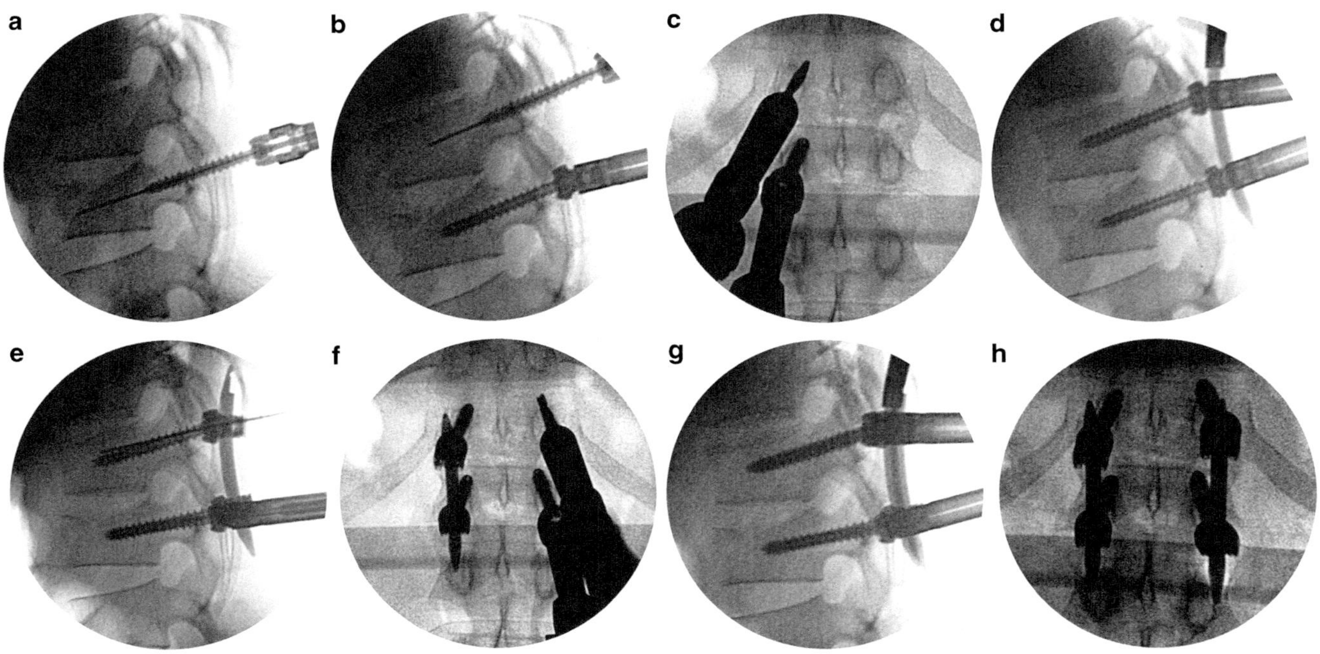

Fig. 13.138 Intraoperative fluoroscopic findings. (**a**): Localization and unilateral placement of L1 screw. (**b**): Localization and unilateral placement of T12 screw. (**c**): Intraoperative orthogonal fluoroscopy. (**d**): Unilateral rod placement. (**e**): Localization and contralateral placement of L1 screw. (**f**): Intraoperative orthogonal fluoroscopy. (**g**): Contralateral rod placement. (**h**): Completion of implant placement

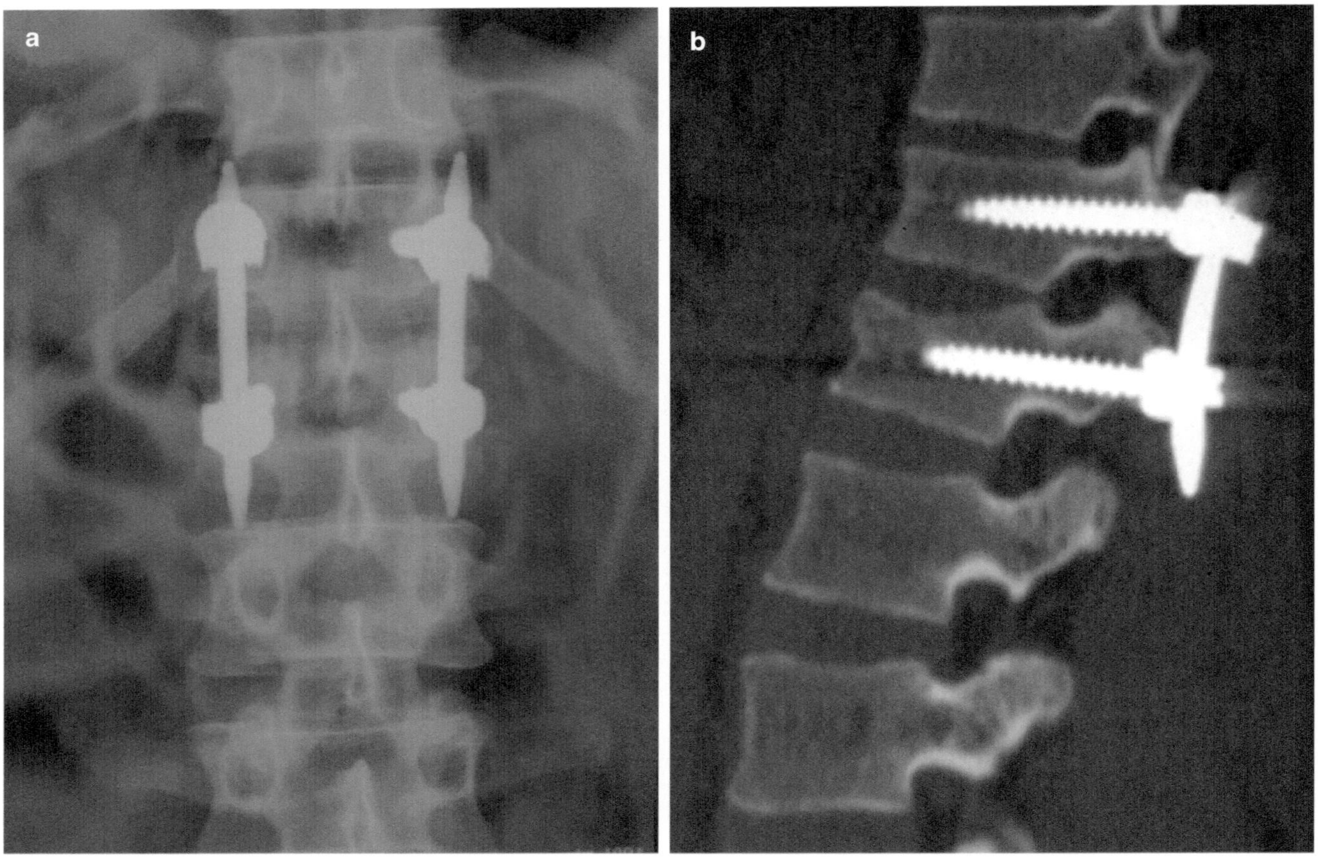

Fig. 13.139 (**a**): Postoperative radiograph (posteroanterior view); (**b**): Postoperative L1 radiograph (lateral view)

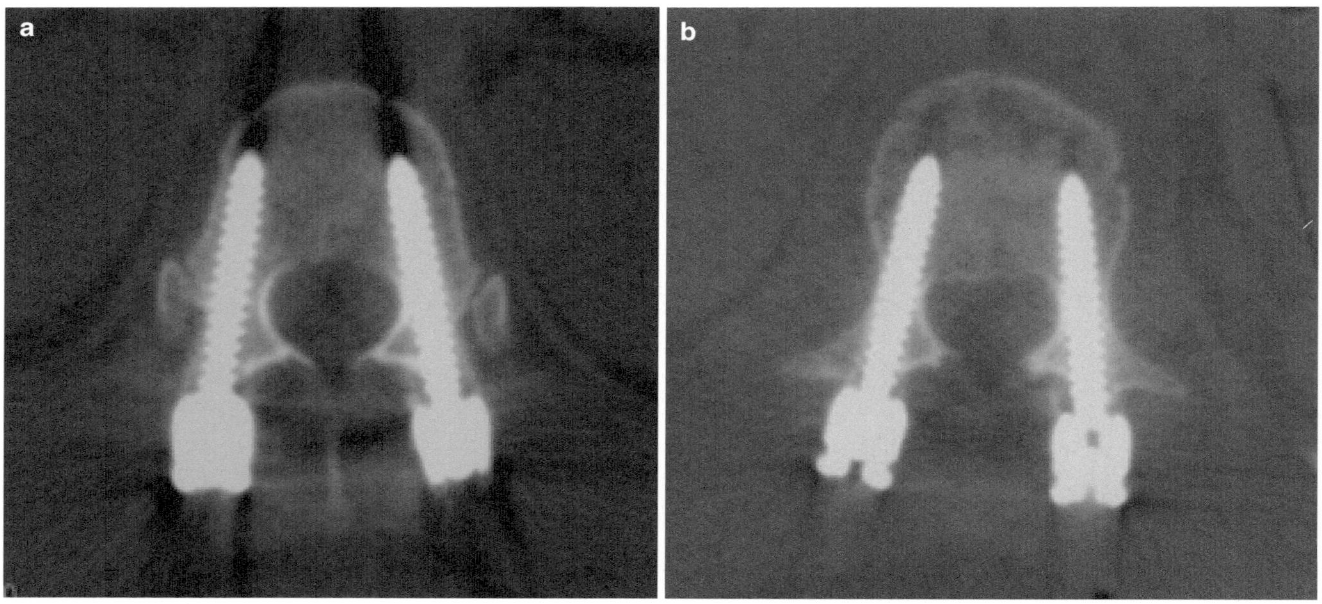

Fig. 13.140 (**a**): Postoperative T12 radiograph (horizontal view); (**b**): Postoperative L1 radiograph (horizontal view)

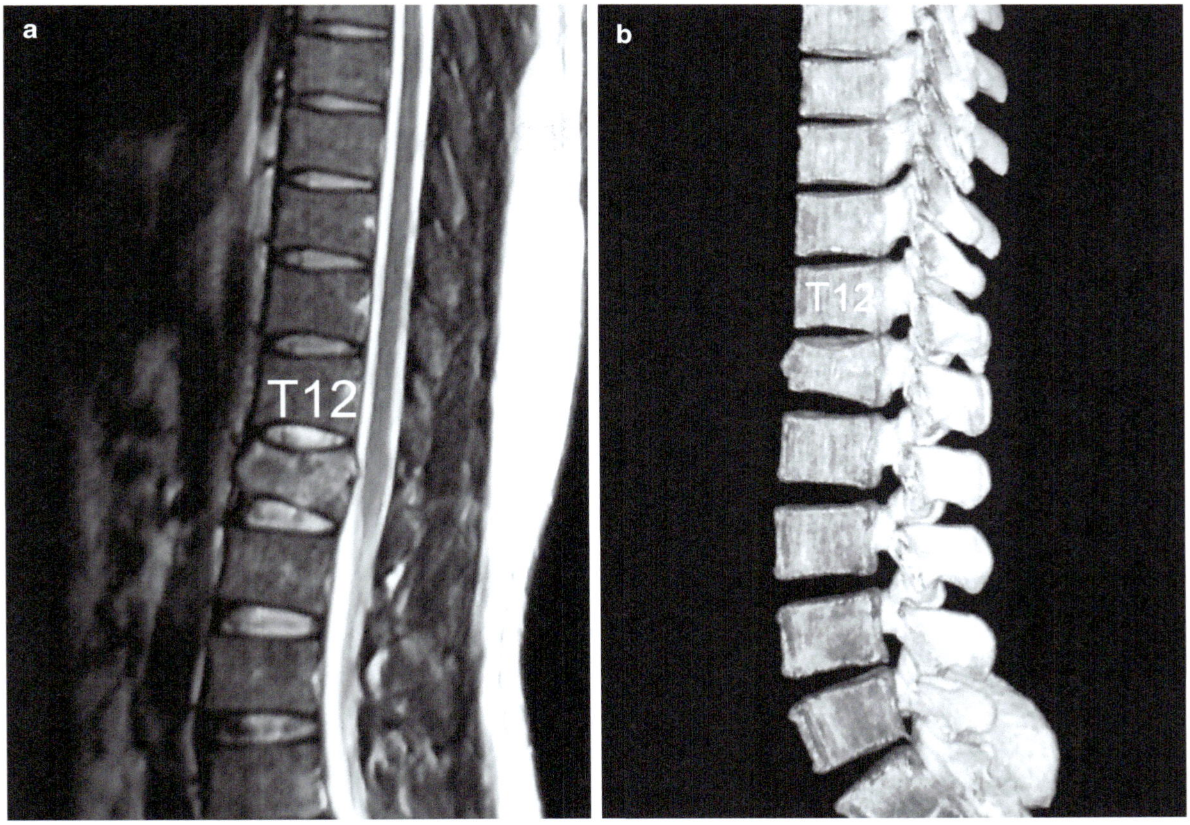

Fig. 13.141 (**a**): Preoperative MRI (sagittal view); (**b**): Preoperative 3D CT reconstruction of the longitudinally split vertebral canal (sagittal view)

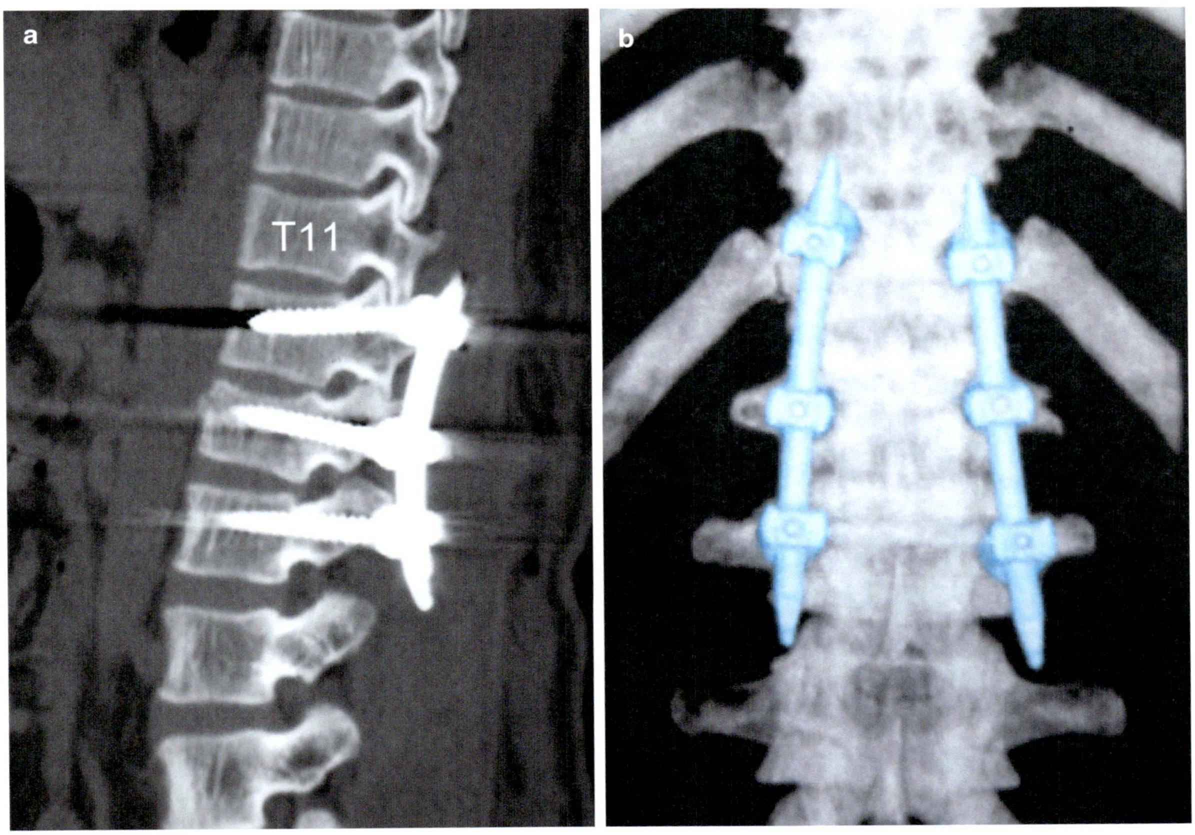

Fig. 13.142 (**a**): Postoperative 3D CT reconstruction (sagittal view); (**b**): Postoperative 3D CT reconstruction (posterior view)

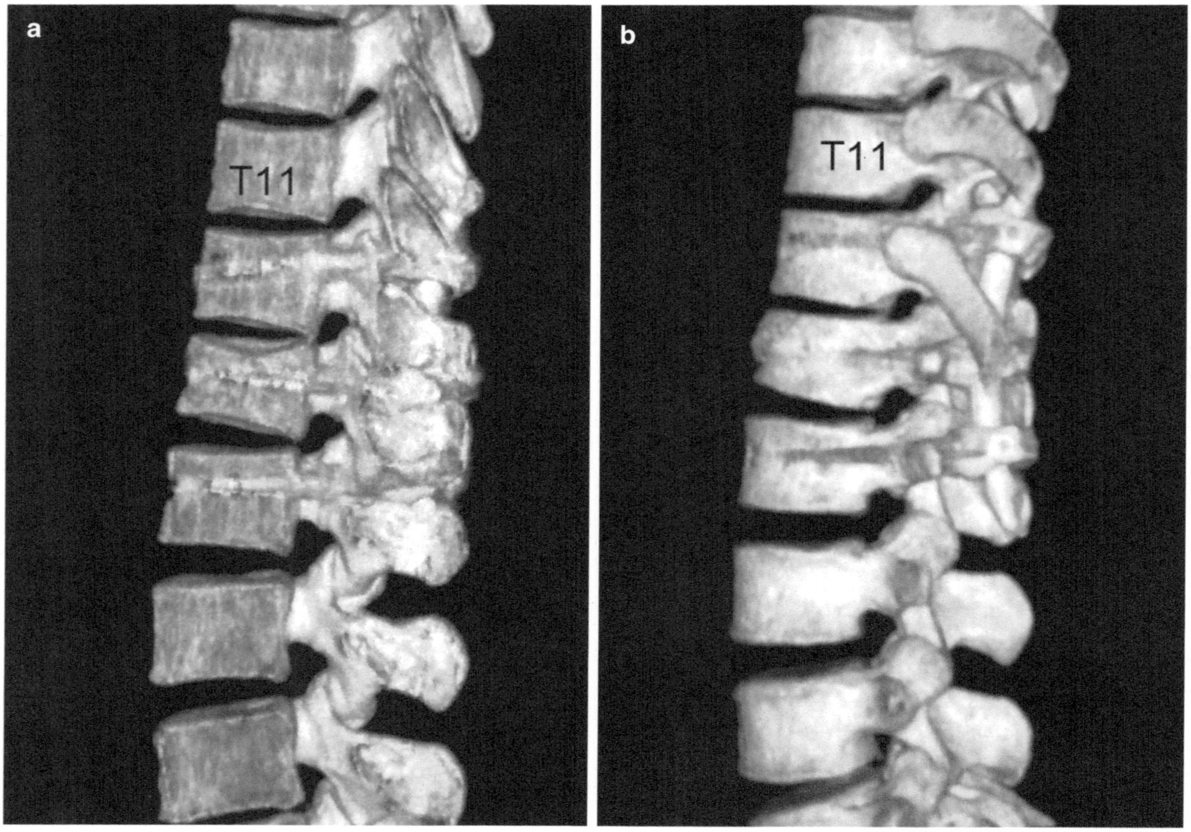

Fig. 13.143 (**a**): Postoperative 3D CT reconstruction of the longitudinally split vertebral canal (sagittal view). (**b**): Postoperative 3D CT reconstruction (lateral view)

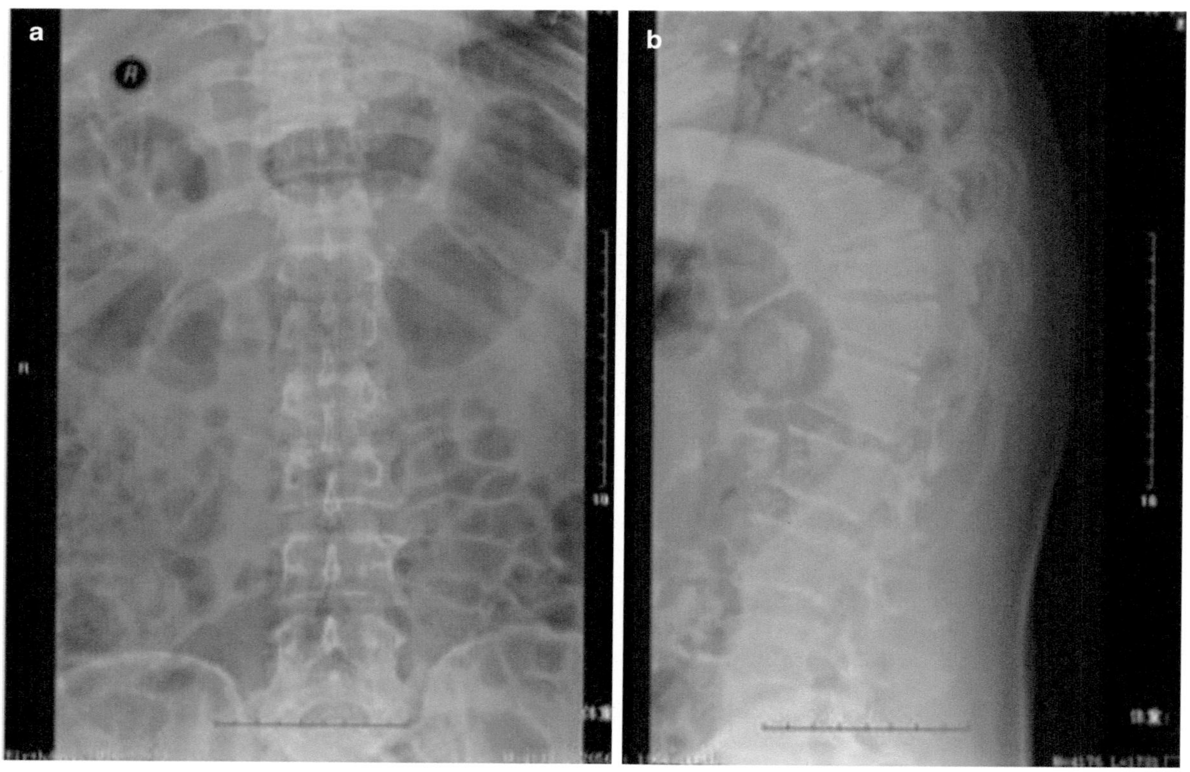

Fig. 13.144 Preoperative X-ray reveals T10–T11 vertebral body compression fracture with local kyphosis. (**a**): Anteroposterior view; (**b**): Lateral view

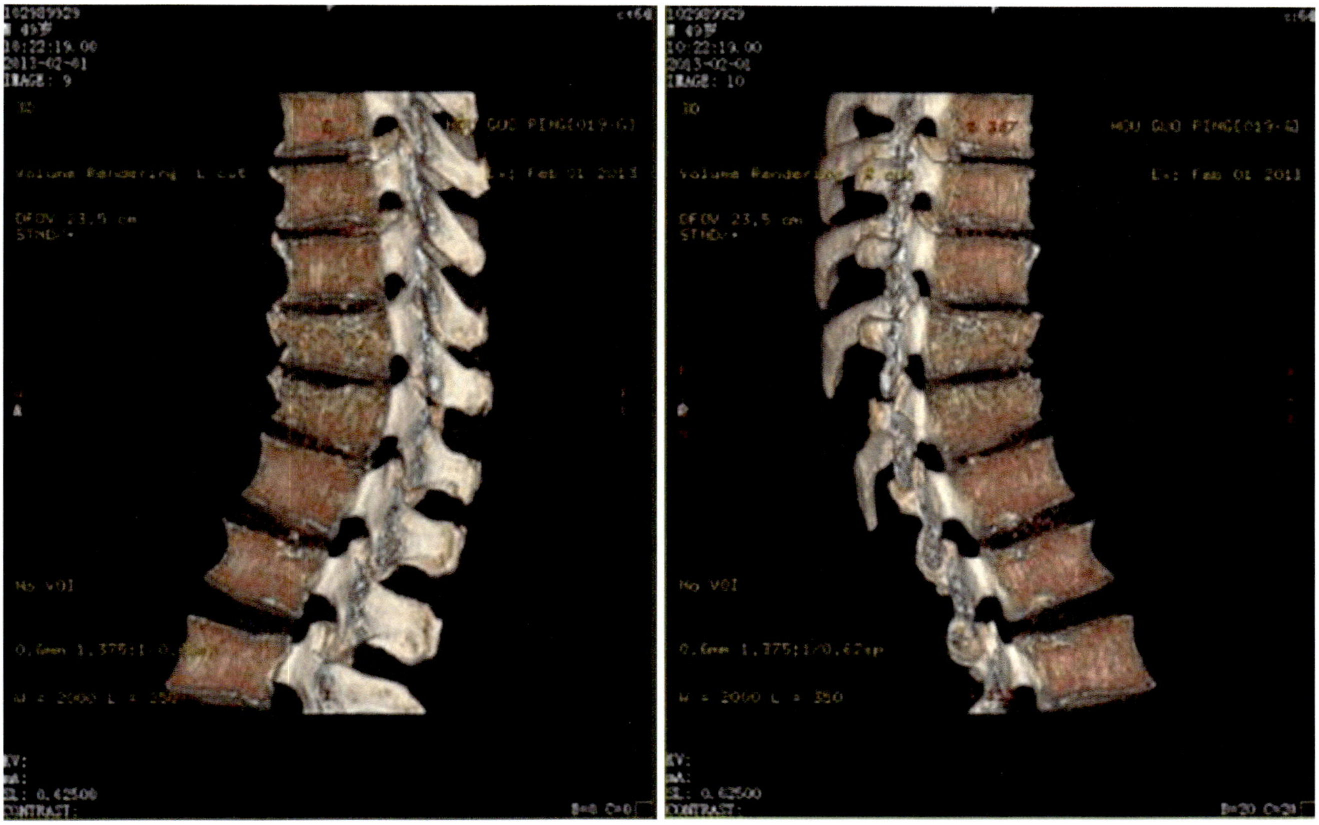

Fig. 13.145 Preoperative 3D CT scan shows no apparent protrusion into T10–T11 vertebral canal

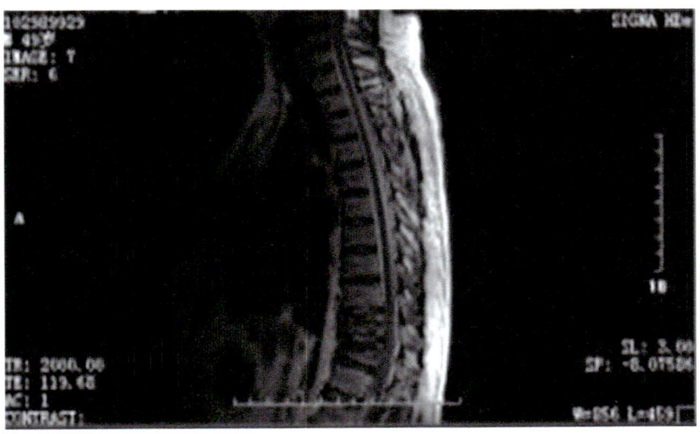

Fig. 13.146 Preoperative MRI shows T10–T11 vertebral body compression

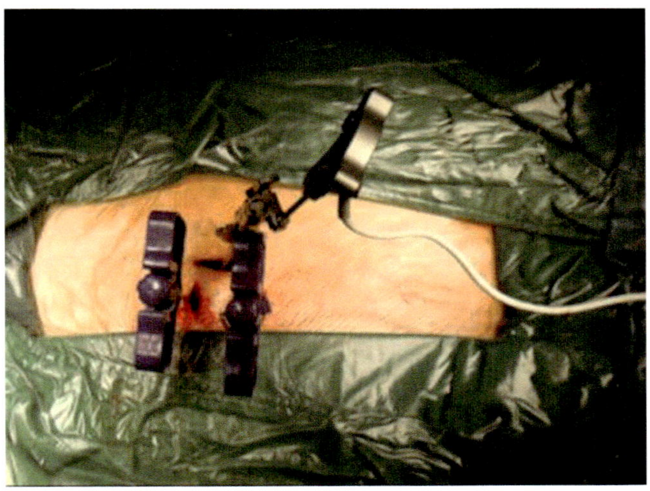

Fig. 13.147 A navigation guide is installed on T9 spinous process

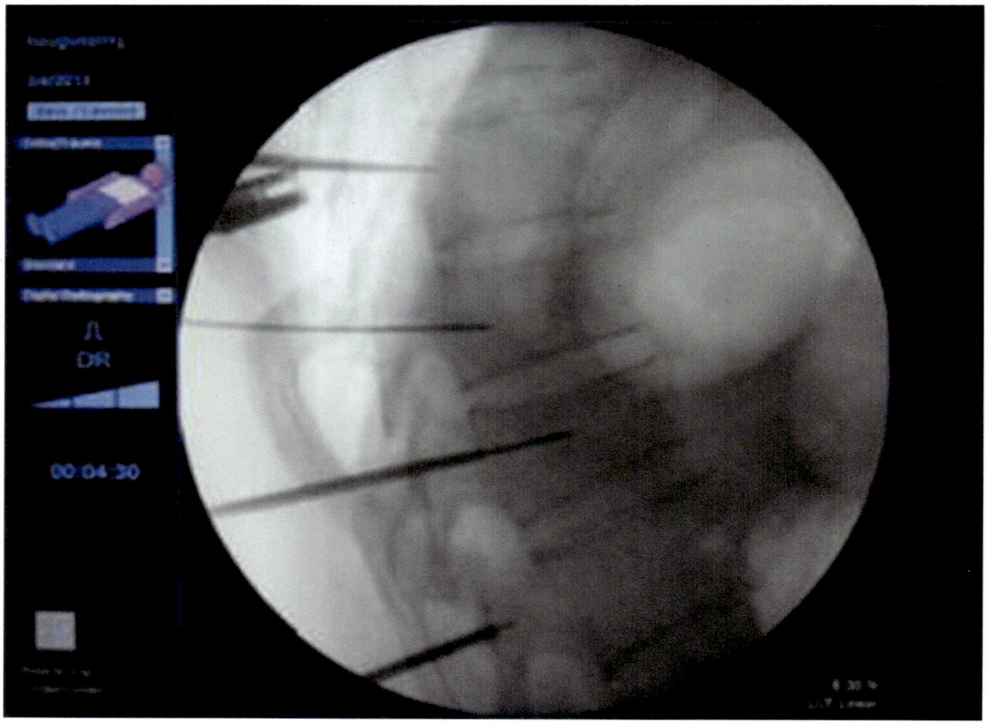

Fig. 13.148 Intraoperative fluoroscopy

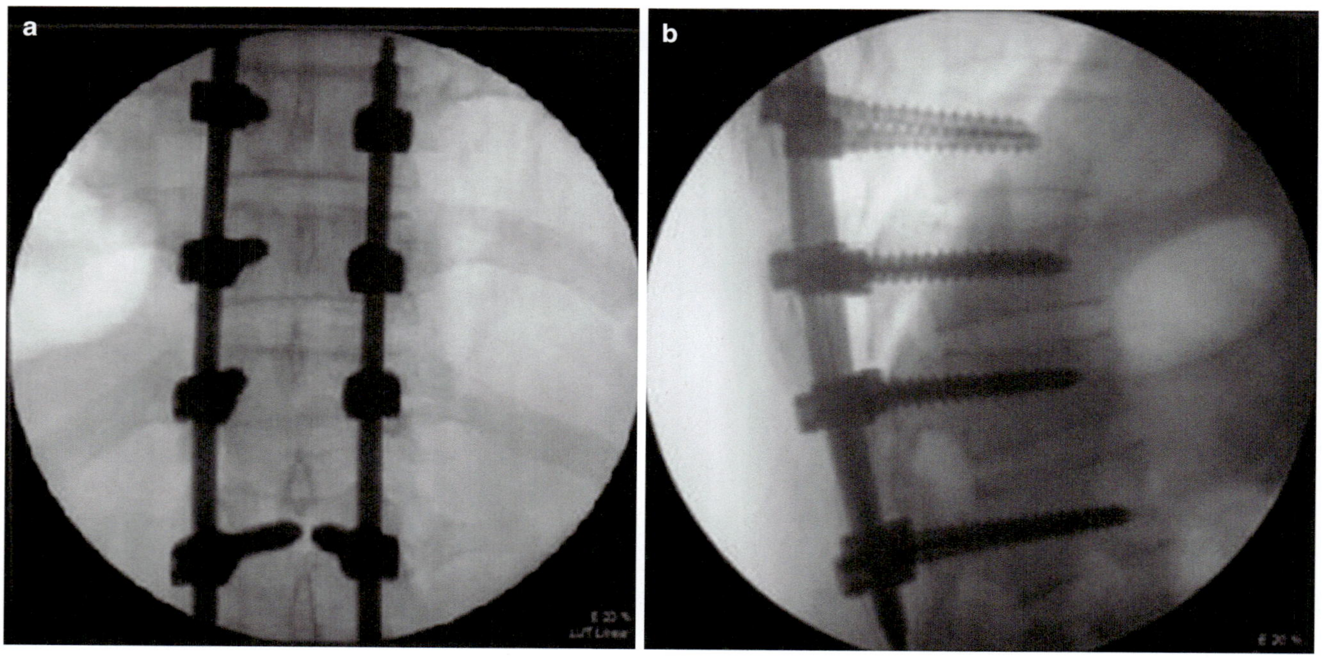

Fig. 13.149 Fluoroscopy image post screw placement. (**a**): Anteroposterior view; (**b**): Lateral view

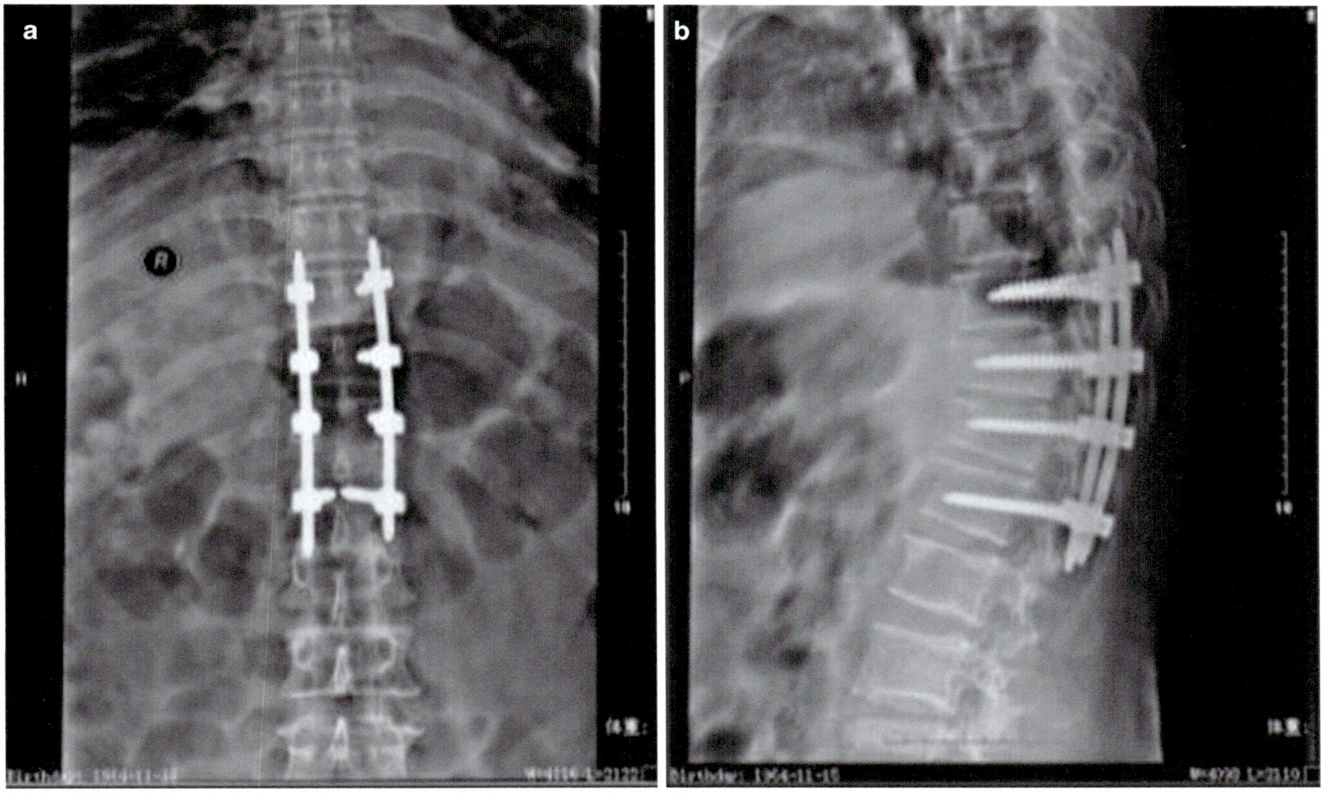

Fig. 13.150 (**a**): Postoperative anteroposterior view and (**b**) lateral view

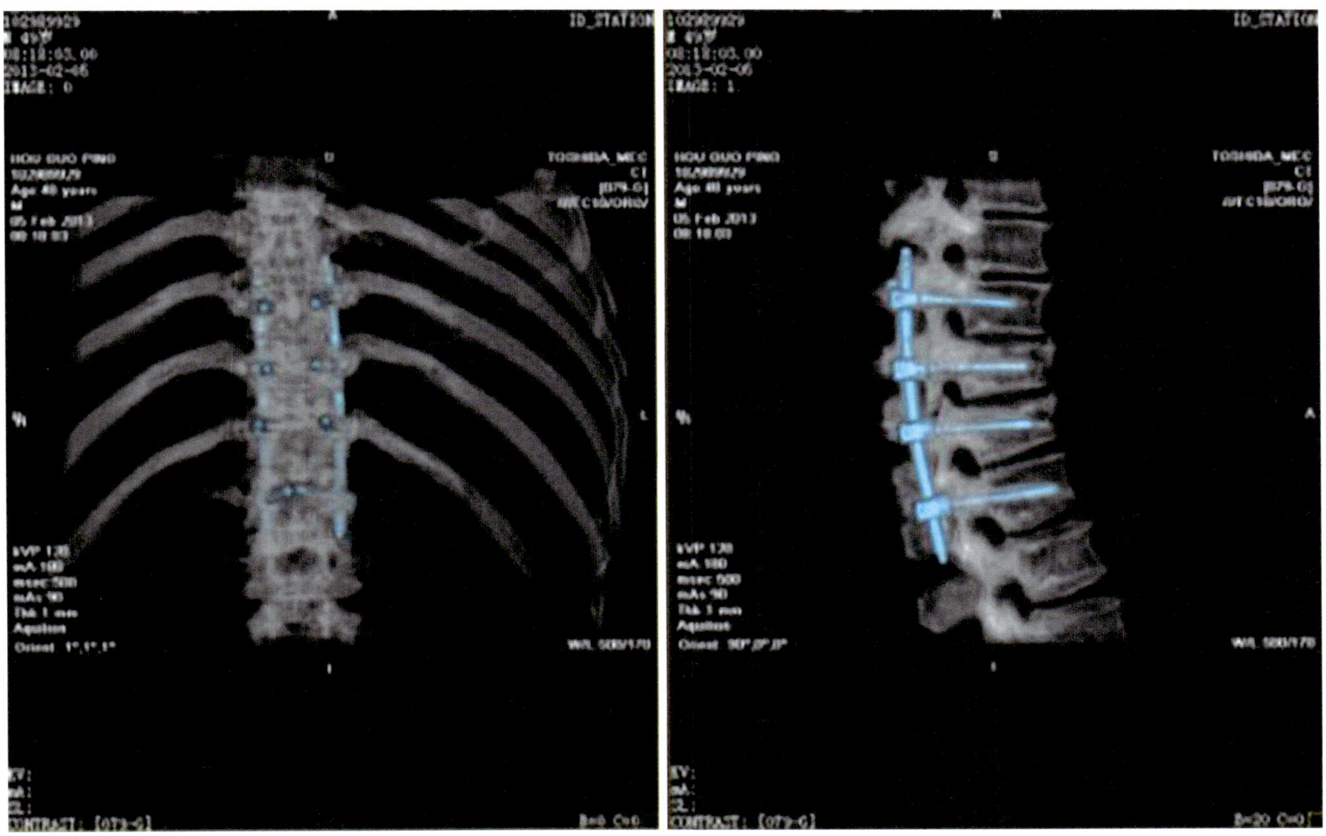

Fig. 13.151 Postoperative 3D CT reconstruction images

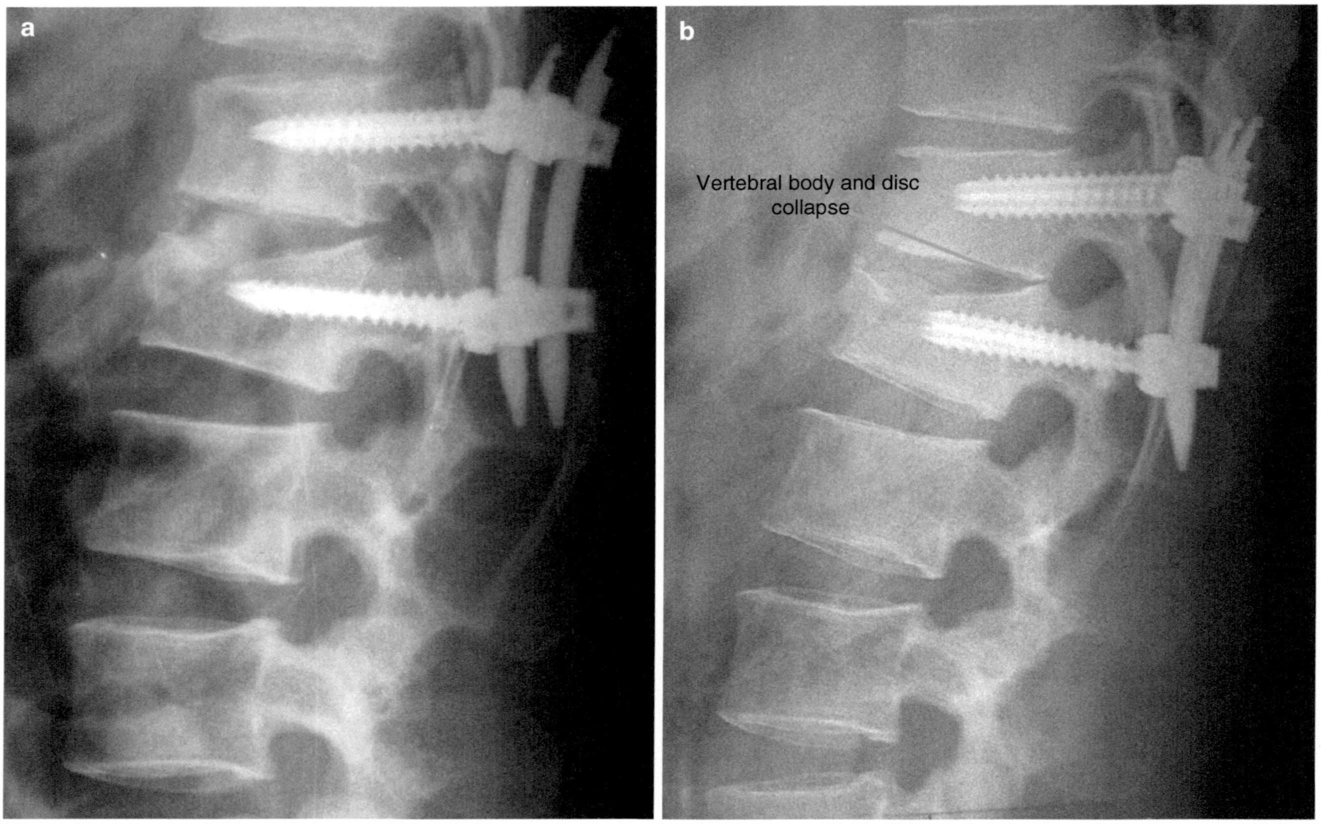

Fig. 13.152 (**a**) X-ray at 3 days postoperatively (lateral); (**b**): X-ray at 3 months postoperatively (lateral)

References

1. Magerl FP. Stabilization of the lower thoracic and lumbar spine with external skeletal fixation. Clin Orthop Relat Res. 1984;189:125–41.
2. Harms J, Rollinger H. A one-stage procedure in operative treatment of spondylolisthesis: dorsal traction–reposition and anterior fusion. Z Orthop Ihre Grenzgeb. 1982;120:343–7.
3. Foley KT, Gupta SK, Justis JR, Sherman MC. Percutaneous pedicle screw fixation of the lumbar spine. Neurosurg Focus. 2001;10:1–8.
4. Court C, Vincent C. Percutaneous fixation of thoracolumbar fractures: current concepts. Orthop Traumatol Surg Res. 2012 Dec;98(8):900–9.

14 Thoracolumbar Percutaneous Vertebroplasty (PVP) and Percutaneous Kyphoplasty (PKP)

Jiang-Jun Zhou, Min Zhao, and Wei Lei

Abstract

Percutaneous vertebroplasty (PVP) and percutaneous kyphoplasty (PKP) are minimally invasive procedures used to treat spinal compression fractures and vertebral body tumor. Both of the two procedures can achieve very good clinical efficacy and improvement in quality of life. Moreover, the pain relief rate reaches above 90% in osteoporosis patients and between 75% and 90% in cancer patients. So PVP and PKP are favored by both the operator and the patient. This chapter shows the specific operation technology through 3D pictures and the corresponding X-ray images, and the 3D profile pictures can show more details about the operation which are easy for surgeons to understand.

Keywords

Thoracolumbar vertebrae · Percutaneous vertebroplasty · Percutaneous kyphoplasty · Minimally invasive

14.1 Percutaneous Kyphoplasty: A Historical Perspective

In percutaneous vertebroplasty (PVP), the needle is placed into the diseased vertebra under direct fluoroscopic monitoring via the pedicle or via the transpedicular approach, and bone cement is directly injected via this route.

In 1984, Galibert and Deramond et al. [1] were the first to carry out PVP in successful treatment of a case of vertebral hemangioma at C2 via injection of polymethyl methacrylate (PMMA) (Fig. 14.1).

In 1994, Garfin and Yuan et al. [2], based on PVP, first proposed the design of percutaneous kyphoplasty (PKP) and applied the technique clinically (Fig. 14.2).

Both PVP and PKP can achieve very good clinical efficacy, and pain relief is immediate in the patients, with improvement in ambulation, reduction in analgesics use, and improvement in quality of life. Moreover, the two surgical methods cause little trauma, scant blood loss, and rapid recovery. Patients readily accept the methods, and the pain relief rate reaches above 90% in osteoporosis patients and between 75% and 90% in cancer patients [3, 4].

14.2 Surgical Techniques of PVP and PKP

14.2.1 Anesthesia

General or regional anesthesia can be used for surgery.

14.2.2 Radiographic Visualization

G-arm or double C-arm fluoroscopy systems are recommended to reduce operative time. G-arm needs to be draped with sterile cover to avoid contamination of the operative field during surgery (Fig. 14.3). Intraoperative standard orthogonal radiographic visualization is done with the spinous process in the center and the superior and inferior endplates in parallel. On lateral visualization, the bilateral pedicles are overlapped and the superior and inferior endplates are parallel. For puncture accuracy, "oval endplates" should be avoided (Fig. 14.4).

J.-J. Zhou · M. Zhao
Department of Orthopedics, The 908th Hospital of Chinese People's Liberation Army Joint Logistic Support Force, Nanchang, China

W. Lei (✉)
Department of Orthopedics, Xijing Hospital, Air Force Medical University, Xi'an, Shaanxi, China
e-mail: leiwei@fmmu.edu.cn

W. Lei, Y. Yan (eds.), *Internal Fixation of the Spine*, https://doi.org/10.1007/978-981-16-1562-7_14

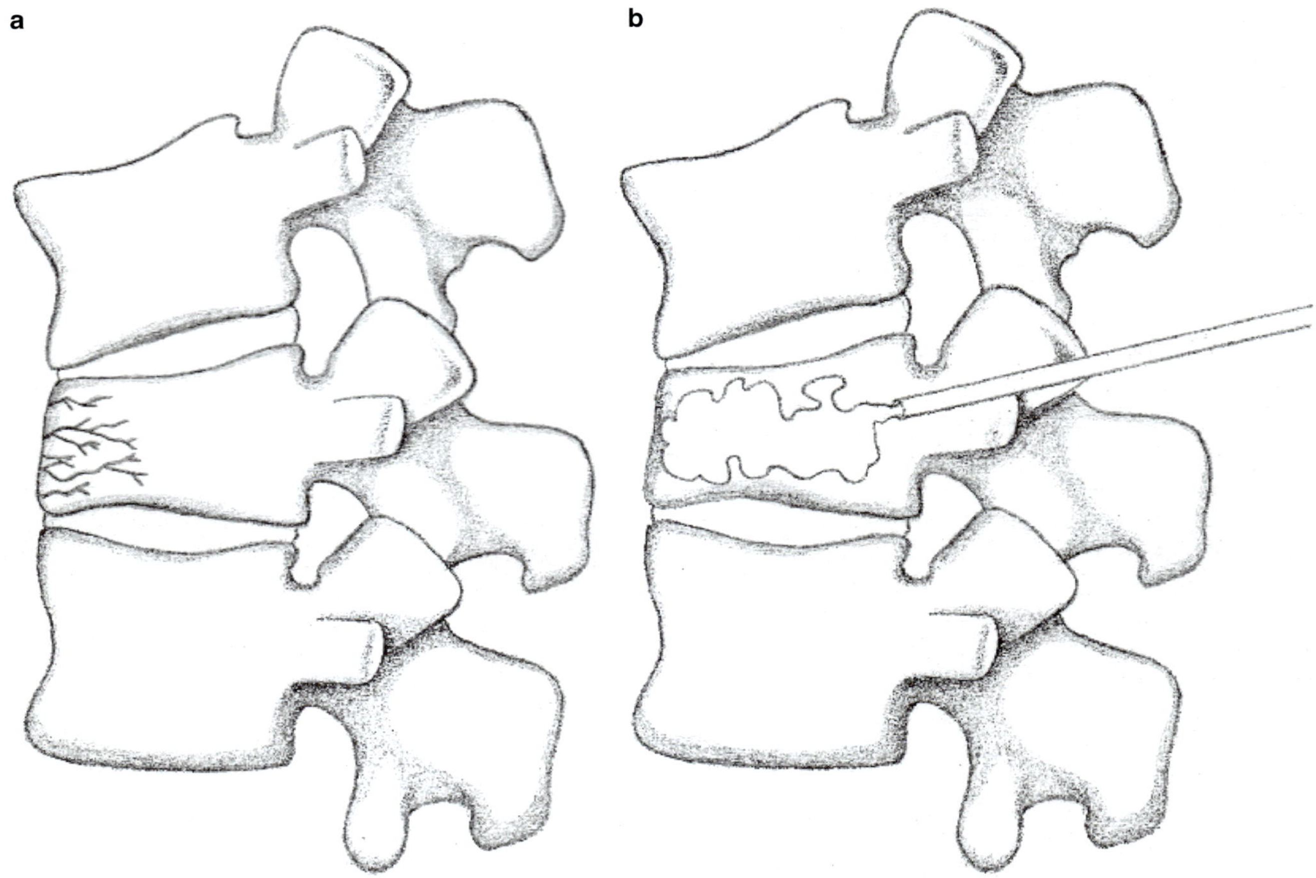

Fig. 14.1 Percutaneous vertebroplasty. (**a**) Vertebral fracture; (**b**) Cement injection

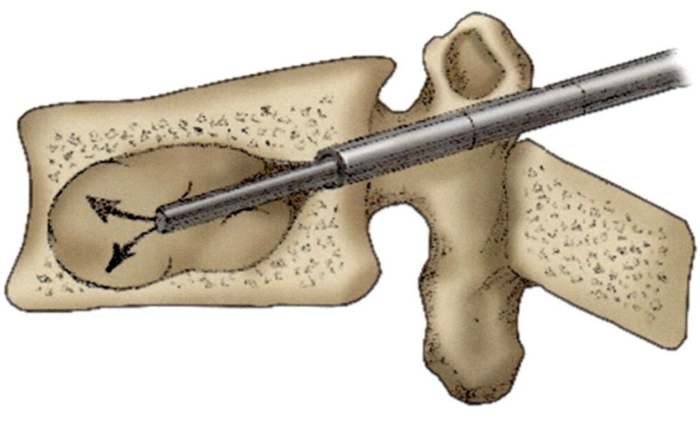

Fig. 14.2 Percutaneous kyphoplasty. The balloon is inflated and the cement is injected into the cavity

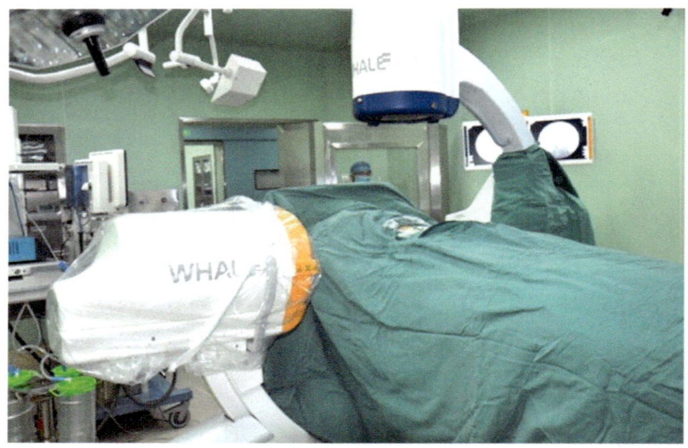

Fig. 14.3 G-arm fluoroscopy. The machine is draped with sterile cover

14.2.2.1 PVP

Determination of Puncture Site

Under orthogonal fluoroscopy, the skin incision is made approximately 1 cm from the lateral border of the projection of the pedicle (Fig. 14.5a, b), and the needle tip is generally located on the superolateral edge of the projection of the pedicle on orthogonal radiograph, equivalent to 2 or 10 o'clock (Fig. 14.6a–e).

Puncture Angle

The thoracic spine is abducted at an angle of approximately 10°–15°, and the lumbar spine approximately 15°–25°.

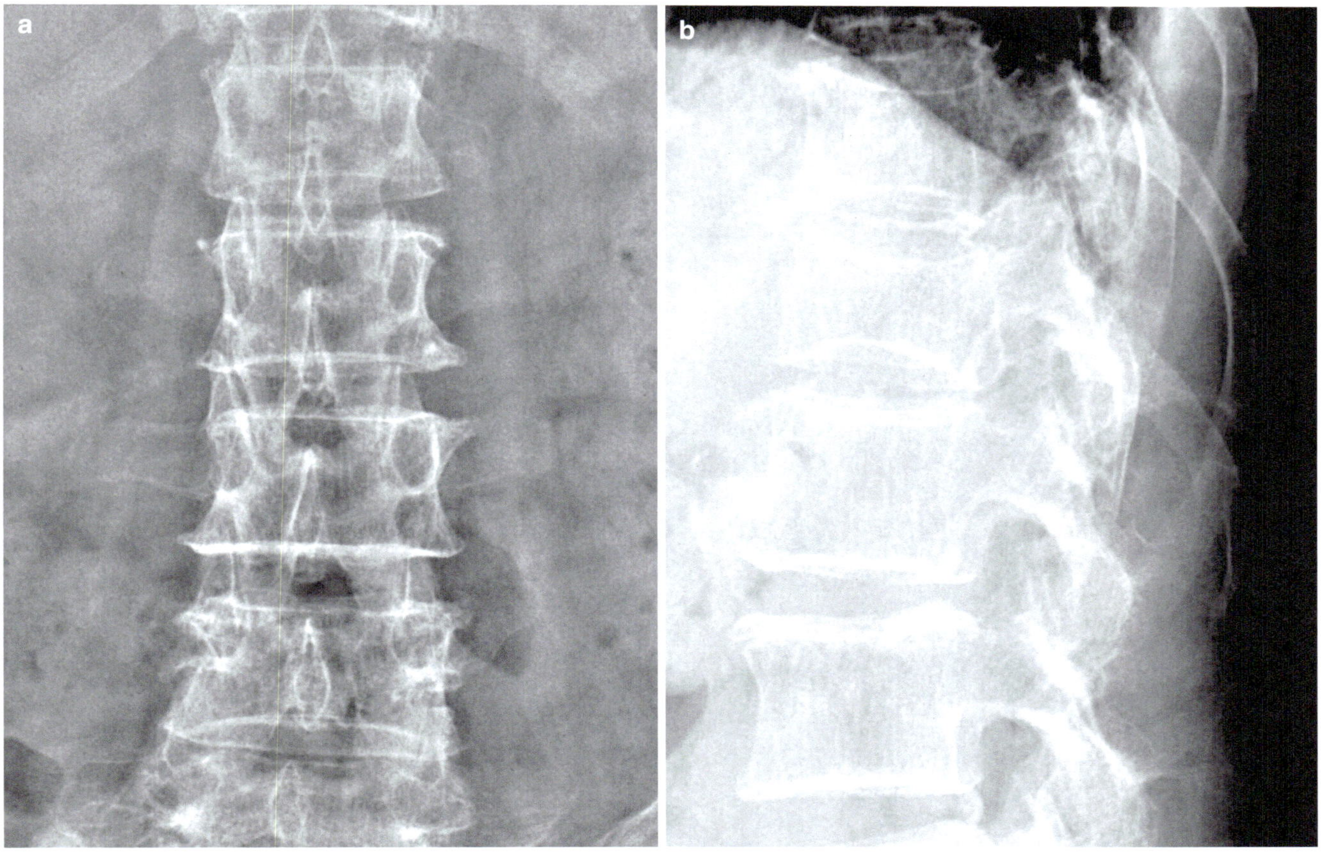

Fig. 14.4 Intraoperative fluoroscopy. (**a**) Orthogonal radiographic view; (**b**) Lateral view

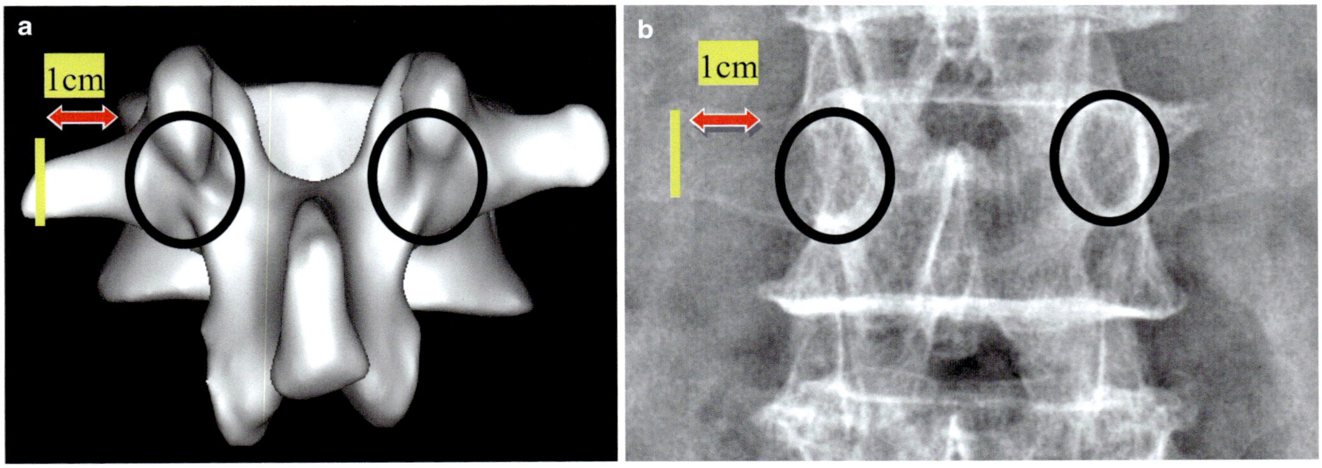

Fig. 14.5 (**a**) 3D image of the L3 vertebral body; (**b**) Anteroposterior radiograph of the L3 vertebral body. The black oval-circle in (a) and (b) are the projections of the pedicles. The incision (yellow vertical line, approximately 0.5 cm long) is located approximately 1 cm from the lateral border of the projection

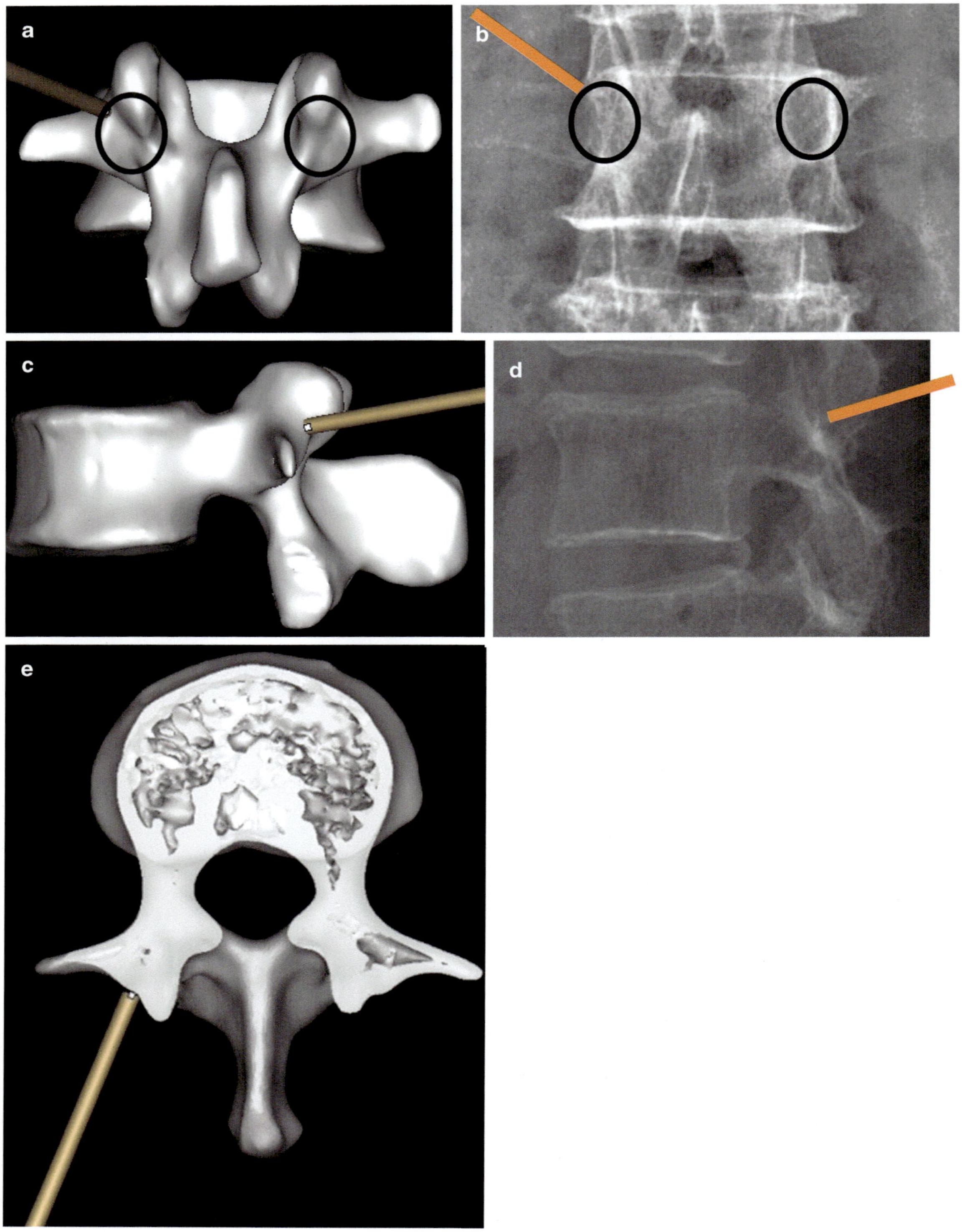

Fig. 14.6 Illustration of the needle entry site. (**a**) The 3D model shows the entry site posteriorly. (**b**) The entry site in the anteroposterior radiograph; (**c**) The 3D model shows the entry site laterally; (**d**) The entry site in the lateral radiograph; (**e**) The 3D model shows the entry angle

Puncture Depth

The needle exceeds the posterior edge of the vertebral body by approximately 2 mm (Fig. 14.7 A–D).

Tailored Adjustment

If the diameter of the pedicle of the thoracic vertebra is too small, a parapedicular approach can be used (Figs. 14.8, 14.9).

Surgical Steps

(a) Bipedicular or unipedicular puncture is made via the conventional posterior approach depending on the tolerability of patients for surgery, pedicle abduction angle, and dexterity of the operators.

(b) Under G-arm fluoroscopy, the projection of the pedicle is marked on the skin using a marker (Fig. 14.10a, b). After conventional sterilization and draping, regional anesthesia is done with 0.05% lidocaine to reach directly the periosteum of the pedicle. A skin incision approximately 0.5 cm in length is made with a sharp scalpel blade.

(c) The beveled bone cement stylet is passed through the pedicle of the diseased vertebra under fluoroscopic guidance (Figs. 14.11 and 14.12).

(d) The needle core is withdrawn and replaced with the guide needle. Then, the soft tissue distractor and the working sleeve are placed along the guide needle. The bone drill then enters the vertebral body approximately 2–3 cm (Fig. 14.13)

(e) Bone cement is prepared until it forms a paste or is "brushed" and then injected into the diseased vertebra (Figs. 14.14 and 14.15).

(f) After confirmation that there is no error, the wound is sutured or pulled together with a Band-Aid.

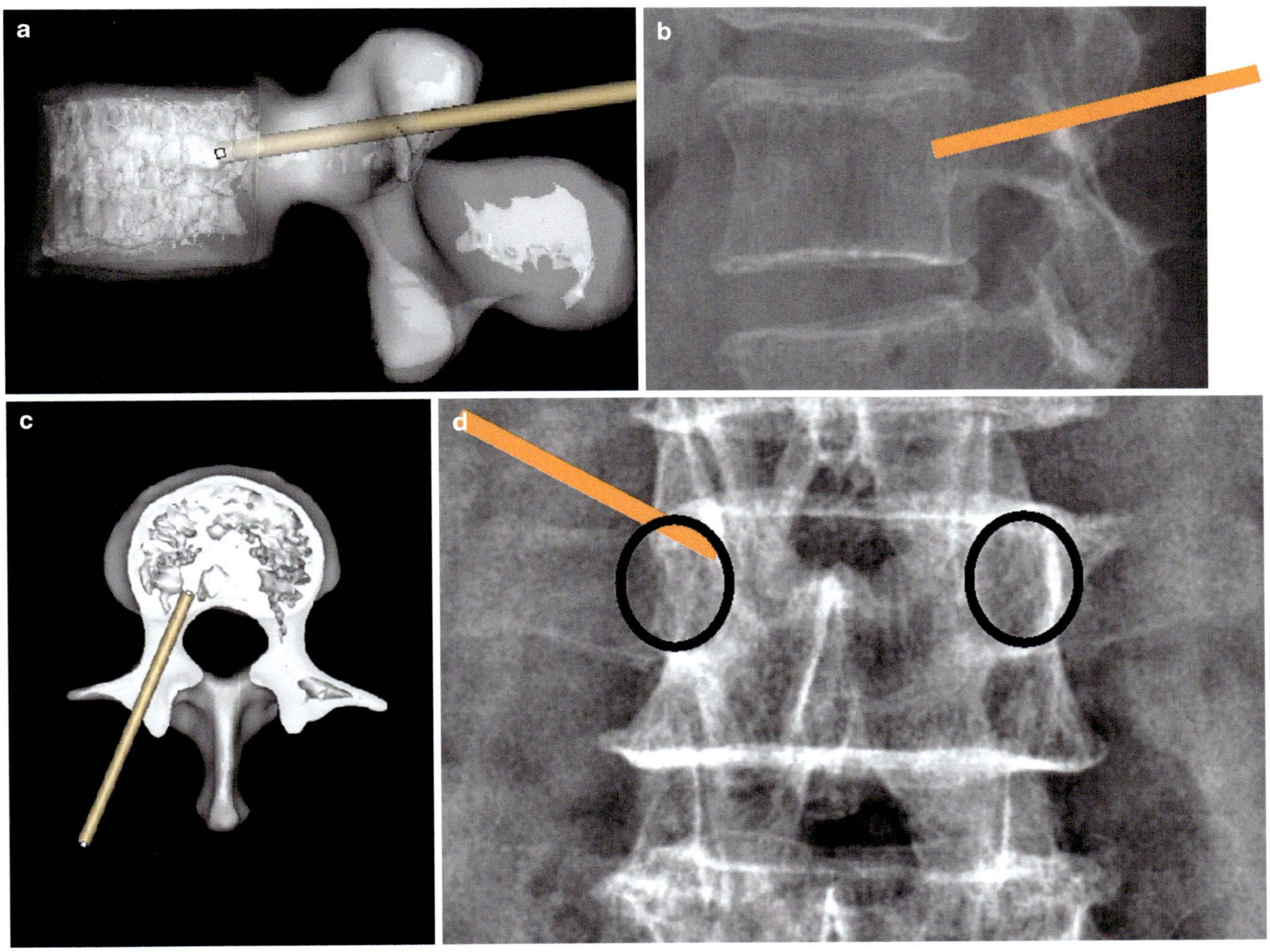

Fig. 14.7 The needle penetrates the posterior wall of the vertebral body by 2 mm. (**a**) The 3D model shows the needle position. (**b**) Needle position in the lateral radiograph; (**c**) The 3D model shows the needle position; (**d**) Needle position in the anteroposterior radiograph

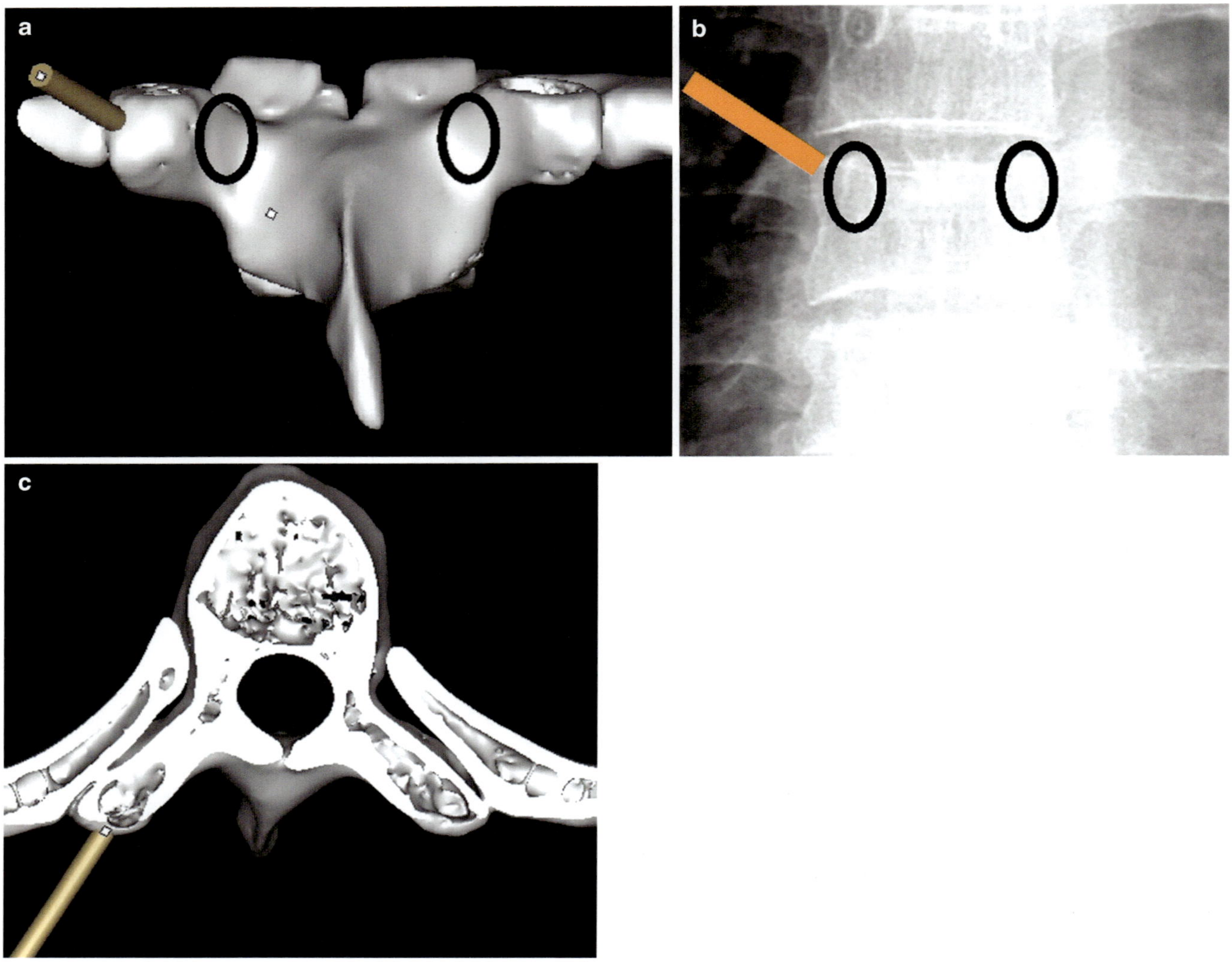

Fig. 14.8 The needle is entered at the lateral edge of the transverse process. (**a**) The 3D model shows the needle position. (**b**) Needle position in the anteroposterior radiograph; (**c**) The 3D model shows the needle angle

14.2.2.2 PKP Technique

Puncture

In PKP, the puncture site, puncture angle and depth, and placement channels are identical to those of PVP. Different from PVP, PKP uses balloon distractor to distract the diseased vertebra and inject bone cement.

Surgical Steps

On the basis of PVP, the working channels are established, and after expansion of the channels with a bone drill, a balloon distractor is placed. Wound preparation is identical to that of PVP.

(a) Balloon distraction is done after confirmation under fluoroscopy that the balloon has passed the working channel (Figs. 14.16 and 14.17). The balloon pressure should be less than 300 PSI, that is, 20 Kpa, and rotating injection can be done to avoid balloon rupture due to rapid rise in pressure. For fresh osteoporotic fracture, balloon pressure should generally be less than 150 PSI (10 Kpa).
(b) The volume of bone cement injected should be largely the same as the size of the distracted balloon. Excessive injection of bone cement should be avoided in order to prevent leakage (Fig. 14.18)

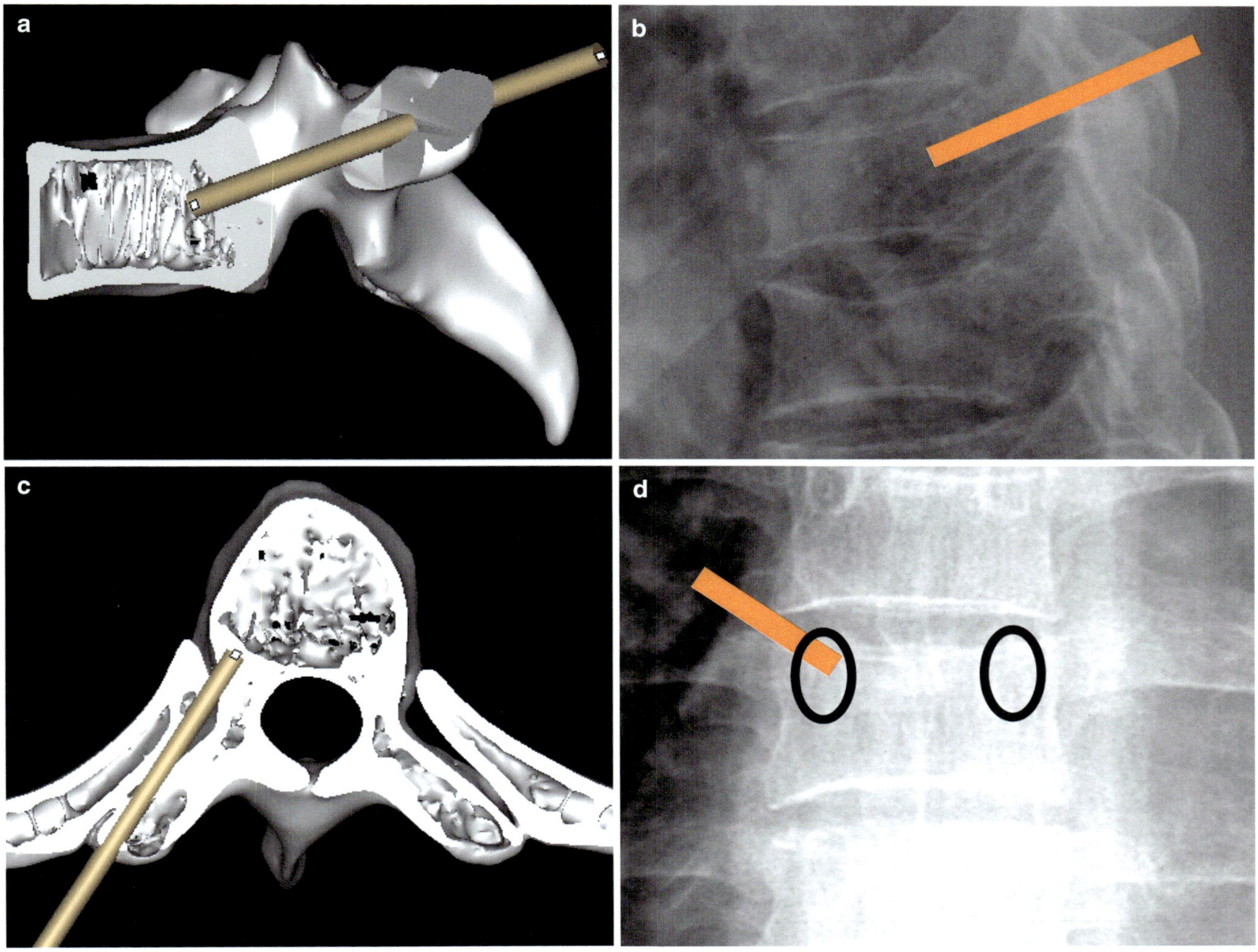

Fig. 14.9 The needle enters via the parapedicular approach. (**a**) The 3D model shows the needle position. (**b**) Needle position in the lateral radiograph; (**c**) The 3D model shows the needle position; (**d**) Needle position in the anteroposterior radiograph

14.3 Clinical Cases

14.3.1 Case No. 1

Patient: An 83-year-old woman with repeated episodes of back pain for years.

Diagnosis: Multiple thoracolumbar compression fractures (T11–L5).

Surgery: Balloon kyphoplasty with injection of bone cement after balloon distraction of T11–L5 vertebral bodies.

Imaging data: Preoperative image is shown in Figs. 14.19 and 14.20, and postoperative images are shown in Fig. 14.21.

14.4 Pearls and Pitfalls

1. Preoperative radiographs should be carefully examined. Surgery should not be performed in cases of severe occupation in the spinal space or manifested nerve compression symptoms.
2. Intraoperative prone position may cause rib fractures in cases of severe osteoporosis.
3. During puncture, the puncture site should be accurately determined in order to avoid inadvertent injury to adjacent tissues such as the spinal cord or the nerve roots, pedicle fracture, and pneumothorax. The stylet should be advanced under fluoroscopy guidance, and the patient

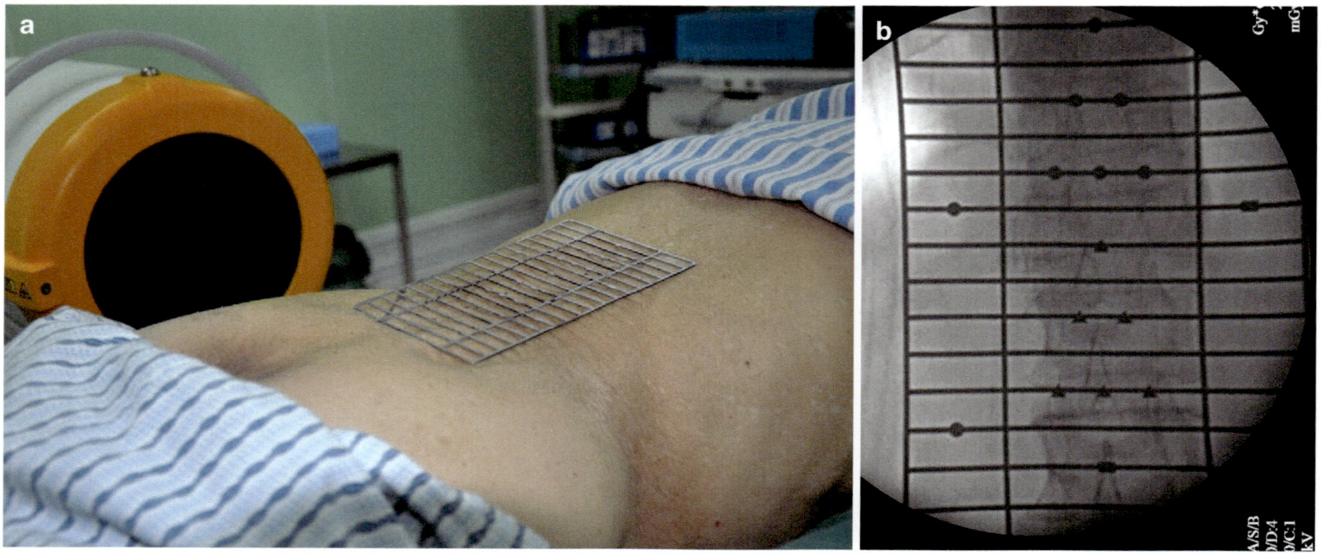

Fig. 14.10 The pedicle is identified and marked (**a**) under C-arm fluoroscopy (**b**)

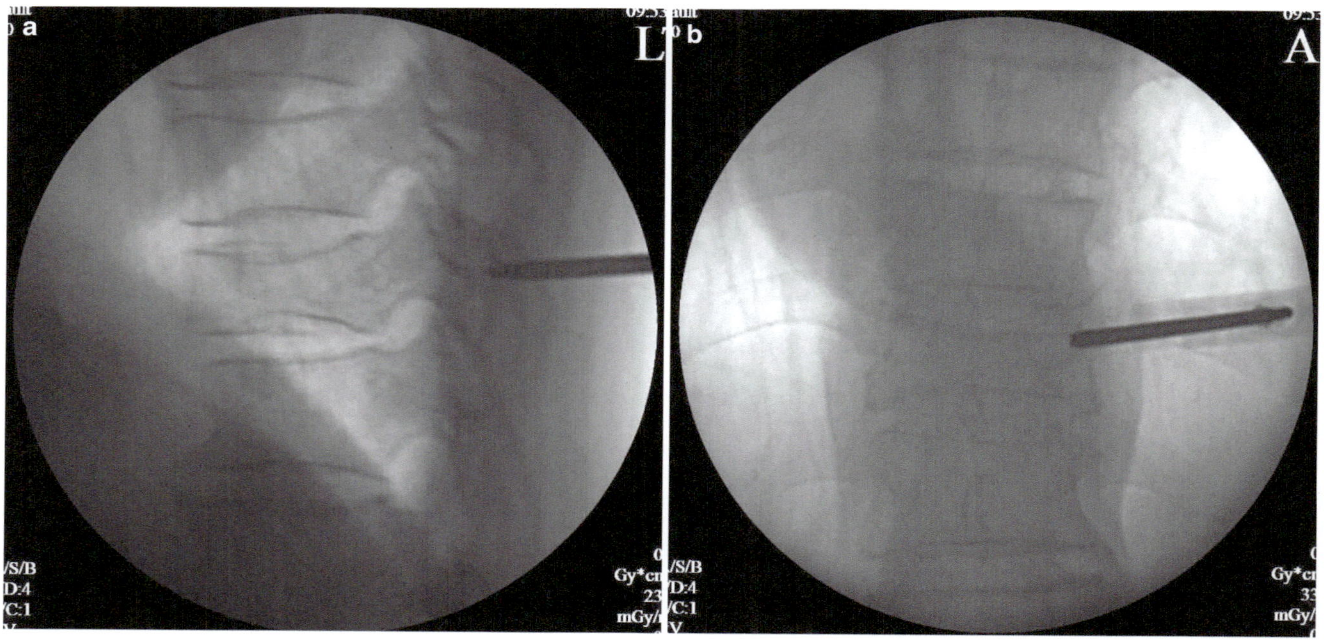

Fig. 14.11 When the stylet reaches the lamina on the lateral radiograph (**a**), it should be positioned at 2 or 10 o'clock at the lateral edge of the projection of the pedicle on the orthogonal radiograph (**b**)

should be asked about presence of any discomforts. Advancement of the stylet is discontinued as soon as nerve system symptoms appear, and the direction of stylet advancement should be changing the needle under fluoroscopy guidance

4. The vertebral bodies are distracted by balloon and the pressure in general should not exceed 300 PSI (20 Kpa); otherwise, severe pain may occur in the patient, and the balloon may also rupture, leading to contrast medium leakage.
5. When the inflated balloon distractor is withdrawn, the pressure should be adjusted to negative. If resistance is encountered, the distractor can be repetitively advanced and withdrawn and then is slowly withdrawn after turning the balloon. The balloon should not be withdrawn by force, which leads to balloon rupture.
6. After bone cement injection, the stylet should be withdrawn after confirmation that the bone cement is completely dry; otherwise, trailing may occur (Fig. 14.22).

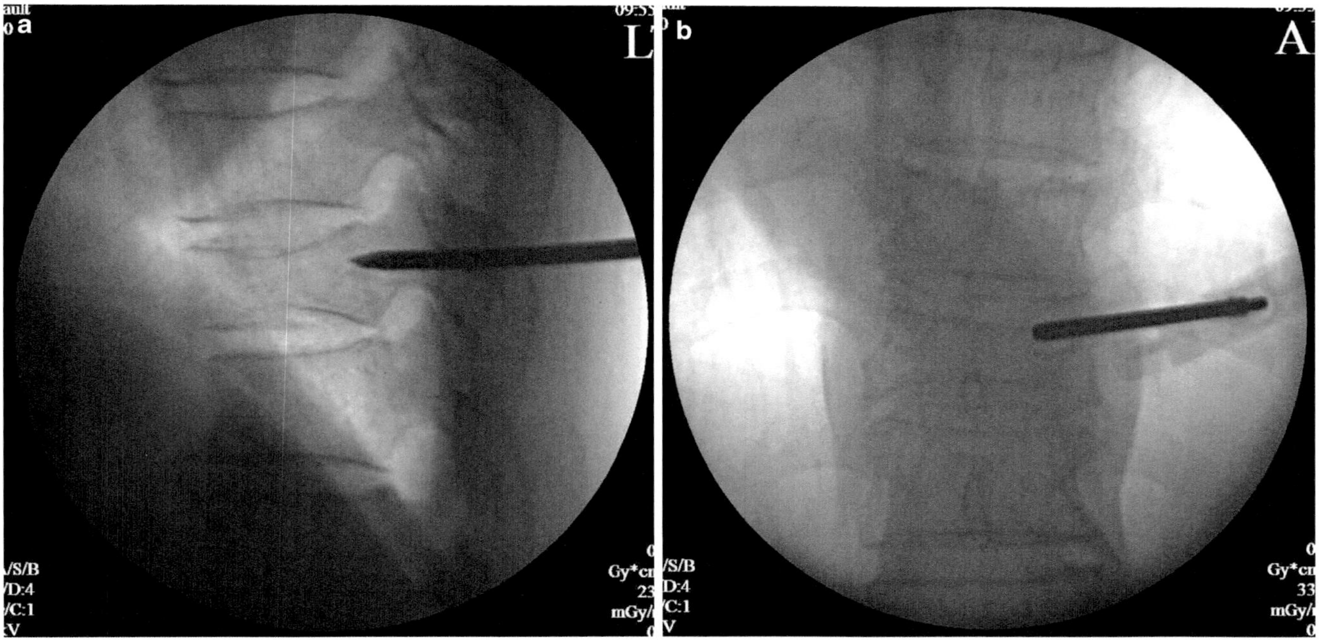

Fig. 14.12 When the stylet passes 2 mm beyond the posterior wall of the vertebral body on the lateral radiograph (**a**), it should be positioned at the medial edge of the projection of the pedicle on the orthogonal radiograph (**b**)

7. Bone cement is generally injected when it appears "brushed" and injection should be slow and at moderate force. Otherwise, bone cement leakage into the vertebral canal, the intervertebral foramen, the intervertebral disc, the paravertebral soft tissue, and the vertebral venous plexus will ensue. If bone cement leaks into the vertebral canal or the intervertebral foramen, it will cause searing injury of the nerve roots and nerve root compression. If this happens, injection should be stopped immediately and laminectomy and nerve decompression should be done. If bone cement leaks into the intervertebral disc, it does not affect the surgical outcome; however, it may increase the risk of fracture of the diseased vertebra or the adjacent vertebrae. If bone cement leaks into the paravertebral soft tissue, it may cause intercostal neuralgia or sciatica.
8. Unilateral or bilateral bone cement injection has no impact on surgical outcome and causes similar symptomatic relief in the patient. The volume of cement should be kept within 3 ml for the thoracic vertebra and 5 ml for the lumbar vertebra, which should be sufficient to increase bone strength. Injection should generally be stopped once the bone cement diffuses to the posterior wall of the vertebral body or leakage occurs.
9. During bone cement injection, reaction to the bone cement should be monitored, and when necessary, dexamethasone can be given intravenously.
10. Depending on the osteoporotic condition, the patient can have bed rest in the supine or prone position for 12 hours to 2 days and thereafter can ambulate wearing thoracolumbar support to reduce the risk of hypostatic pneumonia, venous thrombosis, or kyphosis.
11. Long-term anti-osteoporosis medication should be provided following surgery.

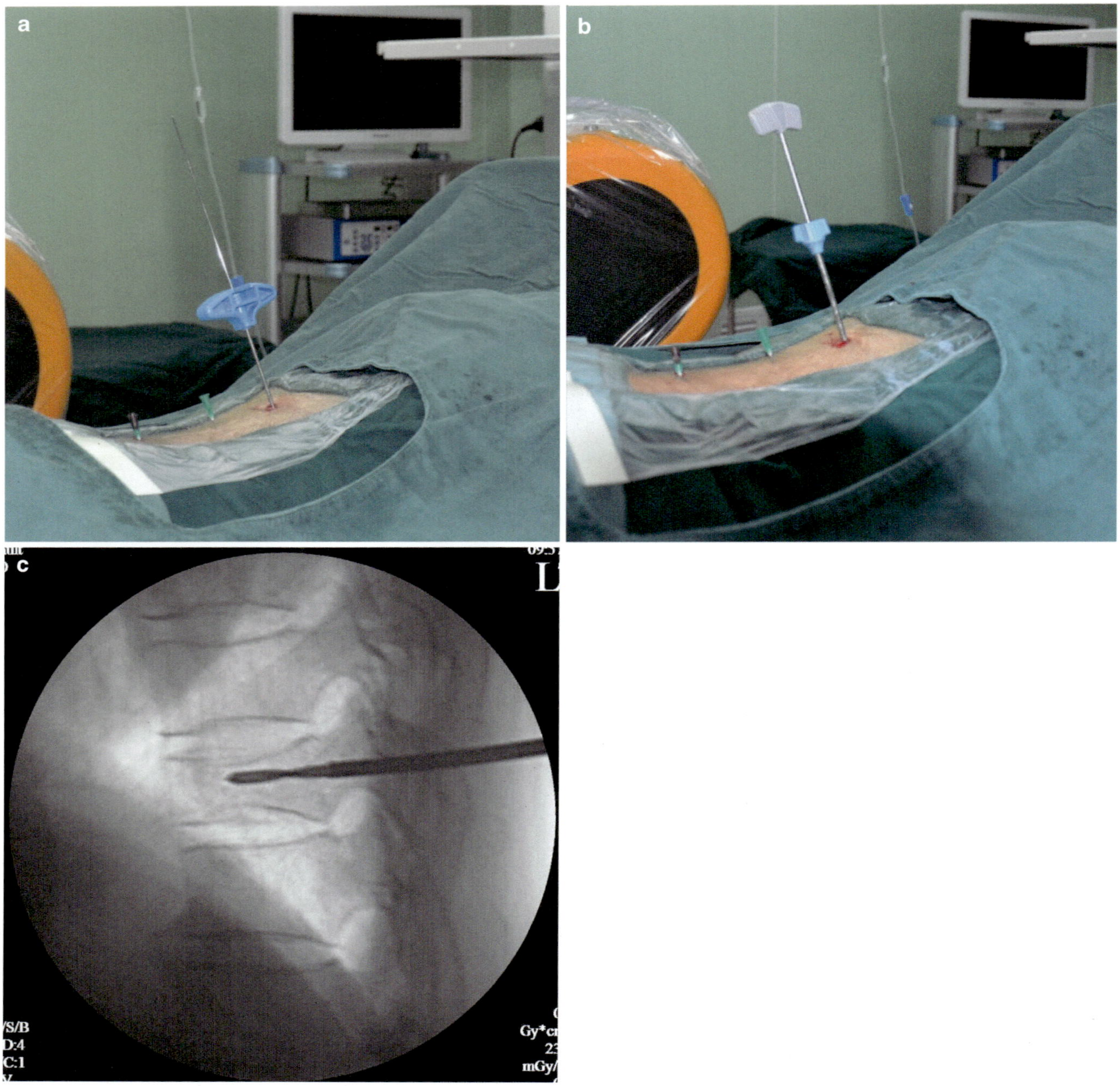

Fig. 14.13 After the needle core is placed (**a**), the working channel is changed (**b**). Then, the bone drill is rotated into the vertebral body (**c**)

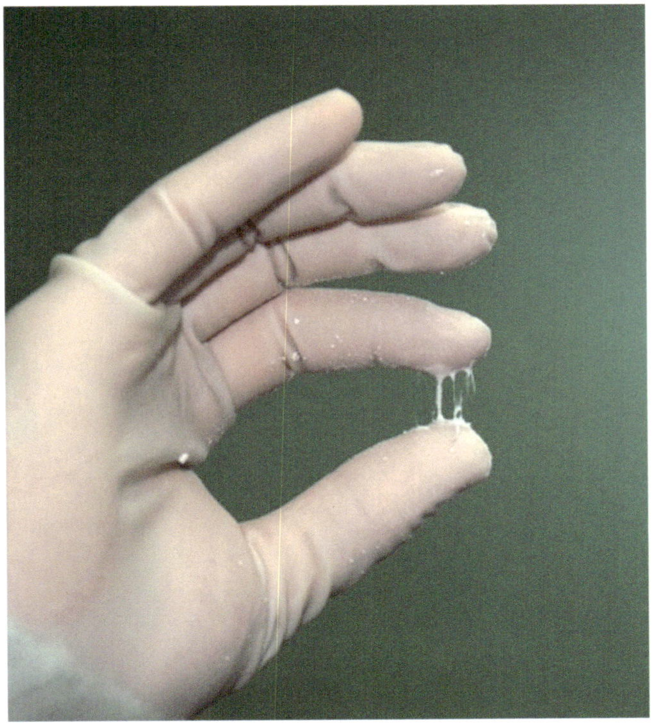

Fig. 14.14 The bone cement appears brushed

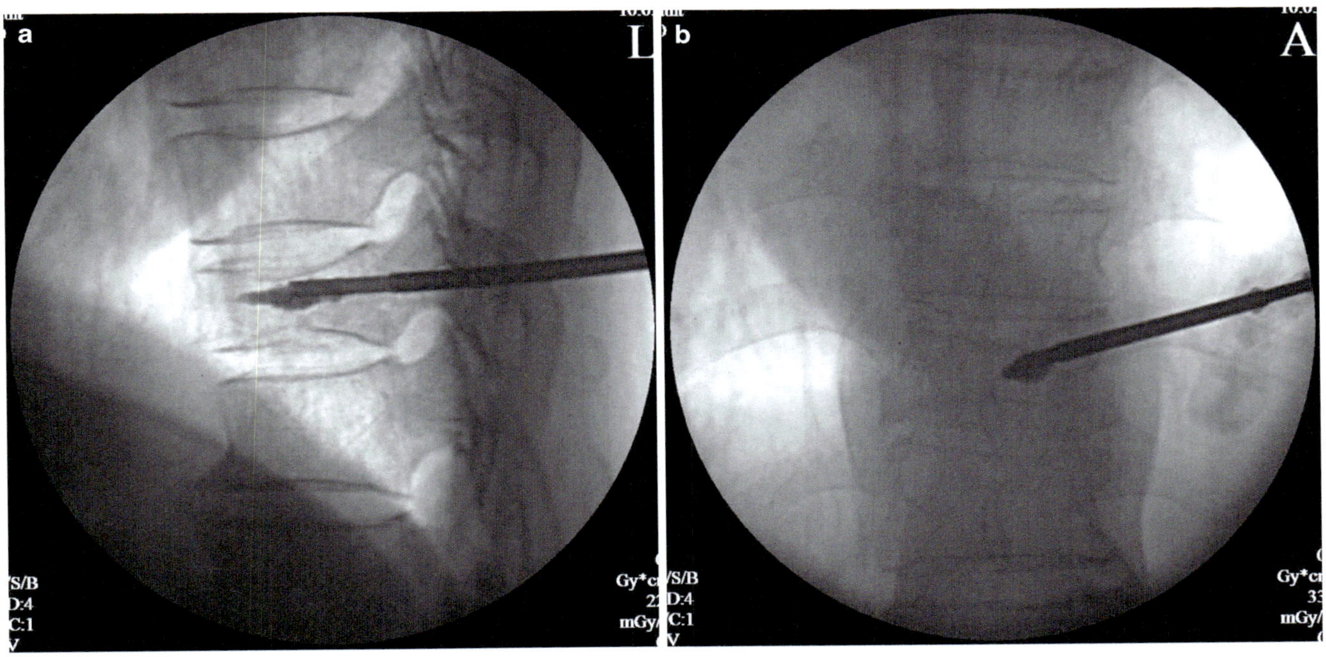

Fig. 14.15 The bone cement is injected. (**a**) Lateral radiograph; (**b**) Anteroposterior radiograph

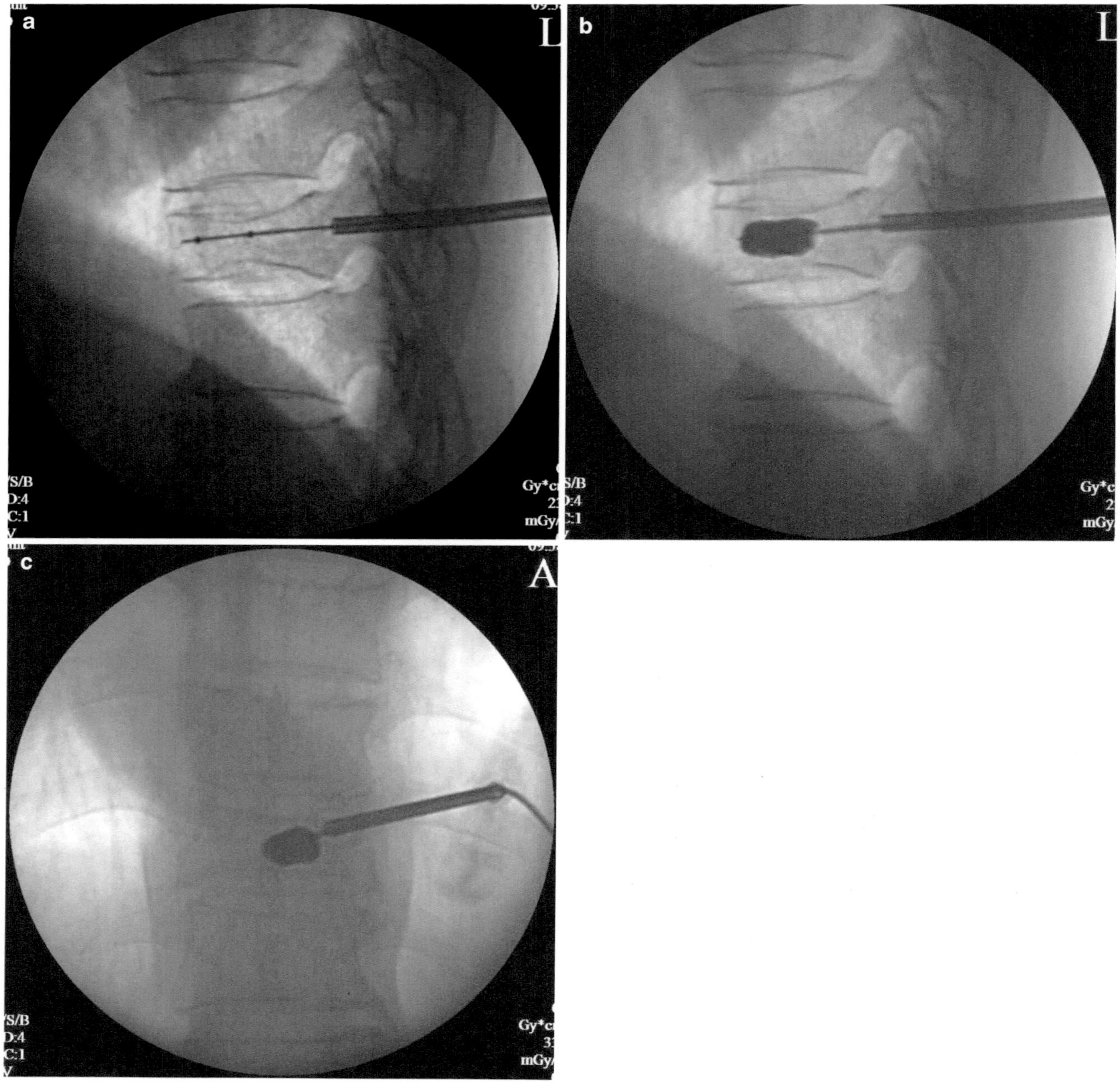

Fig. 14.16 Intraoperative view of the balloon via fluoroscopy. (**a**) Lateral radiograph before the balloon was inflated. (**b**) Lateral radiograph after the balloon was inflated. (**c**) Anteroposterior radiograph after the balloon was inflated

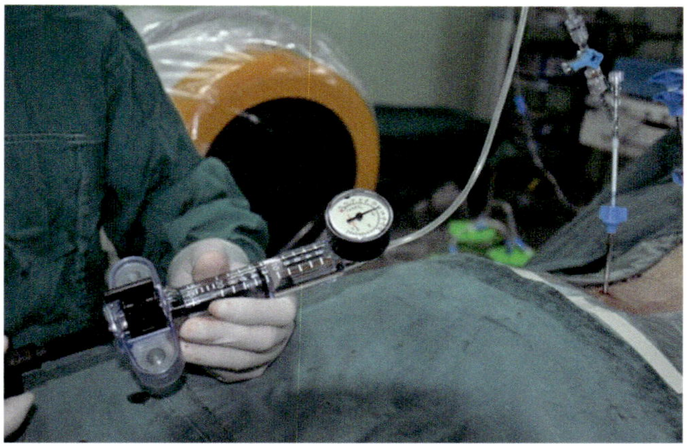

Fig. 14.17 The balloon distractor push bar is slowly turned during the operation

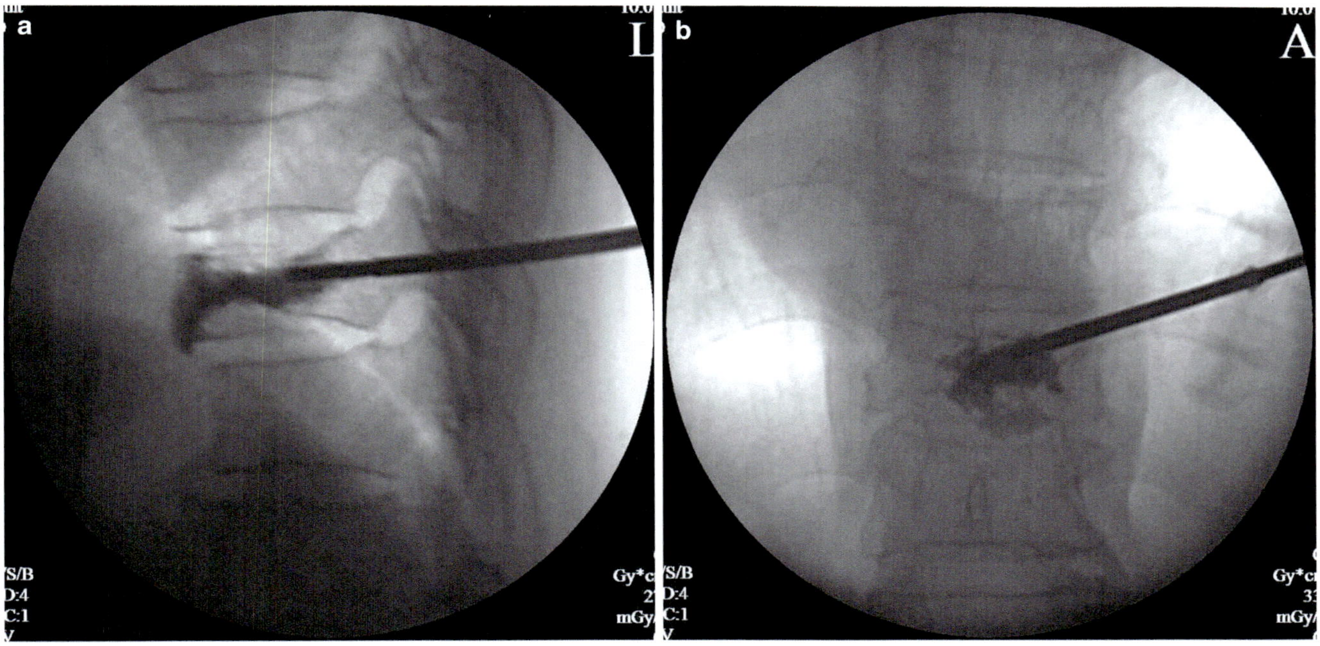

Fig. 14.18 Bone cement is slowly injected. (**a**) Lateral radiograph after the cement was injected. (**b**) Anteroposterior radiograph after the cement was injected

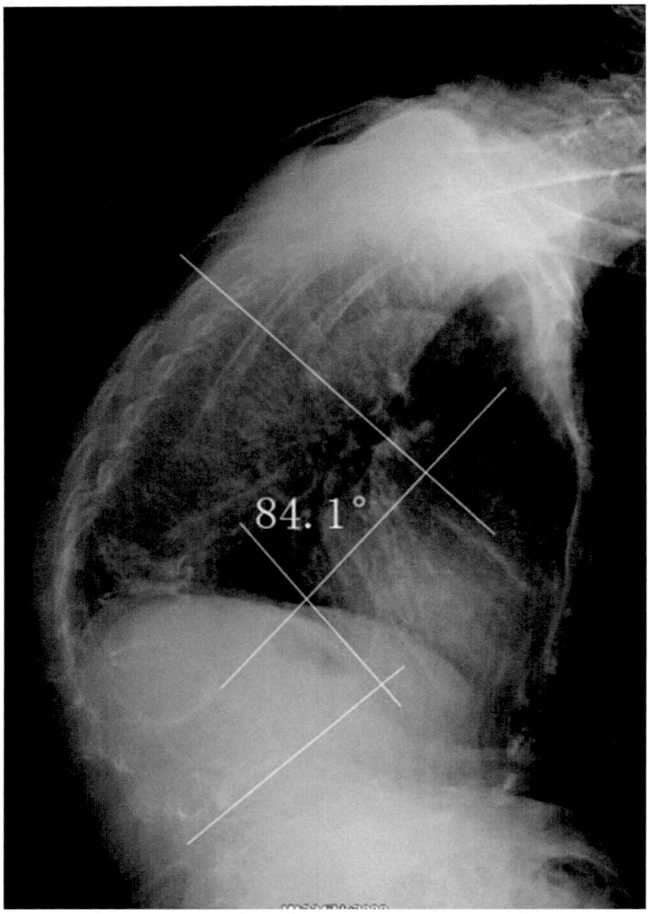

Fig. 14.19 Preoperative X-ray shows multiple thoracolumbar fractures and Cobb's angle is 84.1°

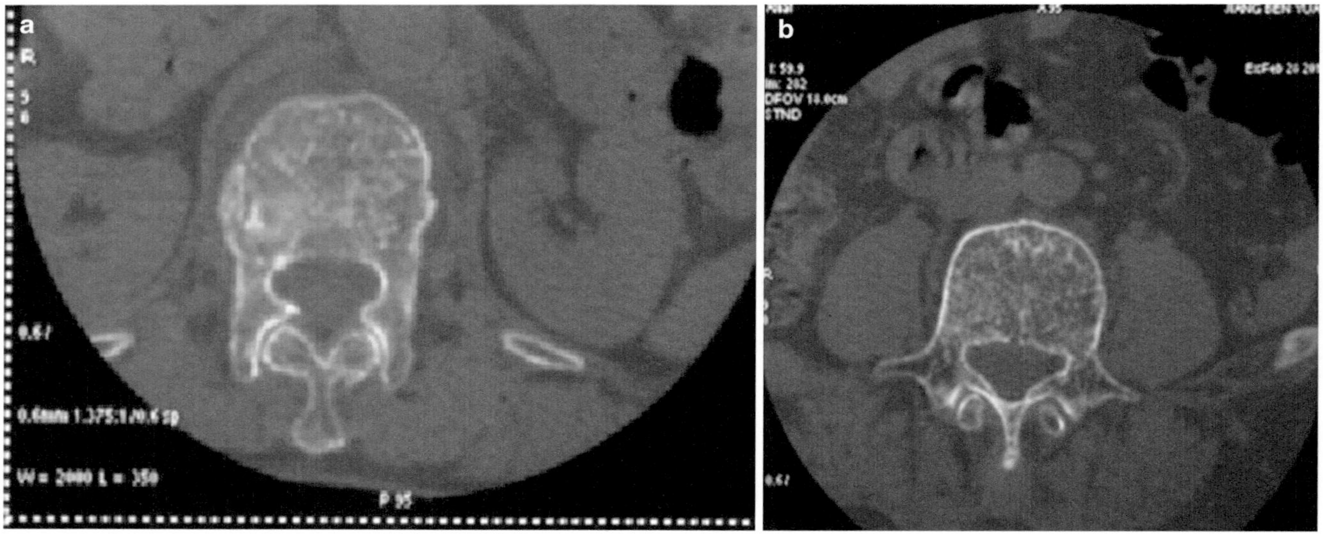

Fig. 14.20 Preoperative CT scan shows severe osteoporosis of the vertebral bodies, and bone absorption is observed in the vertebral body with old fracture. A: T12; B: L5

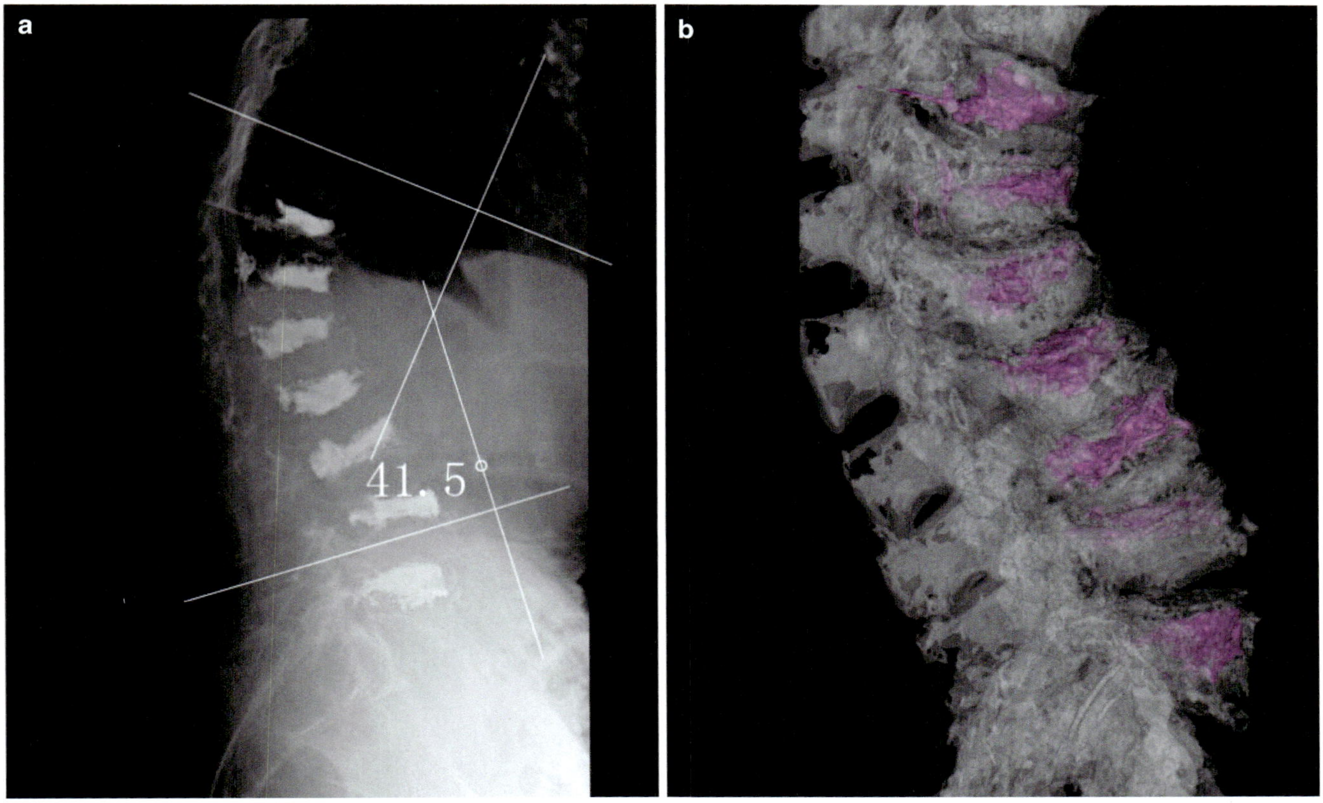

Fig. 14.21 The patient started ambulation 2 days after surgery wearing thoracolumbar support device and lumbar pain completely disappeared. (**a**) Postoperative X-ray shows that Cobb's angle is reduced to 41.5°; (**b**) 3D CT reveals satisfactory bone cement perfusion and no leakage is present

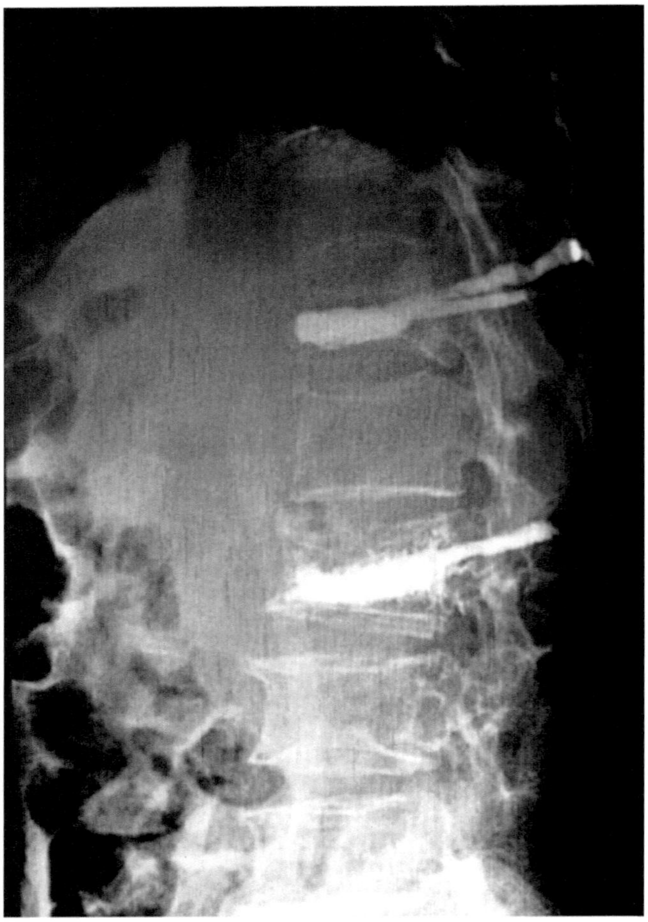

Fig. 14.22 Premature withdrawal of the stylet after bone cement injection readily causes the trailing phenomenon

References

1. Galibert P, Deramond H, Rosat P, et al. Preliminary note on the treatment of vertebral angioma by percutaneous acrylic vertebroplasty [J]. Neurochirurgie. 1987;33(2):1662–8.
2. Heini PF. The current treatment-a survey of osteoporotic fracture treatment: osteoporotic spine fractures: the spine surgeon's perspective. OsteoporosInt. 2005;16:85–92.
3. Bouza C, Lopez T, Magro A, et al. Efficacy and safety of balloon kyphoplasty in the treatment of vertebral compression fractures: a systematic review. Eur Spine J. 2006;21:1–18.
4. Hadjipavlou AG, TzermiadianosMN KPG, et al. Percutaneous vertebroplasty and balloon kyphoplasty for the treatment of osteoporotic vertebral compression fractures and osteolytic tumours. J Bone Joint Surg Br. 2005;87:1595–604.

15 Internal Fixation Technique and Application in the Osteoporotic Spine

YaFei Feng and Wei Lei

Abstract

Pedicle screw fixation is widely used for the stabilization of the thoracolumbar spine in a variety of indications. A typical complication reported in a number of studies is screw loosening, which may be related to the bone quality under osteoporotic and diabetic conditions. Indeed, studies showed a very wide range of failure rates, ranging from less than 1 to 15% in non-osteoporotic patients treated with rigid systems and even up to 60% in osteoporotic subjects. Strategies to limit screw loosening in osteoporotic bone were reported to be generally successful, in comparison with conventional screws. Here in this chapter, we introduced two managements containing expandable and augmented screws that may be a viable option under osteoporosis. Available clinical and biomechanical data show that these methods may be viable options to reduce the risk of screw loosening. The program about the selection of screw within different quality of the bone tissue was also provided. Screw augmentation with bone cement and expandable screws, together with this program, potentially appears to provide a good solution for posterior fixation in osteoporotic patients

Keywords

Osteoporosis · Pedicle screw fixation · Surgical technique

Y. Feng (✉) · W. Lei
Department of Orthopedics, Xijing Hospital, Air Force Medical University, Xi'an, Shaanxi, China
e-mail: leiwei@fmmu.edu.cn

15.1 A Historical Perspective

15.1.1 A Historical Perspective of Osteoporosis Screw Loosening

Screw loosening is a common complication of screw fixation of the spine (Fig. 15.1). Hitherto, many studies have reported cases of spine screw loosening whose incidence varies widely between 1% and 15% among patients with normal bone mass. The causes of loosening include stress occlusion, bone and screw interface strains, surface debris, and local infection. With aging of the population globally, an increasing proportion of elderly osteoporotic patients undergo spine surgery. Meanwhile, the rate of screw loosening noticeably increases in osteoporosis patients due to reduced bone purchase and is reportedly 25%–62.5 clinically.

Current studies on screw stability in osteoporosis patients center around two determinants of screw stability: properties of the screw and bone adjacent to the screw trajectory. More specifically, investigators mainly focus on the development and clinical application of expansive screws and bone cement-augmented screws. The former principally changes the properties of the screw, while the latter increases stability by improving the bone purchase power of the screw trajectory. The current chapter focuses on the clinical application of these two types of screws.

15.1.2 A Historical Perspective of Expansive Screw

In 2000, Cook et al. designed an expansive pedicle screw with a four-petal and groove feature [1].

In 2005, Lei et al. designed an expansive pedicle screw with a two-petal feature [2] and subsequently developed "Lei's modified screw"[3]. These screws use anterior internal expansion technique and have limited expansibility and can be retracted (Fig. 15.2).

W. Lei, Y. Yan (eds.), *Internal Fixation of the Spine*, https://doi.org/10.1007/978-981-16-1562-7_15

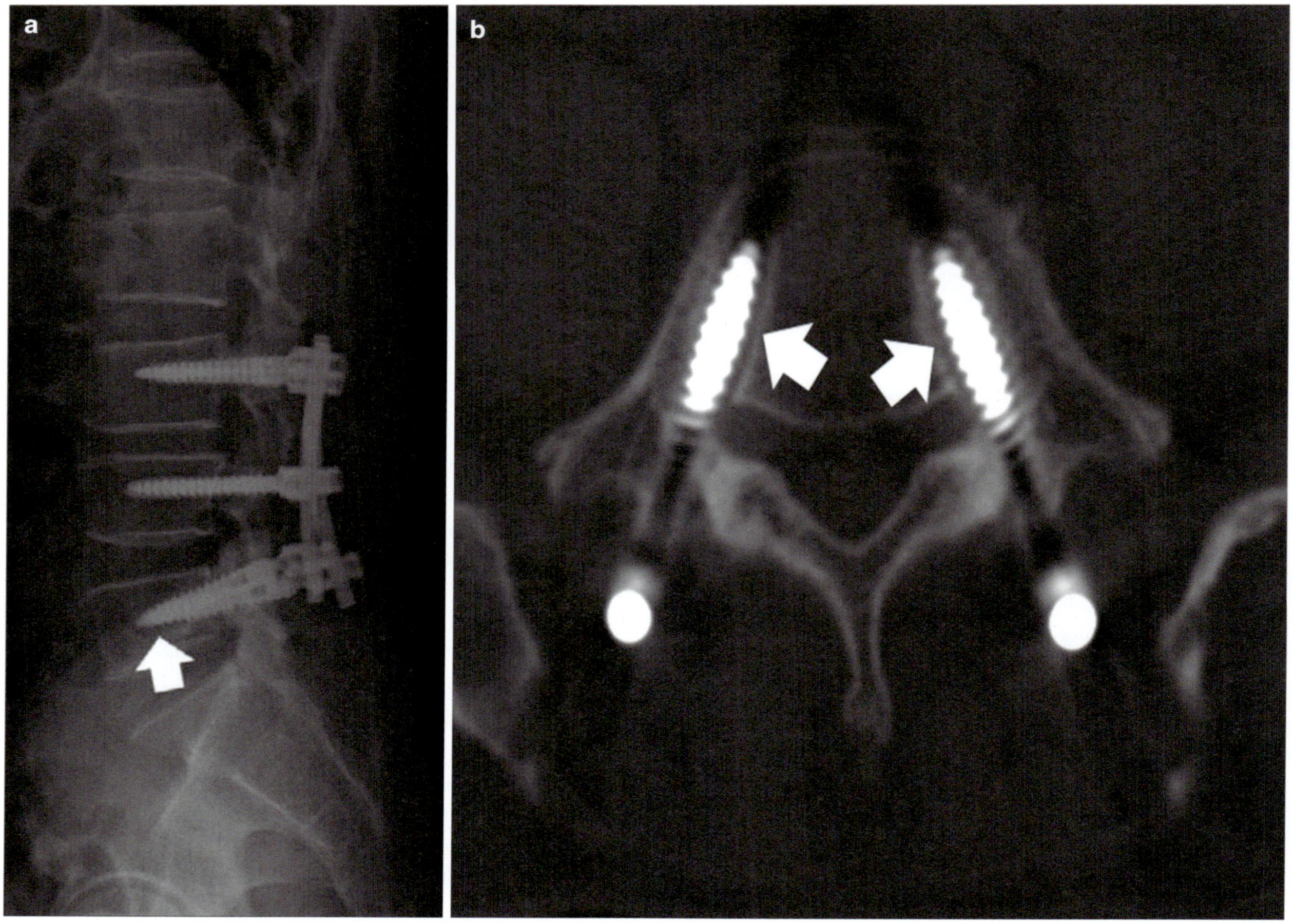

Fig. 15.1 The loosening pedicle screw. (**a**) Lateral view; (**b**) Coronal view

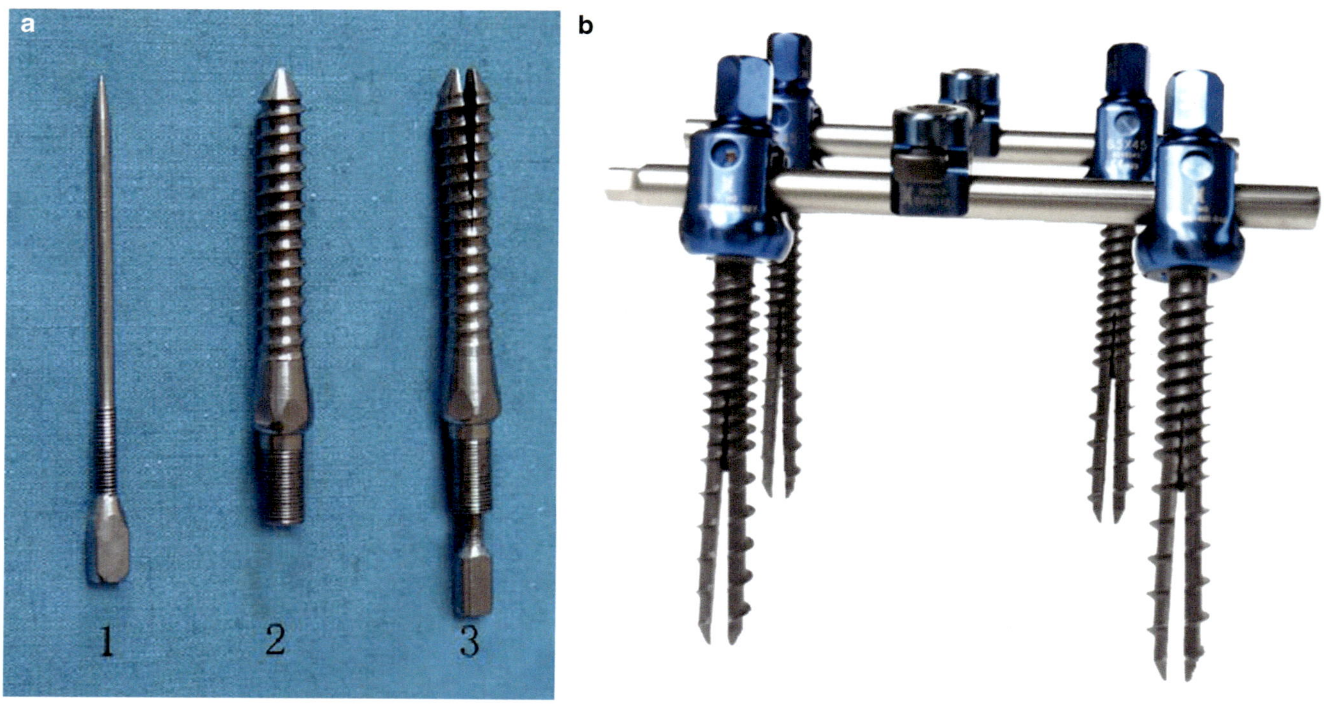

Fig. 15.2 First-generation Lei's modified expansive screw

15.1.3 A Historical Perspective of Bone Cement Screw

In 2013, Chao et al. reported a SmartLoc OMEGA cannulated-fenestrated screw with nine side holes in the anterior [4].

In 2013, Lei et al. developed polymethyl methacrylate (PMMA)-augmented-fenestrated pedicle screws [5] with diameter-tapered lateral perforations, achieving dotted even distribution of bone cement (Fig. 15.3).

15.2 Technical Points

1. Technical procedure for expansive screw fixation: One-step insertion with synchronous distraction (Fig. 15.4 A–D)
2. Technical procedure for bone cement-augmented screw anchor fixation (Fig. 15.5).
3. Stepwise treatment protocol

Based on the above studies, we established standardized treatment protocols for different bone mass conditions as well as principles of implant selection (Table 15.1) in order to provide reliable clinical evidence for a tailored surgical approach for screw fixation.

15.3 Clinical Cases

15.3.1 Expansive Screw Fixation

15.3.1.1 Case No. 1

Patient: A 47-year-old woman with back pain and numbness and pain of the right lower extremity for 1 month.

Diagnosis: Lumbar spondylolisthesis, lumbar degenerative scoliosis, and osteoporosis.

Surgery: Decompression via posterior L4–S1 laminectomy, interbody fusion, spondylolisthesis reduction, and L3–S1 expansive screw fixation. Preoperative (Figs. 15.6, 15.7, 15.8) and postoperative (Figs. 15.9, 15.10) images are shown below.

Imaging data:

15.3.1.2 Case No. 2

Patient: A 39-year-old woman with back pain for 10 years.

Diagnosis: Lumbar degenerative scoliosis and osteoporosis.

Surgery: Posterior correction of scoliosis and T11–S1 expansive screw fixation. Preoperative (Fig. 15.11) and postoperative (Figs. 15.12, 15.13) images are shown below.

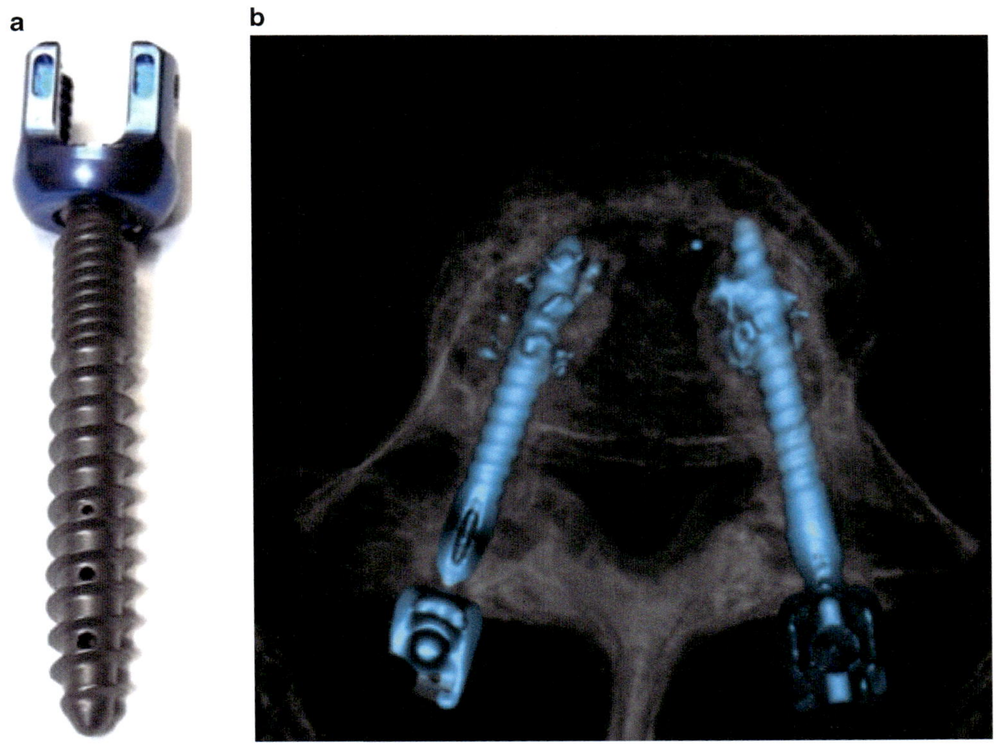

Fig. 15.3 (**a**) The PMMA-augmented-fenestrated pedicle screw; (**b**) 3D CT reconstruction demonstrated the PMMA distribution in the vertebral body

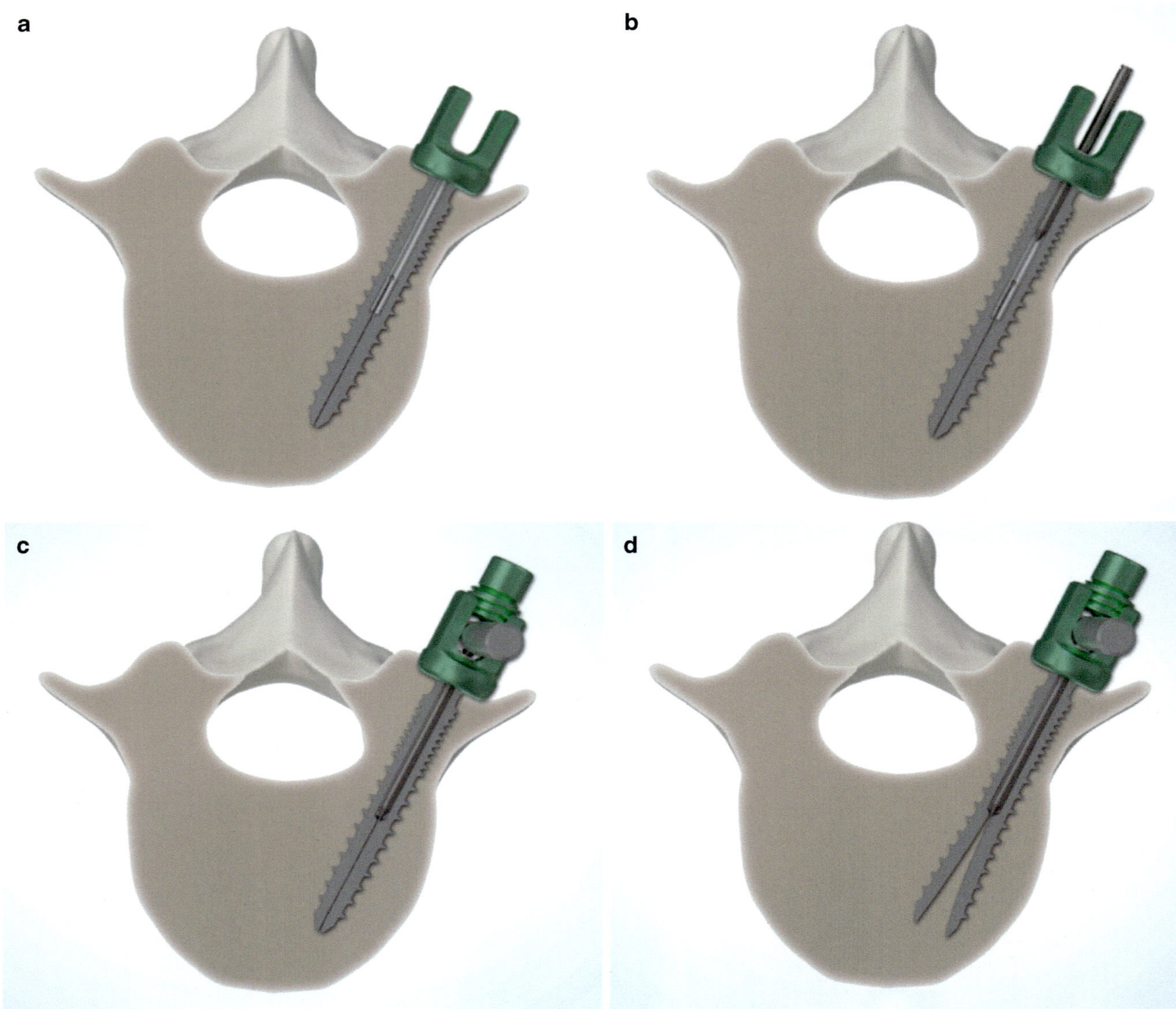

Fig. 15.4 (**a**) Insertion of the screw; (**b**) Insertion of a smaller gauge screw; (**c**) Assembling the rod and screw cap. (**d**) Anterior distraction

15.3.2 Bone Cement-Augmented Screw Fixation

15.3.2.1 Case No. 1

Patient: A 39-year-old man with back pain for 20 years and kyphosis for 10 years.

Diagnosis: Ankylosing spondylitis with kyphosis and severe osteoporosis.

Surgery: Posterior L1–L3 osteotomy and T10–L5 bone cement-augmented screw fixation. Preoperative (Figs. 15.14, 15.15) and postoperative (Figs. 15.16, 15.17) images are shown below.

15.3.2.2 Case No. 2

Patient: An 80-year-old man with back pain for 1 month and 3 months post PKP for L1 vertebra body fracture.

Diagnosis: T12 vertebra body fracture, post L1 PKP, and severe osteoporosis.

Surgery: Posterior T10–L3 bone cement-augmented screw fixation. Preoperative (Fig. 15.18) and postoperative (Fig. 15.19) images are shown below.

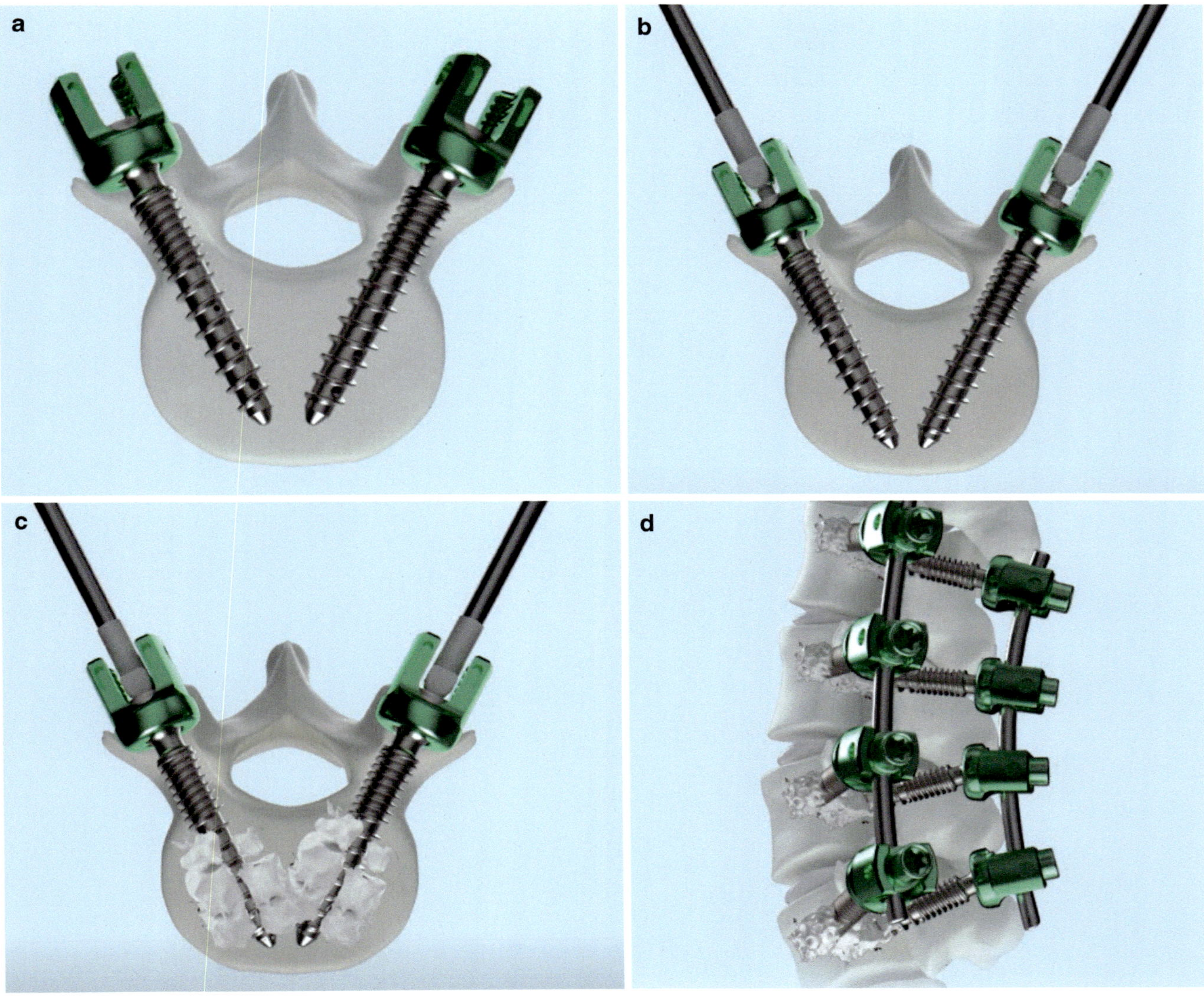

Fig. 15.5 (**a**) Insertion of the screws; (**b**) Insertion of bone cement pushing rod; (**c**) Injecting bone cement. (**d**) The three-dimensional frame structure after rod assembly

Table 15.1 Implant selection for enhanced screw stability under different bone mass conditions

Clinical classification	Bone mineral density	Treatment strategies
Osteoporosis	2.5–3.5 SD	Expansive screw
Severe osteoporosis or revision surgery	>3.5 SD	Bone cement-augmented screw

15.4 Pearls and Pitfalls

1. Surgical indications should be vigorously followed. Excessive use of expansive screws and bone cement-augmented screws should be avoided.
2. When bone cement-augmented screws are used, the inner wall of the screw trajectory should be probed carefully during the operation. Screw location should be confirmed under fluoroscopy, and caution should be exercised to prevent the screw penetrating the anterior vertebra body. The side holes on the screw should surpass the pedicle, and care should be taken to prevent cement leakage into the vertebral canal or the anterior vertebra body.
3. Revision of expansive screws and bone cement-augmented screws is difficult. If screw loosening or breakage occurs, specific revision instruments should be used for revision, and the number of segments for fixation should be extended.

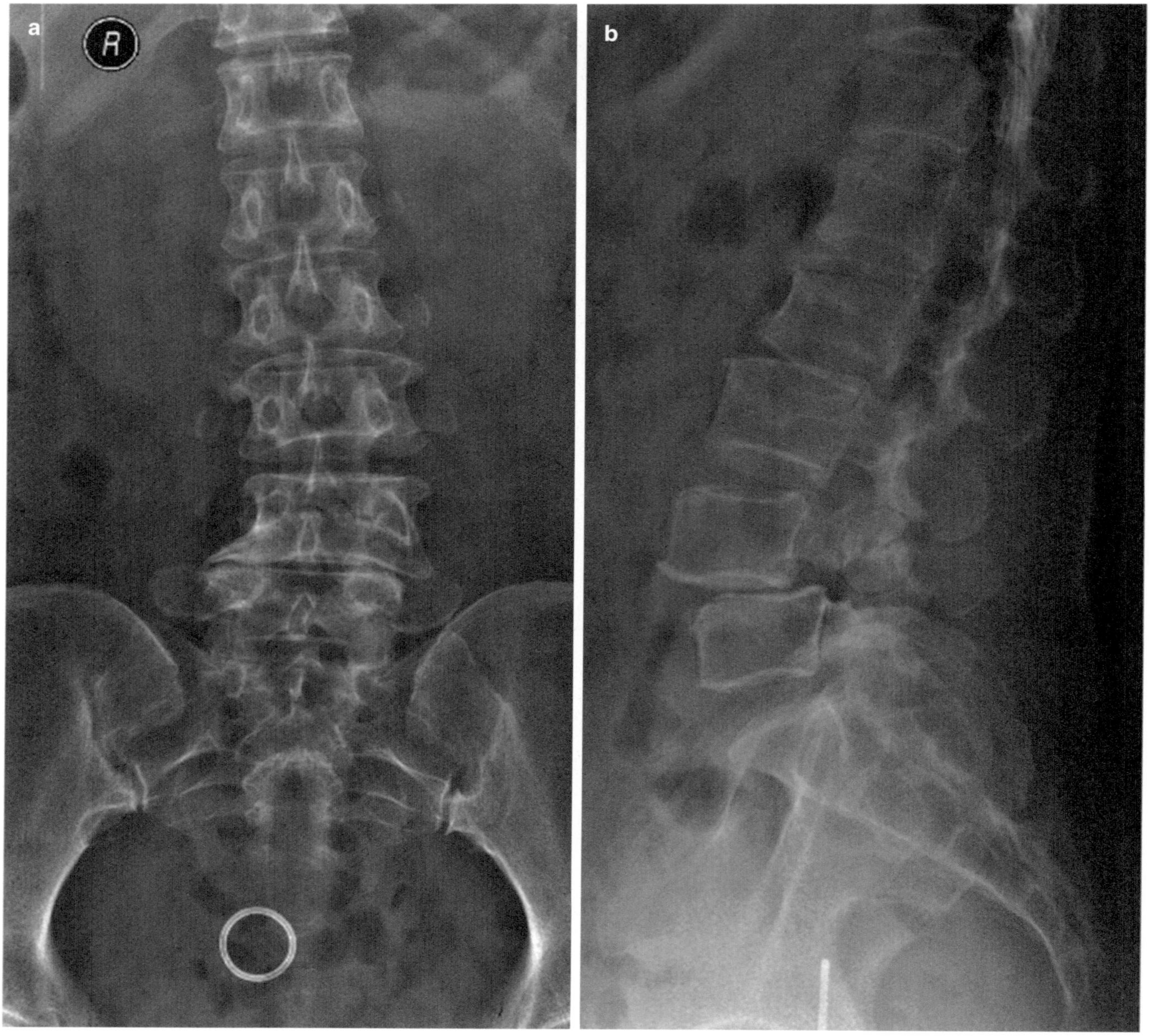

Fig. 15.6 Preoperative radiographs. (**a**) Anteroposterior view; (**b**) Lateral view

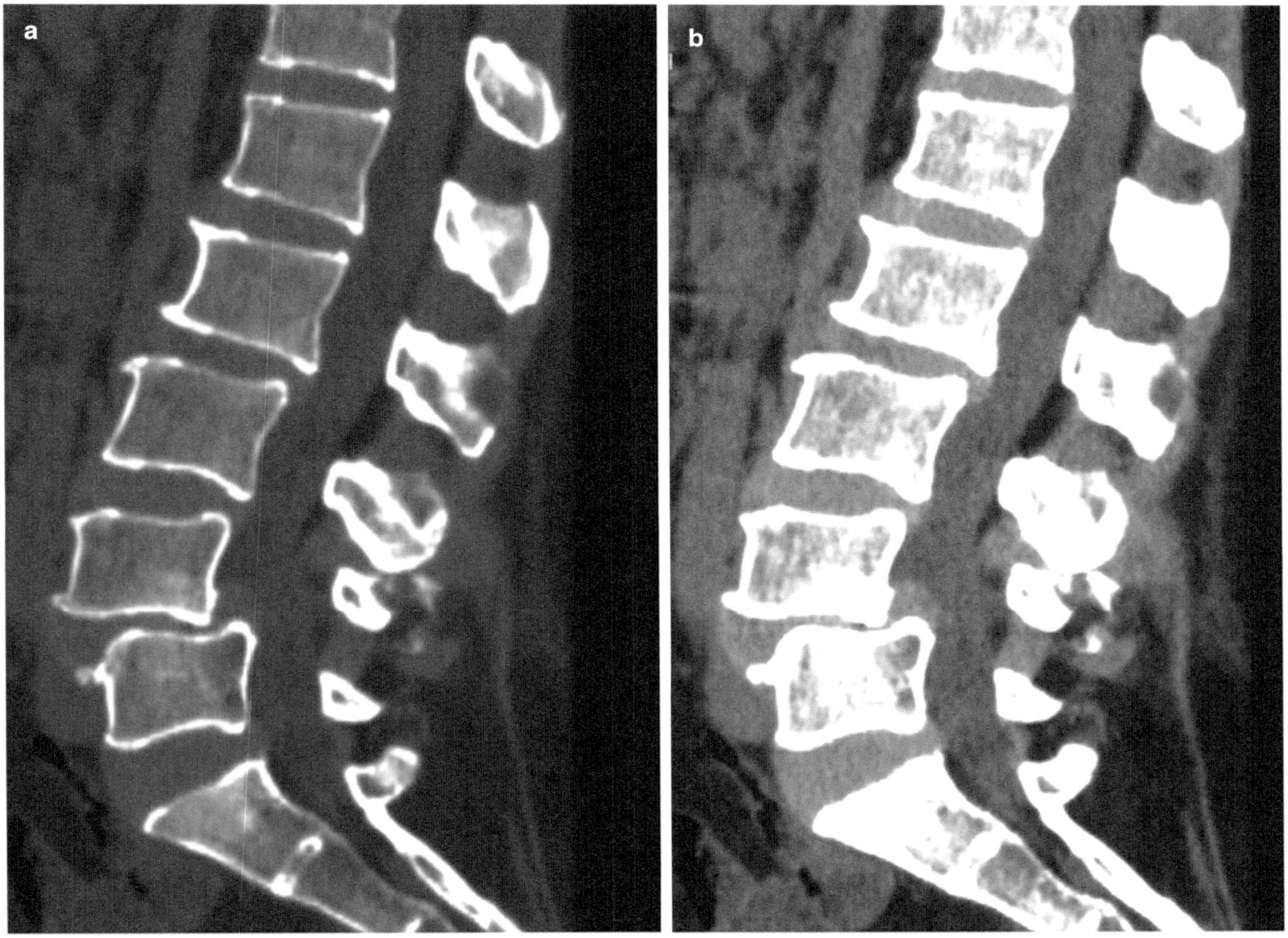

Fig. 15.7 Preoperative CT images. (**a**) Sagittal view showed the bony structure; (**b**) Sagittal view showed the soft tissue

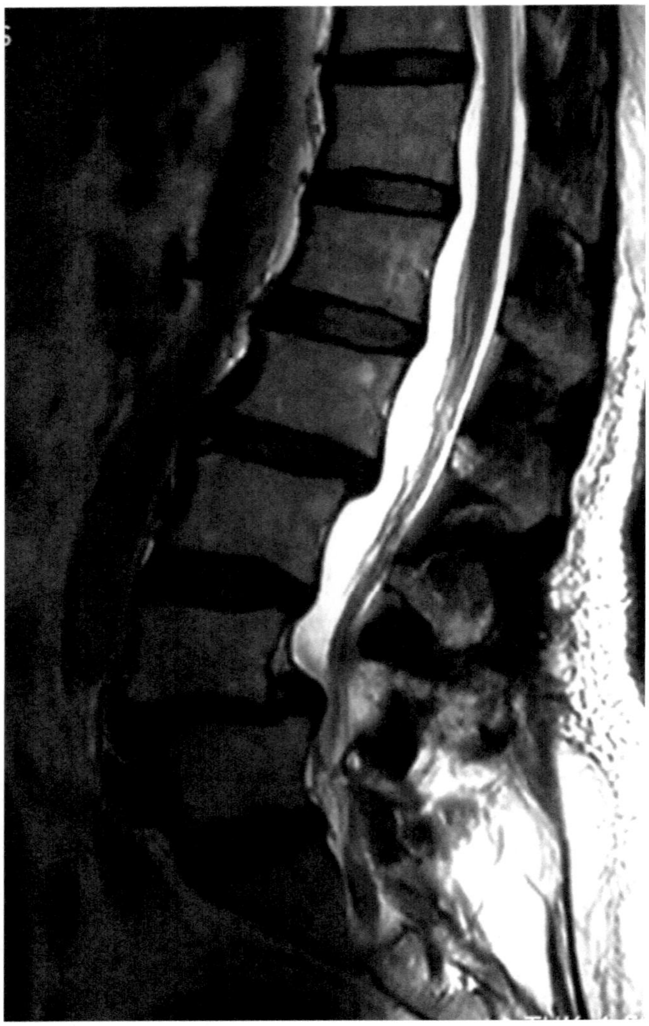

Fig. 15.8 Preoperative MRI

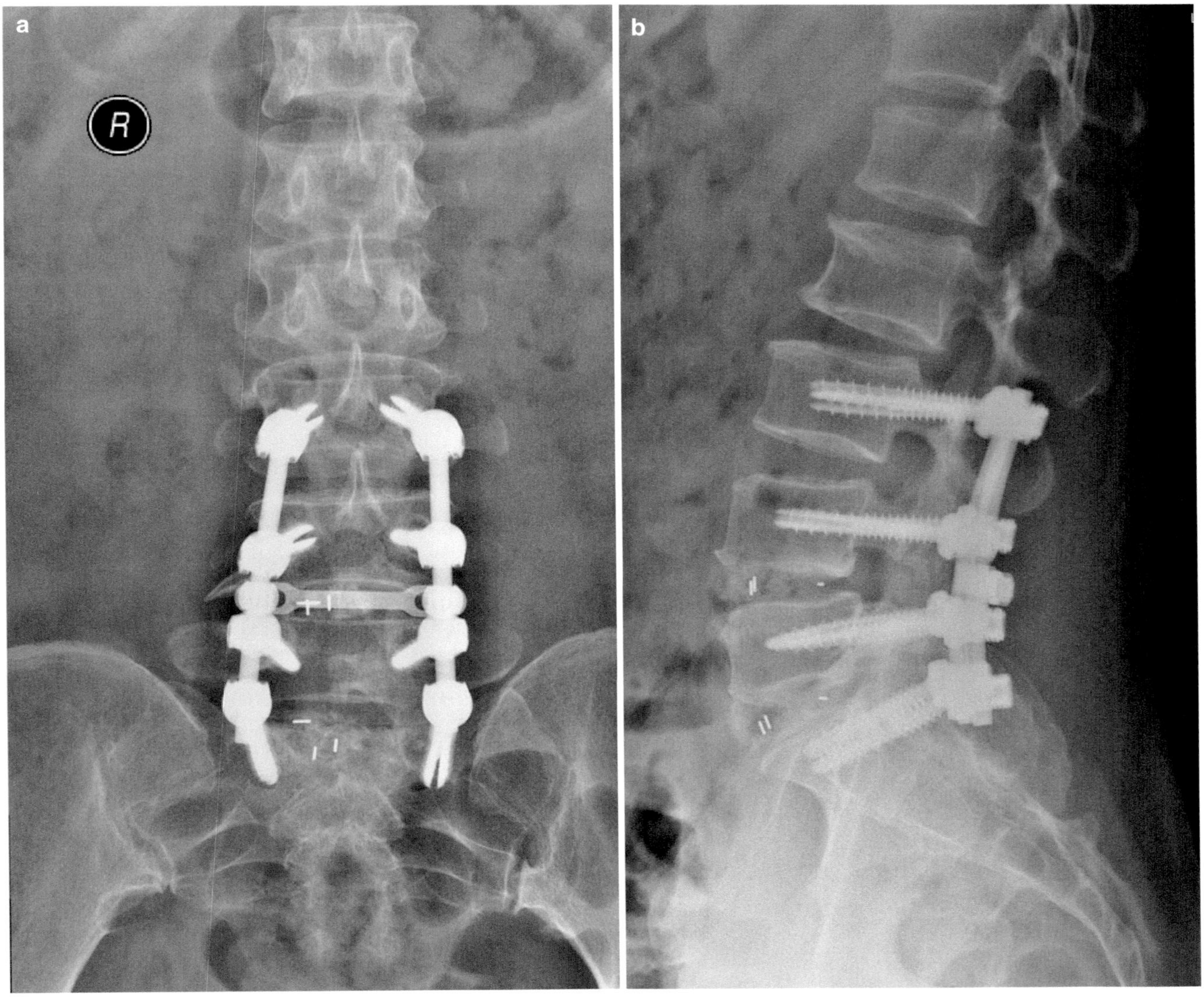

Fig. 15.9 Postoperative radiographs. (**a**) Anteroposterior view; (**b**) Lateral view

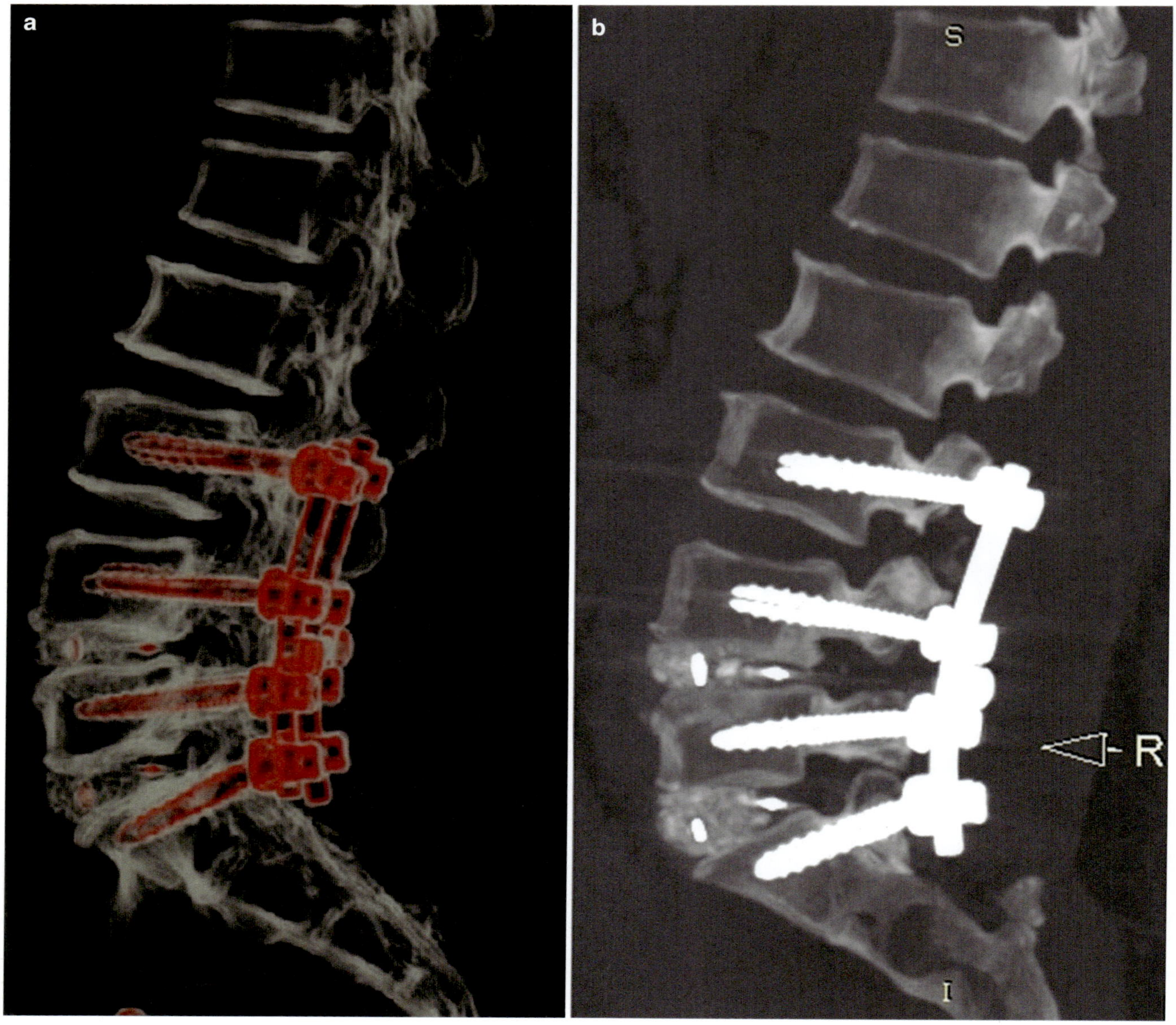

Fig. 15.10 Postoperative CT images. (**a**) 3D CT reconstruction showed the screw and the interbody cage; (**b**) 3D CT reconstruction showed the screw and the interbody cage

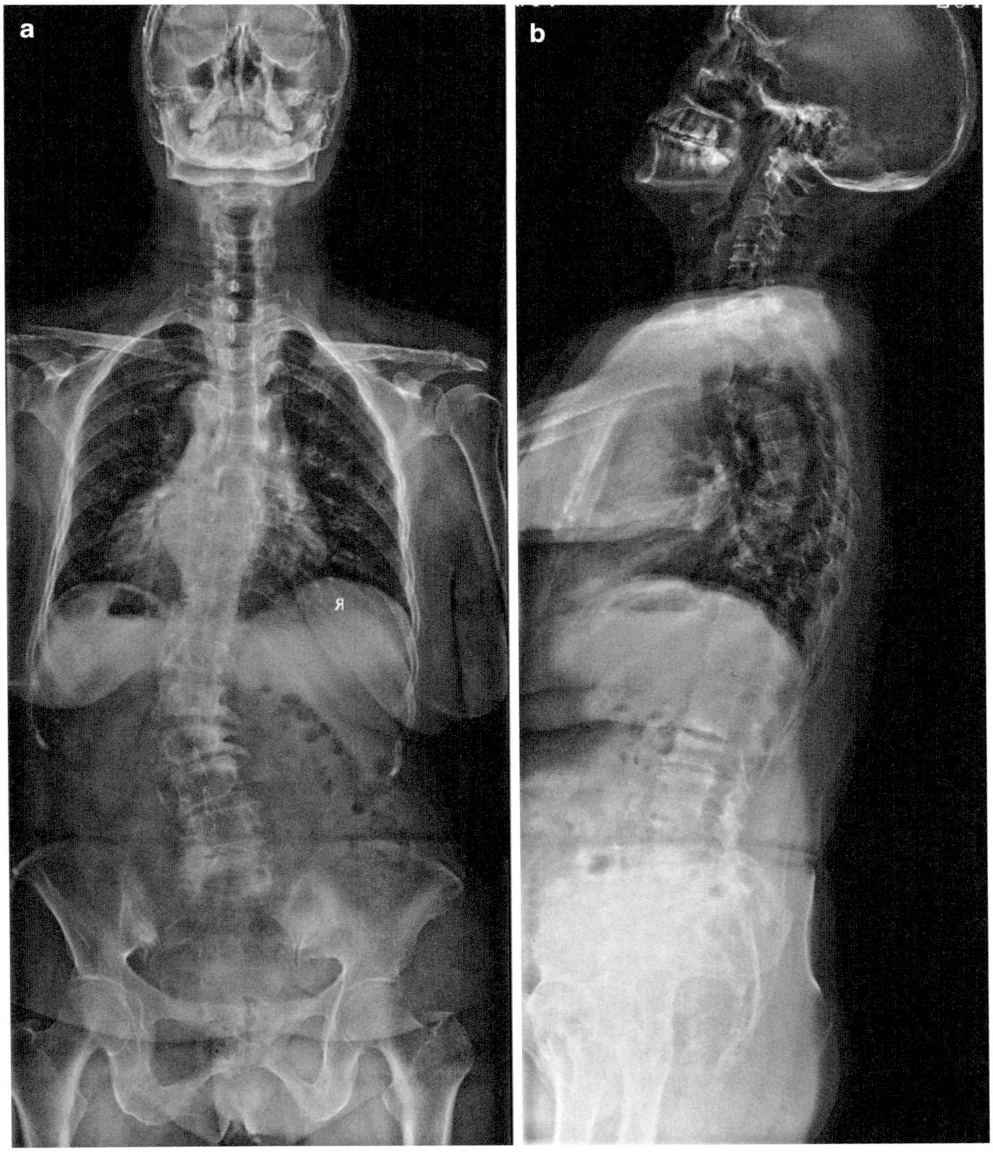

Fig. 15.11 Preoperative radiographs. (**a**) Anteroposterior view; (**b**): Lateral view

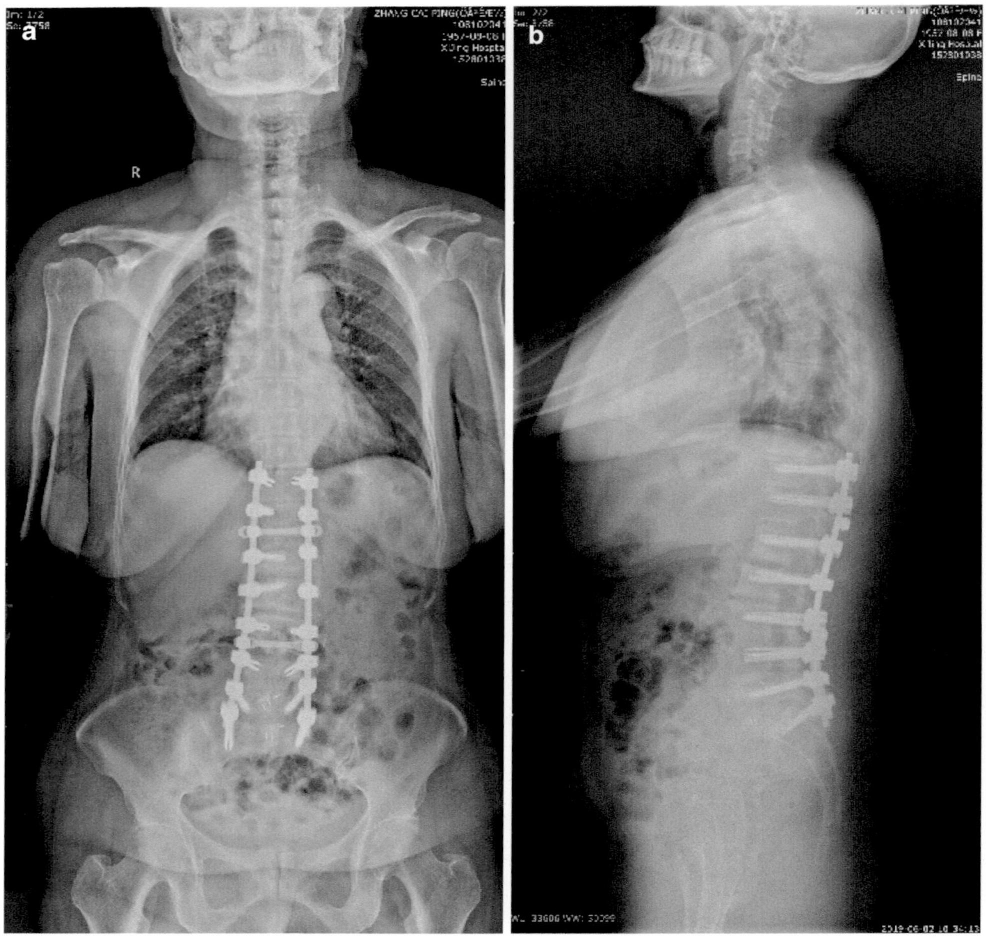

Fig. 15.12 Postoperative radiographs. (**a**) Anteroposterior view; (**b**): Lateral view

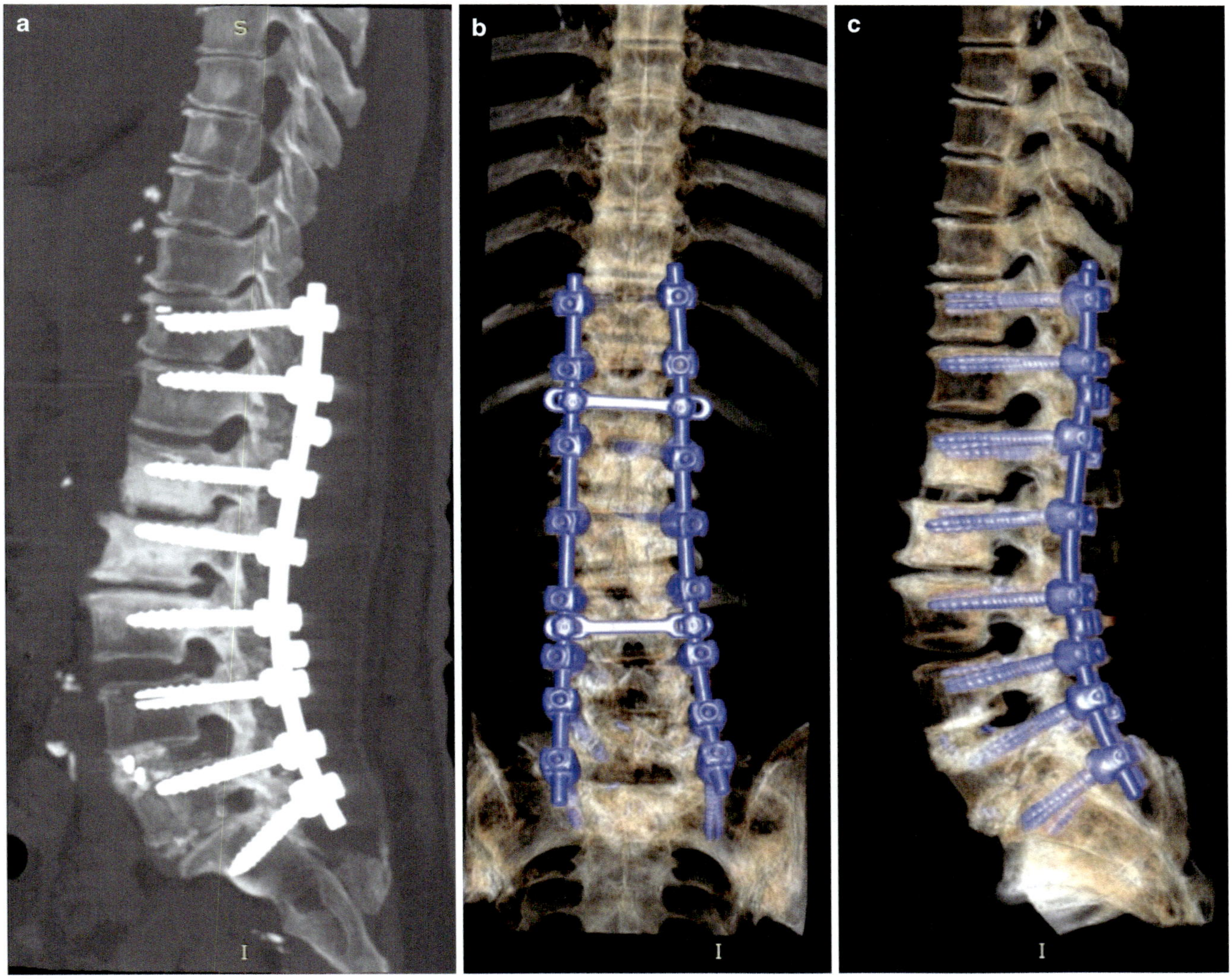

Fig. 15.13 Postoperative CT images. (**a**) 3D CT reconstruction showed the section of pedicle screw; (**b**) 3D CT reconstruction showed posterior view of the construct; (**c**) 3D CT reconstruction showed lateral view of the construct

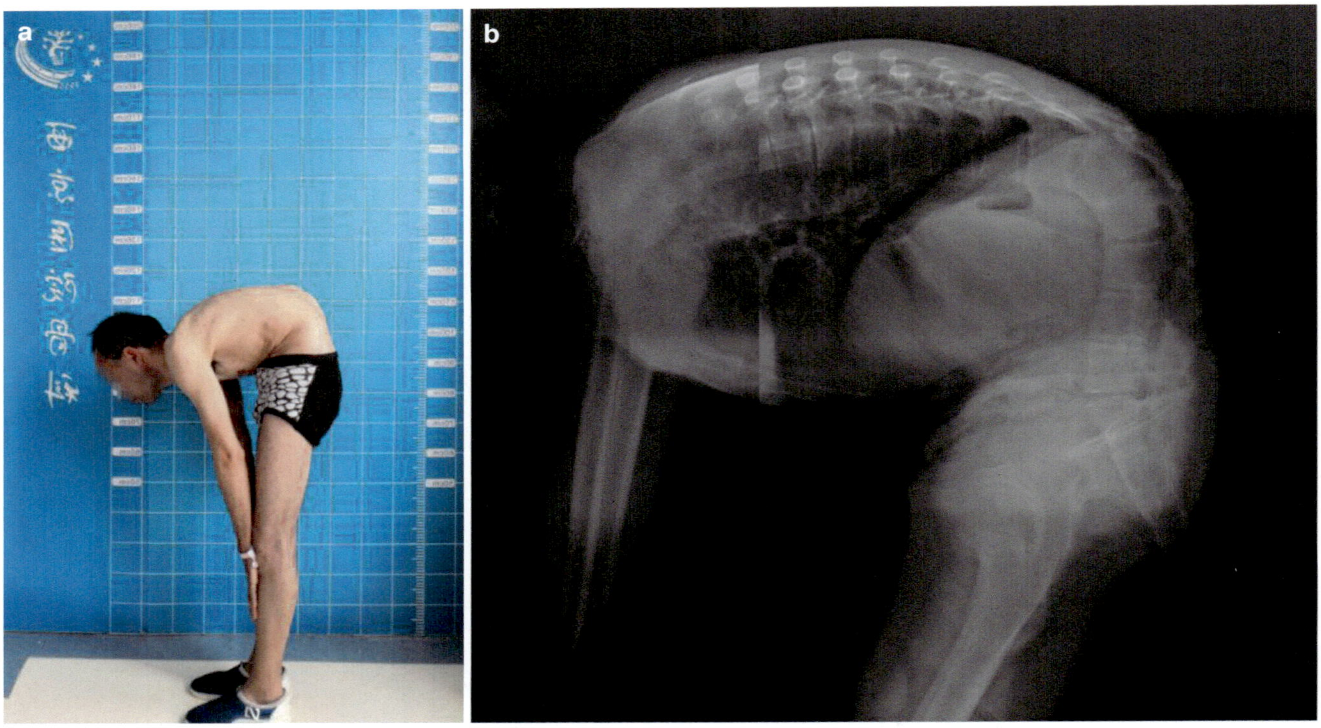

Fig. 15.14 (**a**) Gross photograph and (**b**) preoperative radiograph of the patient

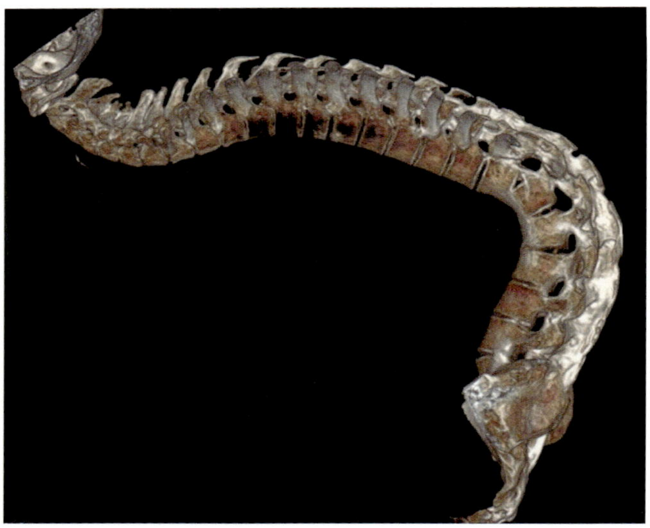

Fig. 15.15 Preoperative CT image

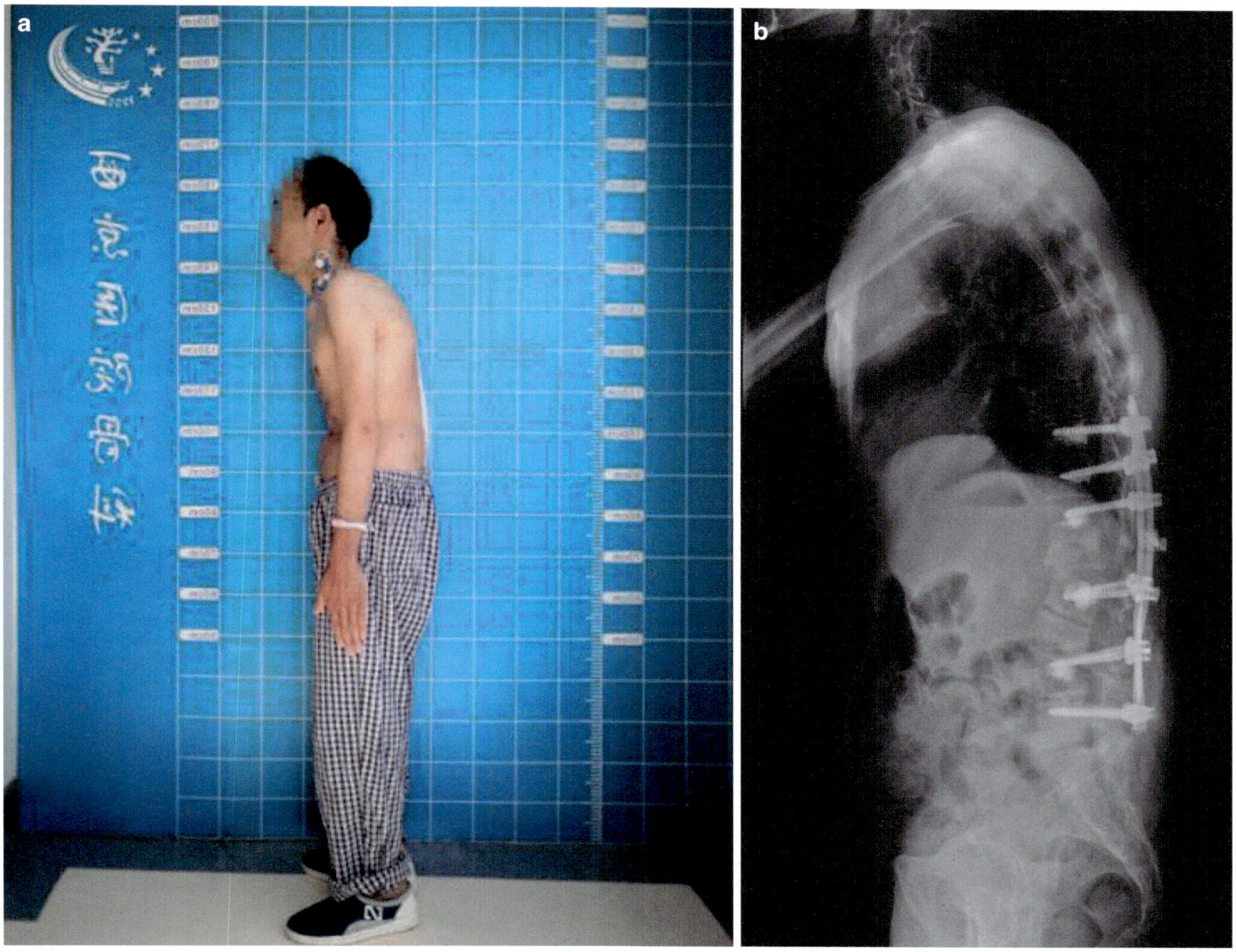

Fig. 15.16 (a) Gross photograph and (**b**) radiograph of the patient after surgery

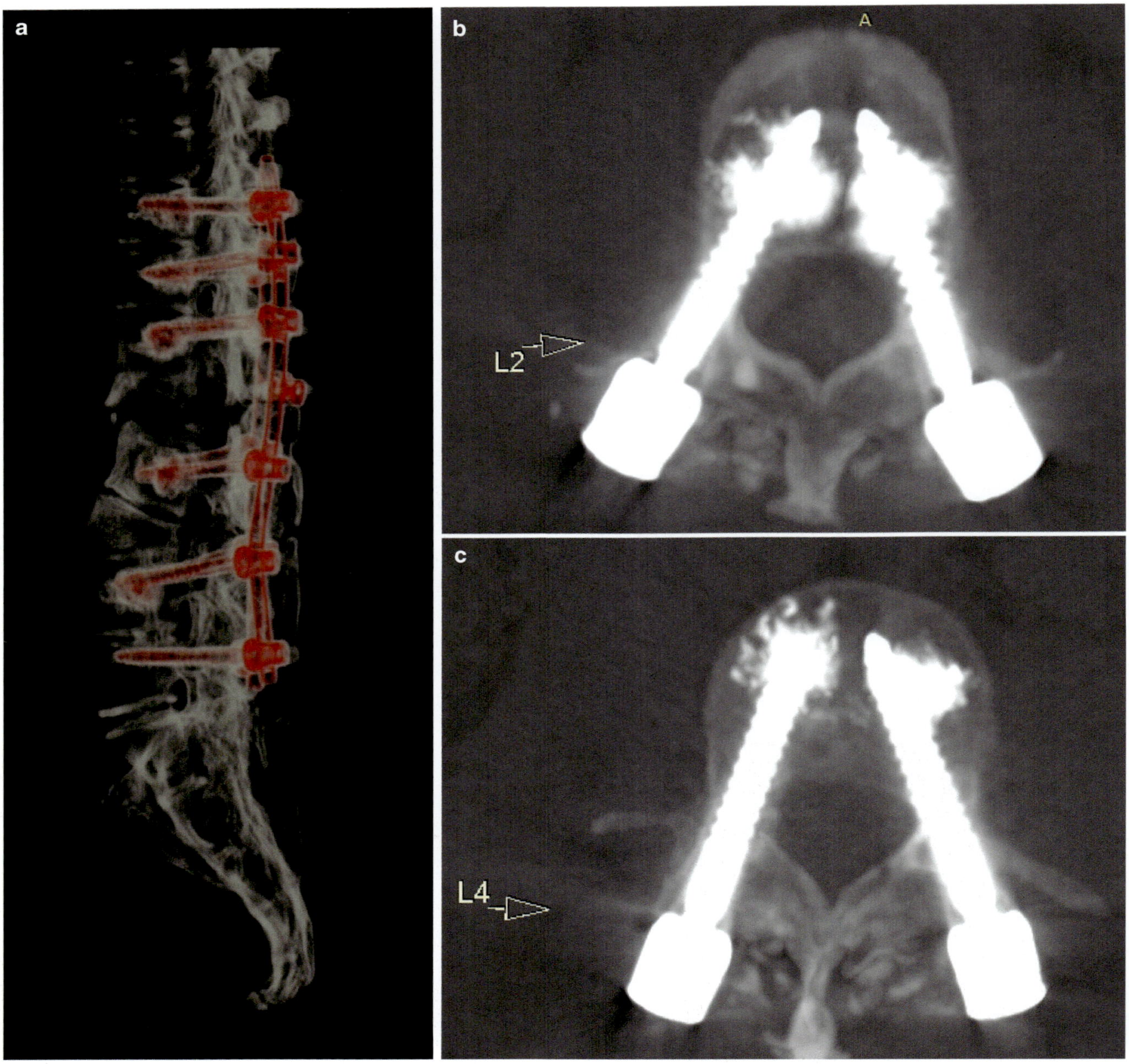

Fig. 15.17 Postoperative CT images. (**a**) 3D CT reconstruction showed the pedicle screw; (**b**) 3D CT reconstruction showed coronal view of the pedicle screw in L2 vertebral body; (**c**) 3D CT reconstruction showed coronal view of the pedicle screw in L4 vertebral body

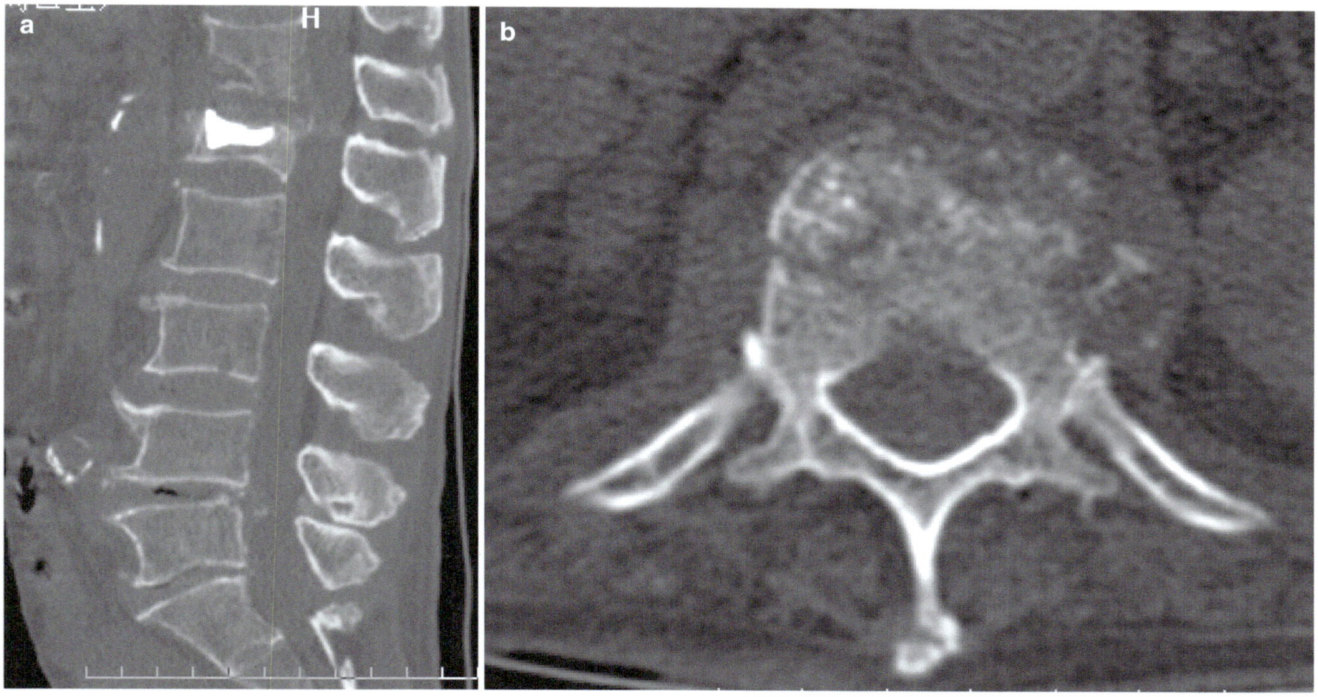

Fig. 15.18 Preoperative radiographs. (**a**) Sagittal CT images showed the bone cement in the L1 vertebral body; (**b**) Coronal CT images showed the T12 vertebral body fracture

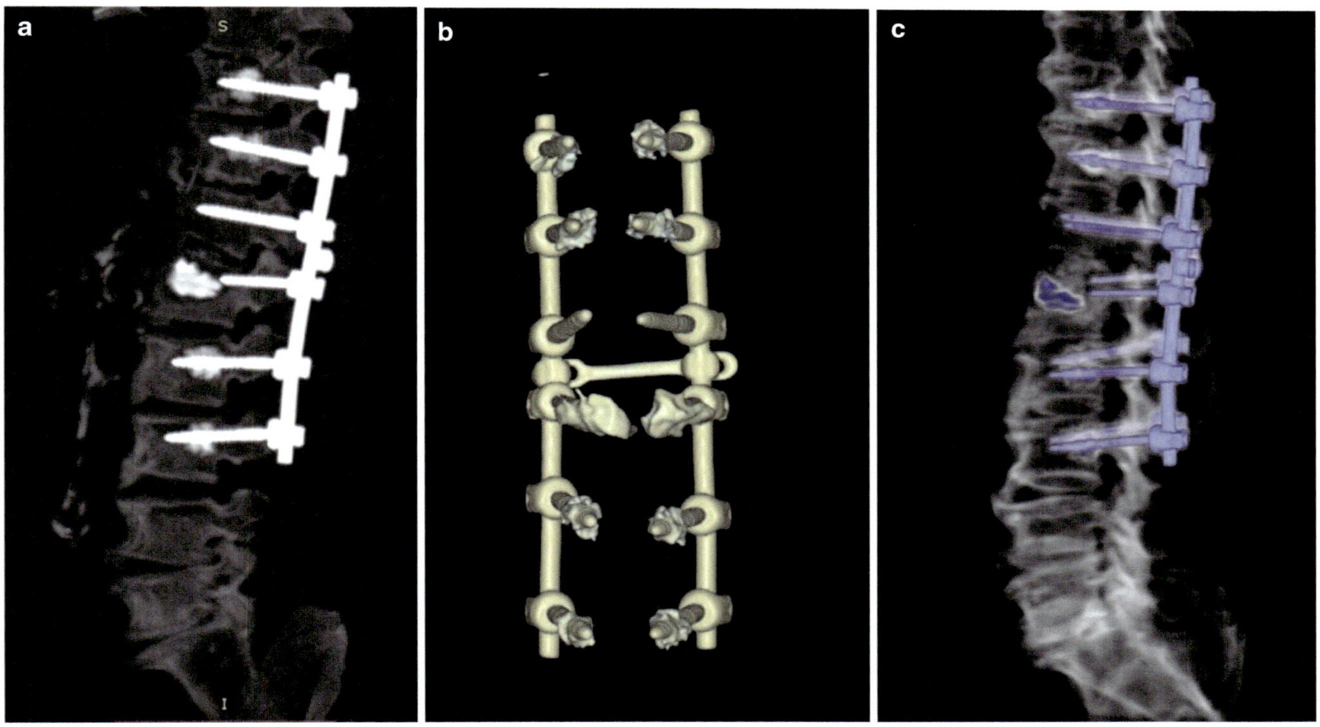

Fig. 15.19 Postoperative CT images. (A): 3D CT reconstruction showed the section of pedicle screw; (B): 3D CT reconstruction showed the construct; (C): 3D CT reconstruction showed lateral view of the construct

References

1. Cook SD, Salkeld SL, Whitecloud TS 3rd, Barbera JJ. Biomechanical evaluation and preliminary clinical experience with an expansive pedicle screw design. Spinal Disord. 2000 Jun;13(3):230–6.
2. Lei W, Wu Z. Biomechanical evaluation of an expansive pedicle screw in calf vertebrae. Eur Spine J. 2006;15:321–6.
3. Wan S, Lei W, Wu Z, Liu D, Gao M, Fu S. Biomechanical and histological evaluation of an expandable pedicle screw in osteoporotic spine in sheep. Eur Spine J. 2010;19:2122–9.
4. Chao KH, Lai YS, Chen WC, Chang CM, McClean CJ, Fan CY, Chang CH, Lin LC, Cheng CK. Biomechanical analysis of different types of pedicle screw augmentation: a cadaveric and synthetic bone sample study of instrumented vertebral specimens. Med Eng Phys. 2013;35:1506–12.
5. Tan QC, Wu JW, Peng F, Zang Y, Li Y, Zhao X, Lei W, Wu ZX. Augmented PMMA distribution: improvement of mechanical property and reduction of leakage rate of a fenestrated pedicle screw with diameter-tapered perforations. Neurosurg Spine. 2016 Jun;24(6):971–7.

Anterior Odontoid Screw Techniques and Application

16

Junxiong Ma, Liangbi Xiang, and Wei Lei

Abstract

Anterior odontoid screw fixation is a commonly used procedure for odontoid fracture. This technique was first proposed by Nakanishi in 1978 and was evolved in the past decades. In this chapter, we thoroughly reviewed the technique development of the anterior odontoid screw fixation technique. Anatomic characters of the axis vertebral body, the entry point, entry angle, entry depth of anterior odontoid screw, and operational details were demonstrated to guarantee the proper position of screw. The characteristics, clinical indications and contraindications, and surgical technique of odontoid screw are introduced in details. The application of these techniques is presented in typical clinical cases.

Keywords

Odontoid fracture · Anterior odontoid screw fixation · Surgical technique

16.1 Anterior Odontoid Screw Fixation Techniques: A Historical Perspective

Nakanishi first proposed the use of anterior odontoid screw technique in 1978 [1].

Subsequently, Bohler et al. independently reported the technique and their experience in JBJS in 1982 [2]. However, the technique can be traced back to 1968.

In 2000, Apfelbaum et al. reported a two-center study of anterior odontoid screw fixation for odontoid fractures with a large population [3]. They also described the surgical indications of the technique, time of surgery, and patient prognosis (Fig. 16.3).

16.2 Anatomy of the Odontoid Process (Figs. 16.1, 16.2, 16.3, 16.4, and 16.5; Table 16.1)

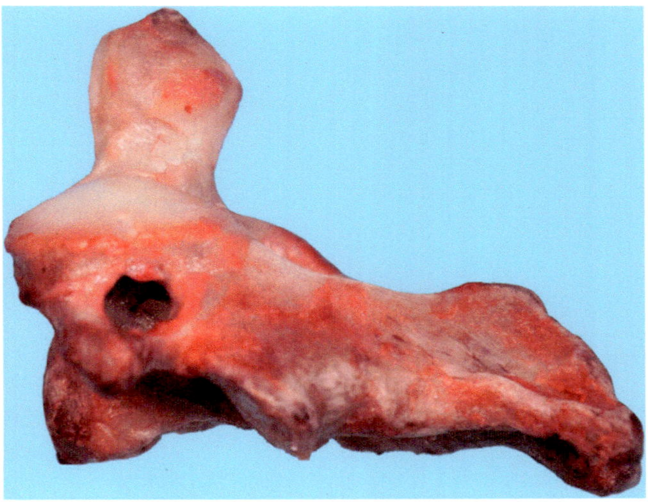

Fig. 16.1 Lateral view of the axis

J. Ma · L. Xiang
Department of Orthopedics, General Hospital of Northern Theater Command, Shenyang, China

W. Lei (✉)
Department of Orthopedics, Xijing Hospital, Air Force Medical University, Xi'an, Shaanxi, China
e-mail: leiwei@fmmu.edu.cn

W. Lei, Y. Yan (eds.), *Internal Fixation of the Spine*, https://doi.org/10.1007/978-981-16-1562-7_16

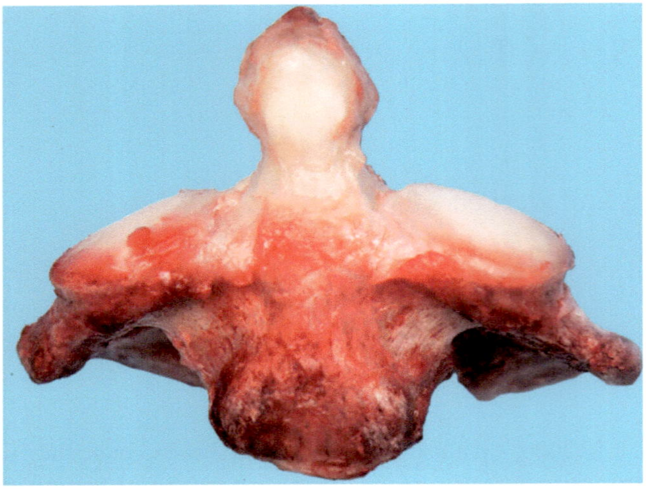

Fig. 16.2 Anterior view of the axis

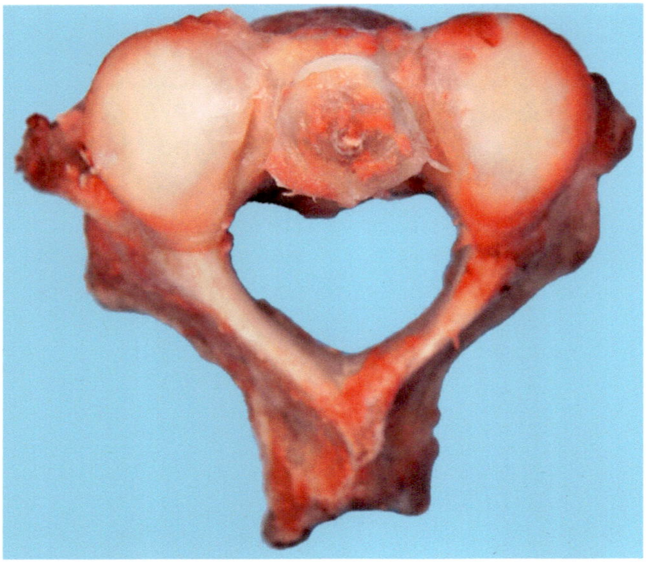

Fig. 16.3 Superior view of the axis

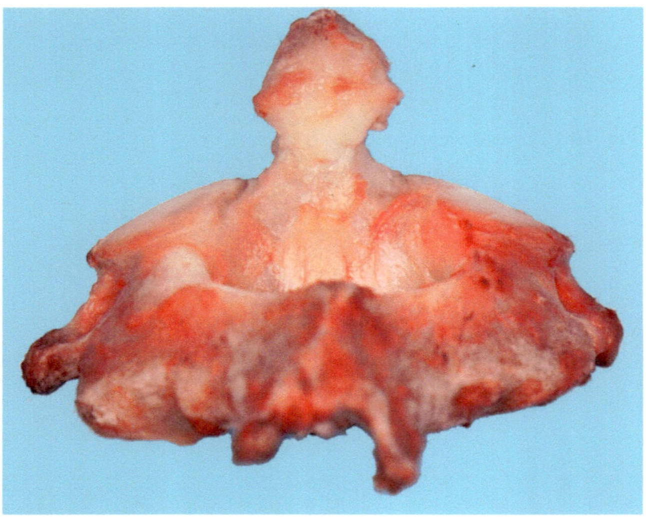

Fig. 16.4 Posterior view of the axis

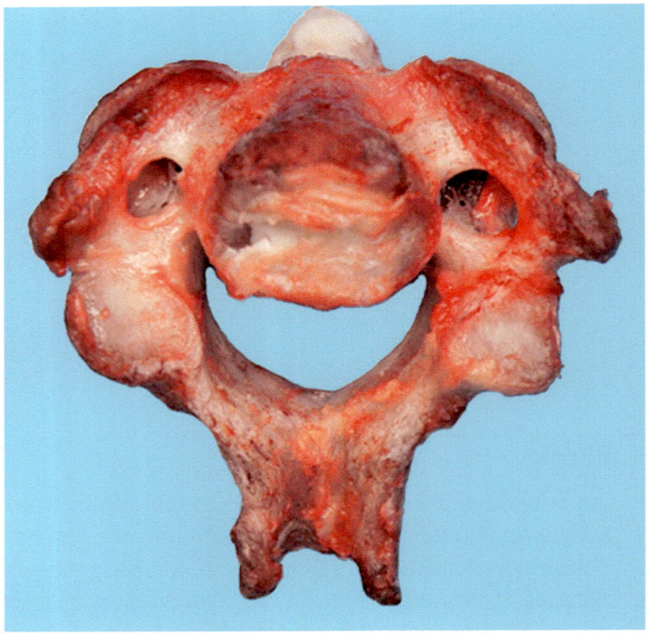

Fig. 16.5 Inferior view of the axis

Table 16.1 Anatomic dimension of the axis in Chinese subjects

Location	Mean ± SD
Height of the odontoid process	14.7 mm ± 1.9 mm
The coronal diameter of the odontoid process	8.3 mm ± 0.6 mm
The sagittal diameter of the odontoid process	10.5 mm ± 1.1 mm
Posterior inclination angle of the odontoid process	10.3° ± 3.5°
Anterior height of the axis body	22.8 mm ± 1.1 mm
Posterior height of the axis body	19.5 mm ± 0.9 mm
Height of the anterior lip of the axis	3 mm ± 0.6 mm

16.3 Key Points of the Odontoid Screw Technique

16.3.1 Screw Entry Site

The entry site of the odontoid screw is the anteroinferior edge of the C2 vertebral body. If one screw is to be placed, the midpoint of the anteroinferior edge of the C2 vertebral body serves as the entry site. If two screws are to be placed, the entry site is 2 to 3 mm from the midpoint on either side.

After the Kirschner (K)-wire is placed into the entry trajectory, an 8-mm hollow hand drill is advanced along the K-wire. The hand drill is then used to create a small groove from the surface of the annulus fibrosus in the intervertebral disc between C3 and C2–C3 to the inferior border of C2 to allow subsequent advancement of the guidewire and drill bit.

16.3.2 Screw Entry Angle

Under fluoroscopy, the screw is entered from the anteroinferior border of C2, passing through C2 vertebral body to reach the vertex of the odontoid process.

16.3.3 Screw Length

Screw length can be measured by two methods: (1) the screw length is measured based on preoperative imaging data and (2) the screw length is measured intraoperatively.

16.4 Surgical Steps (3D Reconstruction Images)

1. Surgical position: The patient is placed supine, with the head and neck in full posterior extension to maximally expose the anterior part of the cervical spine. A circular cushion is used to stabilize the head of the patient. A large bore nasogastric tube is inserted to determine the position of the esophagus and prevent esophagus perforation. The fracture is reduced using skull traction. This technique requires anatomic reduction as much as possible by preoperative skull traction; if full reduction is not achieved, posterior fixation surgery may be considered. Therefore, this should be explained to patients before surgery.
2. Preoperative fluoroscopy: Correct screw placement requires assistance with G-arm fluoroscopy system, and the balloon and tube for fluoroscopy are covered with sterile sheets. Before surgery, a long K-wire is placed on the lateral side of the neck in the same direction of screw insertion, and visual observation via fluoroscopy is done to determine whether the trajectory for maneuvering surgical instruments is blocked or not.
3. Incision and exposure: In our experience, we prefer to make a 5-cm transverse incision on the right C3–C4 intervertebral disc space and reach the cervical spine via an anteromedial approach. Blunt dissection is made in the space between the carotid sheath and the trachea and esophagus and proceeds anterior to the cervical vertebra to reach the inferior border of C2 vertebral body. When C2–C3 is exposed, the superior thyroid artery may need to be ligated. The screw entry site at the anteroinferior C2 vertebral body is determined fluoroscopically.
4. Localization: The screw cap is prone to extend beyond the anterior edge of C2– C3 intervertebral disc, and a small amount of annulus fibrosus and bone is typically removed to create a groove to bury the screw cap. When drilling, a protective plate is used to avoid inadvertent injury to adjacent nerves and vessels. A small cannulated drill bit is used to drill a hole, and a calibrated K-wire 1.2 mm in diameter is inserted toward the posterior tip of the odontoid process in the sagittal plane and toward the midline in the coronal plane (Fig. 16.6a, b). G-arm fluoroscopy is

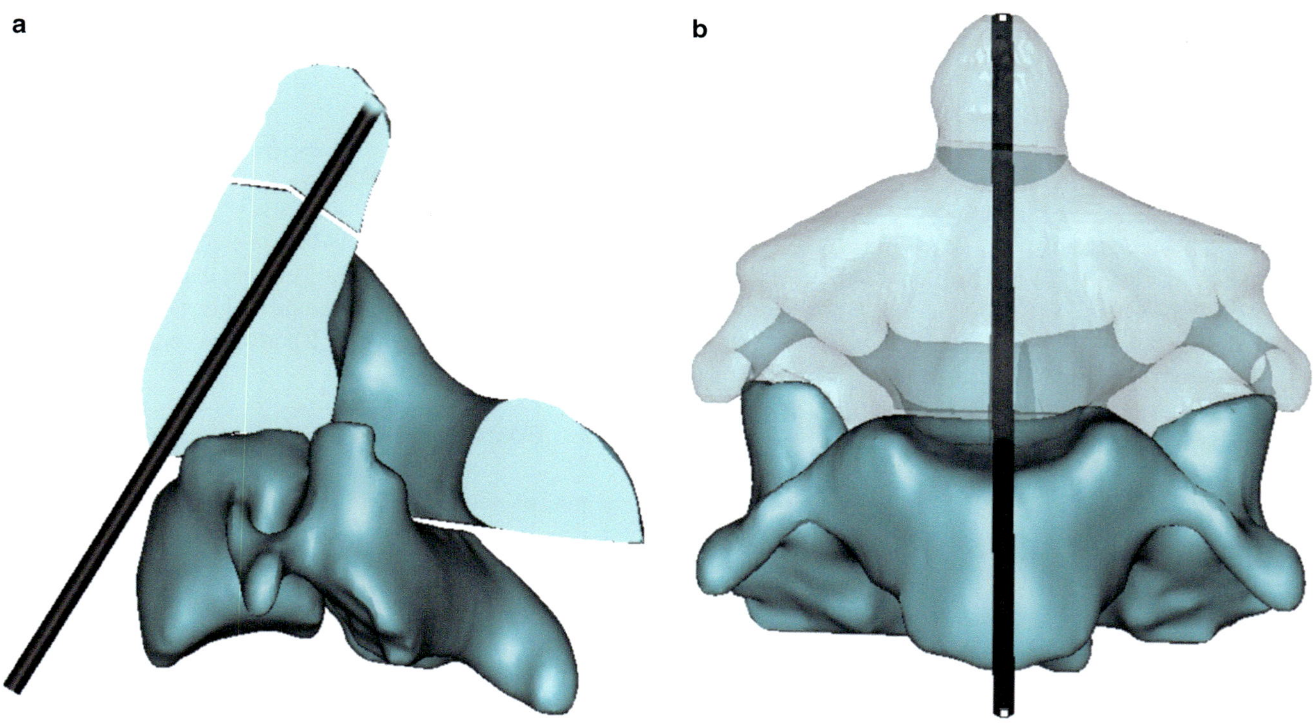

Fig. 16.6 Localization by a stylet. (**a**) Lateral view; (**b**) Orthogonal view

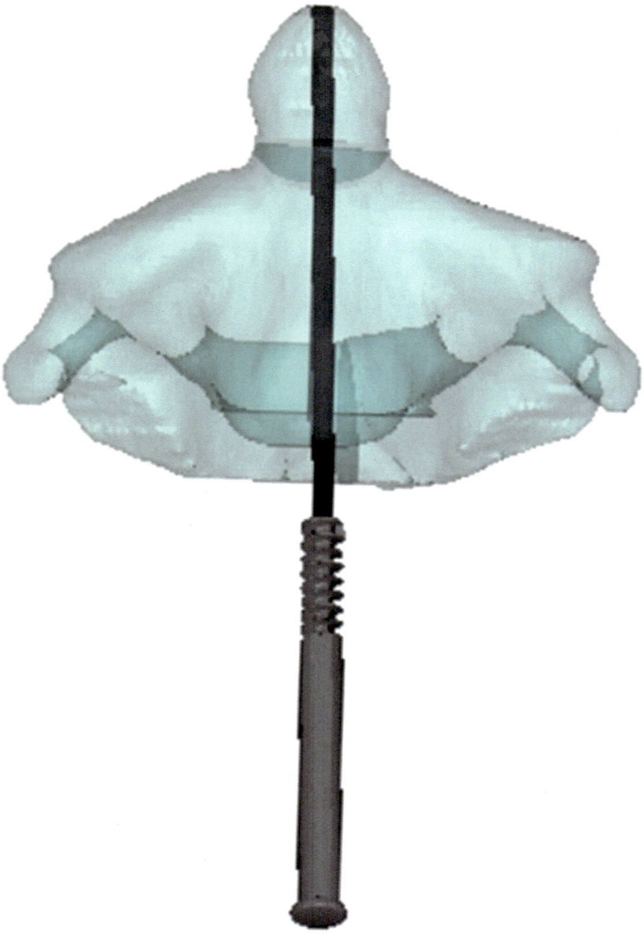

Fig. 16.7 The screw is inserted along the guidewire

used to confirm whether the K-wire has penetrated the cortex of the odontoid process, and whether its position and direction are accurate. Depth is probed using a hollow depth meter, and the trajectory length of the screw should be determined.

5. Screw placement: The penetration depth of the stylet is directly measured. The stylet has a 3.5-mm hollow drill bit; a hole 5 mm in depth is drilled initially (Fig. 16.7). An appropriate length 3.5-mm self-tapping screw is put on the stylet and inserted using a hollow screwdriver. The threaded portion of the tension screw should completely pass beyond the fracture line; otherwise, the tension screw cannot exert its function to assure fracture reduction and fracture separation may even occur (Fig. 16.8).

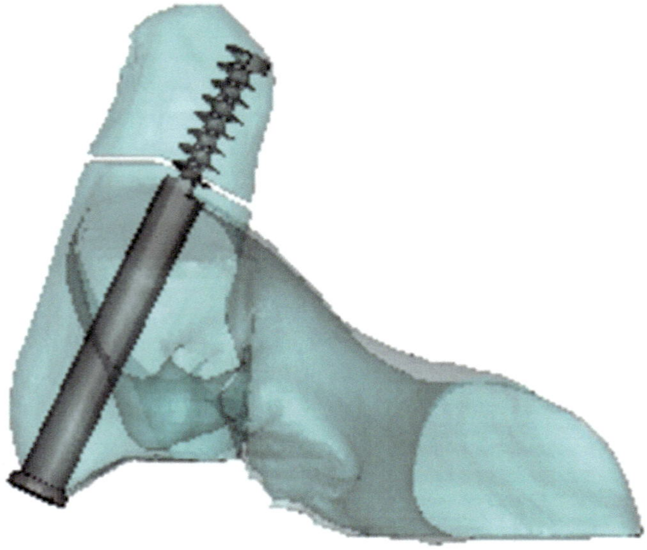

Fig. 16.8 Beware of the position of the screw

16.5 Clinical Cases

16.5.1 Case No. 1

Patient: A 25-year-old woman with neck pain with motor impairment for 5 hours following injury.

Diagnosis: Fracture of the odontoid process.

Surgery: UCSS anterior internal fixation.

Imaging data: Preoperative images are shown in Fig. 16.9, intraoperative images are shown in Fig. 16.10, and postoperative images are shown in Fig. 16.11.

16.6 Pearls and Pitfalls

Placement of each screw should be done under fluoroscopy, and make sure that the stylet is not bent and displaced proximally. Sometimes, the stylet may enter the foramen magnum with the insertion of the screw, which is a horrible scenario (Fig. 16.12).

16.7 Postoperative Care

The patient is observed for 24 hours postoperatively at the ICU. Patient respiration is closely monitored. The neck wears support for 6 weeks, which can be removed while tak-

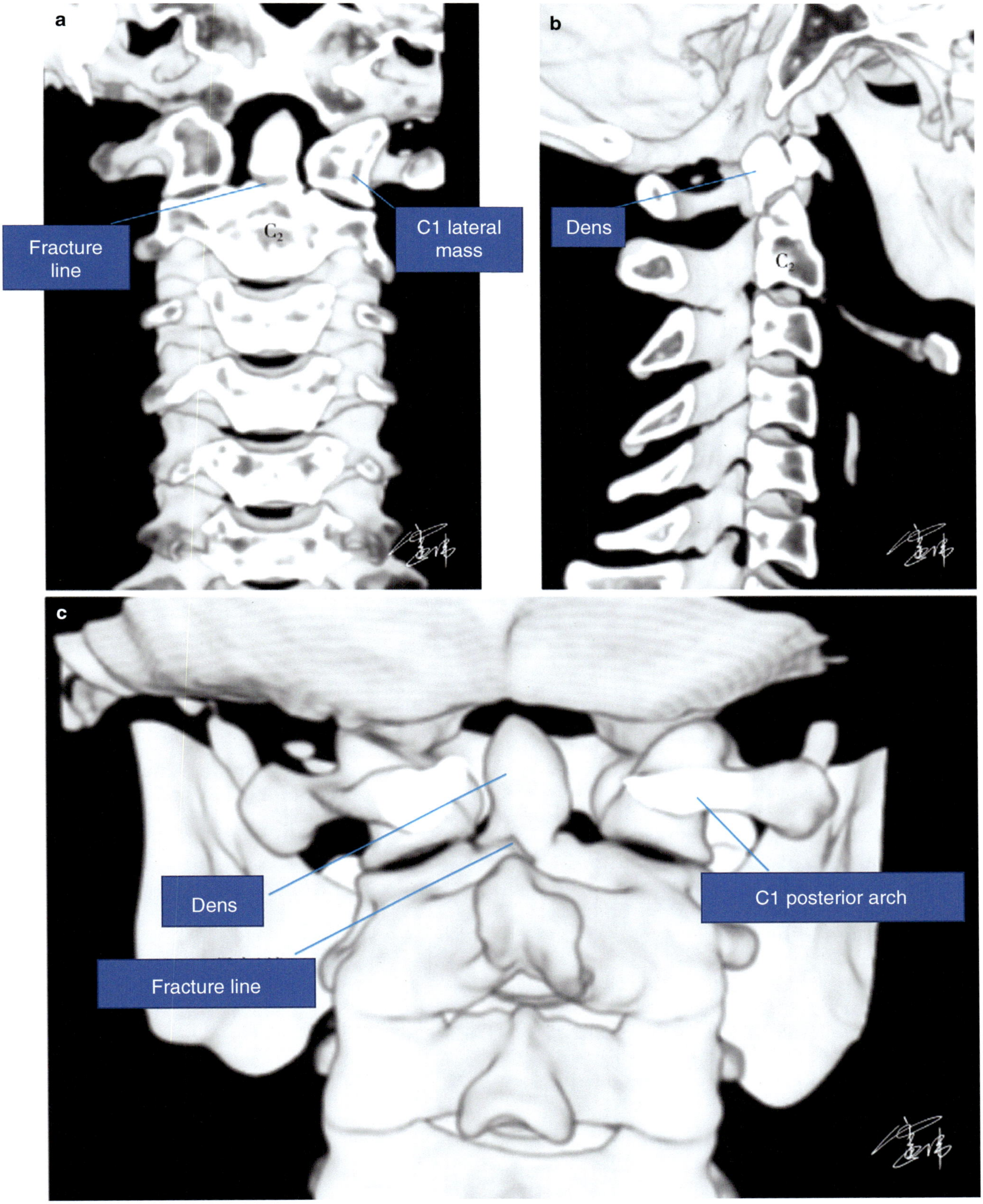

Fig. 16.9 Preoperative images. (**a**) CT 3D reconstruction (anterior view). (**b**) CT 3D reconstruction (lateral view). (**c**) CT 3D reconstruction (posterior view)

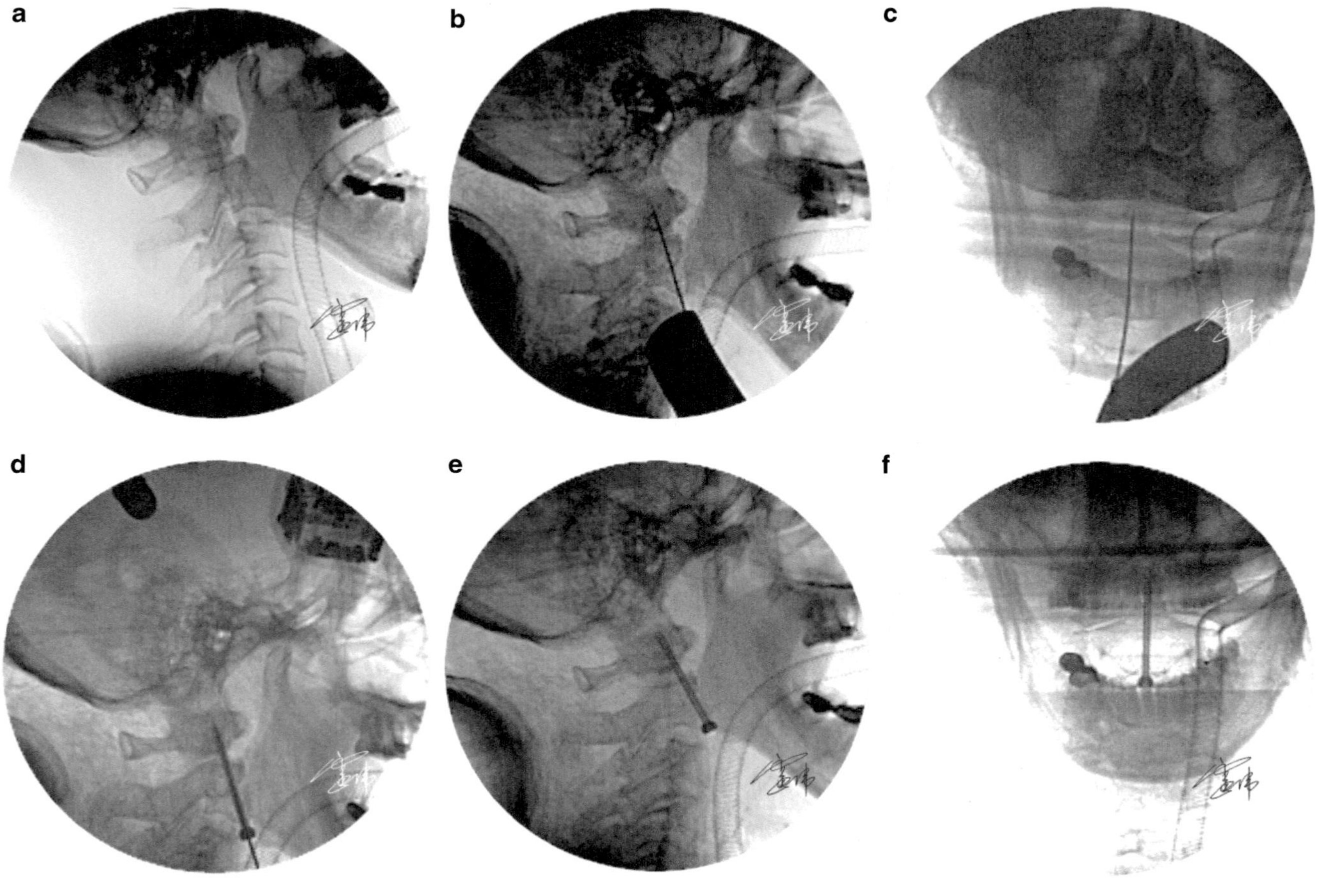

Fig. 16.10 Intraoperative images. (**a**) Before reduction (lateral view); (**b**) Localization by the stylet (lateral view); (**c**) Localization by the stylet (orthogonal view); (**d**) Screw placement (lateral view); (**e**) Completion of fixation (lateral view); (**f**) Completion of fixation (orthogonal view)

ing a shower or rest. Follow-up visit is done at 6, 12, and 24 weeks postoperatively, and healing is studied radiologically.

16.8 Clinical Experiences and Cautions

16.8.1 Surgical Indications of Odontoid Screw Fixation Techniques

(1) Fresh Anderson type II odontoid fracture: The transverse ligament is intact.
(2) Fresh Anderson type III odontoid fracture: If the location of the C2 vertebral body fracture is high and the C2 vertebral body does not have comminuted fracture, and the patient refuses conservative external fixation or dislocation of fracture is present.

16.8.2 Treatment Options for Anteroposterior-Posteroinferior (Reverse Oblique Type) Fracture

The union rate of anterior odontoid screw fixation is comparable to external fixation for anteroposterior-posteroinferior (reverse oblique type) fracture and is approximately 75%. The anatomic union rate is 50%, and the nonanatomic union rate is 25% [3]. Therefore, C1–C2 fixation via the posterior approach is recommended for anteroposterior-posteroinferior (reverse oblique type) fracture, and if anterior odontoid screw fixation is undertaken, postoperative external fixation should be done.

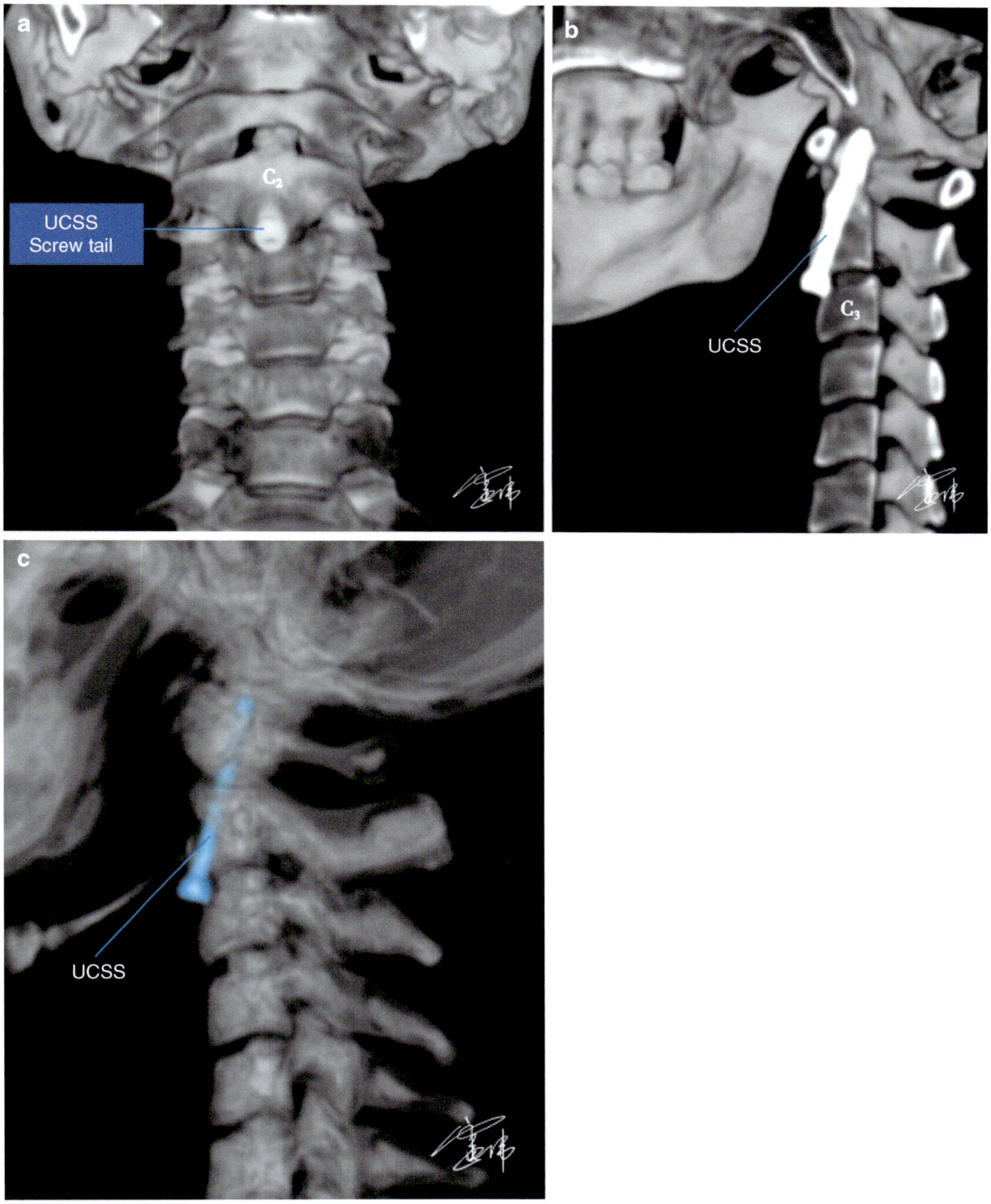

Fig. 16.11 Postoperative images. (**a**) CT 3D reconstruction (anterior view). (**b**) CT 3D reconstruction (sagittal split view). (**c**) CT 3D reconstruction (lateral view)

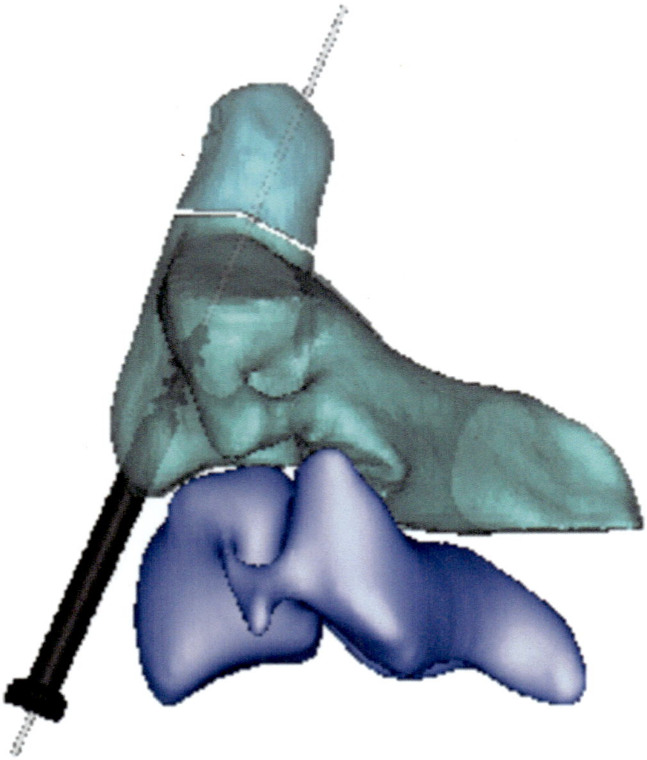

Fig. 16.12 The stylet enters the foramen magnum

16.8.3 Number of Screws

Clinical experiences suggest that there is no difference in overall healing rate of bone fractures with the use of one or two screws [3, 4].

References

1. Chiba K, et al. Anterior screw fixation for odontoid fracture: clinical results in 45 cases. Eur Spine J. 1993;2(2):76–81.
2. Bohler J. Anterior stabilization for acute fractures and non-unions of the dens. J Bone Joint Surg Am. 1982;64(1):18–27.
3. Apfelbaum RI, et al. Direct anterior screw fixation for recent and remote odontoid fractures. J Neurosurg. 2000;93(2 Suppl):227–36.
4. Jenkins JD, Coric D, Branch CL Jr. A clinical comparison of one- and two-screw odontoid fixation. J Neurosurg. 1998;89(3):366–70.

The Interbody Fusion System

17

Yabo Yan and Wei Lei

Abstract

The interbody fusion system is a support used to re-establish the spinal stability in the spinal disorder. It can maintain the intervertebral height and decompress the nerve root. The interbody fusion system included the anterior interbody fusion system, the lateral interbody fusion system, and the posterior interbody fusion system. The materials of interbody fusion system are varied and contained the autograft bone, titanium, PEEK, etc. The functions of various interbody fusion systems are (1) to stabilize intervertebral joint, (2) to increase or maintain intervertebral interval height, and (3) to act as carrier of bone graft material. The chapter introduces the different interbody fusion systems in detail. At the same time, the procedure of insertion of interbody cage in the spine is shown as a step-by-step example. Pearls and pitfalls of the interbody fusion system are summarized at the end of this chapter.

Keywords

Interbody fusion system · Cervical spine · Lumbar spine

Over the recent years, interbody fusion surgery, as an important spine surgery technique, has played an irreplaceable role in the field, especially in the treatment of degenerative spinal diseases. Interbody fusion mainly includes anterior lumbar interbody fusion (ALIF) and posterior lumbar interbody fusion (PLIF). Based on Medtronic Sofamor Danek implants, surgeons in the USA subsequently developed a modified PLIF, namely, transforaminal interbody fusion (TLIF). However, the focal point of orthopedic surgeons has always been increasing the fusion rate and preventing pseudoarthrosis. To achieve this goal, orthopedic surgeons have used multiple internal fixation devices clinically, the most representative of which is the interbody fusion system (Fig. 17.1).

In the 1980s, veterinary orthopedic surgeon Bagby introduced anterior interbody cervical fusion to treat "wobbler's syndrome" in racing horses and achieved satisfactory results. The device was then used in humans, and, thereafter, a variety of interbody fusion systems have entered the field of spine surgery, which have played a critical role in improving the success rate of interbody fusion surgery. The functions of various interbody fusion systems are (1) to stabilize intervertebral joint, (2) to increase or maintain intervertebral interval height, and (3) to act as carrier of bone graft material.

17.1 Devices for Cervical Intervertebral Fusion

17.1.1 Implant

PEEK is an excellent thermoresistant, steam-resistant, radiation-resistant, and durable material, and its main component is polyetheretherketone. PEEK cervical interbody fusion device combines the advantages of superior strength, impact resistance, and radiolucency, allowing observation and evaluation by X-rays and CT scan of implant and bone graft fusion.

(1) The curved surface in anatomic design fits the endplate better.
(2) The surgical steps are the same as the Smith and Robinson technique.
(3) It has good reproducibility. It comes in different dimensions, avoiding the need of intraoperative cropping.
(4) It has an elastic modulus closer to that of the bone tissue and has better biological compatibility.
(5) X-ray titanium rod marker facilitates postoperative evaluation of the position of the prosthesis (Fig. 17.2).
(6) The tools are streamlined in design.

Y. Yan · W. Lei (✉)
Department of Orthopedics, Xijing Hospital, Air Force Medical University, Xi'an, Shaanxi, China
e-mail: leiwei@fmmu.edu.cn

W. Lei, Y. Yan (eds.), *Internal Fixation of the Spine*, https://doi.org/10.1007/978-981-16-1562-7_17

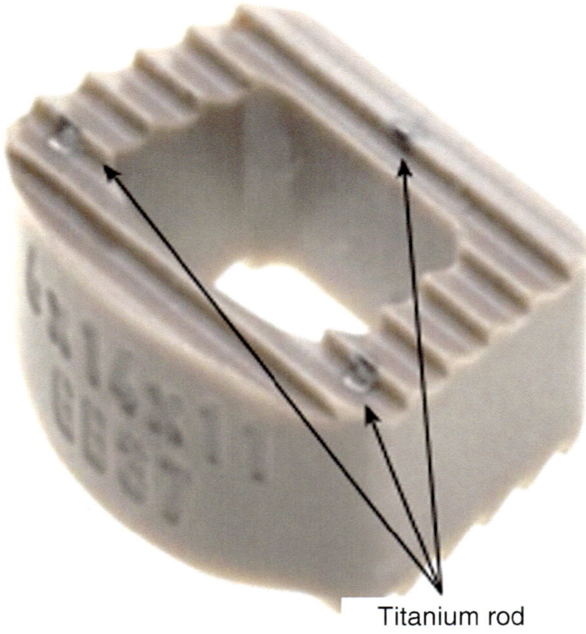

Fig. 17.1 Titanium rod for radiologic marking

17.1.2 Clinical Indications and Contraindications

(1) Indications
   (a) Intervertebral disc herniation, intervertebral disc degeneration, and intervertebral disc space narrowing
   (b) Correction surgery for failed intervertebral disc surgery and postoperative instability
(2) Contraindications

Cervical interbody fusion devices should not be used alone and should be used in combination with anterior steel plate.

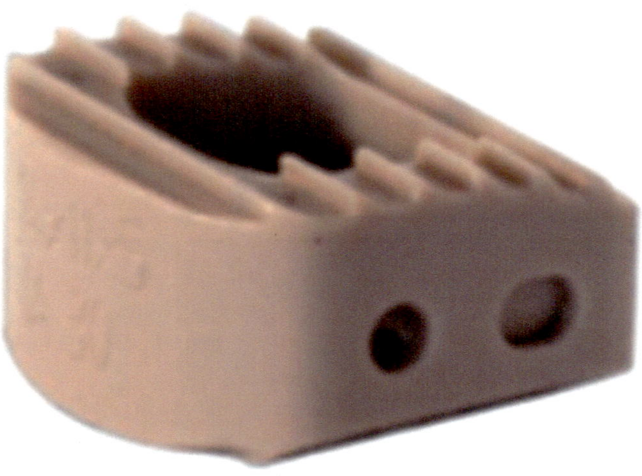

Fig. 17.2 Implant

17.1.3 Surgical Procedures

(1) Exposure

The intervertebral disc is resected by conventional Smith and Robinson technique (Fig. 17.3).

(2) Distraction

Long tail screws are inserted into the anterior surface of the superior and inferior vertebral bodies, and then the CASPAR distractor is placed. The intervertebral space is gradually distracted (Fig. 17.4a, b).

(3) Trial

Appropriately sized prosthesis is chosen for trial (Fig. 17.5).

(4) Preparation of prosthesis

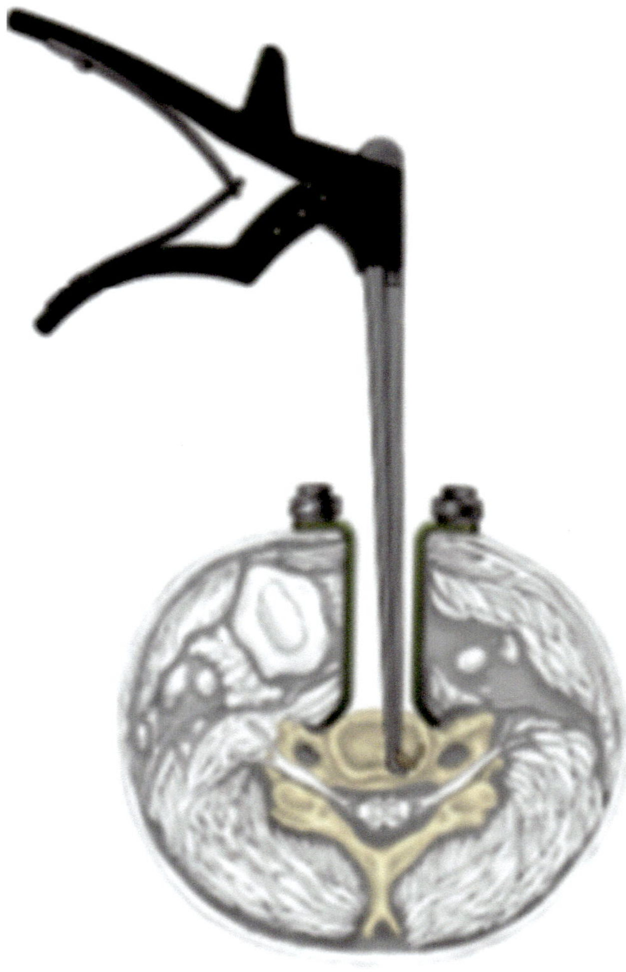

Fig. 17.3 Exposure

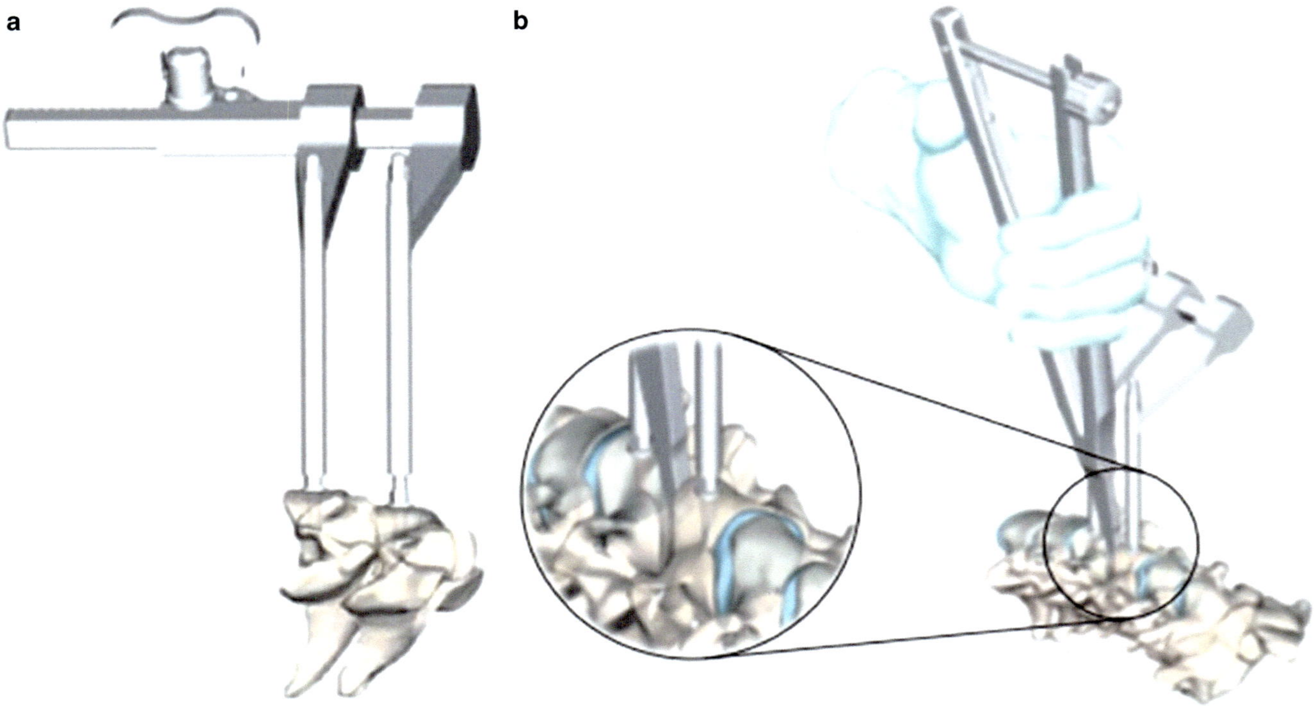

Fig. 17.4 Distraction. (**a**) The distractor is placed. (**b**) The intervertebral space is distracted

Fig. 17.5 Trial

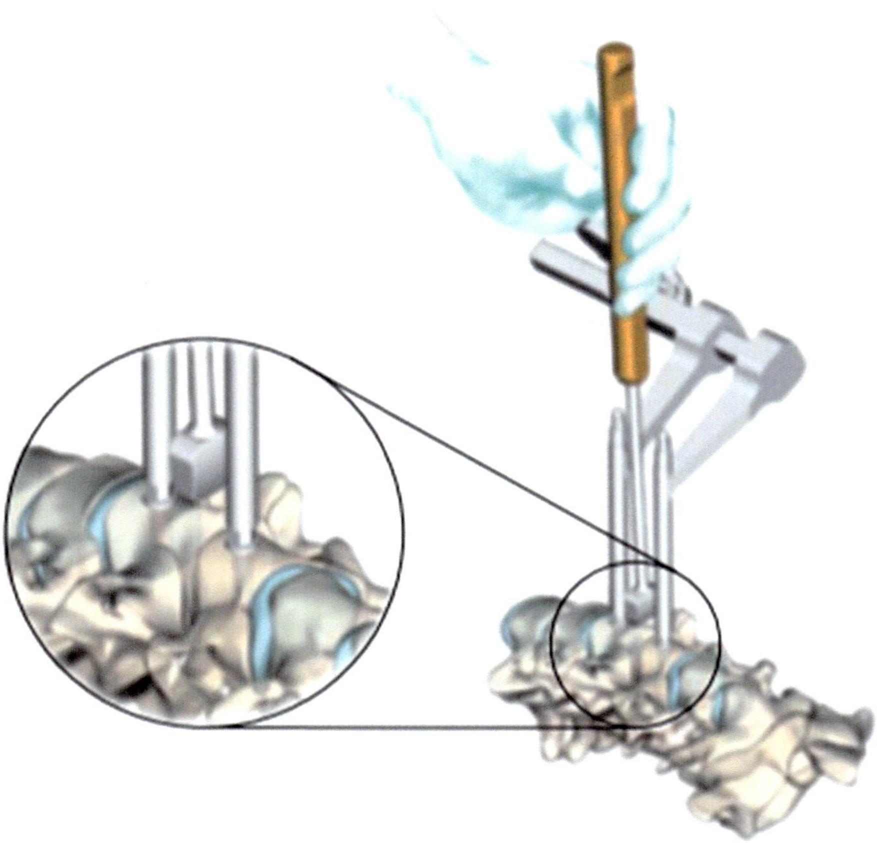

The chosen prosthesis is placed on the prosthesis support, and the morselized bones obtained during decompression or artificial bone materials are added onto the bone graft window of the prosthesis and gently tapped into place (Fig. 17.6).

(5) Prosthesis placement

The prosthesis is put into the processed intervertebral space using a prosthesis holder and stabilized by being gently tapped into the correct place (Fig. 17.7a, b). Correct insertion depth is achieved when the end of the fusion device is reached and is parallel to or slightly lower than the anterior border of the vertebral body. Surgeons should make sure that

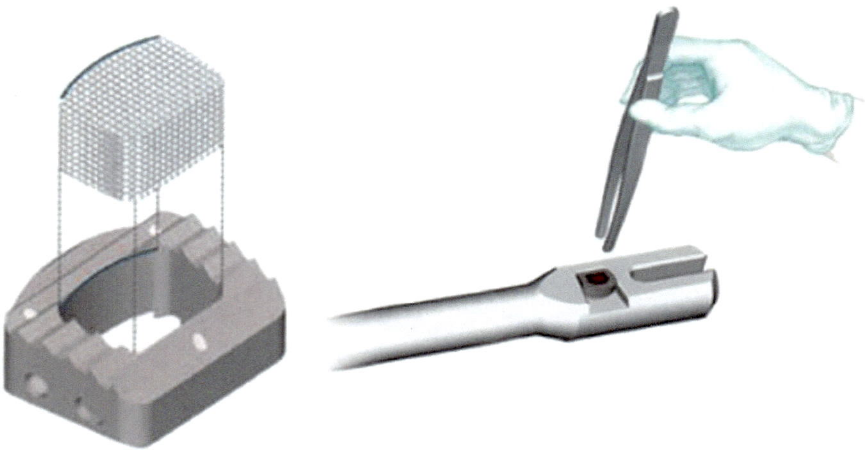

Fig. 17.6 Prosthesis preparation

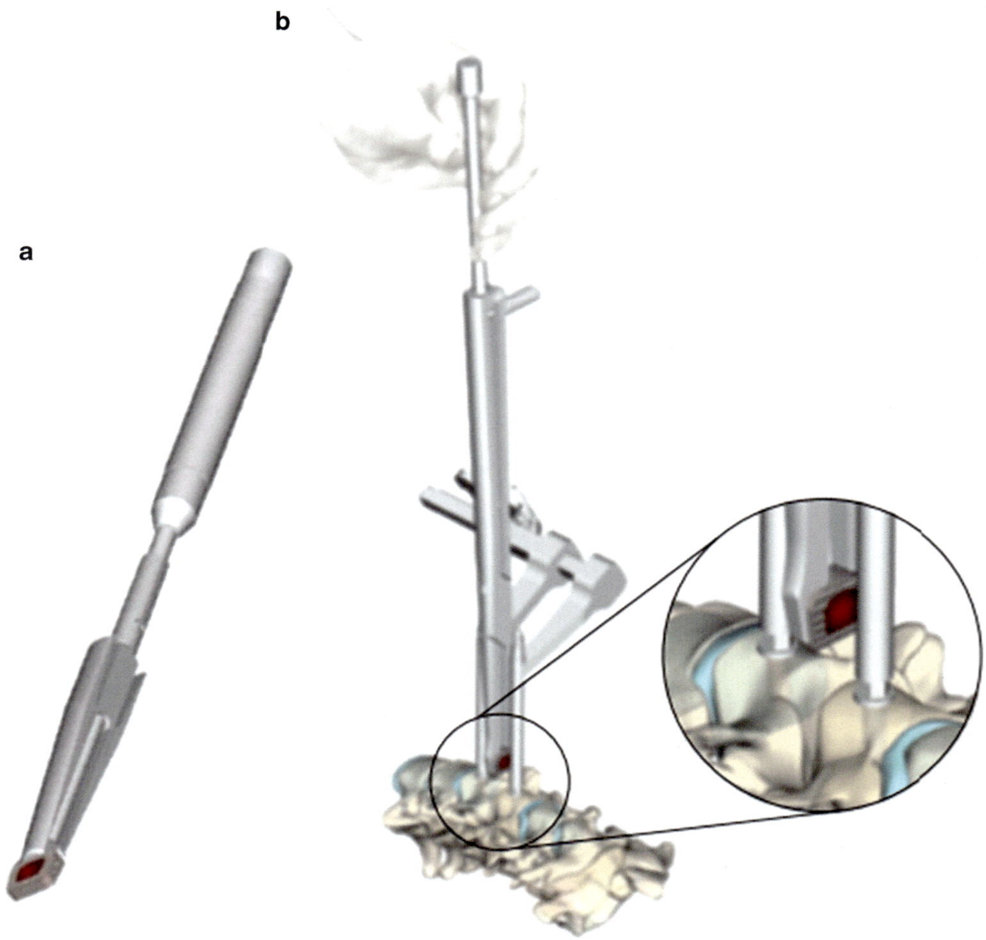

Fig. 17.7 Prosthesis placement. (**a**) The prosthesis is held. (**b**) The prosthesis is put into place

no osteophytes are present in the superior or inferior surface of the disc space to avoid the fusion device being implanted too shallow. Meanwhile, it should be emphasized that the fusion device should not be inserted too deep to avoid severe complications of the nervous system.

Caution: Cervical interbody fusion device should not be used along. It should be used in combination with the anterior steel plate.

17.1.4 Clinical Cases

17.1.4.1 Case No. 1

Patient: A 39-year-old man with left-hand numbness and pain for 1 year with aggravation for 2 months.

Diagnosis: Cervical spondylosis (cervical spondylotic radiculopathy).

Surgery: C5–C6 discectomy and decompression, cervical spine fusion, and cervical anterior steel plate internal fixation.

Imaging data: Preoperative image is shown in Fig. 17.8, and postoperative images are shown in Fig. 17.9a–d.

17.1.4.2 Case No. 2

Patient: A 32-year-old man with sensorimotor impairment of the four extremities for 1 day post injury.

Diagnosis: Cervical spinal cord injury with incomplete paralysis.

Surgery: C3–C4 and C4–C5, C3–C4, and C4–C5 discectomy and decompression surgery and fusion and anterior steel plate internal fixation of the cervical spine.

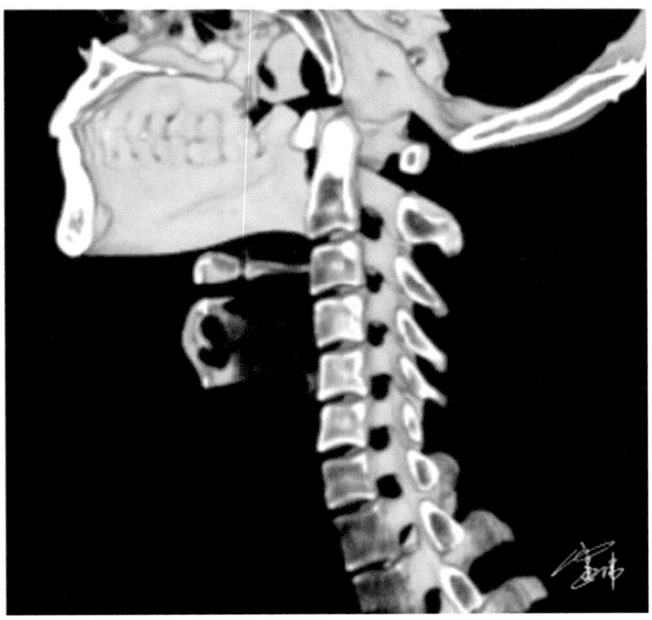

Fig. 17.8 CT 3D reconstruction (sagittal split view)

Imaging data: Preoperative and postoperative comparison is shown in Fig. 17.10a–d.

17.2 Titanium Mesh Cage Fusion Device

17.2.1 Implant

The implant is made of pure titanium and possesses excellent biological compatibility. It comes in a wide variety of diameters for use in the cervical, thoracic, and lumbar spine (Fig. 17.11).

(1) The cylindrical structure of the cage mesh allows omnidirectional bone growth.
(2) Any length can be taken with ease of use.
(3) Contoured edges facilitate handling and rapid insertion.
(4) Apart from its applicability to all types of interbody fusion surgeries, the main advantage of the technique is restoration of the stability of the anterior column following complete or partial corpectomy.
(5) X-ray and MRI images are clear, without artifacts and scattering.

17.2.2 Clinical Indications and Contraindications

(1) Indications

The technique including anterior (ALIF), posterior (PLIF), and transforaminal lumbar interbody fusion (TLIF) and corpectomy is indicated for fixation of cervical, thoracolumbar, lumbar, and lumbosacral segments.

(2) Contraindications

Intervertebral space infection

17.2.3 Surgical Procedures

(1) Anterior spinal reconstruction with a PYRAMESH titanium cage post corpectomy

The surgical procedure is mainly used to restore the height and stability and achieve fusion of the anterior spinal column post total and subtotal corpectomy in patients with spinal tumors, fractures, and spinal cord compression.

(a) The diseased vertebral body is conventionally resected. The goal is complete elimination of symptoms and signs of the disease and full decompression of the spinal cord (Fig. 17.12).

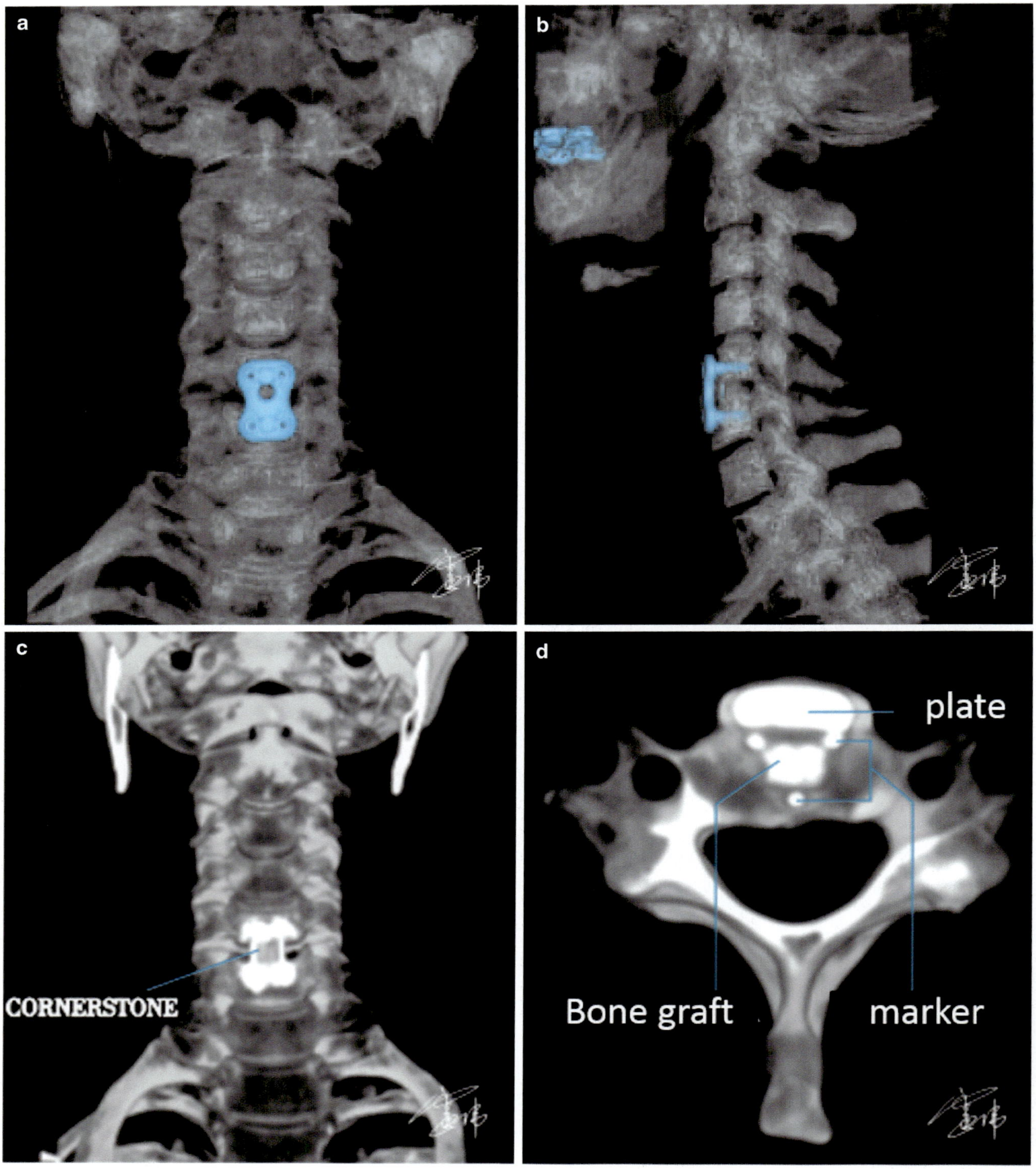

Fig. 17.9 Postoperative images. (**a**) CT 3D reconstruction (orthogonal view). (**b**) CT 3D reconstruction (lateral view). (**c**) CT 3D reconstruction (anterior view, steel plate removed). (**d**) CT 3D reconstruction (horizontal view)

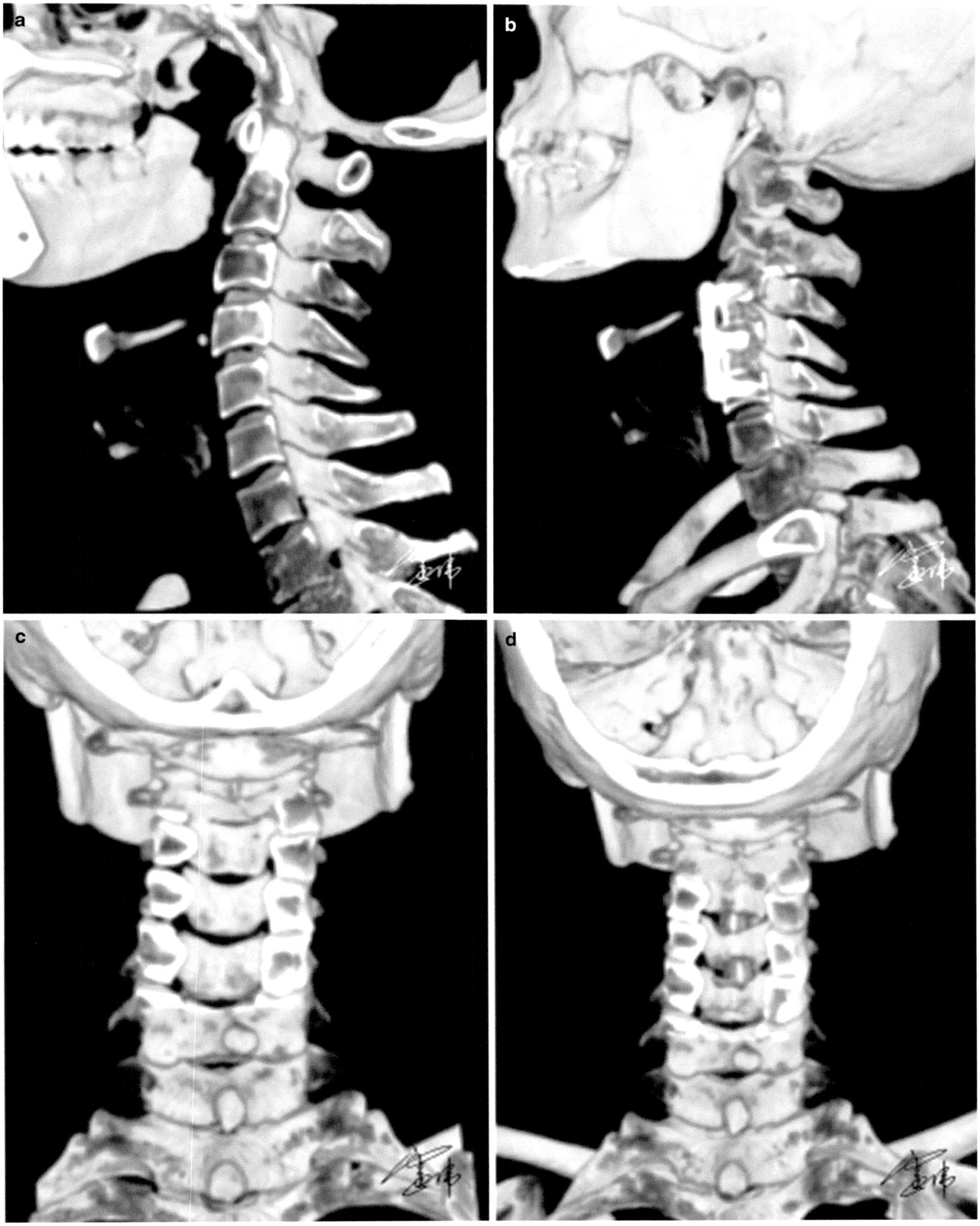

Fig. 17.10 Preoperative and postoperative imaging studies. (**a**) CT 3D reconstruction (preoperative sagittal split view). (**b**) CT 3D reconstruction (preoperative sagittal split view). (**c**) CT 3D reconstruction (preoperative anteroposterior split view). (**d**) CT 3D reconstruction (postoperative anteroposterior split view)

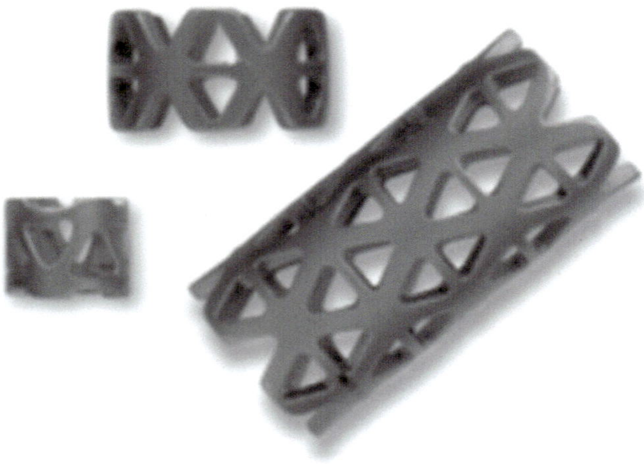

Fig. 17.11 Implants

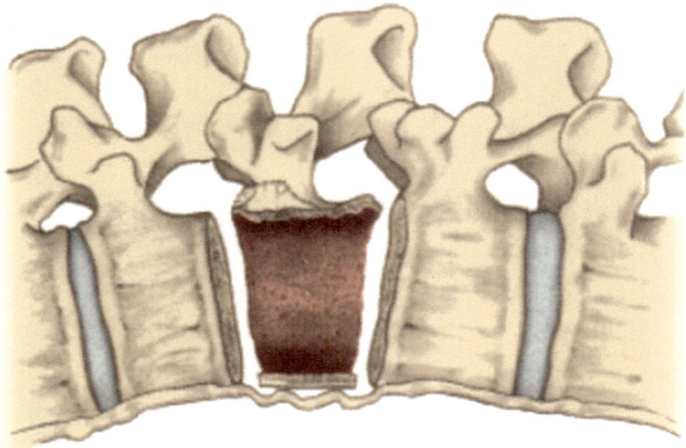

Fig. 17.12 Complete resection of the diseased vertebral body

(b) The height of the anterior column can be restored via manual maneuvering or intervertebral distraction devices (Fig. 17.13).
(c) Identical to conventional interbody fusion surgery, the endplate of the annulus fibrosus and the cartilage on the surface of the superior and inferior endplates of the defect area should be completely removed to facilitate bony fusion.
(d) The span of the interbody defect should be accurately measured, and the titanium mesh cage should be cut at the corresponding length (Fig. 17.14). Then, the titanium mesh cage is filled with bone graft material.
(e) The matching device is used to gently insert the implanted titanium mesh cage into the defect area (Fig. 17.15).
(f) The interbody distraction device is removed and the corresponding assisted internal fixation device such as the Z-plate (Fig. 17.16)

(2) Transforaminal posterior interbody fusion (TLIF)

When interbody fusion devices are used for PLIF, the intervertebral space is generally required to be exposed bilaterally after extensive decompression. The disadvantage of this method is excision of the bilateral articular processes and the increased risk of radical root injuries. Orthopedic surgeons in the USA have started carrying out PLIF via unilateral intervertebral foramen. Meanwhile, TLIF retains the contralateral facet joints and reduces the interference of the operation with the contents in the spinal canal and has achieved good results. The spinal canal is entered via a unilateral approach in the surgery, and there is minimal disruption of the posterior contents with little impact on stability. More bone surface is preserved to allow pedicle screw implantation. Epidural scars are reduced and the operative time is shortened, and intraoperative blood loss and nervous system complications are also decreased.

(a) The pedicle screws are placed in the fusion space in the superior and inferior vertebral body (Fig. 17.17).
(b) The intervertebral space is distracted using the connecting rod between the pedicle screws (Fig. 17.18).
(c) The contralateral laminar space is distracted with a distractor, and the intervertebral space is entered from this side (Fig. 17.19).
(d) The superior and inferior articular processes and the extraneous part of the lamina are excised (Fig. 17.20).
(e) The intervertebral foramen is entered, and the nerve root is retracted upward to expose the intervertebral disc (Fig. 17.21)
(f) The posterior longitudinal ligament and annulus fibrosus are incised, and a window is opened in the intervertebral disc. Then, the nucleus pulposus is removed (Fig. 17.22).
(g) The intervertebral disc is thoroughly cleaned using the matching tool, which should be identical to PLIF (Fig. 17.23).
(h) The prepared anterior intervertebral space is filled with morselized bone and pressed tight (Fig. 17.24)
(i) Appropriately sized fusion devices are chosen according to the height of the intervertebral space and implanted into the intervertebral space as shown in Fig. 17.25.
(j) The connecting rod of the pedicle system is placed and appropriate pressure is applied (Fig. 17.26).

17.2.4 Clinical Cases

17.2.4.1 Case No. 1

Patient: A 29-year-old man with motor sensory impairment of the four extremities for 12 hours after trauma.

Diagnosis: C5 vertebral body fracture.

Surgery: C5 partial corpectomy and decompression and PYRAMESH fusion plus steel plate internal fixation (Figs. 17.27a, b, 17.28a–e).

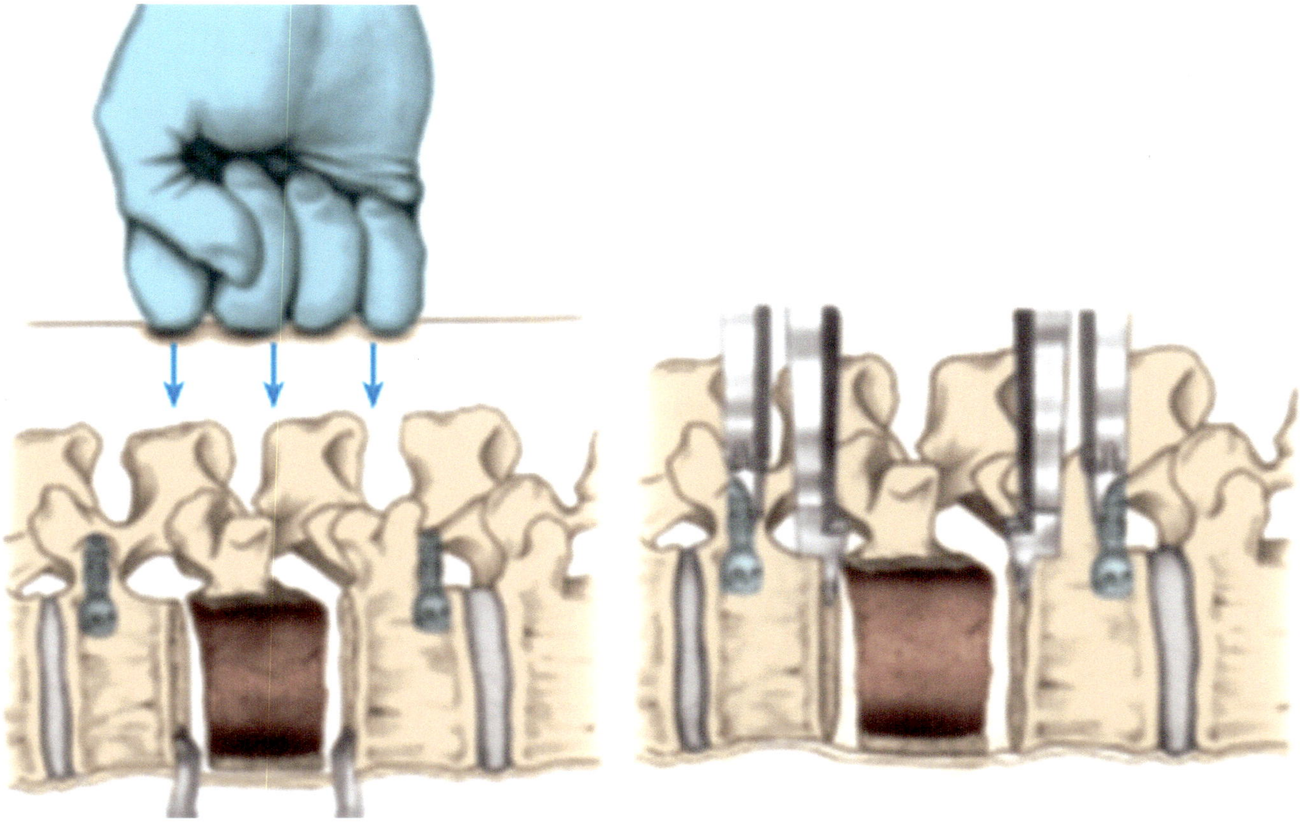

Fig. 17.13 Restoring the height of the anterior column

17.2.4.2 Case No. 2

Patient: A 46-year-old woman was admitted because of numbness of the four extremities and limb weakness on walking for 2 years.

Diagnosis: Cervical spondylosis with ossification of the posterior longitudinal ligament.

Surgery: C4–C5 discectomy and decompression, CONERSTONE fusion, C6 partial corpectomy and decompression, and PYRAMESH fusion plus steel plate internal fixation.

Imaging data: Preoperative image is shown in Fig. 17.29a–e, and postoperative images are shown in Fig. 17.30a–d.

17.2.4.3 Case No. 3

Patient: A 32-year-old man was admitted because of lumbar pain and sensory motor impairment of the lower extremities for 1 day.

Diagnosis: L1 fracture and paralysis.

Surgery: Partial resection of the rib of T12 via an anterior approach, L1 subtotal corpectomy and decompression surgery, and PYRAMESH+ANTARES reduction and internal fixation.

Imaging data: Preoperative images are shown in Fig. 17.31a, b, intraoperative images are shown in Fig. 17.32a, b, and postoperative images are shown in Fig. 17.33a, b.

17.3 Pearls and Pitfalls

(1) Titanium mesh cage assures the restoration of the length and stability of the anterior column of the spine. Therefore, the surgeon should carry out removal of the lesion and spinal cord decompression according to the condition of the disease without worrying about jeopardizing spine stability.
(2) Though applicable to use post corpectomy, titanium mesh cage implantation falls within the category of interbody fusion surgery. Therefore, the treatment of the endplates is identical to that in conventional interbody fusion surgery, which is very critical to postoperative bony fusion.
(3) The purpose of titanium mesh cage is to restore the height and stability of the anterior column of the spine. Therefore, if the local condition allows, titanium mesh

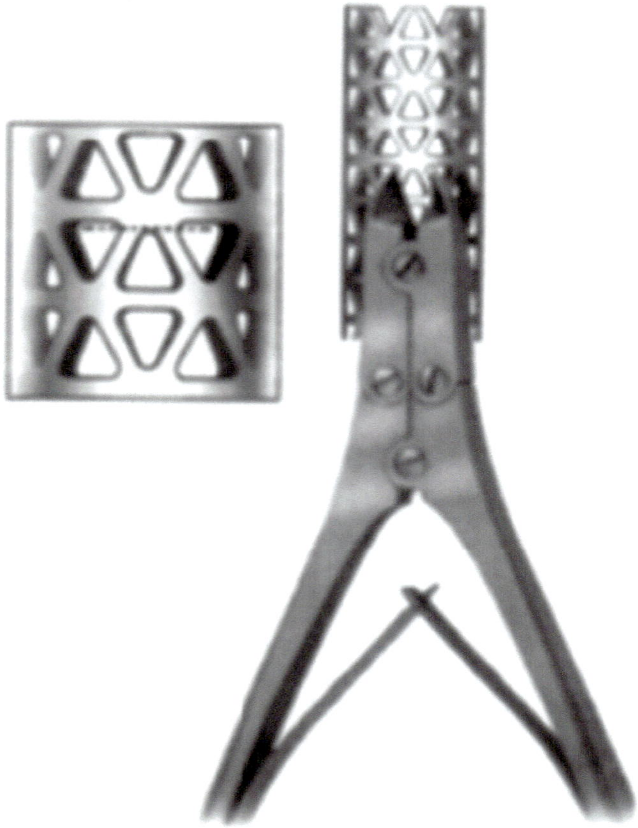

Fig. 17.14 Cutting the titanium mesh cage

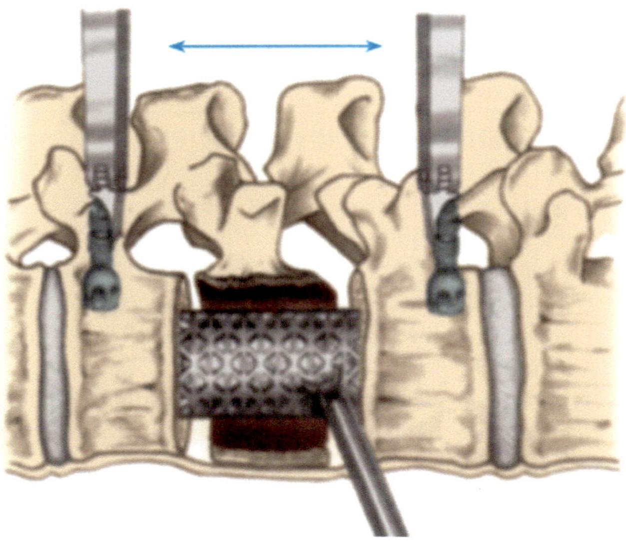

Fig. 17.15 Implanting the titanium mesh cage

cage with the largest diameter should be chosen, which facilitates bony fusion and reconstruction of local stability.

(4) In general, the titanium mesh cage is implanted between two separate vertebral bodies, and its stability depends on compression by the vertebral bodies. Therefore, the titanium mesh cage should be implanted while the intervertebral space is under distraction. The CASPAR distractor is used for the cervical spine, while in the thoracic and lumbar spine, the distractor is loosened after the screws are inserted in the vertebral body to allow intervertebral compression of the titanium mesh cage.

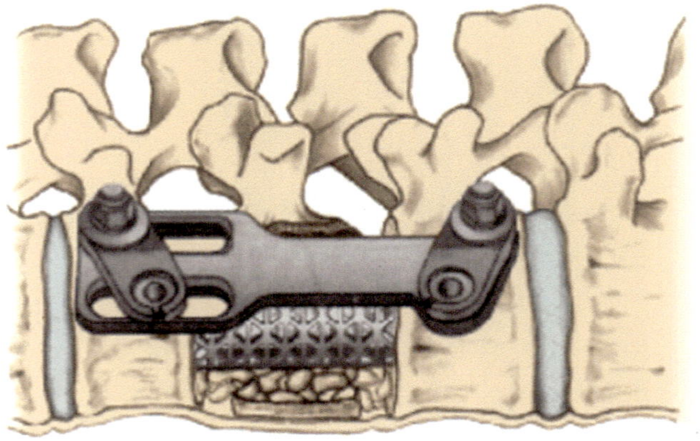

Fig. 17.16 Placing internal fixation device

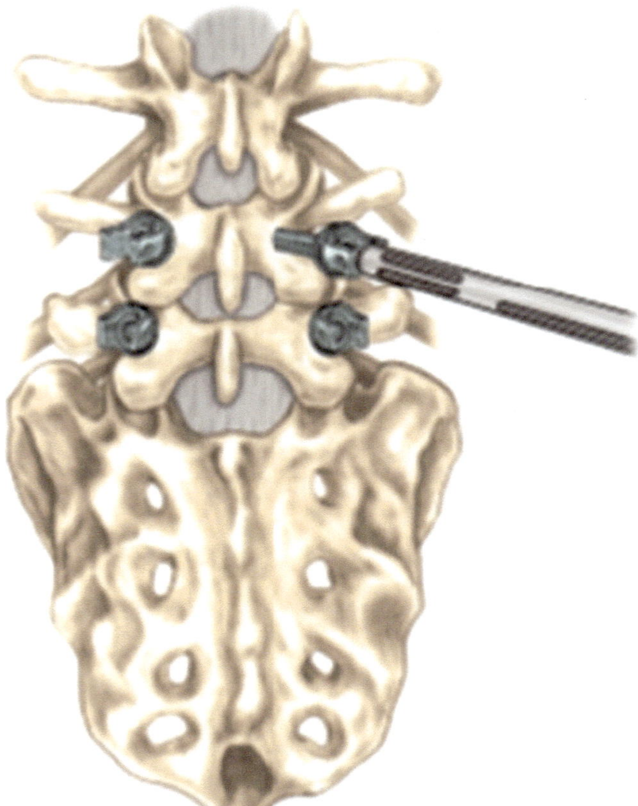

Fig. 17.17 Placing pedicle screws

(5) Despite the intervertebral squeeze effect on the titanium mesh cage that helps regional stability, the titanium mesh cage generally should be combined with other methods of local internal fixation such as anterior

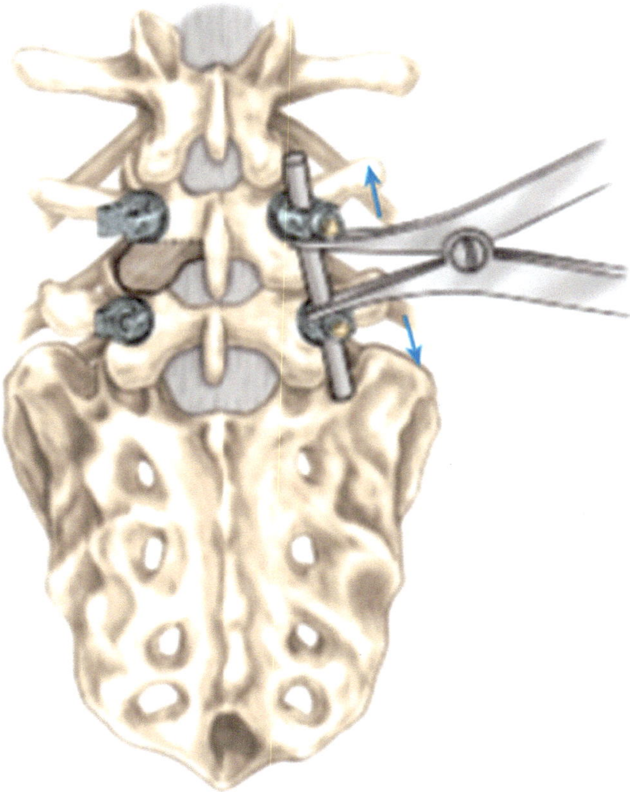

Fig. 17.18 Distraction

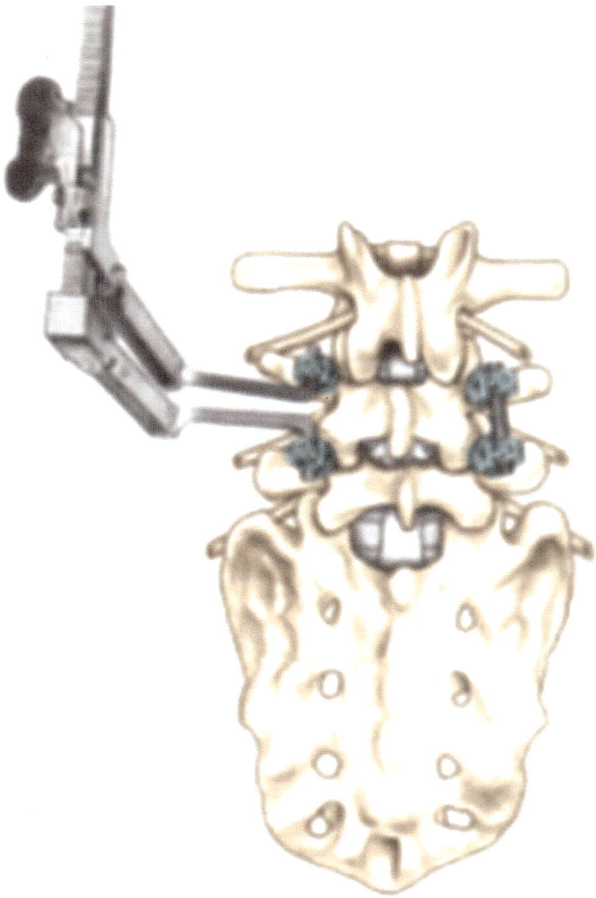

Fig. 17.19 Distraction of the contralateral laminar space

titanium plate of the cervical spine and Z-plate or pedicle screws system for the thoracolumbar spine so that local spine stability can reliably be restored.

(6) Except in cases of advanced malignant tumors, the interior of the titanium mesh cage should be filled with bone graft materials in order to achieve long-term stability.

(7) TLIF is suitable for patients who are surgically indicated for fusion but who do not require extensive spinal canal decompression or only require unilateral decompression so that the articular process is preserved on one side, which is conducive to postoperative restoration of postoperative stability and prevention of breakage of internal fixation. In addition, this effectively reduces surgical interference with the intraspinal contents, thus reducing surgical complications.

(8) TLIF should not be indiscriminatively used in cases requiring bilateral decompression though satisfactory fusion can be achieved. However, clinical symptoms cannot be fully eliminated. Therefore, PLIF should be routinely used for such cases.

(9) The connecting rod of the contralateral pedicle screws and the matching laminar distractor should be effectively utilized to facilitate surgery.

(10) Because the procedure of TLIF is performed more laterally, great care should be taken to avoid inadvertent injury to the nerve roots. Meanwhile, excessive traction of the nerve roots should also be avoided.

(11) Because there is limitation in the size of window in the intervertebral disc, titanium mesh cage smaller in diameter, typically a diameter of 13 mm, is chosen.

(12) Due to the relatively large cross-sectional area of the lumbar intervertebral disc, the anterior intervertebral space should be implanted with large amounts of morselized bone or other graft materials before titanium mesh cage implantation in order to achieve effective fusion area.

(13) Because of the physiologic lordosis of the lumbar spine, titanium mesh cage should be cut into a shape that is high anteriorly and low posteriorly.

(14) After titanium mesh cage implantation, appropriate pressure can be applied using the bilateral pedicle screws, which facilitates local formation of a tension ring as well as prevents posterior displacement.

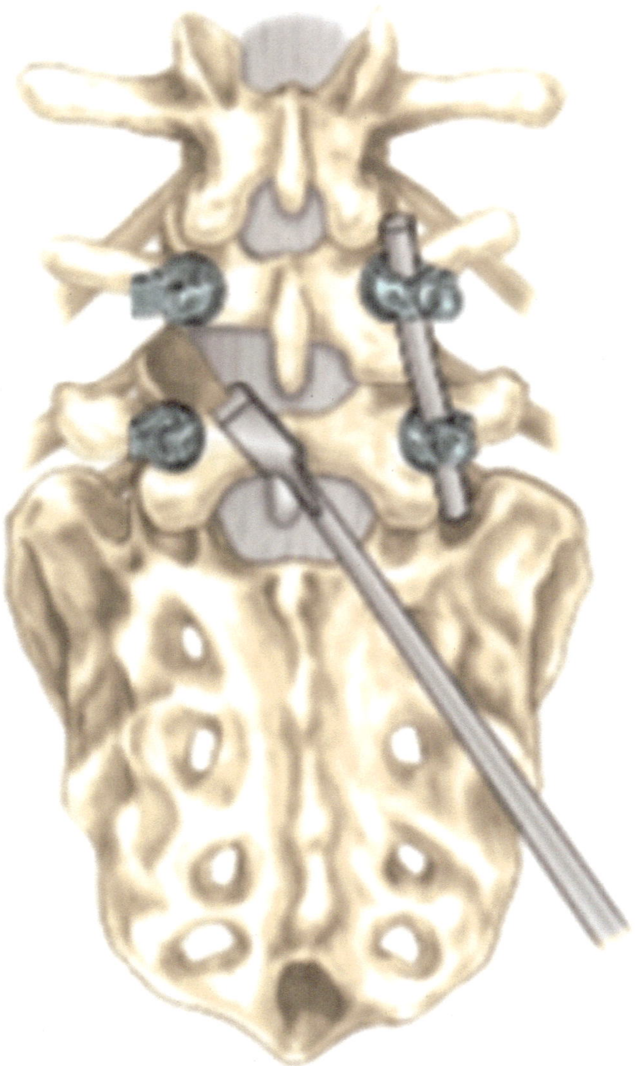

Fig. 17.20 Excision of the superior and inferior articular processes and the extraneous part of the lamina

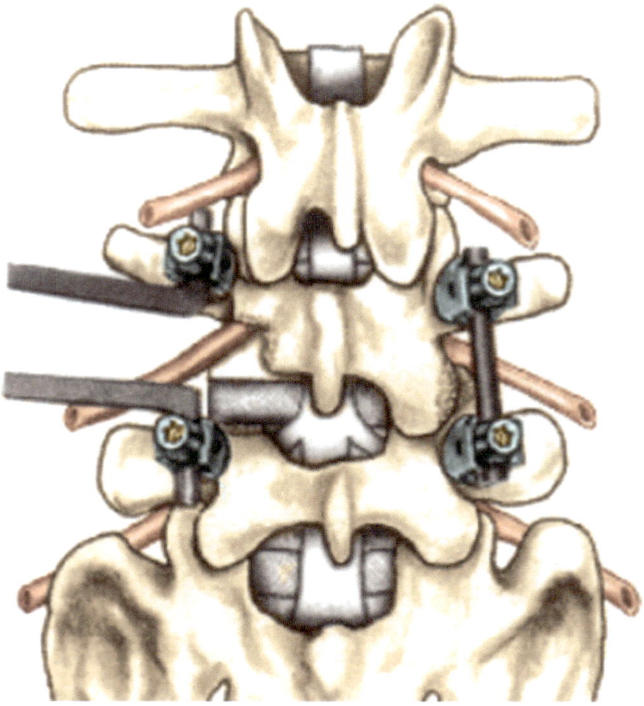

Fig. 17.21 Exposing the intervertebral disc

17.4 Anatomic Lumbar Interbody Fusion Device

17.4.1 Implant (Fig. 17.34)

(1) The contoured surface of the distractor/trial fits the endplate more closely anatomically and facilitates selection of optimally sized implants.
(2) The bullet-like structure has auto-distraction effect and is easy to implant. Moreover, the serrated structures on the surface increase friction and prevent the implant from falling off.
(3) Either unilateral or bilateral fusion device implantation can be undertaken.

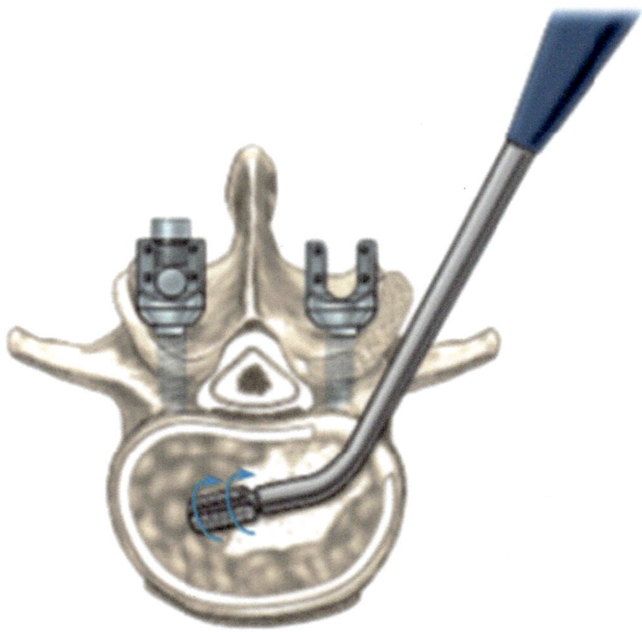

Fig. 17.22 Extracting the nucleus pulposus

(4) The device is suitable for open, small incision, and minimally invasive surgery.
(5) It has a universal implant and tool design and is suitable for surgical entry via multiple approaches.

17.4.2 Clinical Indications and Contraindications

(1) Indications
   (a) Intervertebral disc herniation, intervertebral disc degeneration, and intervertebral space narrowing
   (b) Correction surgery for failed intervertebral disc surgery and postoperative instability
(2) Contraindications

Lumbar interbody fusion device cannot be used singly and should be combined with fixation with posterior pedicle screws.

17.4.3 Surgical Procedures

(1) Unilateral entry

Laminectomy or joint resection and decompression: The superior and inferior articular processes of the diseased segment are excised using osteotomes or drills. Osteophytes can be removed with a burr or drill. In the Kambin triangle, 1-cm square is incised using a scalpel in the annulus fibrosus, and the intervertebral disc is then resected. The main purpose of this step is to excise the ligament protruding into the vertebral canal for nerve decompression. Intervertebral distraction is also undertaken via this entry route to lessen or avoid traction of the nerve root. However, if the intervertebral space is severely collapsed, discectomy should be undertaken following intervertebral space distraction (Fig. 17.35a, b).

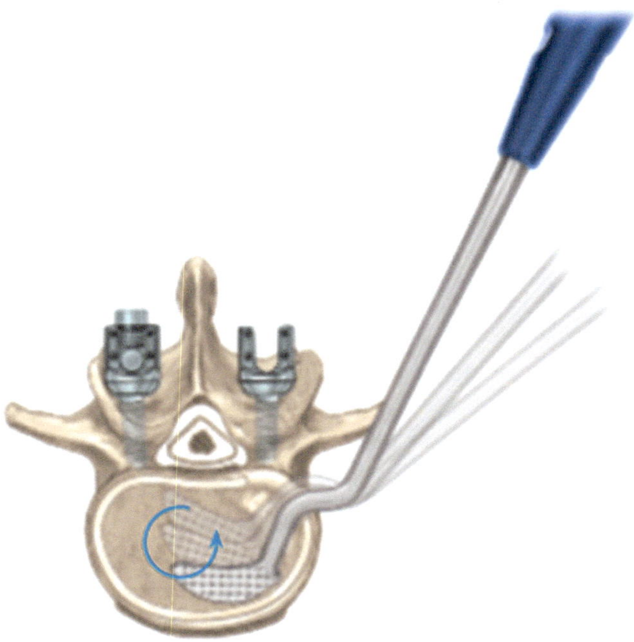

Fig. 17.23 Thorough cleaning of the intervertebral disc

(2)Distraction

The distractor is inserted; its contoured edges sit flush against the endplate. The intervertebral space is distracted in sequence until the satisfactory intervertebral space and intervertebral foramen height have been achieved. The screw and rod system is inserted on the contralateral side. In the process of preparing the endplate, distraction should be maintained and the screw and rod system is temporarily locked (Fig. 17.36).

(3) Preparing the intervertebral space

The intervertebral disc is resected using a straight or curved scraper. The head or side blade of the scraper is turned for safer operation, either manually or using an electric system (Fig. 17.37a, b).

(4) Preparing the endplate

Various specially designed angled intervertebral tools are available that facilitate preparing the endplate ipsilateral or contralateral to the side of discectomy (Fig. 17.38a, b).

(5) Inserting the trial

The trial is inserted until the right intervertebral height is reached. The location and direction of the trial are confirmed by orthogonal and lateral fluoroscopy (Fig. 17.39a, b, c).

(6) Lumbar vertebra fusion device implantation

Based on the trial, an appropriately sized implant is chosen and held by holding pliers. Before implantation of the lumbar vertebra fusion device, the anterior and lateral vertebral body is filled with autologous bone graft, and the central hollow area of the implant is filled with bone grafts. The implant is gently tapped into place, and the posterior of the implant is 3–4 mm below the annulus fibrosus. The implant should be satisfactorily positioned (Fig. 17.40a, b).

(7) Completing the final structure

When the entire structure is installed, pressure is applied contralaterally, and load is applied to the anterior column to restore the lordosis of the lumbar vertebra. The epidural space and the intervertebral foramen are probed to assure that nerve decompression is complete. The pedicle screw and rod system is similarly implanted contralateral to the side of surgery to stabilize the entire structure (Fig. 17.41).

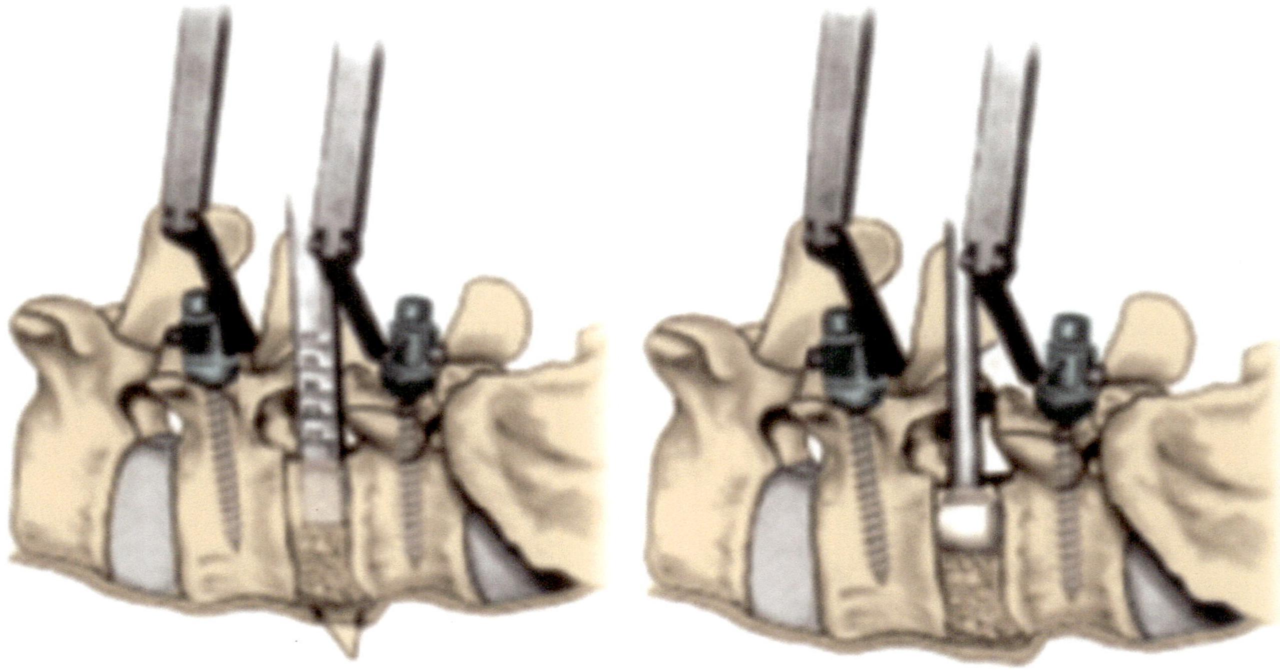

Fig. 17.24 The morselized bone is implanted and pressed tight

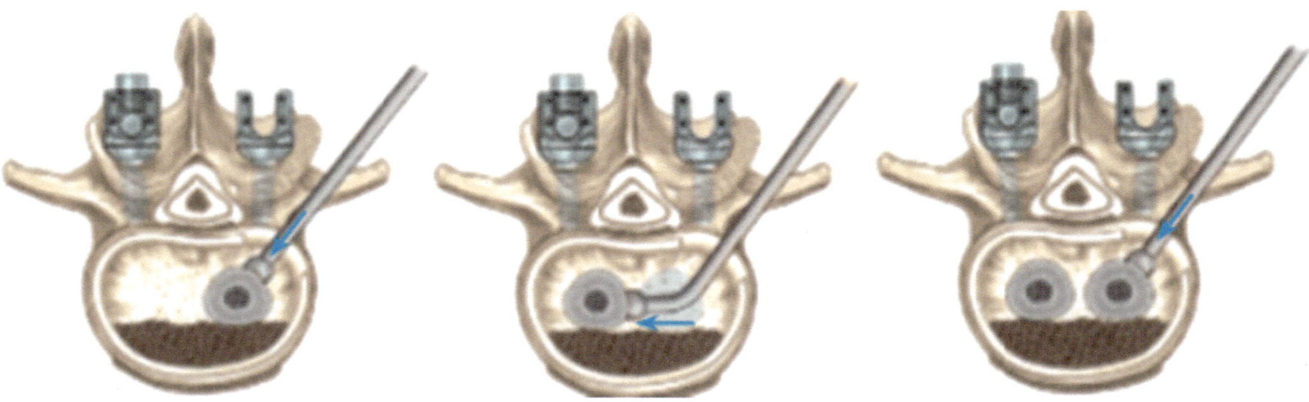

Fig. 17.25 Implanting the PYRAMESH

(8) The bilateral approach is done by referencing to the unilateral approach (Fig. 17.42a, b).

17.5 Clinical Cases

17.5.1 Case No. 1

Patient: A 46-year-old man with pain of the lower extremities and difficulty in walking for 2 years.

Diagnosis: L5–S1 intervertebral disc herniation.

Surgery: Bilateral fenestration of L5–S1 intervertebral space, nucleus pulposus extraction, intervertebral space bone graft, lumbar vertebra fusion device implantation, and L5–S1 pedicle screw internal fixation.

Imaging data: Preoperative image is shown in Fig. 17.43a–d, and postoperative images are shown in Fig. 17.44a–d.

17.5.2 Case No. 2

Patient: A 57-year-old woman with back pain and radiating pain of the left lower extremity for 1 year and worsening for 3 months.

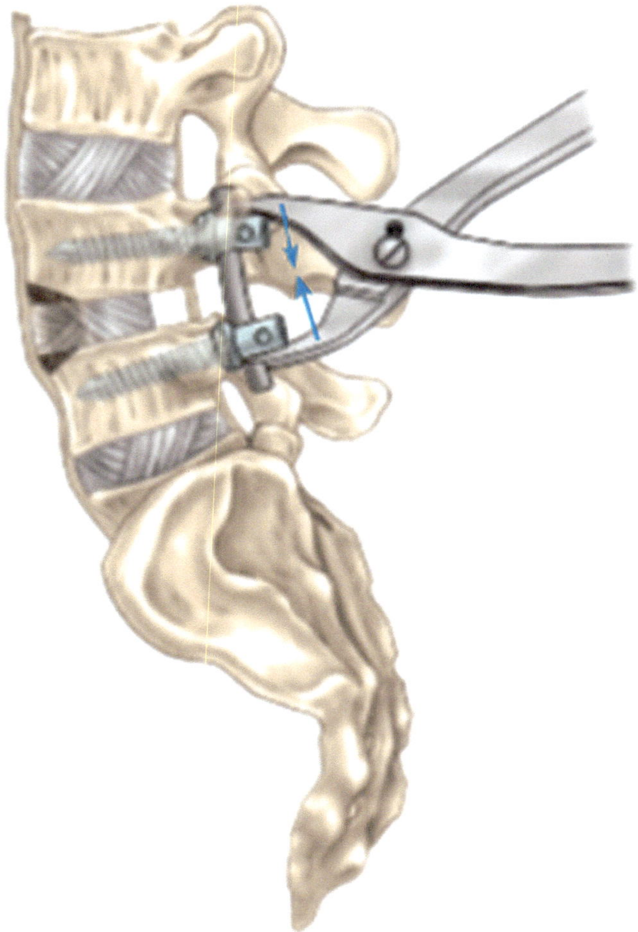

Fig. 17.26 Placement of the connecting rod. Appropriate pressure is applied

Diagnosis: L5 isthmic spondylolisthesis.

Surgery: L5–S1 left intervertebral disc fenestration with removal of nucleus pulposus from the intervertebral disc, intervertebral space bone graft, lumbar vertebra fusion device implantation, interbody fusion surgery, spondylolisthesis reduction, and L5 and S1 pedicle screw internal fixation.

Imaging data: Preoperative images are shown in Fig. 17.45a, b, and postoperative images are shown in Fig. 17.46a–e.

17.5.3 Case No. 3

Patient: A 62-year-old woman with back pain and radiating pain of the left lower extremity for 2 years and worsening for 2 months.

Diagnosis: L5 isthmic spondylolisthesis.

Surgery: L5–S1 left intervertebral disc fenestration with removal of nucleus pulposus from the intervertebral disc, intervertebral space bone graft, lumbar vertebra fusion device implantation, spondylolisthesis reduction, and L5 and S1 pedicle screw internal fixation.

Imaging data: Preoperative images are shown in Fig. 17.47a–d, and postoperative images are shown in Fig. 17.48a–e.

17.6 Pearls and Pitfalls

1. Implantation of the lumbar vertebra fusion device preserves the bone integrity of the superior and inferior endplate. The strength of distraction is powerful; therefore, it should be used with caution in cases with a too narrow intervertebral space.
2. The lumbar vertebra fusion device is tapped into the intervertebral space. Therefore, before tapping the device, osteophytes in the posterior edges of the vertebral body should be removed in order to minimize the tapping force and lessen irritation of adjacent nerve structures.
3. Because the lumbar vertebra fusion device has surface contact with the superior and inferior endplate, intervertebral stabilization is relatively poor. Therefore, in principle, it should be combined with the pedicle fixation.
4. Because the lumbar vertebra fusion device is made of high-strength carbon fiber and has good radiolucency, bony fusion can be examined radiologically following surgery.
5. Because the lumbar vertebra fusion device has non-screw contact with the superior and inferior endplate, the endplate should be prepared thoroughly when the lumbar vertebra fusion device is to be used. Otherwise, bony fusion will be delayed or fusion may fail. The matching tool set facilitates transverse and lateral preparation of the superior and inferior endplates.

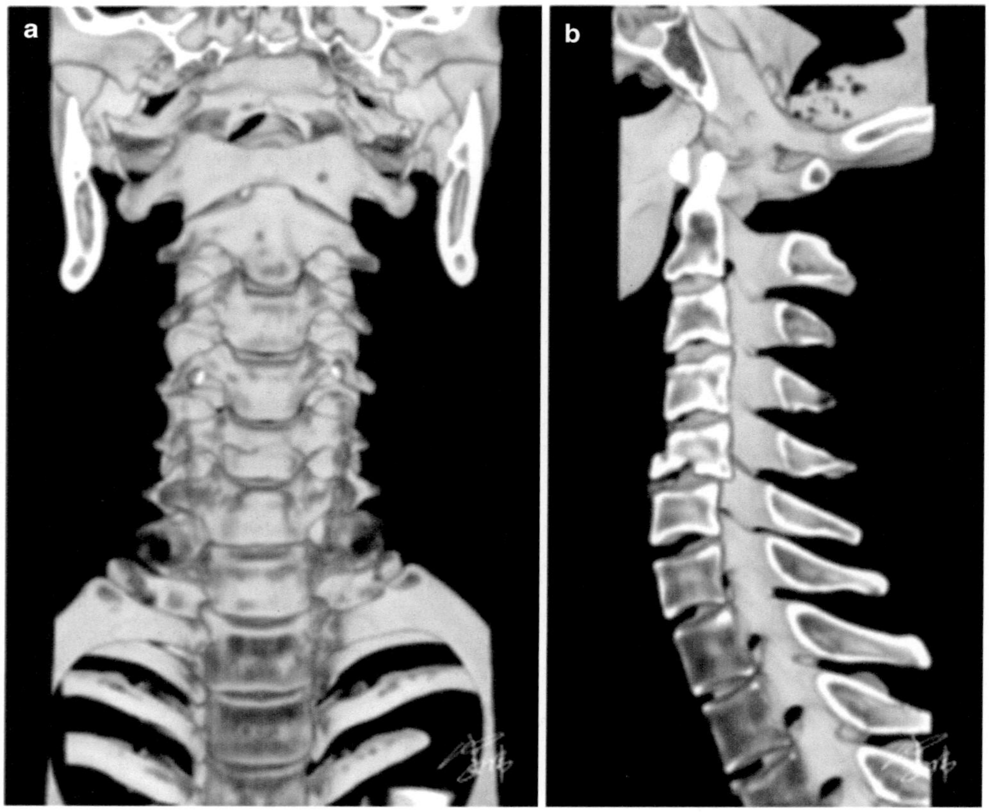

Fig. 17.27 Preoperative images. (**a**) CT 3D reconstruction (orthogonal view). (**b**) CT 3D reconstruction (sagittal split view)

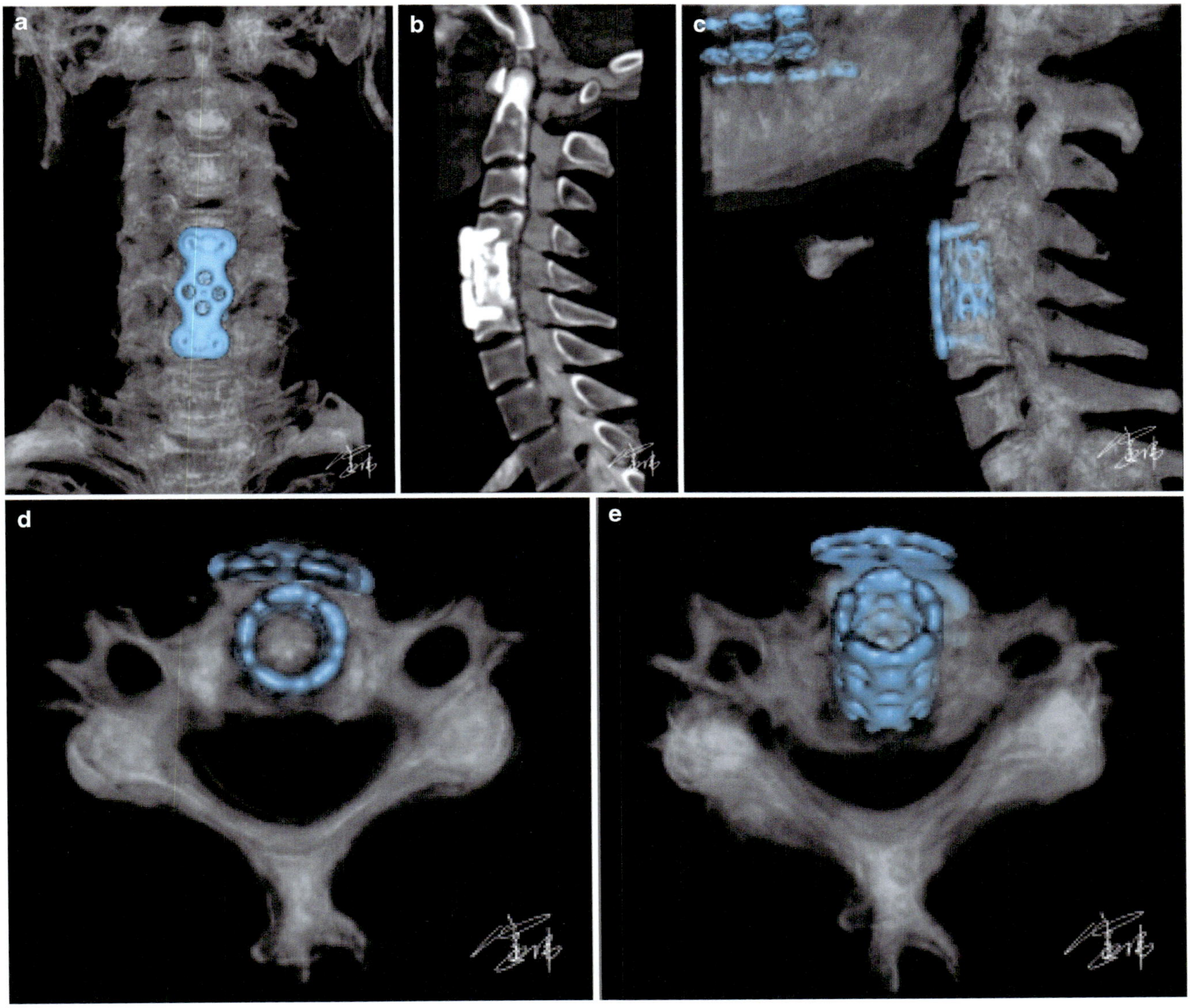

Fig. 17.28 Postoperative images. (**a**) CT 3D reconstruction (orthogonal view). (**b**) CT 3D reconstruction (lateral view). (**c**) CT 3D reconstruction (lateral view). (**d**) CT 3D reconstruction (horizontal view). (**e**) CT 3D reconstruction (horizontal view, anterior tile 40°)

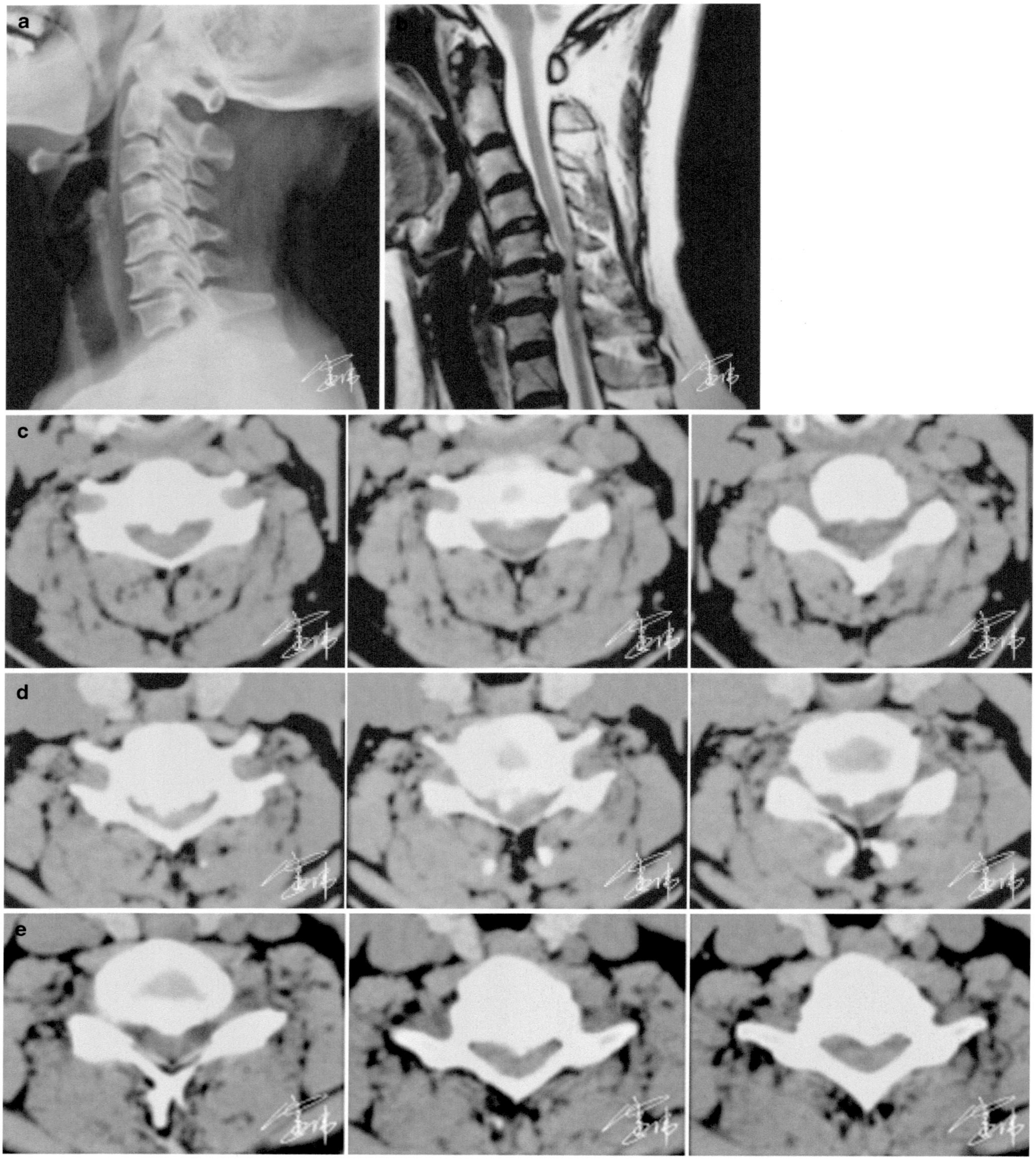

Fig. 17.29 Preoperative images. (**a**) X-ray radiograph (lateral view). (**b**) MRI (sagittal view). (**c**) C4–C5 intervertebral space. (**d**) C5–C6 intervertebral space. (**e**) C6–C7 intervertebral space

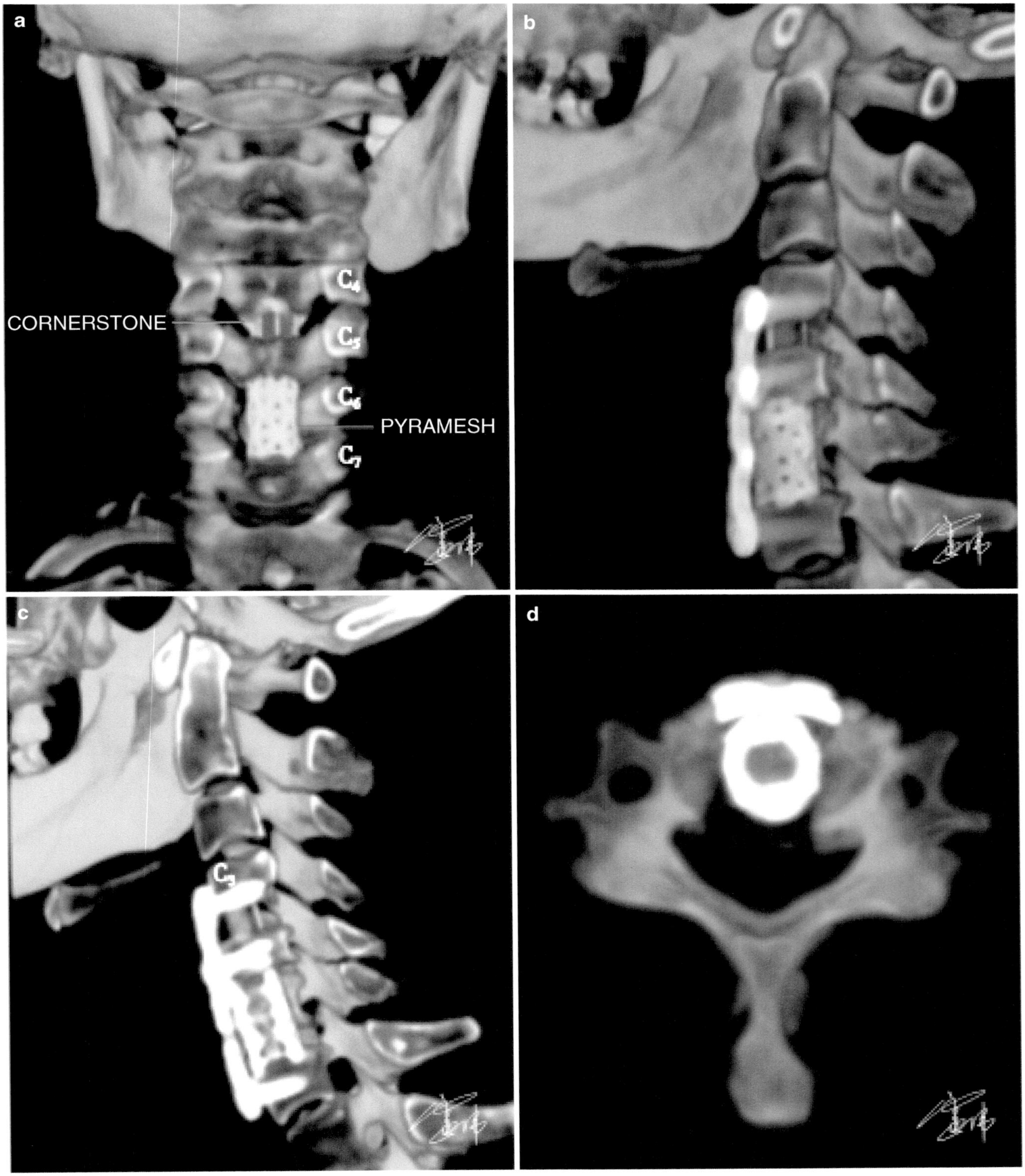

Fig. 17.30 Postoperative images. (**a**) CT 3D reconstruction (posterior split view). (**b**) CT 3D reconstruction (sagittal split view). (**c**) CT 3D reconstruction (sagittal split view). (**d**) CT 3D reconstruction (horizontal view)

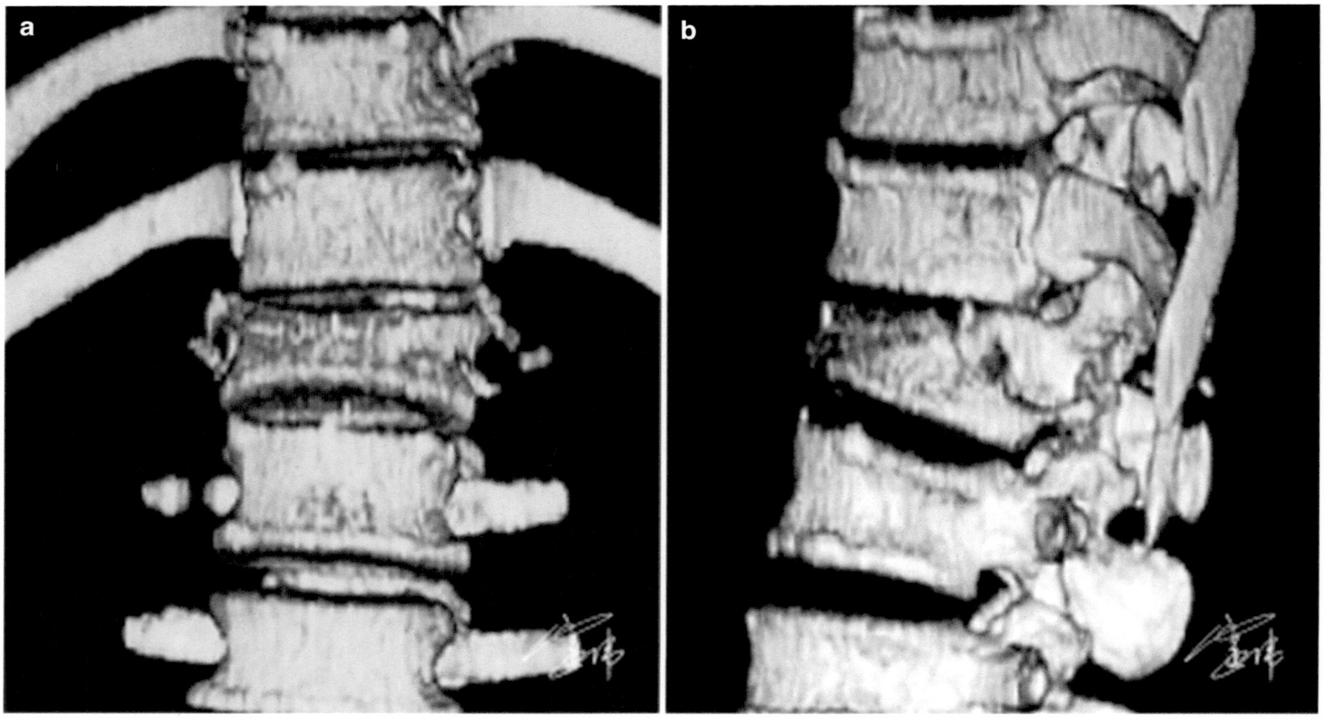

Fig. 17.31 Preoperative images. (**a**) CT 3D reconstruction (orthogonal view). (**b**) CT 3D reconstruction (lateral view)

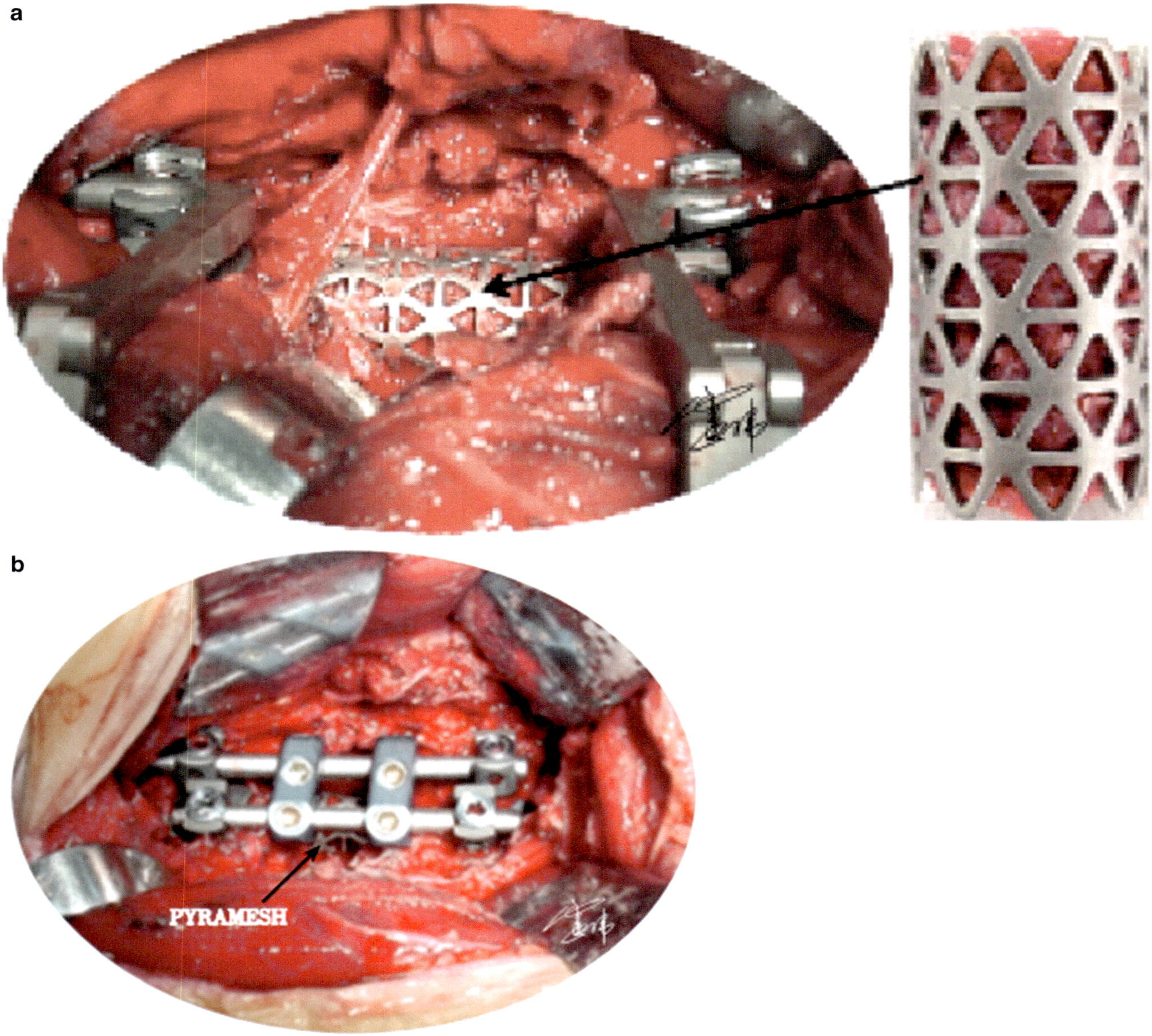

Fig. 17.32 Intraoperative images. (**a**) PYRAMESH bone graft and reconstruction of stabilization via an anterior approach. (**b**) ANTARES internal fixation

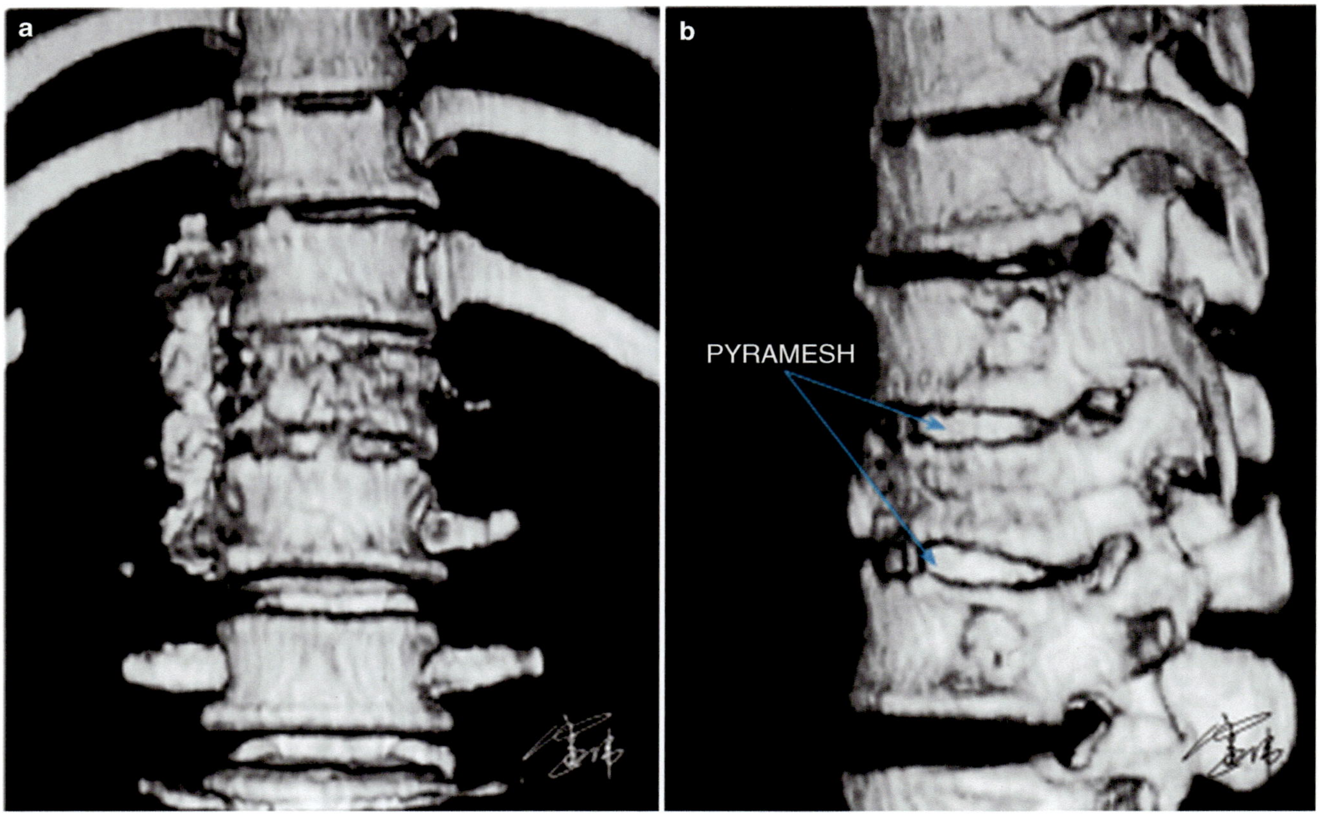

Fig. 17.33 Postoperative images. (**a**) CT 3D reconstruction (orthogonal view). (**b**) CT 3D reconstruction (orthogonal view)

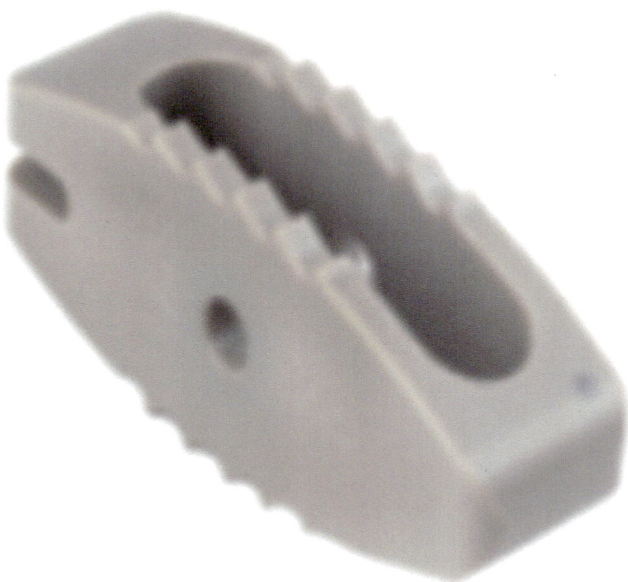

Fig. 17.34 Implant

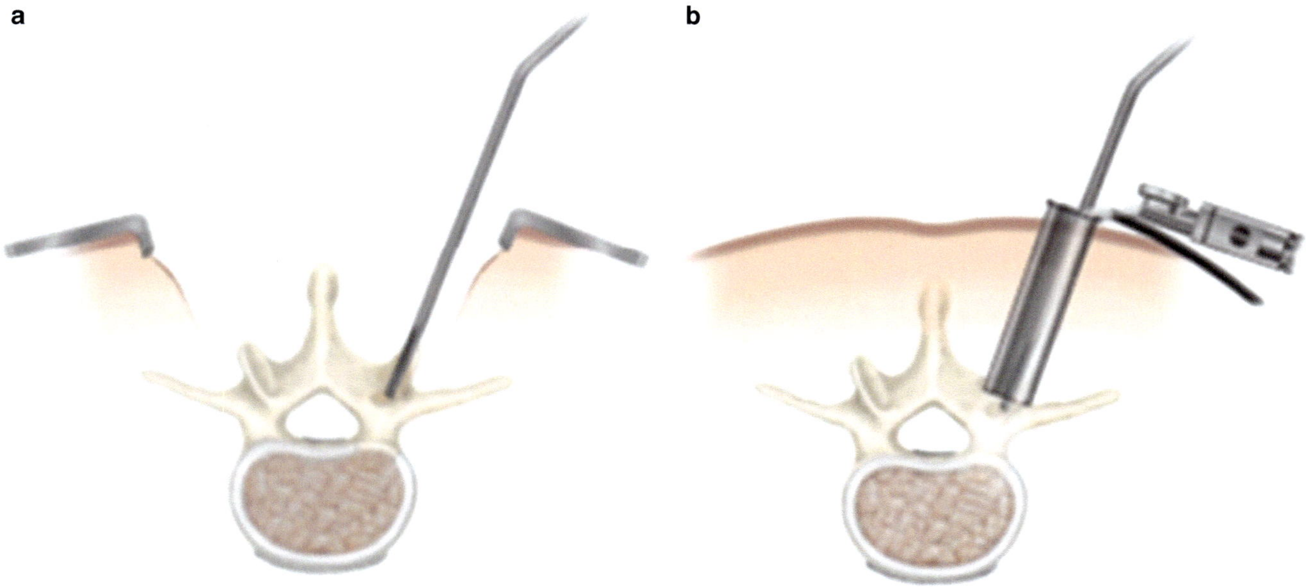

Fig. 17.35 Unilateral entry. (**a**) Open surgery. (**b**) Minimally invasive surgery

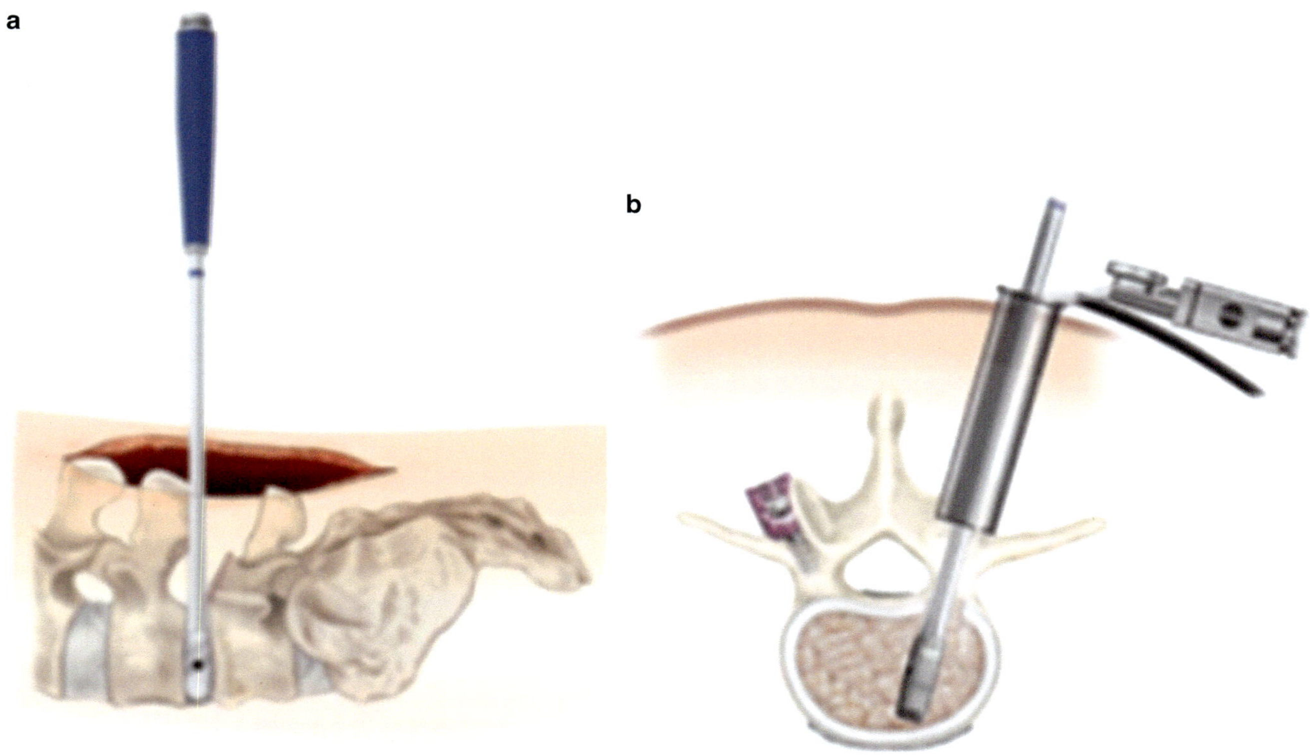

Fig. 17.36 Distraction. (**a**) Open surgery. (**b**) Minimally invasive surgery

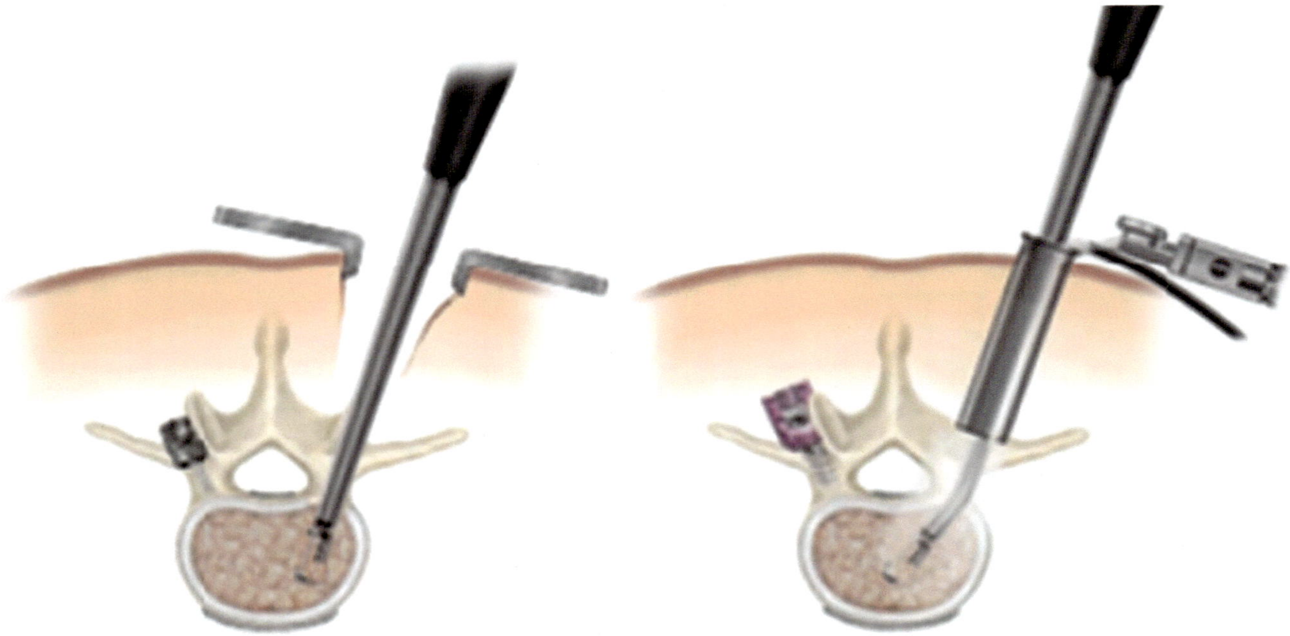

Fig. 17.37 Preparing the intervertebral space. (**a**) Open surgery. (**b**) Minimally invasive surgery

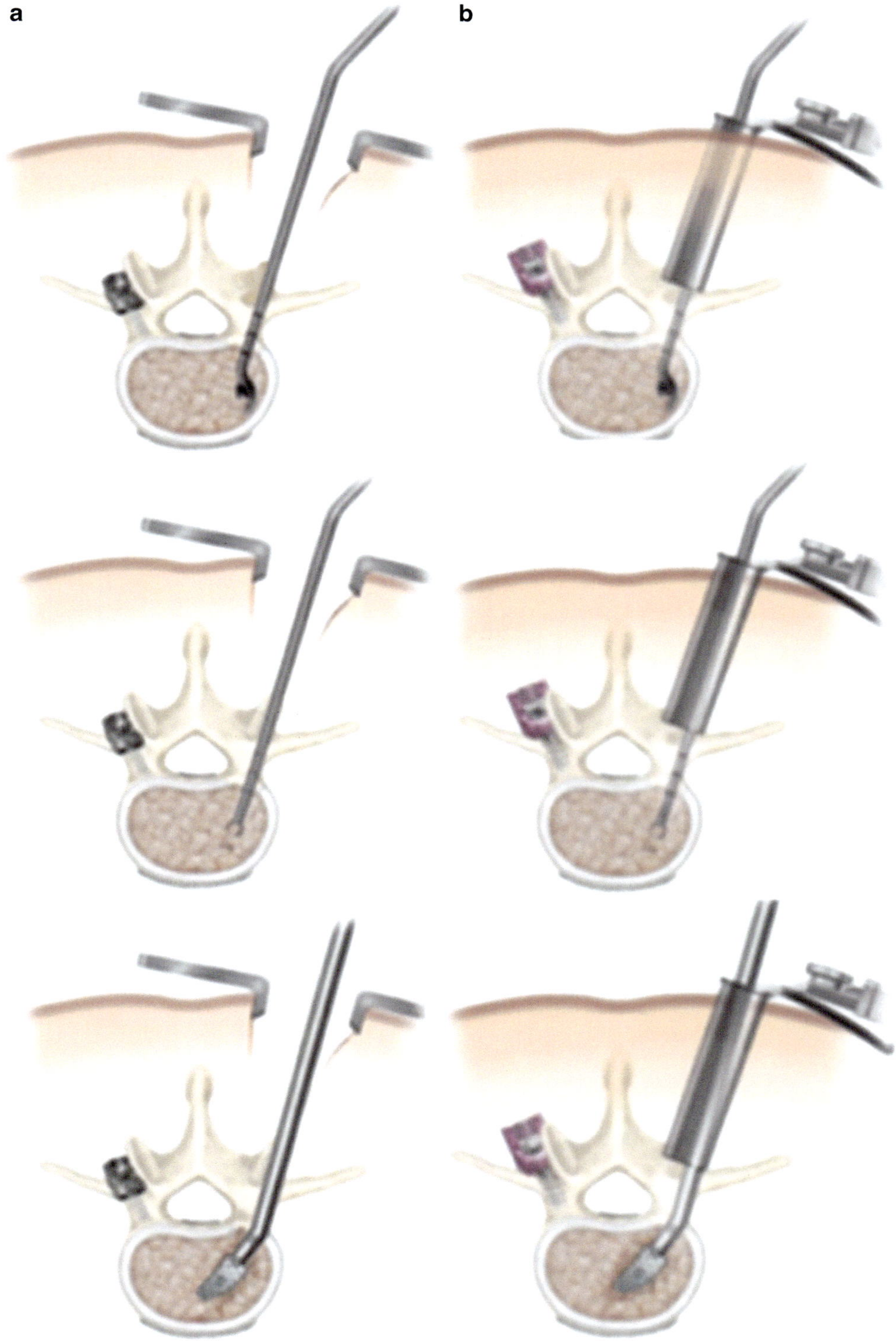

Fig. 17.38 Preparing the endplate. (**a**) Open surgery. (**b**) Minimally invasive surgery

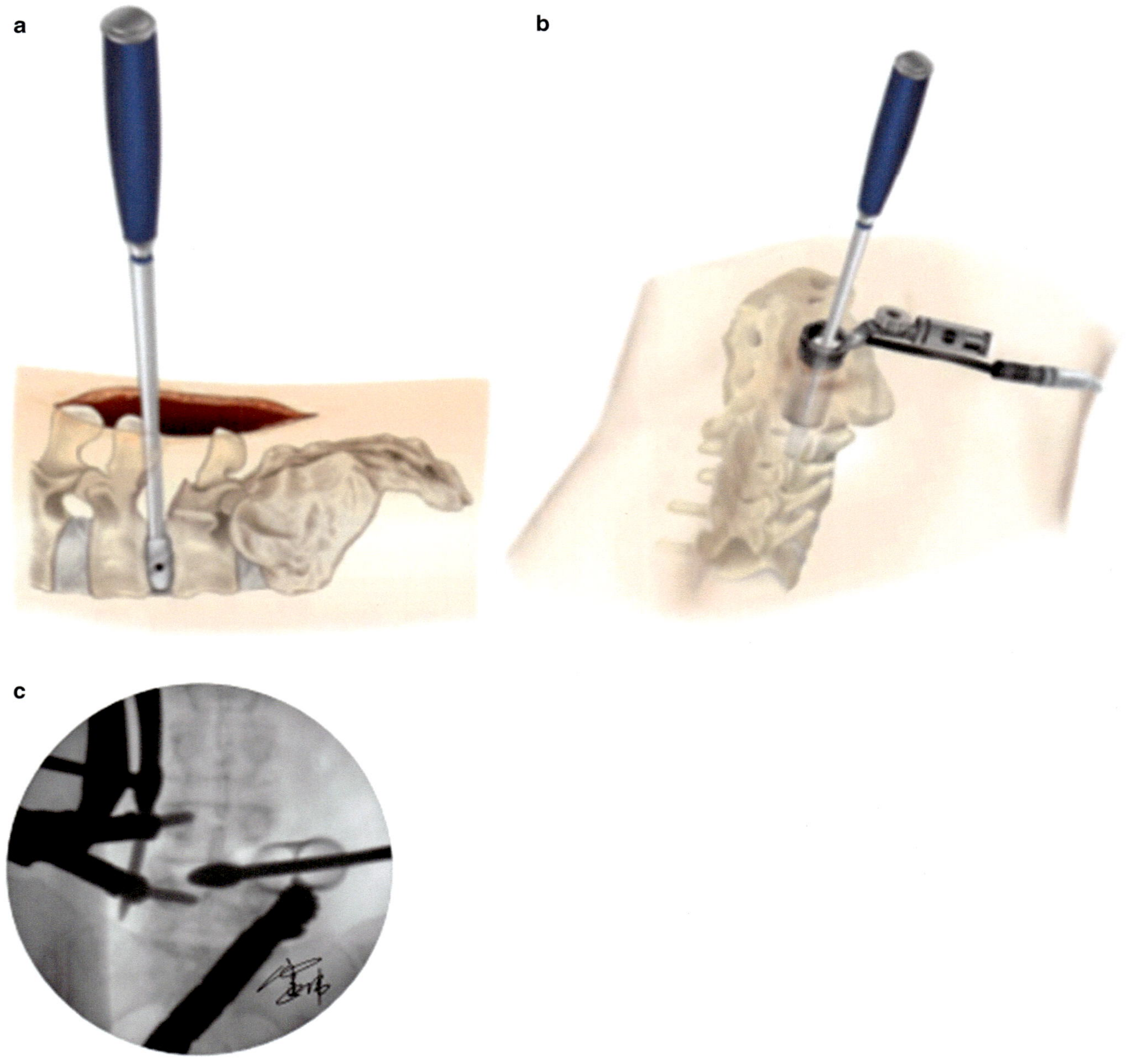

Fig. 17.39 Inserting the trial. (**a**) Open surgery. (**b**) Minimally invasive surgery. (**c**) Confirmation by fluoroscopy

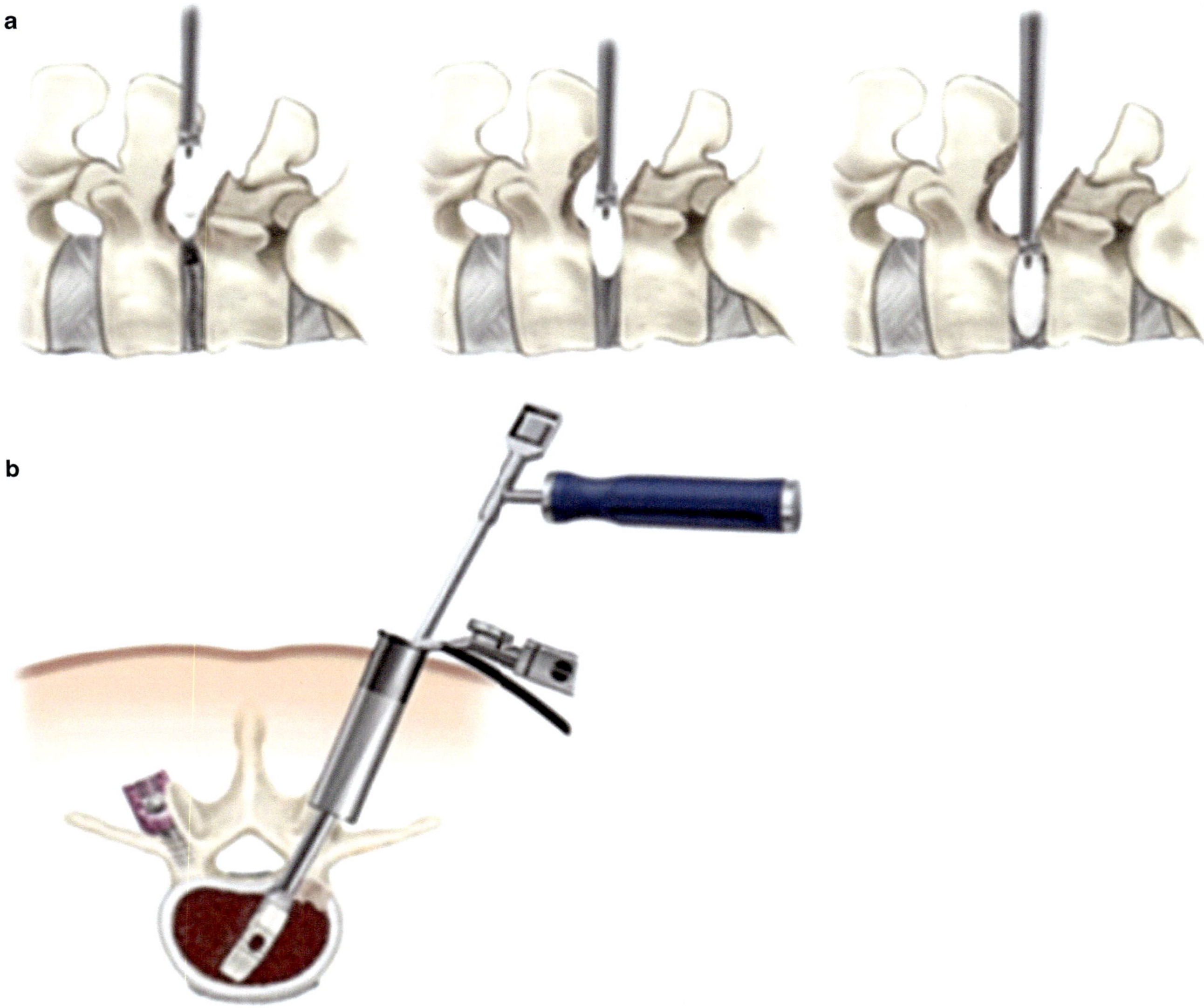

Fig. 17.40 Lumbar vertebra fusion device implantation. (a) Open surgery. (b) Minimally invasive surgery

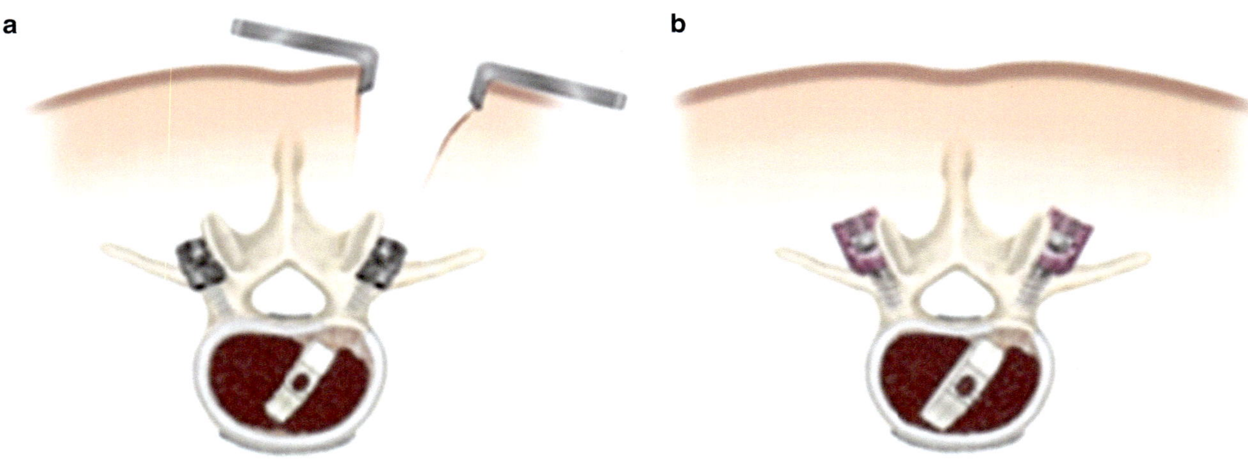

Fig. 17.41 Completion of the implantation. (a) Open surgery. (b) Minimally invasive surgery

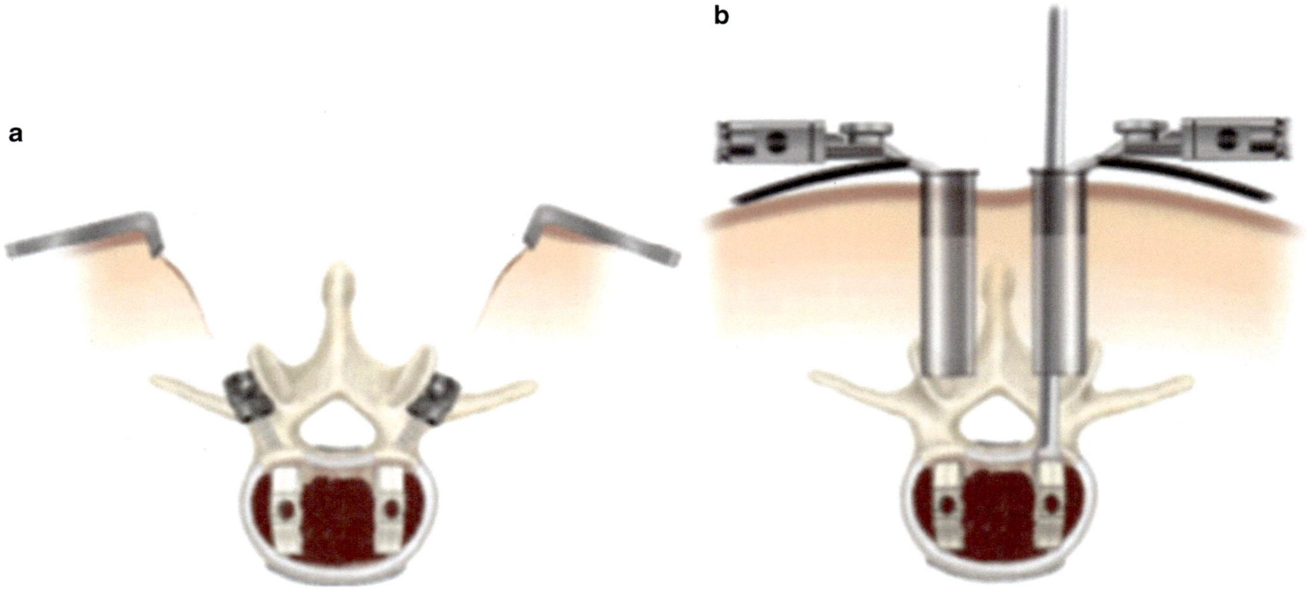

Fig. 17.42 The bilateral approach. (**a**) Open surgery. (**b**) Minimally invasive surgery

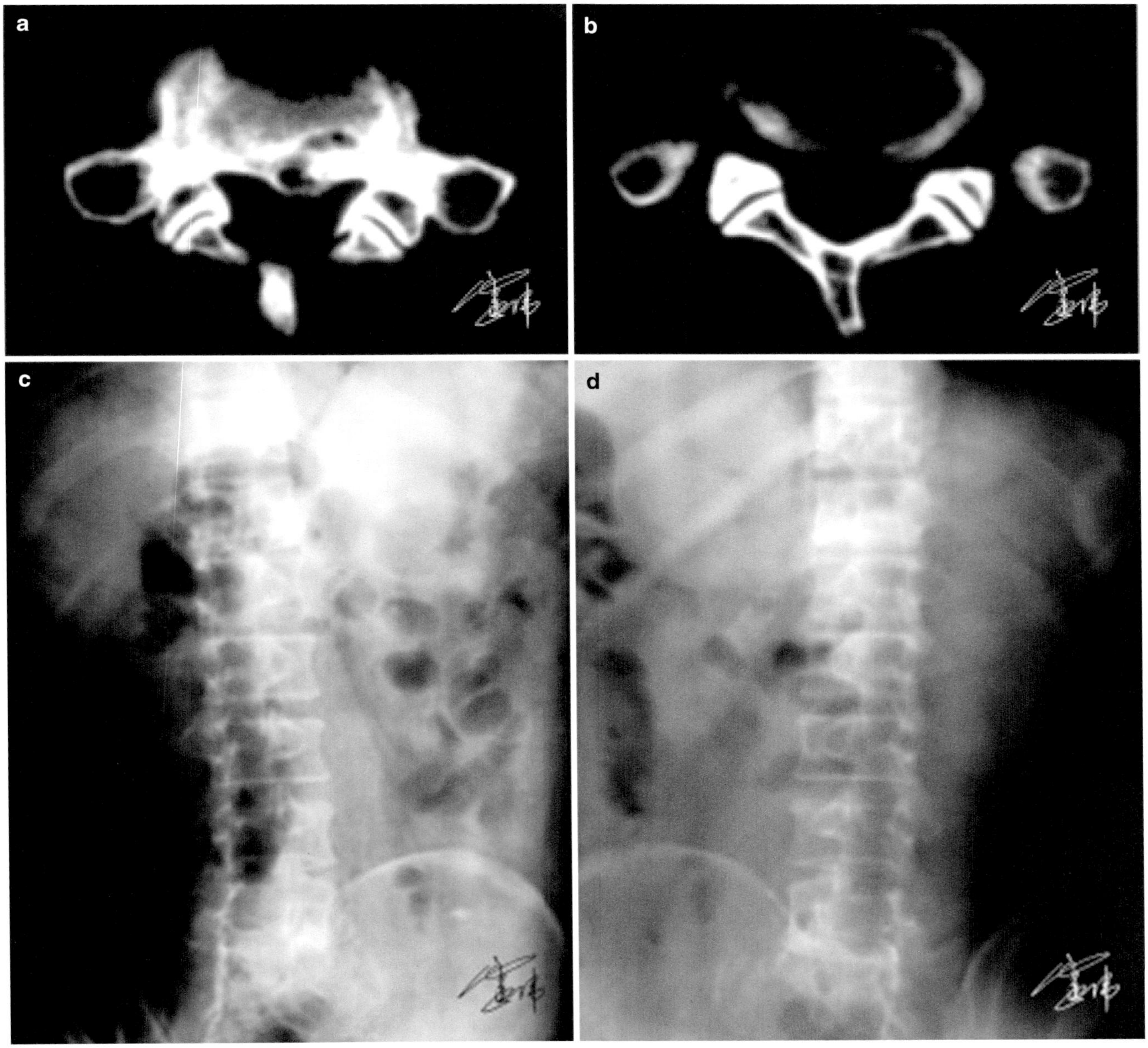

Fig. 17.43 Preoperative images. (**a**) L5–S1 intervertebral space. (**b**) L4–L5 intervertebral space. (**c**) Radiograph (right oblique). (**d**) Radiograph (left oblique)

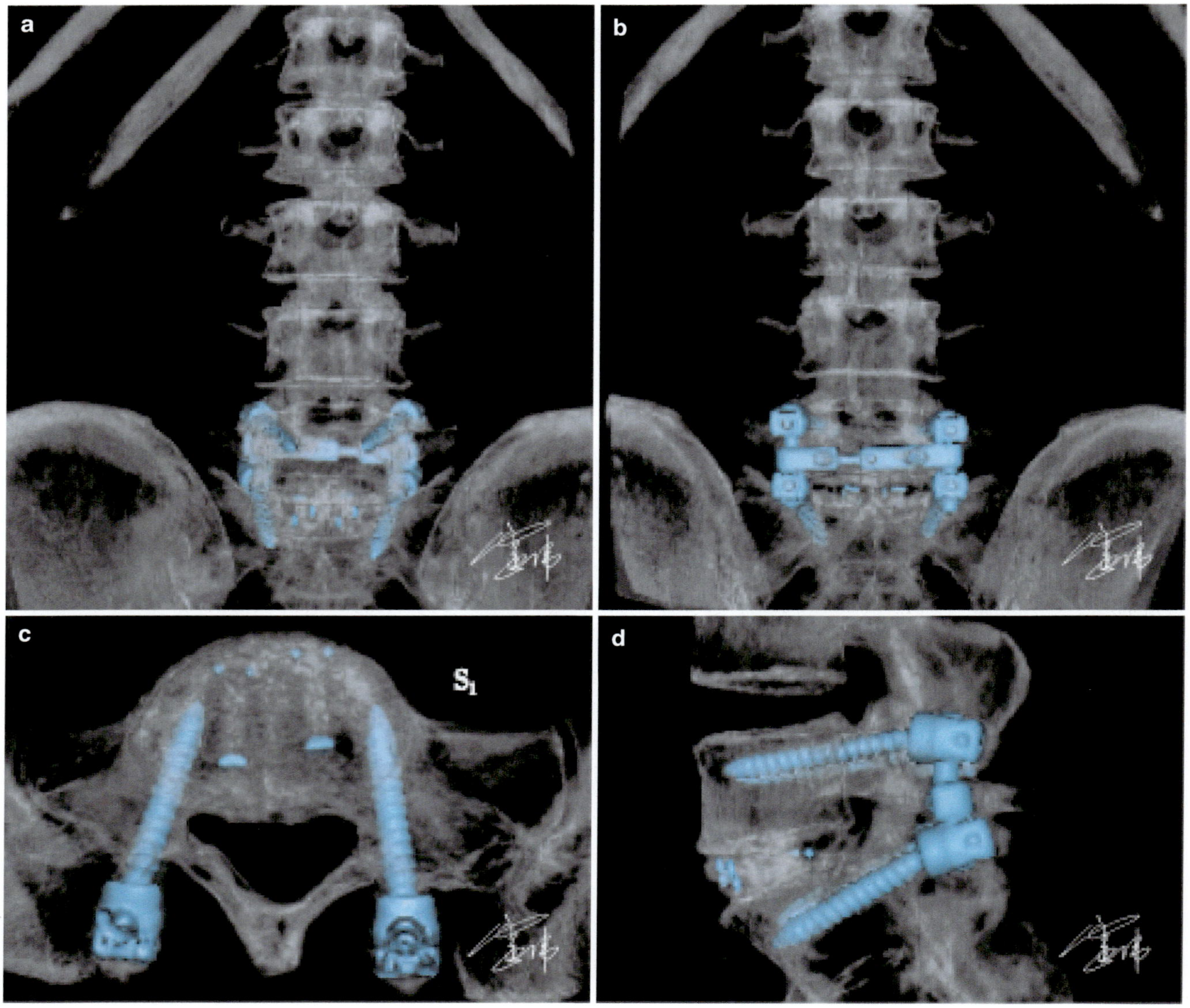

Fig. 17.44 Postoperative images. (**a**) CT 3D reconstruction (anteroposterior view). (**b**) CT 3D reconstruction (posteroanterior view). (**c**) CT 3D reconstruction (horizontal view). (**d**) CT 3D reconstruction (lateral view)

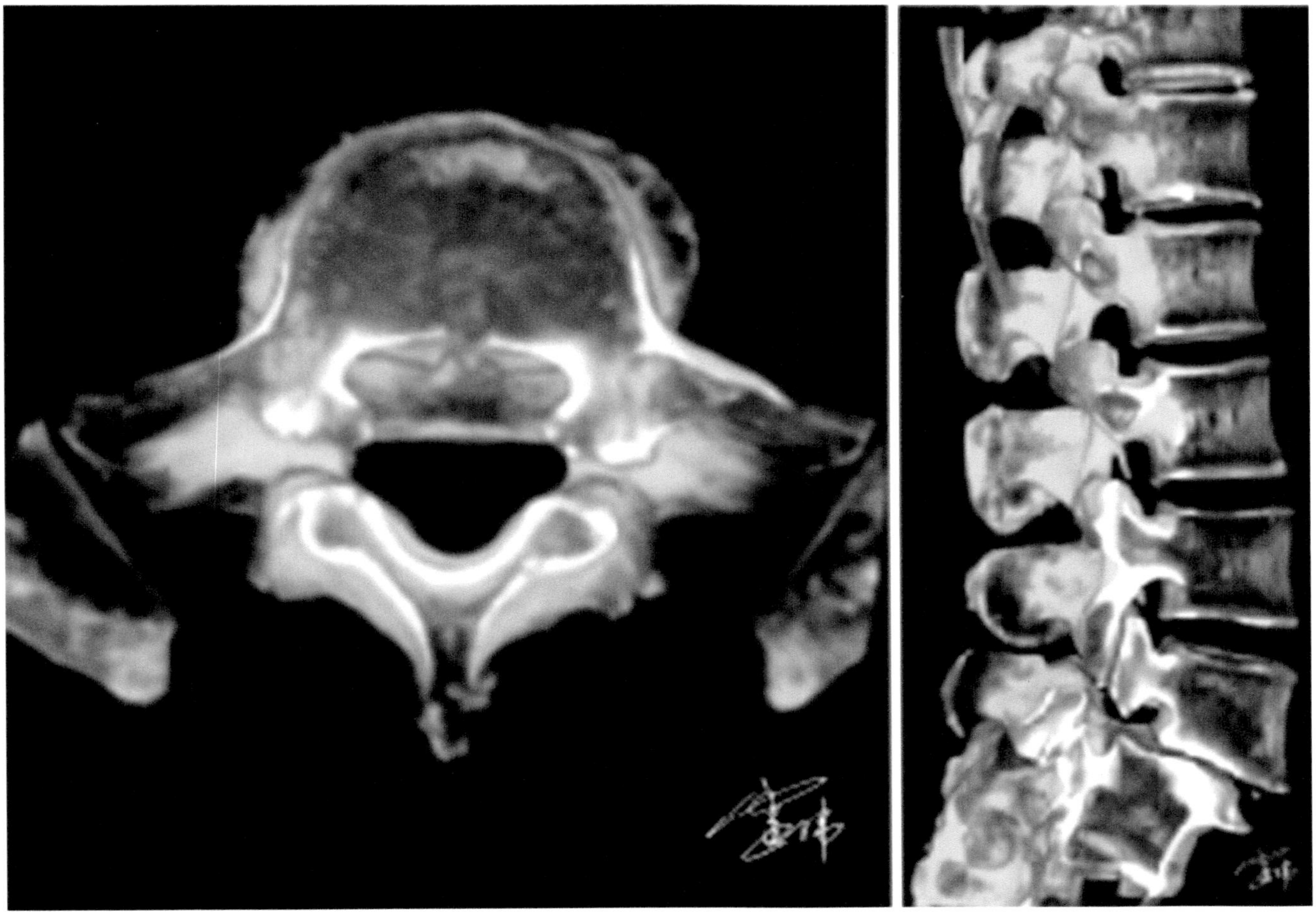

Fig. 17.45 Preoperative images. (**a**) CT 3D reconstruction (horizontal view); (**b**) CT 3D reconstruction (lateral view)

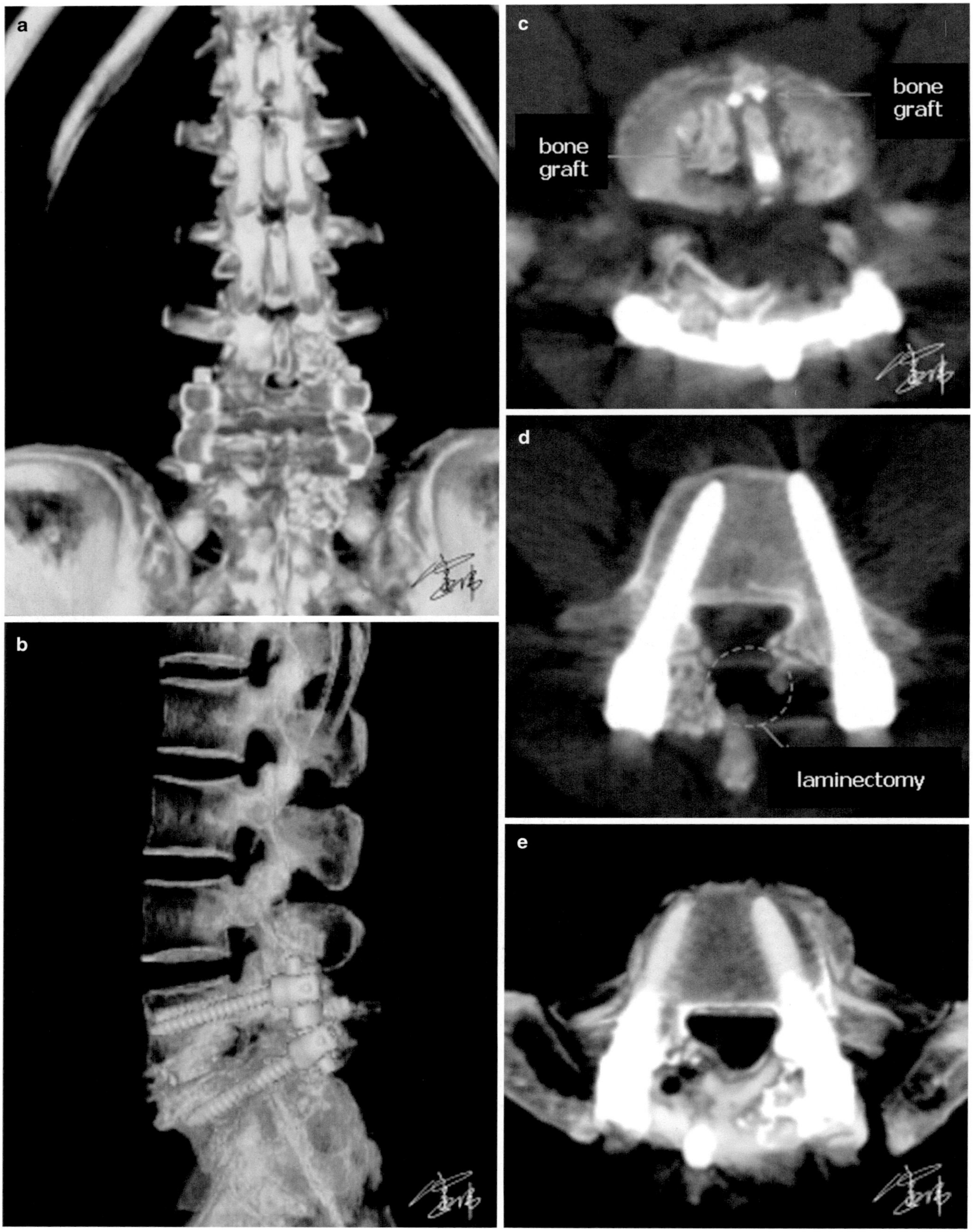

Fig. 17.46 Postoperative images. (**a**) CT 3D reconstruction (posteroanterior view); (**b**) CT 3D reconstruction (lateral view); (**c**) CT 3D reconstruction (horizontal view); (**d**) CT 3D reconstruction (horizontal view); (**e**) CT 3D reconstruction (horizontal view, showing full spondylolisthesis reduction)

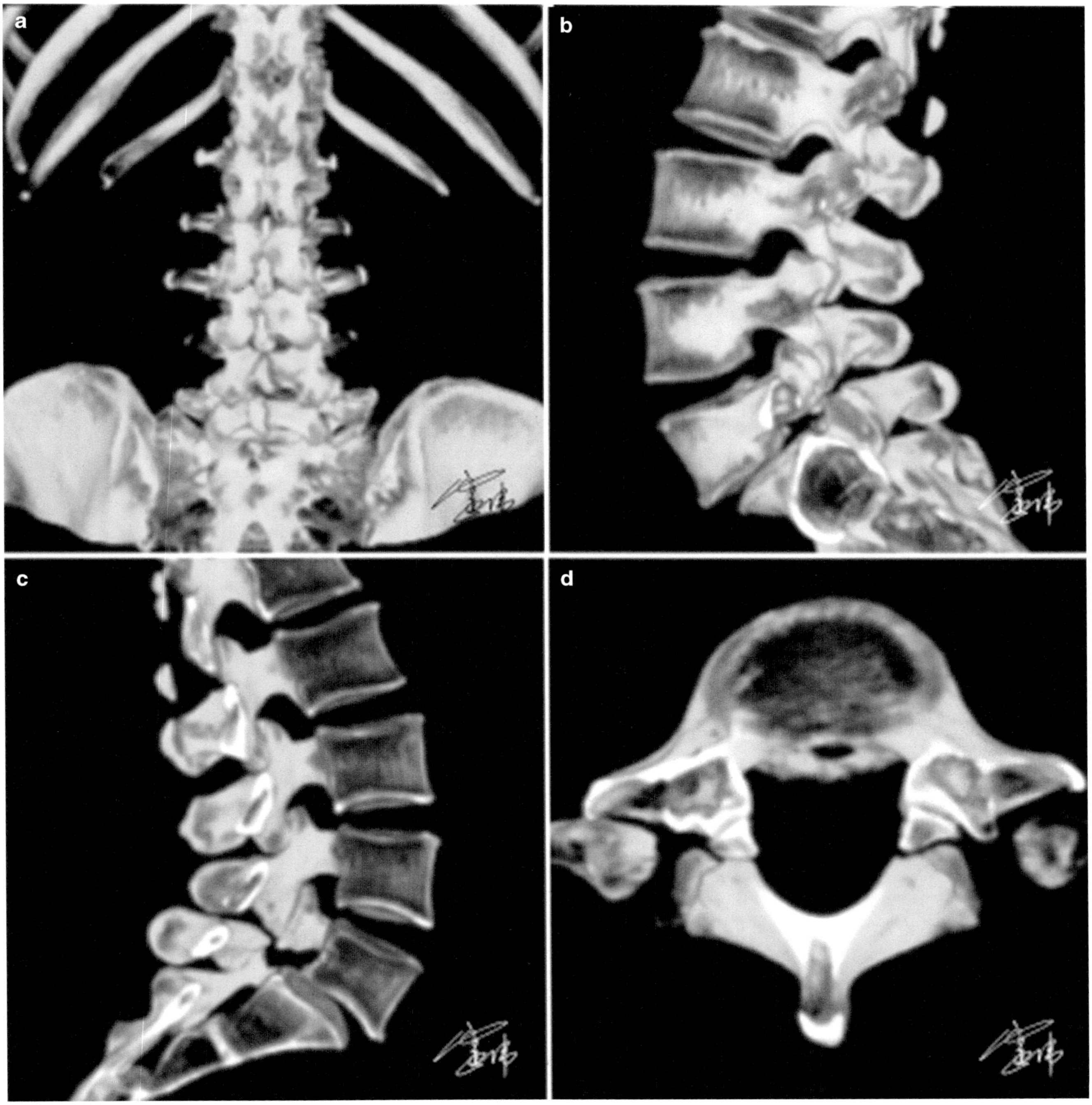

Fig. 17.47 Preoperative images. (**a**) CT 3D reconstruction (posteroanterior view); (**b**) CT 3D reconstruction (lateral view); (**c**) CT 3D reconstruction (sagittal view); (**d**) CT 3D reconstruction (horizontal view)

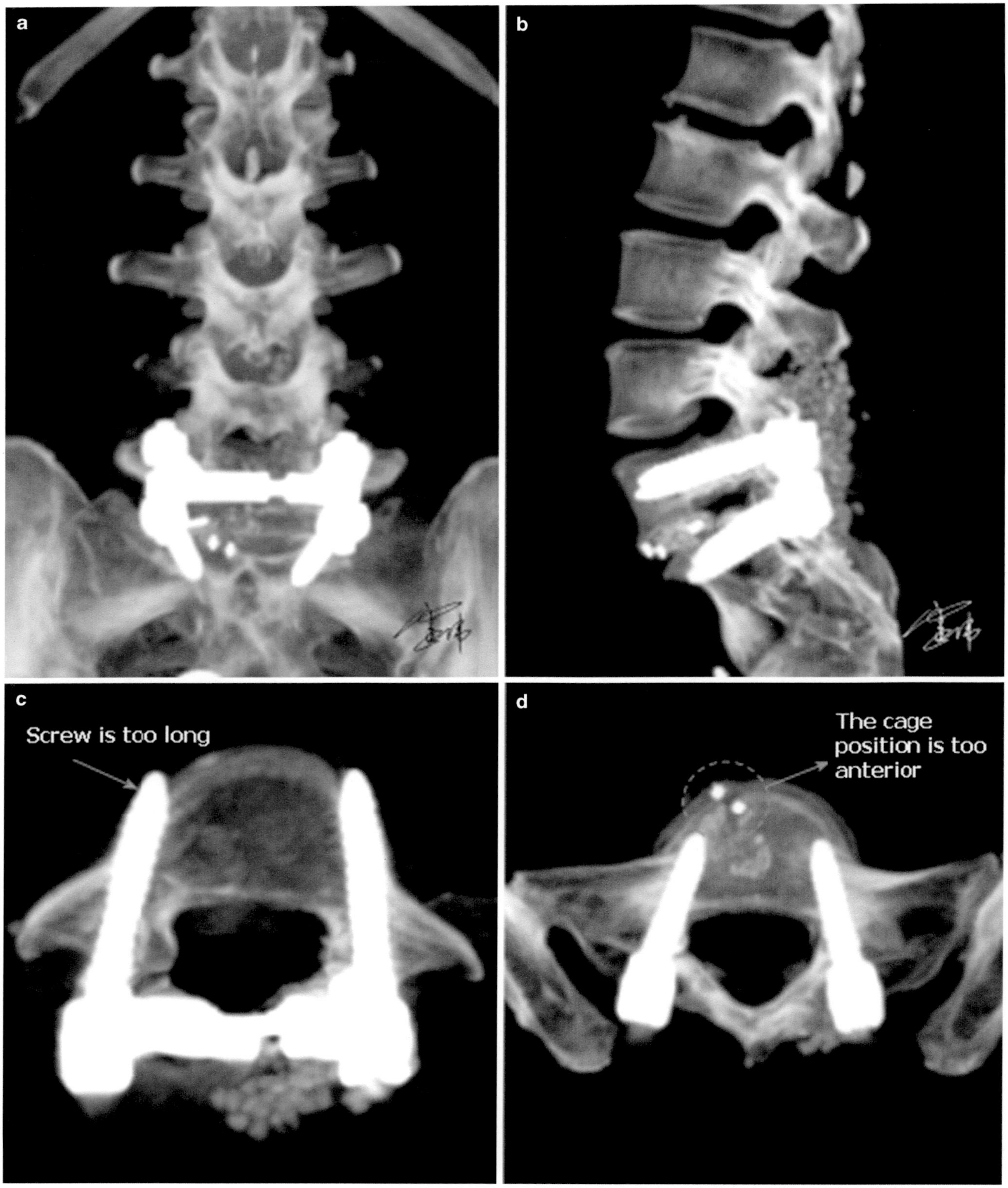

Fig. 17.48 Postoperative images. (**a**) CT 3D reconstruction (posteroanterior view); (**b**) CT 3D reconstruction (lateral view); (**c**) CT 3D reconstruction (horizontal view); (**d**) CT 3D reconstruction (L5 horizontal view). (**e**) CT 3D reconstruction (S1 horizontal view)

Printed by Printforce, the Netherlands